Gynecology

THIRD EDITION

Condensed from
Jones and Jones:
Novak's Textbook of Gynecology,
Tenth Edition

Gynecology

THIRD EDITION

Georgeanna Seegar Jones, M.D.

Professor of Obstetrics and Gynecology
Eastern Virginia Medical School
Norfolk, Virginia

Howard W. Jones, Jr., M.D.

Professor of Obstetrics and Gynecology
Eastern Virginia Medical School
Norfolk, Virginia

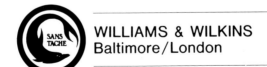

WILLIAMS & WILKINS
Baltimore/London

Copyright © 1982
Williams & Wilkins
428 East Preston Street
Baltimore, MD 21202, U.S.A.

Made in the United States of America

First Edition, 1971
Asian Edition, 1972
Portuguese translation, 1974
Spanish translation, 1975
Second Edition, 1975
Reprinted 1977
Reprinted 1978
Reprinted 1979
Reprinted 1980
Third Edition, 1982
Reprinted 1983

Library of Congress Cataloging in Publication Data

Main entry under title:

Gynecology.

   Condensed from Novak's Textbook of gynecology, 10th ed.
   Edition for 1975 by E. R. Novak.
   Includes bibliographies and index.
   1. Gynecology. I. Jones, Georgeanna Seegar, 1912–   . II. Jones, Howard Wilbur, 1910–   . III. Novak, Edmund R. Gynecology. IV. Novak, Edmund R. Textbook of gynecology. [DNLM: 1. Genital disease, Female. WP 100J77s]
RG101.N692 1981   618.1   80-29004
ISBN 0-683-04467-2

Composed and printed at the
Waverly Press, Inc.
Mt. Royal and Guilford Aves.
Baltimore, MD 21202, U.S.A.

Preface

Tragedy has accompanied the preparation of the 10th edition of this text. Nine editions had the guiding experience of a Novak—first that of Emil, clinician and gigantic pioneering gynecological pathologist and, following his death in 1957, that of Edmund who followed his father's footsteps. The untimely death of Edmund occurred in the Spring of 1979 just as the tenth revision was to begin. However, he had already started and his final scientific effort is the revision of Chapter 20 on tuberculosis, a problem of very personal interest to him, for early in his career he was hospitalized with this disease for almost 2 years.

In order to secure a prompt and contemporary revision, and with an eye to the future, a young and vigorous mini-team of collaborators was recruited for the tenth edition. The two senior authors were pleased and proud to include Dr. Conrad Julian, Resident of Hopkins and for several years a member of its staff, and later Professor of Obstetrics and Gynecology at Vanderbilt University in Nashville. Dr. Anne Colston Wentz, also Hopkins trained, and now Professor of Obstetrics and Gynecology at the Vanderbilt University in Nashville, and Dr. Howard Jones, III, trained at the University of Colorado and the M. D. Anderson Hospital in Houston, and now Assistant Professor of Obstetrics and Gynecology at the Vanderbilt University in Nashville. It was believed that this group of active clinicians would provide a contemporary and youthful view, and it was hoped that the senior authors would provide a desirable homogeneity.

It is necessary to record that after completing most of the work on Chapters 1, 16, 17, 22, 23, and 24, Conrad Julian died suddenly and unexpectedly in late November 1979. These chapters were finalized by the other authors.

Except for the chapter on unchanging anatomy and portions of others, the book has been essentially rewritten with a view to emphasizing current views of contemporary gynecology.

It is interesting to read Emil Novak's preface to the first edition. He was among the pioneers to realize that the then emerging field of gynecological endocrinology was here to stay, and the first edition emphasized this subspecialty. Through the revisions, that feature has continued and expanded with the development of knowledge. About one-third of the chapters of the tenth edition concern not only the physiology of the reproductive process which now extends from the brain to the pelvis, but also with the still growing aspects of abnormalities of these mechanisms.

An emphasis on pathology was another original feature of this textbook. This has been continued because more than a mere acquaintance with pathology is an absolute requirement for the superior practice of gynecology. It is fortunate, and indeed not coincidental, that the younger and newer collaborators have a special interest in this aspect of our specialty.

For whatever reason, the time allocated to gynecology (and obstetrics) has tended to be curtailed in the curricula of several medical schools in the United States. Fortunately, this has been less so elsewhere in the world. Such a change has required an abbreviated approach to learning the specialty dictated by the development of a core curriculum (which means leaving

v

out something), the development of terminal objectives, enabling objectives, multiple choice examinations, and the other requirements of an abbreviated mass approach. For these reasons, this condensed version of the full text is provided in paperback for students whose principal interest may be in other specialties.

A more complete edition is available in hardback and is intended for students with a deeper interest and for practitioners. It includes, of course, not only all material suggested in the various core curricula, but other material necessary for a comprehensive coverage of general gynecology, gynecological oncology, and gynecological endocrinology. While familiarity with, and reference to, original sources are essential components of scholarship, the approach in this book is unshamedly tempered by years of clinical experience. This simply means that attitudes have been molded by reference to the most instructive and important original source of all—the patient.

The authors are grateful to colleagues and friends who have supplied illustrative and other material. We must expecially mention Dr. Edward F. Lewison, world authority on the breast, who has provided in a section of one chapter a definitive view of the gynecologist's role in the diagnosis and treatment of diseases of this important reproductive organ.

Dr. Donald Woodruff, a long-time friend and collaborator of the senior authors, has contributed a superlative chapter on diseases of the vulva and an equally comprehensive and useful chapter on the vagina. These two chapters by an international authority in these areas greatly strengthen the book.

We are especially grateful to Mrs. Nancy Gilliam, Mrs. Linda Lynch, Ms. Sandra Horn, Ms. Victoria Johnston and Ms. Patsy Burnside, our secretaries, who have so efficiently checked the references, corralled the figures, typed the manuscripts and attended to the innumerable details associated with an author's effort.

This is also an opportunity to acknowledge the courtesies of the staff of The Williams & Wilkins Company who helped overcome the sadness surrounding the tenth edition by a cooperative spirit which in the end made this tenth edition a pleasure to produce.

Contributors

Georgeanna Seegar Jones, M.D., Professor of Obstetrics and Gynecology, Eastern Virginia Medical School, Norfolk, Virginia

Howard W. Jones, Jr., M.D., Professor of Obstetrics and Gynecology, Eastern Virginia Medical School, Norfolk, Virginia

Howard W. Jones, III, M.D., Department of Obstetrics and Gynecology, Vanderbilt University School of Medicine, Nashville, Tennessee

Conrad G. Julian, M.D.†, Professor of Obstetrics and Gynecology, Vanderbilt University, School of Medicine, Nashville, Tennessee

Edmund R. Novak, M.D.†, Associate Professor of Gynecology and Obstetrics, The Johns Hopkins University, School of Medicine, Baltimore, Maryland

Anne Colston Wentz, M.D., Professor of Obstetrics and Gynecology, Vanderbilt University, School of Medicine, Nashville, Tennessee

J. Donald Woodruff, M.D., Professor Emeritus, Gynecology and Obstetrics, The Johns Hopkins University, School of Medicine, Baltimore, Maryland

† Deceased.

Contents

CHAPTER 1

Anatomy

The female reproductive organs are divisible into two groups, the external and internal. The former comprise the vulva and vagina; the latter the uterus, tubes, and ovaries (Fig. 1.1).

THE VULVA

The vulva, representing the part of the genital apparatus visible externally, is a composite structure (Fig. 1.2).

Labia Majora

The labia majora are two longitudinal raised folds of adipose tissue covered by skin which is rather heavily pigmented. Before puberty the vulva is rather flat, and the labia minora are much more conspicuous than the labia majora. In the postpubertal female, the latter extend posteriorly toward the perineum. On separating them posteriorly, a slightly raised connecting ridge, the *fourchette*, is seen. Just anterior to this, between it and the vaginal orifice, is a shallow, boat-shaped fossa, the *fossa navicularis*. The external surface of the labia shows a heavy growth of hair, usually curly, but the hair on the inner surface is much more sparse.

The substance of the labia majora is adipose tissue, although it contains also a light fascial layer. The labia themselves are to be looked upon as corresponding to the scrotum of the male.

Mons Pubis

The mons pubis is a mound of fat covered by hair, situated just above the level of the symphysis pubis, at the lowest portion of the anterior abdominal wall.

Labia Minora

The labia minora are two firm pigmented folds which extend from the clitoris posteriorly to about two-thirds of the distance toward the perineum. Anteriorly they subdivide, one fold covering the clitoris to form its prepuce, the other passing beneath the glans to form, with its fellow of the opposite side, the frenulum clitoridis.

The skin covering the labia minora is devoid of hair follicles, but is very rich in sebaceous glands.

Clitoris

The clitoris is a small, cylindrical, erectile organ corresponding to the male penis. Like the latter it consists of a glans, a corpus or body, and the crura. Only the *glans clitoridis*, about 6 to 8 mm in diameter, is visible externally between the two folds into which the labia minora bifurcates anteriorly, the upper fold forming the *prepuce* and the lower the *frenulum* of the clitoris. The *body* extends upward toward the pubis beneath the skin dividing into two *crura* which are attached to the pubic bones. The clitoris is made up of erectile tissue, with many large and small venous channels surrounded by large amounts of involuntary muscle tissue. The erectile tissue is arranged into corpora cavernosa, and there is no corpus spongiosum as in the case of the male organ.

Vestibule

The vestibule is the boat-shaped fossa which becomes visible on separation of the labia. In it are seen the vaginal orifice and, anterior to this, the urinary meatus. In the virgin the former is partly occluded by the

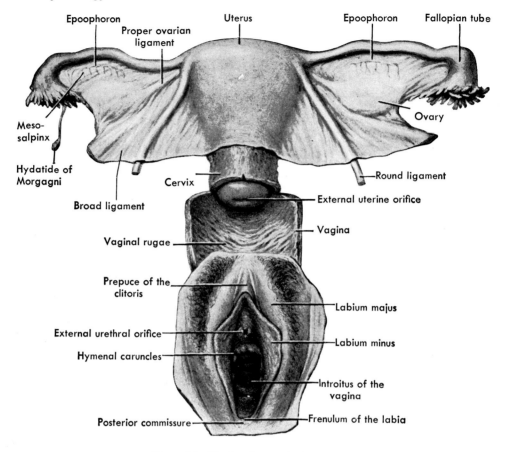

Figure 1.1. The female reproductive organs.

hymen, a rather rigid membrane of firm connective tissue covered on both sides by stratified squamous epithelium.

Urethra

The urethral meatus is the small slitlike or triangular external orifice of the urethra. It is visible in the vestibule, at about two-thirds of the distance from the glans clitoridis to the vaginal orifice. At each side of the meatus one usually sees a small pitlike depression in which there are a number of mucous glands, called the lesser glands of the vestibule, to distinguish them from the greater glands (Bartholin).

Just below the outer part of the meatus are the orifices of the *paraurethral* or *Skene's ducts*.

The *female urethra*, opening externally at the meatus, is lined proximally by a stratified transitional type of epithelium, whereas its distal portion is covered with stratified squamous epithelium. The canal is surrounded by a labyrinth of *paraurethral glands*, the homologues of the male prostate.

Vulvovaginal or Bartholin's Glands

The vulvovaginal or Bartholin's glands are lobulated racemose glands situated one on each side of the vaginal orifice, at about its middle, deep in the perineal structures.

The main duct of the gland is lined by a stratified transitional type of epithelium, except for a very short distance within the orifice. As the ducts become smaller and smaller, the epithelium is flatter and flatter, so that in the finest branches it consists of a single layer of flat cells. The acini are lined by a layer of cuboidal cells with basal nuclei. The function of the gland is the secretion of mucus for lubrication of the vaginal orifice and canal, especially during coitus.

THE VAGINA

The vagina is a musculomembranous canal which connects the vulva with the uterus. It

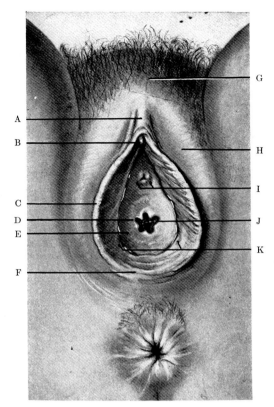

Figure 1.2. The vulva: *A*, prepuce; *B*, clitoris; *C*, labia minora; *D*, hymen; *E*, vestibule; *F*, posterior commissure; *G*, mons pubis; *H*, labia majora; *I*, opening of Skene's ducts; *J*, vagina; and *K*, vulvovaginal (Bartholin's) glands.

is about 9 or 10 cm in length, and, in the erect position of the woman, its direction is in general upward and backward from its vulvar to its uterine end. Its upper end expands into the cup-shaped *fornix*, into which the cervix uteri is fitted. The portions of the fornix in front of, behind, and at the sides of the cervix are designated as the anterior, posterior, and lateral fornices.

In the virgin, the *mucous membrane* of the anterior vaginal wall is horizontally corrugated, with a central vertical ridge, thus producing the arbor vitae appearance. These ridges are absent in the widened canal of the woman who has borne children.

The mucous membrane of the vagina is reddish pink, and is lined by a stratified squamous epithelium into which project many tiny subepithelial papillae of the subjacent fibrous tissue. In the young child the epithelium shows only perhaps six or eight layers of cells, but in the postpubertal phase many more layers are present.

Beneath the mucous membrane is the muscular coat, made up of an inner circular and an outer layer. The outermost layer is the fibrous, derived from the pelvic connective tissue.

CERVIX

The cervix is separated from the corpus externally by a slight constriction corresponding to the region of the internal os. The portion of the cervix above the level of the vagina is the supravaginal portion, that protruding into the vagina is the *pars* or *portio vaginalis*. The *cervical canal* is somewhat spindle-shaped, terminating below at the *external os*, a small round or transversely slitlike opening averaging in the nulliparous woman about 5 mm in diameter. At its upper end the cervical canal communicates with the uterine cavity through a constricted orifice called the *internal os*.

The *mucous membrane* covering the external or vaginal surface is of the stratified squamous variety, a continuation of that covering the adjacent vagina. The cervical canal, on the other hand, is lined by an entirely different type of mucous membrane, the endocervix, which is distinguished by the following features.

1. A tall, "picket" variety of columnar epithelium, with deeply stained nuclei placed close to the basement membrane, and a cytoplasm which is rich in mucin:
2. Glands of the racemose variety, lined by epithelium like that found on the surface: studies by Fluhmann indicate that there is in reality a complex system of tunnels and clefts that appear like glands (Fig. 1.3).
3. Stroma of fibrous tissue type, rich in spindle cell elements.

The muscular coat of the cervix is well developed in the region of the internal os, but becomes increasingly sparse at a lower level, so that only a thin outer layer is present in the lower portion of the cervix, with a corresponding increase in the proportion of connective tissue. Glandlike vestiges of the mesonephric duct are occasionally observed deep in the cervical musculature.

THE UTERUS

The uterus is a hollow, thick-walled muscular organ which is situated in the pelvis,

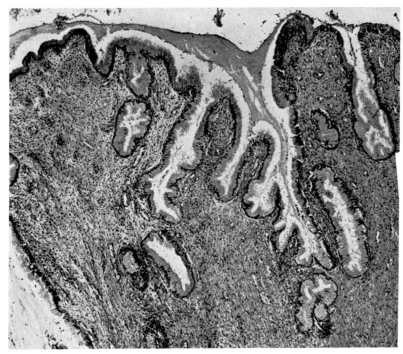

Figure 1.3. Microscopic appearance of cervix, showing characteristic "picket" gland epithelium, racemose glands, and spindle-celled fiborous stroma.

between the bladder anteriorly and the rectum posteriorly. It is placed almost at right angles to the vagina, with the bladder below and in front of it. It is somewhat pear-shaped, and measures in the nulliparous woman about 8 to 9 cm in length, 6 cm in its widest portion, and about 4 cm in thickness. It is divisible into a *corpus* and *cervix*. The upper domelike portion of the corpus is called the *fundus*, whereas the angle marking the attachment of the tube at each side is the *cornu*. The *uterine cavity* is rather conical, with the base above at the fundus and the apex, corresponding to the narrow internal os, leading into the cervical canal. Externally the corpus is covered with peritoneum.

The mucous membrane of the uterine body is the *endometrium*. This varies in thickness not only in individual women, but even more at different phases of the menstrual cycle.

The *stroma* is a characteristic immature type of connective tissue, made up of a homogeneous mass of small cells with round or slightly oval nuclei and, in the early stages of the cycle, almost no cytoplasm. They are supported by an almost invisible light fibrillary supporting structure. The vascular supply of the endometrium is through two sets of vessels, the spiral or coiled arterioles and the basal arterioles. The latter are the chief nutritional vessels, supplying especially the basal layers. The spiral arterioles, on the other hand, play an important part in the mechanism of the menstrual cycle and especially in menstrual bleeding.

The *muscular* coat of the uterus is made up of involuntary muscle fibers arranged in an interlacing fashion which, at least in the non-pregnant woman, is not disposed in any definite layer pattern. The serous coat consists of the peritoneum, which covers the entire corpus uteri.

Ligaments of the Uterus

Broad Ligaments

Each of these consists of a broad double sheet of peritoneum which extends from the lateral surface of the uterus outward to the pelvic wall. At its upper border the broad ligament encircles the fallopian tube, and beyond the tube continues on the pelvic wall as the *infundibulopelvic ligament*, through which the ovarian vessels make their way toward the tube and ovary. From the lower edge of the tube the broad ligament extends downward to surround the round ligament, this portion constituting a sort of tubal mesentery, or *mesosalpinx*. In this portion is found the parovarium (epoophoron or organ of Rosenmüller), which represents the lateral portions of the vestigial remains of the mesonephric tubules. To its medial side lies the paroophoron, likewise made up of vestigial mesonephric tubules, which, like those of the epoophoron, empty into the main mesonephric, or Wolffian, duct. It is the latter which in the male develops into the vas deferens. At its lower border the broad ligament is thickened, with a condensation of connective tissue and some muscle fibers, forming the thonglike *cardinal ligament* or *ligamentum colli of Mackenrodt* (Fig. 1.1).

Uterosacral Ligaments

The uterosacral ligaments fuse with the posterior fibers of the cardinal ligaments medially to blend with the fascial encasement of the upper vagina and cervix. The uterosacral ligaments proceed posterolaterally to again blend with the fibers of the endopelvic fascia anterior to the lateral aspects of the sacrum at about the junction of the second and third sacral vertebrae. In their course posteriorly they describe an arclike curve, the concavity of which is directed toward the midline.

Pubocervical Ligaments

These consist of two bands of connective tissue that pass from the posterior aspect of the pubis to the anterolateral aspects of the cervix. They blend with the fascial covering of the neck of the bladder medially to which they give some support.

The Round Ligaments

These are two round, muscular bands which arise from the lateral aspect of the fundus on each side, a short distance below and anterior to the insertion of the tube. They course outward between the broad ligament layers in a curved fashion to the internal inguinal ring, passing then through the inguinal canal, and spreading out in a fanlike fashion to fuse with the subcutaneous tissue of the labia majora. The thickness of these ligaments is very variable, but averages about 5 to 6 mm. They are made up of involuntary muscle continuous with that of the uterus itself, and their function seems to prevent retrodisplacement (Fig. 1.1).

Blood Supply

The blood supply of the uterus is derived from the ovarian and uterine arteries. The former, which correspond to the spermatic arteries of the male, arises from the abdominal aorta, passing down behind the peritoneum to the infundibulopelvic ligament, through which it enters the mesosalpinx to supply the tube and ovary, finally anastomosing with the uterine artery to complete the utero-ovarian vascular arch.

The uterine artery arises from the anterior branch of the hypogastric artery, passing toward the uterus through the parametrium. It turns upward about 1.5 or 2 cm lateral to the cervix, coursing upward in an extremely tortuous fashion to anastomose with the ovarian and giving off many branches to the uterine wall as it courses upward. As it turns upward at the level of the cervicovaginal juncture it is in close relation to the ureter, which passes *downward and inward*, behind the artery, on its course to the bladder (Fig. 1.4).

Because of the occasional problem that the clinician encounters with regard to the management of hemorrhage resulting from trauma or disease affecting the branches of the hypogastric artery, it is worthwhile to spend a little time in understanding the collateral circulation and flow characteristics of these vessels. The hypogastric artery provides most of the blood supply to the pelvic viscera and the pelvic musculature. It also provides a significant blood supply to the hip and the musculature involved in hip and thigh motion. Conceptually, it is convenient to divide it into two major divisions. The posterior division supplies parietal branches only, while the anterior division provides both visceral and parietal blood supply, but is mainly involved in visceral supply. The external iliac artery runs along the medial aspect of the psoas muscle, following the pelvic brim. The internal iliac, or hypogastric artery, arises as a branch from it, in front of the sacroiliac joint, and at this point, it is crossed anteromedially by the ureter which maintains its position attached to the parietal peritoneum of the pelvis. At the upper border of the greater foramen it divides into the posterior and anterior branches. For the most part, the parietal branches are given off early in the course of the posterior division of the artery and these include the iliolumbar, laterosacral and superior gluteal. As the artery

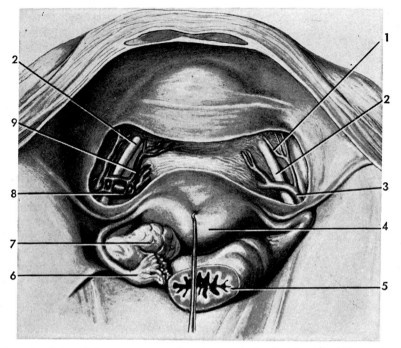

Figure 1.4. The topic relationship between ureter and uterine vessels. On the *left side* both the arteries and veins are drawn; on the *right side*, only the arteries: *1*, cervical branch of uterine artery; *2*, ureter; *3*, uterine artery; *4*, uterus; *5*, rectum; *6*, fallopian tube; *7*, ovary; *8*, uterine veins; and *9*, vesical vein.

proceeds as the anterior division, it gives off most of its parietal branches early and these include the inferior gluteal, pudendal and obturator. From this point onward, the visceral branches include the vaginal, inferior vesicular, uterine and finally the superior vesicular. The middle hemorrhoidal artery frequently arises as a common trunk with the pudendal from the posterior aspect of the anterior division.

The veins correspond in a general way with the arteries. The ovarian veins, on their way from the hilum of the ovary toward the vena cava, form, between the layers of the broad ligament, a rich network called the *pampiniform plexus*. On the right side the ovarian vein empties into the inferior cava itself, on the left into the left renal vein. The uterine veins follow the arteries and empty into the internal iliac veins.

Nerve Supply of the Female Genitalia

The genital tract is supplied by branches of both the autonomic and spinal nerve pathways. In the human certain higher centers as well as the *tuber cinereum* are of importance in regulating various sexual and menstrual functions, and one must always be cognizant of the highly important hypothalamic-hypophysial domination of ovarian function.

Various sympathetic and parasympathetic fibers of the *autonomic* system below the bifurcation of the aorta form the superior hypogastric plexus or presacral nerve, which is the chief supply of the uterus. As they pass caudal, they form the ganglion of Frankenhäuser or uterovaginal plexus located near the base of the uterosacral ligaments.

The ovary is supplied not by the sacral fibers, but rather by branches of the renal and aortic plexuses which are located in the suspensory ligaments of the ovary.

The pudendal nerve of the *spinal* nervous system is the primary source of motor and sensory activation of the lower genital tract. This is derived from roots of the second, third, and the fourth sacral nerves. It passes out of the pelvis via the greater and lesser *sciatic foramina*, and enters the pudendal canal of the *obturator fascia*. Various branches supply vulva, vagina, and perineum. Other nerves such as the ilioinguinal, genitofemoral, and cutaneous femoral nerve also contribute to the lower genital tract and perineum, but for details one is urged to consult appropriate neuroanatomical texts (Fig. 1.5).

THE FALLOPIAN TUBES

The tubes are two musculomembranous canals which transport the ova from the ovaries to the uterus. They are about 11 or 12 cm in length, and are divisible, for purposes of description, into four parts. (1) The *interstitial portion* is the narrow portion contained in the muscular wall of the uterus, which the tube penetrates to reach the uterine cavity. (2) The *isthmus* is the narrow portion of the tube close to its insertion into the uterine cornu. (3) The *ampulla* is the wider, baggier middle portion of the tube. (4) The distal third or so is the *fimbriated extremity*, which is rather funnel-shaped, the small orifice being surrounded by a number of peaked fringes or fimbriae.

Histologically, the tube consists of three coats, as follows: (1) the *serous coat*, which is formed by the encircling peritoneum of the upper margin of the broad ligament; (2) the *muscular coat*, arranged for the most part in an inner circular and an outer longitudinal layer; and (3) the *mucosa*, or endosalpinx, which is disposed in longitudinal folds or rugae, usually only three or four in number at the isthmus, but branching and subbranching longitudinally toward the fimbriated extremity, so that a cross section of the latter presents a very arborescent appearance as compared with the few folds at the isthmus. The lining *epithelium* is composed of a single layer of cells, superimposed on a rather cellular tunica propria. Like the uterine epithelium, the epithelium of the tube undergoes definite cyclical changes.

THE OVARIES

The ovaries are two ovoid bodies which constitute the genital glands of the female. They are placed, one in each side of the pelvis just below the tubes, the outer ends of which are curved over them in an arclike fashion. They measure about 3.5 by 2 by 1.5 cm, although there is considerable variation. Anteriorly, the ovaries are set in the posterior surface of the broad ligament much as a diamond is set in a ring. At the line of attachment is the *hilum*, through which blood vessels and nerves enter and leave the ovary.

The *external surface* of the ovary is of dull, whitish, opaque appearance. The ovary is attached to the uterus by a well developed *ovarian ligament*, while the upper outer pole is suspended to the side of the pelvis by that portion of the broad ligament beyond the tube (infundibulopelvic ligament or suspensory ligament of the ovary).

On section, the ovary is divisible into an outer cortex and a central portion or medulla. Covering the cortex is the so-called *germinal epithelium*, made up of a single layer of cu-

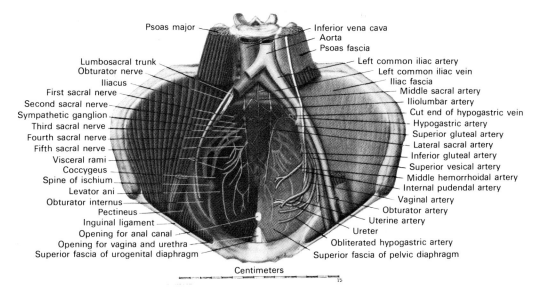

Figure 1.5.   The vessels and nerves of the female pelvis. On the *left half* the fascia is intact, on the *right* it has been removed.

boidal epithelium. It is usually unapparent in the adult ovary, but often appears in the presence of chronic inflammation. Under such conditions the epithelium may show metaplastic changes. Beneath the epithelium is the cortical stroma, which, just beneath the epithelium, shows a slightly condensed layer called the *tunica albuginea*. The stroma itself is made up of compactly placed spindle cell connective tissue cells, in which are seen the follicular elements and their derivatives.

In the ovary of the young child the follicles are exceedingly numerous, being estimated at about 1,000,000 in number in the ovary of the newborn child, but becoming progressively less numerous after puberty. The histological structure of the mature follicle, as well as of the *corpus luteum* in its various stages is described in Chapter 3 under "Cyclic Changes in the Ovary." Only a small proportion of primordial follicles reach full maturity, the majority being blighted at various phases of development by the process known as *atresia folliculi*. This is characterized by death of the ovum, followed by degeneration and disappearance of the granulosa, so that in this *cystic stage* the atretic follicle appears as a tiny cyst, with or without a lining epithelium. With increasing age, the follicle count drops progressively as indicated by Winter.

Hilus Cells

In the hilus of the ovary one not infrequently finds small nests and occasionally rather large fields of ovoid or polyhedral cells, usually arranged in rather mosaic fashion. They were originally spoken of by Berger as sympathicotrophic cells, but these hilus cells, as they are more commonly designated, are now looked upon as the homologues of the interstitial or Leydig cells of the testis, which they indeed resemble histologically. The peculiar rectangular crystalloids of Reincke may be found in both, although by no means invariably. There is remarkable similarity, if not identity, between hilus and theca cells (as discussed by Loubet and Loubet) and they both represent modified stromal cells.

The Pelvic Floor and Perineum

This is described in the section on relaxations and fistulas (Chapter 13).

References and Additional Readings

Berger, L.: La glande sympathicotrope du hile de l'ovaire; ses homologies avec la glande interstitielle due testicule; les rapports nerveuses des deux glandes. Arch. Anat. (Strasb.), *2:* 255, 1923.
Dallenbeck, F. D., and Vonderlin, D.: Innervation of the endometrium. Arch. Gynaekol., *215:* 365, 1973.
Fluhmann, C. F.: The developmental anatomy of the cervix uteri. Obstet. Gynecol., *15:* 62, 1960.
Forsberg, J. G.: Cervico-vaginal epithelium; its origin and development. Am. J. Obste. Gynecol., *115:* 1025, 1973.
Huffman, J. W.: Detailed anatomy of paraurethral ducts in adult female. Am. J. Obstet. Gynecol., *55:* 86, 1948.
Huffman, J. W.: Mesonephric remains in cervix. Am. J. Obstet. Gynecol., *56:* 23, 1948.
Huffman, J. W.: Mesonephric remains in human female. Q. Bull. Northwest Univ. Med. Sch., *25:* 1, 1951.
Loubet, R., and Loubet, A.: Le systeme des cellules hilaires de l'ovaire: hyperplasies et tumeurs. Soc. Franc. Gynecol., *33:* 589, 1963.
Pearl, M., and Plotz, E. J.: Supernumerary ovary. Obstet. Gynecol., *21:* 253, 1963.
Rubin, I. C., and Novak, J.: *Integrated Gynecology, Principles and Practice,* Vol. 1. Blakiston Company, Division of McGraw-Hill Book Company, Inc., New York, 1956.
Snell, R. S.: *Clinical Anatomy for Medical Students.* Little, Brown, Boston, 1973.
Weed, J. C.: Pelvic anatomy from the point of view of a gynecologic surgeon. Clin. Obstet. Gynecol., *15:* 1035, 1972.
Winter, G. F.: Follicle counts in the ovaries of healthy nonpregnant women. Zentralbl. Gynaekol., *84:* 1824, 1962.
Zacharin, R. F.: The anatomic supports of the female urethra. Obstet. Gynecol., *32:* 754, 1968.

CHAPTER 2

Physiology of Menstruation and Pregnancy

CURRENT STATUS OF THE PHYSIOLOGY OF MENSTRUATION

Sexual maturation is apparently a gradual, not a cataclysmic, process which is dependent upon development of the central nervous system. Specifically, it involves the concentration of adrenergic and cholinergic neurotransmitters in the hypothalamus. This is accomplished by transmission of the neurotransmitters, norepinephrine, dopamine and/or serotonin from the site of origin, along nerve tracts which have their endings in the hypothalamus.

The hypothalamus has two anatomically distinct nervous systems: (1) The essentially nonmyelinated nerve fibers with neurons which originate in the hypothalamus. These are the peptidergic neurons with the function of synthesizing the characteristic hypothalamic peptides, and the tuberohypophyseal dopamine system, (Table 2.1) and (2) the myelinated nerve fibers with cell bodies outside the hypothalamus and axons only within the hypothalamus. These are transmitting noradrenergic or serotonergic impulses to the peptidergic neurons for increase or decrease of synthesis of peptide hormones (Fig. 2.1).

Maturation of Hypothalamus

Neurotransmitters are concentrated in the hypothalamus from the source of synthesis in the cortex and sensory organs. The concentration of these neurotransmitters in the hypothalamus, as in the cerebral cortex, can be shown to increase with the age of the individual, presumably related to the quality or quantity of sensory stimuli exposure (Fig. 2.2). The noradrenergic nervous system is the only part of the nervous system which has the ability to grow postnatally and actively regenerate by sprouting after injury. Growth can also be stimulated in a dose-dependent relation by nerve growth factor. These characteristics of ontogenicity and plasticity have led Ruf to hypothesize that when the adrenergic neurons reach the limit of their growth potential, puberty is initiated by the adult level of terminal arborization of adrenergic neurons synapsing with hypothalamic peptidergic neurons (Fig. 2.3).

Lulibern (LRH, luteinizing-releasing hormone) is the hypothalamic hormone which stimulates synthesis and release of pituitary gonadotropins, FSH and LH. LRH is a decapeptide, it is not species specific, and is active by all routes of of administration. LRH synthesis is apparently stimulated by norepinephrine and perhaps inhibited by serotonin. An axon-axonal stimulus from dopaminergic neurons in the hypothalamus may cause release or inhibition of release of LRH into the pituitary portal vessels. The LRH release is pulsatile, apparently dependent upon the catecholamine control stimulus. The differential in FSH and LH baselines which allows the orderly development of ovarian function is dependent upon the difference in the clearance rates of these two pituitary hormones in relation to the secretory pulse. The lower clearance rate of FSH with the similar secretory pulse results initally in a higher circulating FSH than LH. The pulsatile secretory pattern is related to the catecholamine stimulation of LRH. As the FSH stimulation reaches sufficient levels to cause ovarian LH sensitivity and concomitant estrogen produc-

Table 2.1
Secretory Products of Hypothalamic Peptidergic Neurons[a]

Anterior Pituitary Effectors	Posterior Pituitary Hormones	Hormone Carriers	Tuberohypothalamic Dopamine System
LRH (GnRH)	Oxytocin	E-Neurophysin	Dopamine (PIF?)
Substance P	Vasopressin	N-Neurophysin	
GRH			
GIH			
TRH			
CRH			

[a] LRH, luteinizing-releasing hormone (gonadotropin-releasing hormone); PIF, prolactin-inhibiting factor; GRH, growth factor-releasing hormone; GIH, growth factor-inhibiting hormone; TRH, thyrotropic-releasing hormone; CRH, corticotropin-releasing hormone, E, estrogen; N, nicotine.

tion, the positive estrogen feedback at the hypothalamic and pituitary levels causes increased pituitary "sensitivity" and increased gonadotropin release. This eventuates in the LH "ovulatory" surge.

Modulation Pathways

Modulation of hypothalamic function occurs in three ways. (1) *Steroid feedback, the long loop*: This is illustrated by the positive and negative *estrogen* feedback described above. In addition, *testosterone* feeds back at the arcuate nucleus on the tonic LRH control and *inhibin*, the protein hormone from the granulosa cells of the follicle, feeds back to inhibit FSH preferentially over LH. (2) *Pituitary feedback, the short loop*: LH has been shown by Kuhl and Taubert to cause decreased LRH by a stimulatory effect upon L-cystine arylamidase, an enzyme which destroys LRH. Since this enzyme is activated by estrogen, it is not present in high concentration in the postmenopausal women and, therefore, the short loop feedback is ineffective under these circumstances. (3) *The intrapituitary feedback, the ultrashort loop*: LRH can desensitize its own receptors on the pituitary gonadotropins.

Basal LH Control: Negative Estrogen Feedback

Although the CNS is the primary source of stimulation to development of reproductive organs, the final key to this development is a normal ovary. Estrogen from the ovary modulates the pituitary FSH and LH levels through a negative feedback on the basal levels and a positive feedback on the cyclic surge. Basal gonadotropic control by the hypothalamus is dependent upon peptinergic neurons in the posterior hypothalamus in the region of the arcuate nucleus which synthesize LRH. The negative estrogen feedback whereby estrogen reduces secretion of FSH and LH is probably modulated by estrogen receptors in the LRH neurons.

LH Surge: Positive Estrogen Feedback

The control of the cyclic gonadotropic function, the midcycle LH surge, in the rat, is through neurons in the anterior hypothalamus in the suprachiasmatic or supraoptic nuclei. These cells, in addition to containing estrogen receptor protein, have the capability of aromatizing C_{19} steroids to estrogens and metabolizing estradiol to catechol estrogens. Recent experiments by Kérdelhue et al. and by Vijayan and McCann indicate that substance P, an undecapeptide synthesized in neurons of the suprachiasmatic nucleus, inhibits the action of LRH on pituitary LH and FSH release in animals under estrogen stimulation. Substance P could, therefore, be a gonadotropin cell membrane stabilizer which is, itself, inhibited by estrogen.

A working hypothesis is that in the absence of a high estrogen milieu, there is a stable *gonadotropic* membrane; the cell is accumulating FSH and LH. As the estrogen rises and the critical dose and duration of estrogen exposure is attained, the membrane stabilizer is inhibited. The now permeable gonadotropic membrane releases its accumulated LH and the preovulatory LH surge occurs. Thus, the "positive" estrogen feedback may well be explained on the basis of a double negative effect, the inhibition of an inhibition.

Integration with Ovarian Function

The functional hypothalamic unit therefore requires peptidergic neurons which are

AT BIRTH

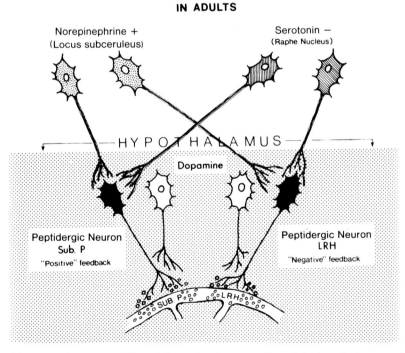

IN ADULTS

Figure 2.1. Diagrammatic representation of the anatomic composition of the hypothalamus and the relation of the aborization of the adrenergic nervous system at birth (*top*), and in adulthood (*bottom*), to maturation of the hypothalamus. Axons from extrahypothalamic neurons of the adrenergic system located in the locus subceruleus (norepinephrine), and the raphe nucleus (serotonin), compose some of the myelinated fibers of the hypothalamus. Norepinephrine is thought to *stimulate* function and serotonin *inhibit*. These axons terminate on the intrahypothalamic peptidergic neurons and control synthesis of peptides, as illustrated by substance P (Sub. P) and luteinizing-releasing hormone (LRH). The tuberohypophyseal dopamine system, completely within the hypothalamus, in addition to inhibiting pituitary prolactin secretion may also control the release of other hypothalamic hormones into the portal vessels of the median eminence. Axons of both the intrahypothalamic peptidergic and dopanergic neurons are unmyelinated.

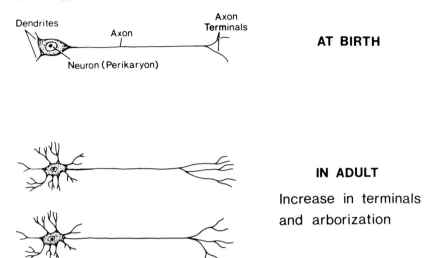

AT BIRTH

IN ADULT

Increase in terminals
and arborization

Figure 2.2.   Maturation of adrenergic nervous system. Diagram of increased numbers of dendrites and terminal aborization of axons in the adrenergic nervous system from birth to adulthood. The ontogenicity and plasticity of these cells allows increased activity with age.

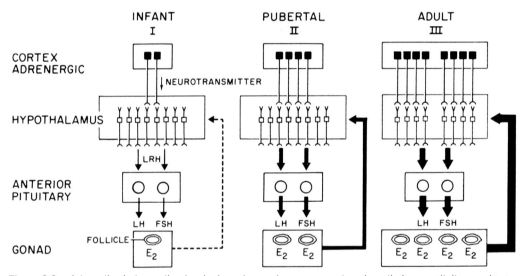

Figure 2.3.   Interaction between the developing adrenergic nervous system, hypothalamus, pituitary and ovary from infancy to adulthood. (Derived from K. B. Ruf: *Zeitschrift fuer Neurologie, 204:* 95, 1973.)

programmed to synthesize hypothalamic hormones, neurotransmitters to regulate the synthesis by both stimulus and inhibition, and a third set of neurons with axon-axonal junctions to initiate the release of the hormones. This third set of neurons comprises the tuberohypophyseal dopamine system. The peptidergic neurons must also contain steroid receptor proteins to allow for modulation by the long loop steroid feedback.

LH and FSH are secreted by the pituitary in an episodic fashion related to episodic LRH secretion. There is no LRH surge in midcycle to account for the LH surge. Rather

it is related to a change in the pituitary release mechanism which in turn is related to the ovarian estrogen.

Two circumventricular organs outside of the blood brain barrier (Table 2.2), the **median eminence** and the **organum vasculosum lamina terminalis (OVLT)** might indeed furnish access of estrogen in the general circulation to the hypothalamus. The **tanycyte**, which is the specialized cell of the third ventricle, increases its absorption surface in relation to the amount of circulating estrogen. It could theoretically, therefore, transport estrogen from the vessels of the median emi-

Table 2.2
Circumventricular organs: Hypothalamic
Appendages Outside Blood Brain Barrier

Organ	Function
Pineal	Integration of reproductive function with external environmental factors, sun and moon cycles, gravity
Median eminence (infundibulum)	Junctions of axons from hypothalamic peptidergic neurons with the hypothalamic pituitary portal vessels. Tanycytes, specialized third ventricle ependymal cells, span the entire median eminence reaching from the vessel walls to the ventricle. The absorptive surfaces of these cells are estrogen sensitive. The median eminence may be an area especially important in estrogen feedback to the luteinizing-releasing hormone (LRH) neurons in the arcuate nucleus
Organum vasculosum lamina terminalis (OVLT)	Thought to contain LRH neurons. Because of its blood supply and its connection with the suprachiasmatic and supraoptic nuclei of the anterior hypothalamus, it is suspected that it may have a role in estrogen feedback to the suprachiasmatic area. Destruction does not influence the cycle in the rhesus monkey
Area postrema	Initiates vomiting due to systemic vs. central factors. Thought to influence changes in blood pressure and fluid intake
Subcommissural organ	Function unknown

nence to the ventricle and from the ventricle to the neurons in the arcuate nucleus. Another source would be the caudal branch of the arterial vessel which supplies the median eminence and sends branches into the arcuate nucleus. The blood supply to the OVLT is by way of the internal carotid system and blood from the portal system of the OVLT drains in both directions between the OVLT and the median preoptic nucleus. Neurons in this area synthesize substance P. Although neurons in the OVLT have been said to secrete LRH, this secretory function of the organ is little understood.

Follicular Growth

Follicular growth which will result in ovulation of a single active follicle begins 2 to 4 days prior to the menstrual bleeding episode which will precede the ovulatory event. At this time in the cycle, estrogen and progesterone are reaching their nadir, and with the falling steroid milieu, and in the absence of follicular *inhibin*, FSH begins to rise. It is this FSH stimulation which causes the flurry of follicular activity which signals the growth of the cohort follicles for the next cycle. FSH continues to rise during the first 7 to 10 days of the follicular phase associated with a slightly delayed LH rise. The rising LH in the first part of the follicular phase is responsible for the production of estrogen by the theca surrounding the developing follicles. However, during this phase of the cycle estrogen remains relatively low. The follicle, which is to become the active follicle, will be the one which is able to concentrate the greatest amount of estrogen and therefore become independent of FSH stimulation. As the follicles grow they secrete increasing amounts of *inhibin* and therefore after the 7th day of a 28-day cycle, FSH begins to fall. Only the follicle which has accumulated sufficient high affinity estrogen-binding protein to become autonomous can survive. The remaining follicles, without sufficient FSH support, begin to become atretic.

Ovulation

During the preovulatory swelling phase, 4 days prior to ovulation, a rapid increase of estrogen occurs. This estrogen surge is from the active follicle, and triggers the LH surge and release of prostaglandin $F_{2\alpha}$. Although the preovulatory LH surge initiates luteinization of the granulosa cells and corpus luteum formation, ovulation per se is dependent upon a vascular phenomenon, formation of the **stigma**. In experimental animals, and by inference in the human, it can be shown that prostaglandin $F_{2\alpha}$ is responsible for orientation of the follicle to the exterior of the ovarian cortex, stigma formation and eventual ovulation. However, although ovulation apparently will not occur in the absence of prostaglandin, the LH surge may also contribute to the ovulatory process.

The LH surge initiates a number of reactions in the ovary which lead to progesterone production by the corpus luteum, and a shift in the estradiol precursor pathway from the

Δ^5 dehydroandrosterone to the Δ^4 progesterone substrate described by Ryan and Coronel. The LH surge is also important in oocyte maturation and resumption of meiosis. Following the initial stimulatory phase of the LH surge, with cyclic AMP accumulation and increased steroid production, a "desensitization" occurs. As high cyclic AMP levels inhibit ovulation by inhibition of prostaglandin, this desensitization phase is necessary for ovulation and explains the decreased estrogen synthesis following the LH surge. Decreased estrogen may also be important for ovulation as collagenase and plasminogen are inhibited by estrogens and these enzymes may be necessary to digest the basement membrane of the follicle at the stigma during ovulation.

Corpus Luteum Function

After ovulation, the ensuing corpus luteum function results in production of sufficient estrogen to inhibit the posterior hypothalamic LRH neurons, decreasing pituitary FSH and LH synthesis and release. As the corpus luteum regresses, approximately 2 to 4 days prior to menstruation, steroid levels reach a sufficiently low concentration to allow the pituitary to increase FSH secretion. This initiates the growth of follicles and the cycle begins all over again.

The normality of corpus luteum function depends upon the initial programming of the granulosa cells to contain proper FSH receptor sites and the necessary enzymes for progesterone production, a proper FSH stimulation, beginning in the prior cycle, to initiate normal numbers and composition of granulosa cells, and finally adequate residual LH stimulation for a 14-day luteal span. It is as yet unresolved whether the corpus luteum fixed life span depends upon its failing response to minimal LH perhaps due to receptor loss, or upon some active luteolytic factor. Prostaglandin $F_{2\alpha}$ is perhaps the cause of the final denouement of the corpus luteum (see Aksel).

Summary. The ability of the ovary to respond to the pituitary gonadotropins with follicle growth, estrogen production, ovulation, corpus luteum formation, and progesterone production depends primarily upon the normality of the chromosomal content. In the absence of two normal X chromosomes, it has been shown that, as oocytes begin to go into meiotic division during the second or third month of embryonic life, the germ cells disappear from the genital ridge leaving only stroma and forming a "streak ovary" (Chapter 8). Given two normal X chromosomes and a normal complement of oocytes, the eggs organize around them the granulosa cells. This follicular envelope allows arrest of meiosis in the diplotene stage by oocyte maturation inhibitor (OMI). The granulosa cells of these primordial follicles increase in number, forming a primary follicle. The primary follicle induces the theca cell differentiation from the ovarian stroma, thus completing the Graafian follicle. The estrogenic potential of the ovary is then established. For growth to an antrum follicle and steroidogenesis, however, stimulation by pituitary gonadotropins is necessary. The normally programmed granulosa cells contain FSH receptor sites. FSH initiates: (1) LH receptors in both granulosa and probably theca cells; (2) a high affinity estrogen-binding protein, which allows the granulosa cells to concentrate estrogen, the true follicle growth hormone; (3) inhibin, the protein hormone which suppresses FSH preferentially over LH; and (4) synthesis of the mucopolysaccharides, the ground substances of the follicular fluid, and the basement membrane.

Granulosa cells, in the first half of the cycle, during the follicular phase, do not have a steroidogenic function, nor do they have a blood supply, but receive their nourishment from the systemic system through diapedesis across the basement membrane. Theca cells, on the other hand, with a good blood supply and access to LH, develop a steroidogenic function as the LH receptors are induced. The theca cells concentrate estrogen precursors, dihydroepiandrosterone and androstenedione and aromatize them into estradiol. This estrogen is then concentrated in the granulosa cells by high affinity estrogen-binding protein. It is estrogen which initiates DNA replication and multiplication of the granulosa cells. The preovulatory estrogen surge by the active follicle not only stimulates the LH surge, but also production of prostaglandin. Once ovulation has occurred, vascularization of the luteinized granulosa cells takes place rapidly. Following a brief LH desensitization stage, steroidogenesis is resumed, and now the luteinized granulosa cells are producing progesterone. Thus, they have changed their formerly predominant protein synthesis capacity to steroid synthesis. One of the first manifestations of this change is the appearance of an activated 3β-ol-dehydrogenase enzyme. Estrogen continues to be produced by the luteinized theca cells. However, with the availability of progesterone, there is a shift of the steroidogenic pathway from the Δ^5 pathway, to the Δ^4 pathway.

In the luteal phase of the cycle, the active follicle is still responsible for the major estradiol production as well as for the entire ovarian progesterone production. Luteinized theca cells have never been shown to produce progesterone, but they continue to produce estradiol.

The normality of corpus luteum function depends first upon the initial programming of the granulosa cells to contain proper FSH receptors, and the necessary enzymes for progesterone production, secondly upon a proper FSH stimulation, beginning in the prior cycle, to initiate normal numbers and composition of granulosa cells, thirdly upon an adequate LH surge to induce granulosa luteinization, and finally upon adequate residual tonic LH stimulation during the luteal phase to ensure an adequate 14-day span. The final denouement of the corpus luteum is caused by the flood of prostaglandin $F_{2\alpha}$ produced under the stimulus of the luteal steroids. In the absence of prostaglandin, Halban's disease, or persistent corpus luteum, occurs.

CHEMISTRY OF STEROID HORMONES

Nomenclature

The ovarian, testicular, and adrenal hormones are steroids derived from the same basic molecular structure of cholesterol. The steroid nuclei from which these hormones derive their names, estrane, androstane, and pregnane, with the designation of the rings and the numbering of the carbon atoms, are shown in Figure 2.4. The major structural differences are the absence of the side chain (C_{20} and C_{21}) in the androstane nucleus, from which the androgens are derived, and the absence of both the side chain and a methyl group at C_{19}, in the estrane nucleus, from which the estrogens are derived. Progesterone and the adrenal corticoids belong to the pregnane series.

Stereoisomerism can occur at any of the asymmetric carbon atoms, 5, 8, 9, 10, 13, and

PREGNANE

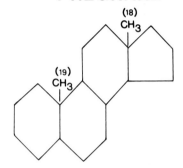

ANDROSTANE

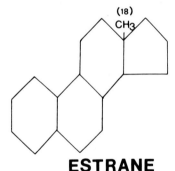

ESTRANE

Figure 2.4. The steroid hormone parent nuclei from which the nomenclature is derived. The ring designations and the carbon atom numbers are shown in the pregnane nucleus. Hydrogen atoms are not shown on the androstane or estrane nuclei.

14, and is important as it affects the biological activity of the compound. The Greek letters alpha, α, and beta, β, are used to designate the stereometric position of the hydrogen atom or substituents in relation to the angle of the methyl groups at carbon atom 18 or 19 or both, β being in the same plane and α in the opposite. When drawn on a formula, solid lines are used for the β position and dotted lines are used for the α position. The β position, which is present in biologically active steroids, is also referred to as *cis* while the α position may be called *trans*. The terms *allo* and *epi* are sometimes used to denote the α and β positions. However, *allo* is used only in relation to the hydrogen atom at C_5, while *epi* can be used in relation to any carbon atom.

The presence of a double bond is noted in the nomenclature by changing the suffix "ane" to "ene." Two double bonds are denoted by the suffix "diene" and three by "triene." The number of the lowest sequential carbon designates the position of the bond, and this number should be placed between the name of the parent nucleus and the prefix. The Greek letter delta, Δ, placed before the parent nucleus name with the superior carbon number, Δ^5, has also been used for this purpose.

The presence of a hydroxyl group is denoted by the prefix "hydroxy" or the suffix "ol" and a ketone group by the prefix "oxo" or the suffix "one." The absence of a substituent group or a carbon is designated by the prefixes "des" or "nor."

Biosynthesis

The ovary, adrenal, and testis all possess capabilities for biosynthesis of all steroids. Utilizing cholesterol as a substrate (Fig. 2.5) after hydroxylation at C_{20} and C_{22}, the side chain is split off with the formation of pregnenolone and isocaproic acid. Reduced nicotinamide adenine dinucleotide phosphate (TPNH) is an essential cofactor. TPNH is usually necessary wherever an hydroxylation occurs. Nicotinamide adenine dinucleotide (DPN) is essential for the dehydrogenase reactions, removal of hydrogen.

Two major pathways have been shown to exist from cholesterol to either testosterone or estrogen; the Δ^4 pathway, via progesterone, and the Δ^5 pathway by way of dehydroepiandrosterone (DHEA). Progesterone is formed from pregnenolone by removal of the hydrogen at the three position and shifting of the double bond from the B ring to the A Ring (Fig. 2.6). The first reaction utilizes a 3β-hydroxydehydrogenase which is catalyzed by DPN. The isomerization reaction, which shifts the double bond from the Δ^5 to the Δ^4 position, can be accomplished either enzymatically or chemically.

Following the formation of 17α-hydroxy- progesterone, the side chain can be removed, forming Δ^4-androstene-3,17-dione, which can be converted readily to either testosterone or estrogens (Fig. 2.7). For aromatization at ring A, three additional hydroxylations, two at C_{19} and one at C_2, must be accomplished prior to inserting the two additional double bonds into the structure of ring A.

The second pathway, the Δ^5 pathway, is through pregnenolone to dehydroisoandrosterone (DHA) rather than to progesterone. The dehydroisoandrosterone pool in the blood represents a constant source of steroid substrate.

The Δ^5 pathway, directly through DHA, is most active in estrogen production by the theca and interstitial cells of the ovary during the proliferative stage of the cycle, while the Δ^4 pathway, through progesterone, is the one of choice following luteinization and corpus luteum formation.

The final steroidogenic synthetic potential of the adrenal, ovary, or testis depends upon the substrate and the amount of enzymes and cofactors present. In addition to these organ sources, peripheral conversion of androstenedione to estrogens and androgens occurs in the skin and appendages. The presence of subcutaneous fat has a positive influence on the efficiency of these mechanisms.

HORMONE CONTENT OF TISSUE AND BODY FLUIDS: METABOLISM, FUNCTION, MECHANISMS OF ACTION

Definitions. The secretion rate equals the estimated hormone contribution of a gland to the total blood hormonal concentration. The production rate equals the total blood hormone concentration from whatever source. Metabolic clearance rate equals the volume of blood which is cleared of hormone per unit of time.

Estrogens

Tissue Content and Metabolism

Appreciable amounts of estrogens have been recovered from follicular fluid and human placenta, as well as from urine, blood, feces, and bile of pregnant and menstruating women. Since estrogen receptors are present in relatively high concentrations in brain and pituitary as well as in breasts, it would be

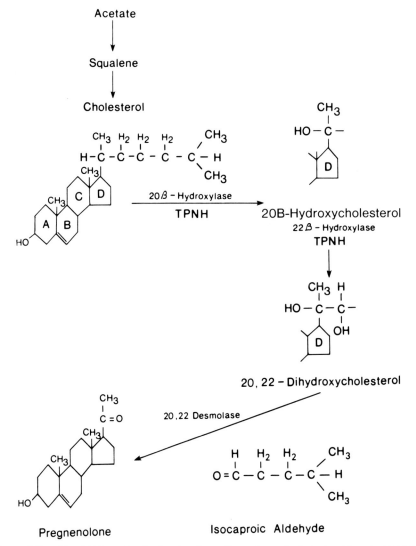

Figure 2.5.   Steroid biosynthesis showing the pathway through cholesterol to pregnenolone.

assumed that these tissues would also contain measurable amounts of estrogens. Circulating estrogens are bound to a specific estrogen binding-protein for transport and are conjugated in the liver for excretion into the urine or feces as glucuronides or sulfates.

The endometrium, an estrogen target organ, also has the ability to conjugate estrogen and may well control its own growth in this fashion. Thus, the more mature the endometrium, the less biologically active the estrogen to which it is exposed.

The liver and brain metabolize estradiol to catechol estrogens, C_2-methoxy and C_2-hydroxy, metabolites (see Fig. 2.10). Catechol estrone may be biologically active in the cen-

tral nervous system but does not bind or translate in the periphery as estrogen. The metabolic pathway to catechol estrogen is therefore the major pathway of inactivation of estrogens at the peripheral target organs. In pregnancy, the fetal placental unit through the fetal liver, metabolizes estradiol to estetrol and it is this pathway by which estrogen is inactivated in pregnancy.

Estradiol and estrone are the major components of Graafian follicle fluid; estriol represents the largest urinary estrogen component. Although all three major estrogens have been identified in placental extracts, estriol seems to be the predominant placental estrogen.

Steroid Biosynthesis of Androgen

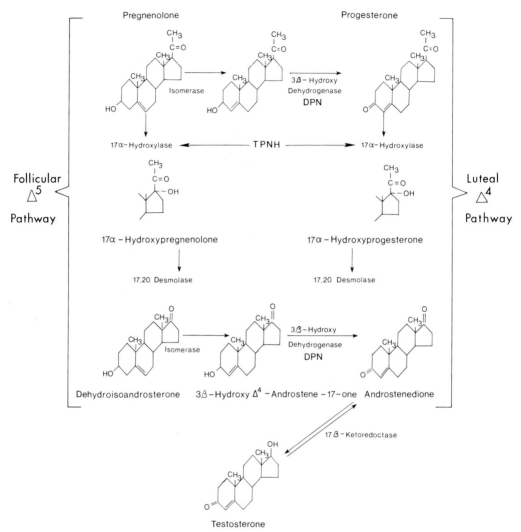

Figure 2.6. Steroid biosynthesis showing the pathway from pregnenolone through progesterone to androstenedione or testosterone.

Ovary

Follicular Fluid. Estradiol from follicular fluid is the most potent naturally occurring ovarian estrogen. Estrone is also found in the follicle, but in lesser amounts, and since the conversion reaction between the two hormones is reversible, an equilibrium is probably established.

Blood production and ovarian secretion rates (Fig. 2.8) calculated from simultaneous comparison of peripheral and ovarian vein bloods with follicular fluid estrone and estradial values (Table 2.3) in the normal menstrual cycle are shown.

Blood

Estrone and estradiol in the normal menstrual cycle in relation to other steroids, as well as to pituitary FSH and LH have been measured by radioimmunoassay. The range for estradiol is between 20 and 500 pg/ml and for estrone between 50 and 400 pg/ml. Menopausal values for estradiol are below 10 pg/ml and below 30 pg/ml for estrone. Male values are between the range of 15 through 25 pg/ml for estradiol and 40 through 75 pg/ml for estrone.

The metabolic clearance rate of estradiol is reported by Longcope et al. to be 1360 L/day

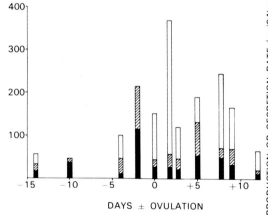

Androstenedione   Testosterone

17β – Ketoreductase

19 Hydroxylase   ⟶ TPNH ◄

Aromatization

17β – Ketoreductase

Estrone   Estradiol

Figure 2.7. Steroid biosynthesis showing the pathway from androstenedione to estrone and estradiol. Androstenedione may be derived from either progesterone through the 17α-hydroxyprogesterone or from dehydroepiandrosterone.

for females and 1600 L/day for males, while the clearance rate of estrone is the same for males and females, approximately 2000 L/day.

Urine

Urinary metabolites of estradiol are conjugated as glucuronides or sulfates or double conjugates, glucuronide:sulfates. Some idea about the relative importance of each metabolite can be obtained by the classic work of Gallagher and associates who measured the various urinary fractions after administering radioactive carbonlabeled estradiol (Fig. 2.9). Catechol estrogens comprise up to 10% of urinary metabolites. The urinary estrogen curve parallels the serum levels. The amounts of estriol, estrone, and estradiol recoverable from the urine during the various phases of the menstrual cycle can be seen in Table 2.4.

The metabolites in the estriol pathway are all active at the peripheral target organs, as they all bind to estradiol receptor protein and transcribe the estrogen message. However, the affinity and retention times are different. Estradiol is the most efficient, and estriol the least. Both the liver and the central nervous system metabolize estrogen to 2-hydroxy and 2-methoxy estrogens. These metabolites are apparently inactive at the peripheral target tissues, but are active in the central nervous

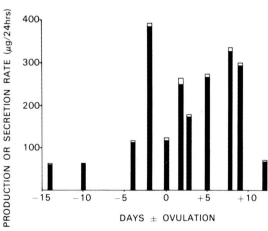

Figure 2.8. (*Left*) Blood production rate for estrone or ovarian secretion rate. (*Right*) Estradiol (E_2) throughout the normal menstrual cycle. Values have been plotted by the estimated day of ovulation (0) for each subject. Total blood production rate for each subject is indicated by the height of the bar. The amount of estrone (E_1) or estradiol from each steroid is indicated by the corresponding codes:

Estrone:

■ = ovarian E_1
□ = E_1 derived from E_2
□ = E_1 derived from other sources

Estradiol:

■ = ovarian E_2
□ = E_2 derived from E_1

(From D. T. Baird and I. S. Fraser: *Journal of Clinical Endocrinology & Metabolism, 38:* 1009, 1974.)

Table 2.3

Concentration (ng/100 ml) of Estrone (E₁) and Estradiol (E₂) in Follicular Fluid

Patient No.	Right Ovary		Left Ovary	
	E₁	E₂	E₁	E₂
1	—	—	2.86[a]	1144[a]
2	2.40[a]	44.1[a]	1.04	10.19
	6.39[a]	130.7[a]	—	—
	8.95[a]	166.0[a]	—	—
	5.90	88.63	—	—
	5.37	83.12	—	—
3	—	—	4.94[a]	127.5[a]
4	—	—	1.55	7.35
5	0.33	2.23	0	0.80
6	0	1.46	0	0
7	0.42[a]	12.78[a]	—	—
8	24.41[a]	380.5[a]	—	—
9	16.5[a]	375.0[a]	—	—

[a] All follicles of diameter 1 cm or greater. (From D. T. Baird and I. S. Fraser: *Journal of Clinical Endocrinology & Metabolism, 38:* 1009, 1974.)

system, inducing the LH surge (Naftolin et al., 1975) the positive estrogen feedback effect, but not the negative, LH suppression (Gethmann et al., 1978). The ratio of estradiol and estrone to catechol estrogens, varies in certain metabolic disease states such as obesity, anorexia, or thyroid disease (Chapter 30). Catechol estrogen content of brain is not depleted by ovariectomy, although peripheral estrogen target organs are depleted of their estrogen stores. Estrogen induced cAMP accumulation in the hypothalamus is inhibited by catechol estrogens, but such an antiestrogen is not apparent in the peripheral target tissues.

A third metabolic pathway for inactivation of circulating estrogen is present during pregnancy. Estradiol is converted only by the fetal liver to estetrol, E₄ (Tulchinsky et al.).

Bile and Feces

The recovery of substantial amounts of estrogen from the feces has been reported following estrogen administration. Siebke and Schuschania reported equal amounts of estrogen in the feces and the urine of normally menstruating women. Autopsy findings indicate that the liver of pregnant women is high in estrogen content, and Cantarow et al. report that the bile content is 3 times that of the blood in human term pregnancy. These combined experimental observations suggest an enterohepatic estrogen circulation. A consideration of the enterohepatic circulation is of importance in determining the biologic effect of estrogenic drugs. Either the mode of administration or the chemical configuration

of the drug can change the circulation time and thereby the access of the steroid to liver cells.

Skin and Appendages: Contribution of Androgenic Steroids to Estrogen Milieu

Testosterone is secreted presumably by the hilus cells of the ovary. Abraham has confirmed a midcycle peak and slightly higher values in the luteal phase as compared to the follicular phase (Fig. 2.10). The range for normal menstruating females is between 20 and 50 μg/ml. The ovarian contribution to the peripheral testosterone value is estimated at 33% during the follicular and luteal phases and 60% at the midcycle. The remainder is due to adrenal function. Testosterone contributes relatively little to the ovarian E₂ blood production rate.

Androstenedione (ADD) is the steroid preferentially secreted by the ovarian stromal cells. The range for normal menstruating females is between 100 and 220 μg/ml. An appreciable amount of ADD is also secreted by the adrenal but, under normal conditions, the contribution of the ovary makes up as much as 70% of peripheral ADD at midcycle (Table 2.5). ADD is an important steroid, as it is a precursor for estrone. In the menopause, little or no estrogen is secreted by the ovary. All of the serum estrone is derived by peripheral conversion of ADD, which at this time of life is thought to come mainly from the adrenal.

ADD can also be aromatized to estrogen by cells of the anterior, but not posterior, hypothalamus, furnishing the ovary with a differential feedback control mechanism of the cyclic and tonic gonadotropic centers.

Summary. The theca cells of the ovarian follicles synthesize estradiol, which is immediately in equilibrium with estrone. Estrogen is transported to its target organs by conjugation with a specific estrogen binding protein, rendering it biologically inactive. It is conjugated to sulfate and/or glucuronide in the endometrium, and in the liver, kidney, and gut. It is further metabolized by the liver to estriol through the 16-keto-estrone pathway. In the central nervous system, as well as in the liver, estrogens are also metabolized to catechol estrogens, by hydroxylation and/or methylation in the C₂ position. These metabolites, unlike the estrogens in the estriol pathway, are biologically inactive in the peripheral target organs, as they are not recognized

ESTROGEN METABOLITES

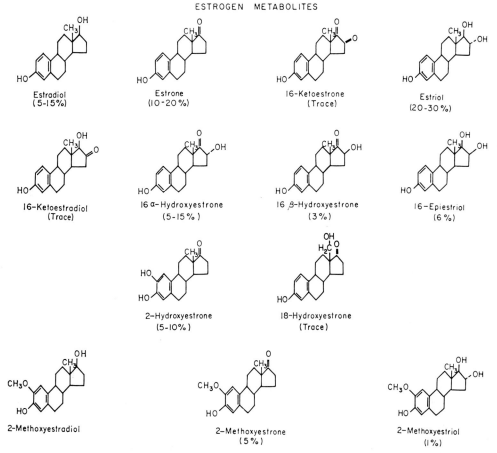

Figure 2.9. Human urinary metabolites of estrogen with the estimated total urinary radioactivity found on recovery experiments. (Compiled with the assistance of F. Gallagher.)

Table 2.4
Estrogen Levels Found at Various Times during Menstrual Cycle

Time in Cycle	Estrogens Excreted (μg per 24 hr)					
	Average			Range		
	Estriol	Estrone	Estradiol	Estriol	Estrone	Estradiol
Onset of menstruation	6	5	2	0–15	4–7	0–3
Ovulation peak	27	20	9	13–54	11–31	4–14
Luteal maximum	22	14	7	8–72	10–23	4–10

(From J. B. Brown: *Lancet, 1:* 320, 1955.)

by the estrogen receptors. They are, however, active in the central nervous system. All of these estrogen conjugated metabolites are excreted in the urine. A substantial amount of estrone is excreted in the bile and appears in the feces as estrone sulfate or a double conjugate estrone glucuronide-sulfate.

An additional contribution is made to the total body estrogen pool by the peripheral conversion of androstenedione. This precursor steroid is synthesized by both the adrenal and the ovarian stromal cells. It is converted to estrone by the skin and its appendages and is the major source of estrogen in the menopausal woman.

Functions

Estrogen is commonly regarded as the "female sex hormone" as it is indeed responsible for many of the typical female characteristics:

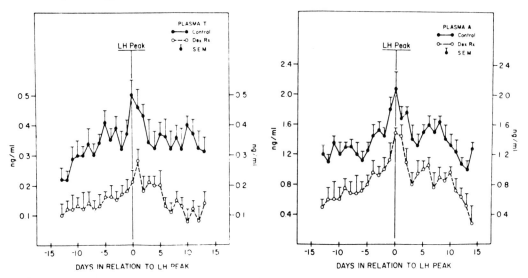

Figure 2.10.   Patterns and levels (mean ± SEM) of serum testosterone (*T*) and adrostenedione (*A*) during two consecutive menstrual cycles in six menopausal women. The first cycle served as control and the adrenal cortex was suppressed with dexamethasone (*Dex Rx*) during the second cycle. LH, luteinizing hormone. (From G. E. Abraham: *Journal of Clinical Endocrinology & Metabolism, 39:* 340, 1974.)

Table 2.5
Ovarian and Adrenal Contribution to Peripheral Androgens (ng/ml)[a]

Steroid	Ovarian Contribution[b]			Adrenal Contribution
	F	M	L	
T	0.1 (33%)	0.3 (60%)	0.1 (33%)	0.2 (40–66%)
DHT[c]		0.1 (50%)		0.1 (50%)
A	0.5 (45%)	1.5 (70%)	0.8 (60%)	0.6 (30–55%)
DHEA[c]		0.8 (20%)		3.2 (80%)
DHEA-S	80 (4%)	200 (10%)	80 (4%)	2000 (90–96%)

[a] F, early folicular; M, midcycle; L, late luteal phase; T, testosterone; A, adrostenedione; DHT, dihydrostestosterone; DHEA, dehydroepiandrosterone; DHEA-S, dehydroepiandrosterone sulfate.
[b] Numbers in parentheses are percent contribution calculated by comparing control cycles with a cycle in which the adrenal cortex was suppressed by dexamethasone.
[c] Ovarian contribution not influenced by phase of menstrual cycle.
(From G. Abraham: *Journal of Clinical Endocrinology & Metabolism, 39:* 340, 1974.)

fat deposition, breast growth and development, and the external female genitalia. It also has a selective growth effect upon all tissues derived from the Müllerian ducts. In addition to these specific sex-related actions estrogen exerts an effect on general physiology, controlling blood proteins and lipids, and influencing supportive tissues, specifically the vascular and skeletal systems. Different tissues show different sensitivity to similar "estrogen" doses. Therefore, it is important to define a dose response in terms of a specific tissue.

Vagina

The cornification of the vagina described many years ago by Stockard and Papanicolaou is so characteristic of estrogenic activity that it has been used to define an estrogen. These changes are described in Chapter 3, "Cyclic Cytology and Histology of the Genital Tract."

Uterus

Under estrogen stimulation the cervix becomes patulous, the os open, and the mucus abundant, acellular, and fluid, with ferns of crystallization, and capable of supporting sperm motility. There is a marked increase in the size of the uterus, which comprises both the endometrium and the uterine musculature. This growth effect is associated with an increase in the blood supply of the affected tissues. The rhythmic contractility of the uterine musculature reaches its peak under estrogen dominance.

Fallopian Tubes

The motility of the fallopian tubes is also under the control of estrogen, the greatest activity being in the estrogen dominant phase.

Ovary

Estrogen is perhaps the true "growth hormone" for the Graafian follicle, the major function of pituitary FSH being to induce synthesis of a high affinity estrogen-binding protein which can concentrate estrogen in the granulosa cells. It is this estrogen per se then which stimulates the follicular DNA system necessary for cellular replication.

In addition to its role as a follicular growth stimulant, estrogen stimulates the synthesis of ovarian prostaglandins, which facilitate ovulation in the late follicular phase of the menstrual cycle and cause luteolysis of the corpus luteum in the premenstrual phase.

Breasts

The growth of the duct system of the breast is stimulated by estrogen. The nipple erectility and pigmentation of the areolae are also estrogen-dependent.

Pituitary

The presence of specific estrogen receptor proteins in the cytosol of pituitary gonadotrophs indicates that there is probably an action of estrogen at the pituitary level.

The most striking effect of estrogen on the pituitary is seen in the lactotrophic cells. Prolactin secretion is enhanced by estrogen. This stimulation accounts for the increased size of the pituitary gland during pregnancy, as the "pregnancy cells" are, in fact, lactotrophs.

Assay of somatotropin, a pituitary growth hormone (Merimee et al.), indicates that estrogen stimulation enhances the pituitary response of this hormone to any inciting stimulation. The effect may be mediated through the hypothalamus and an effect upon somatostatin has not been precluded.

Hypothalamus

The Positive and Negative Estrogen Feedback on Gonadotropin Control. The positive and negative estrogen feedback modulation of pituitary gonadotropins, FSH and LH secretion, although once considered a direct effect upon the pituitary, is now thought to be mediated initially through the hypothala-
mus. The negative feedback is clearly at the hypothalamic level, on the LRH neurons in the region of the arcuate nucleus. As estrogen rises, LRH is inhibited, as evidenced by decreased LH, in a linear dose-dependent relationship. The results of this effect are seen in the luteal phase of the cycle when the estradiol is highest over the longest time span, resulting in the lowest LH basal levels during the cycle.

The explanation of the positive estrogen feedback is more complicated and controversial. This estrogen effect is not dose-related but depends upon a critical estrogen stimulation over an exposure time of from 36 to 72 hours in duration. This time lag seems to mediate against a direct pituitary effect, and makes it more likely that the effect upon the pituitary is secondary and mediated through the hypothalamus. Furthermore, the effect of estradiol in pituitary cell cultures is to stimulate cell synthesis but not release of LH.

Hypothesis. The best evidence at present is that the "positive feedback" on LH secretion is indeed a double negative effect, an inhibition of an inhibition. Substance P, a hypothalamic peptide secreted in neurons of the anterior hypothalamus in the region of the suprachiasmatic nucleus, is apparently an LRH inhibitor. One can consider this a gonadotropic LH release inhibitor and an inducer of a cell membrane stabilizer. Thus, substance P may act on the gonadotropins as dopamine does on the lactotrophs. If estrogen inhibits substance P, the LH release inhibitor, the release of LH would be favored over accumulation. The LH surge would then represent the amount of LH which the cell is capable of releasing when the membrane has maximal *permeability*, in relation to the amount of LH which it has stored during the follicular phase when the membrane has maximum *stability* (Fig. 2.11).

Just prior to and after the LH surge, the LRH stimulus is reduced by the negative estrogen feedback. Synthesis and release of LH are therefore minimal, resulting in the low LH baseline seen during the luteal phase of the cycle. If, however, an exogenous LRH pulse is given in this phase, the percentage response of LH over the baseline is increased as compared to the follicular phase response (Fig. 2.12). In the luteal phase of the cycle, the pulsatile LH response to endogenous LRH is also exaggerated as shown by Santen

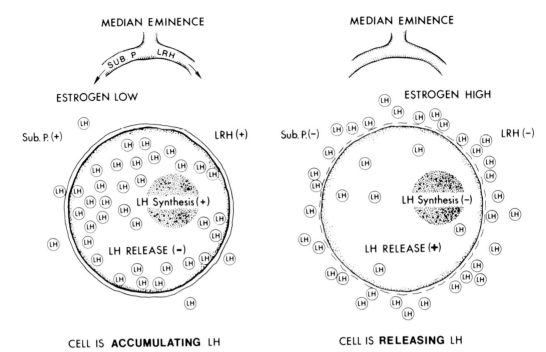

Figure 2.11. Diagram of pituitary gondotroph illustrating the hypothetical effect of estrogen on luteinizing hormone (LH) release and synthesis based on the assumption that substance P (*Sub. P.*) induces inhibition of LH release at the level of the cell membrane. Estrogen inhibits luteinizing-releasing hormone (LRH) from the hypothalamus in a linear dose relationship. If estrogen also inhibits substance P, but only after a specified time exposure to a specific dose level, depolarization of the gonadotropic cell membrane would allow a sudden release of accumulated LH. Thus, the ''positive'' estrogen feedback may be due to an inhibition of an inhibition.

and Bardin. This indicates a permeable cell membrane with maximum release.

Neurophysin. The most convincing estrogen effect upon the hypothalamus is its ability to increase estrogen-dependent neurophysin, the hypothalamic peptide which may be the LRH protein carrier. Using a dynamic estrogen stimulation test and measuring the response of neurophysin, one can demonstrate the integrity of at least this one function of the hypothalamus.

Enzymes. Two hypothalamic enzymes are also stimulated by estrogen, oxytocinase, which degrades oxytocin, and L-cystine arylamidase, important in the degradation of LRH.

Thyroid

The clinical observation that women are more prone to hyperthyroidism and myxedema than men and that these conditions often have their onset at puberty, in pregnancy, or at the menopause has fostered the belief among gynecologists and obstetricians that there is a close relationship between thyroid and ovarian function. Thyrotropic-stimulating hormone (TSH) has a limited cross-reactivity with LH, both immunologically and biologically, and this may help to explain some of these apparent relationships (Fig. 2.13). The LH-like action of TSH is seen only when excessively high values of TSH are present. The biologic cross-reactivity may explain the hyperestrogenism which is occasionally associated with thyroid pathology. If in addition to an elevated pituitary TSH, there is also an elevated TRH, prolactin production with lactation may occur due to the prolactin stimulating effect of TRH (see Chapter 30). Such a TRH elevation usually is present only with severe hypothyroidism.

Estrogens also cause an increase in the serum thyroxin-binding globulin, thus increasing the amount of bound thyroxin circulating. The bound hormone, however, is inactive and, therefore, this mechanism has little significance in abnormal physiologic states.

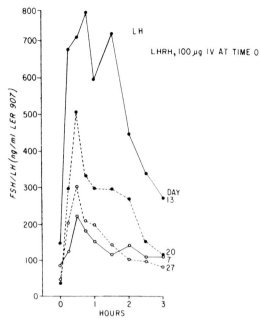

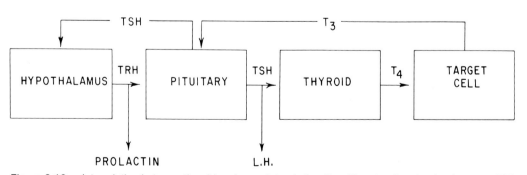

Figure 2.12. Luteinizing hormone (LH) response of a normal woman to an acute luteinizing hormone-releasing hormone (LHRH) stimulation of 100 μg intravenously, given weekly during a normal menstrual cycle, at 0 hour. The response in relation to baseline is greatest at midcycle, day 13, and midluteal phase, day 20, when estrogen exposure is highest. At day 20 the LH baseline is the lowest, 40 ng/ml, but the response is greatest. There is a rise to slightly over 500 ng/ml, which is 12 times the baseline, as compared to 6.5 times the baseline on day 13. The low baseline in the luteal phase signals an active negative estrogen feedback with low production of LHRH and LH synthesis, while the brisk response to LHRH indicates a permeable cell membrane with maximum LH release. FSH, follicle-stimulating hormone.

Hyperthyroidism in turn also increases the estrogen-binding protein, causing an apparent increase in the estrogen if total serum estrogen blood levels are assayed. It also shifts estrogen metabolism to the catechol estrogen pathway from the estriol pathway. This decreases the peripheral biologic activity and perhaps increases some central nervous system estrogen activity. Hypothyroidism, on the other hand, decreases the sex hormone-binding globulin, and therefore increases the biologically active estrogens. It also increases the conversion of androstenedione to estrogens by way of testosterone, and shifts the metabolic pathway from catechol estrogens. All of these changes can result in increased estrogen stimulation and chronic anovulation with dysfunctional uterine bleeding.

Adrenal

Estrogen increases the cortisol-binding protein, transcortin, and therefore causes an increased circulation of bound cortisol.

Pancreas

Houssay, a number of years ago, reported a marked improvement in experimental diabetes in the rat after estrogen administration. Funk et al. found that estrogen enhanced the production of insulin probably through a pituitary pathway. However, Barnes and his associates demonstrated that estrogen will check glycosuria in a pancreatectomized dog or monkey, indicating that the effect may be through the liver rather than by an increased insulin output. Kirchick and associates have

Figure 2.13. Interrelation between thyroid and gonadotropic function. Thyrotropic-releasing hormone (TRH) stimulates prolactin which usually inhibits luteinizing hormone (LH). However, if thyrotropic-stimulating hormone (TSH) is unusually elevated an LH-like effect will be induced because of the chemical similarity between TSH and LH.

found a decreased pituitary sensitivity to estrogen in alloxan-treated diabetic rats. This decreased sensitivity results in a lack of response to LRH stimulation and failure of LH surge and ovulation. The administration of insulin corrects this defect.

Thymus

Atrophy of the thymus following estrogen administration has been described by Selye.

General Systemic Effects

Skeletal Growth. Estrogen has a marked effect on skeletal growth, estrogen stimulation being associated with epiphysial closure at puberty and estrogen deprivation with osteoporosis. This is characterized by increased bone resorption and hypercalcemia.

Proteins. Estrogen augments the amount of many specific blood proteins; the thyroxin-binding globulin, transcortin, angiotensin, aldosterone-binding protein, coagulation factor IX renin substrate and plasma fibrinogen among those studied.

Vascular. The effect on lipid metabolism and the circulatory system has been of interest in relation to the possible role estrogens may play in protecting against arteriosclerotic cardiovascular disease. In the rat they have been shown to enhance the respiration of the aorta and to decrease experimentally produced atherosclerosis in the cardiac but not thoracic arteries. Colburn and Buonassisi have identified estrogen receptors on vascular endothelial cells, thus confirming their involvement in hormone action.

Miller and Miller have shown that estrogens specifically cause an increase in the high density lipoprotein (HDL), and a decrease in the low density lipoprotein (LDL). The function of the low density lipoprotein which carries the major cholesterol seems to be to carry cholesterol into the cells for repair of cell membranes; it also exerts a feedback mechanism to inhibit the endogenous production of cholesterol (Goldstein and Brown). It is apparent that, until all of these functions and interrelations have been properly worked out, the interpretation of the results of increasing or decreasing any one of these substances will not be understood.

Hematology. Estrogen administration predisposes to thromboembolic phenomena (see Chapter 32). Ambrus et al. in a study of patients on oral contraceptives found that these steroids increased the clotting factors II,

VII, IX and X when given to patients with increased platelet adhesiveness. This is associated with a decreased fibrinolytic activity in the vein walls. Therefore, patients with impaired defense systems are at risk if the clotting factors are increased by estrogen administration. Witten and Bradbury in 1951 reported a definite decrease in blood volume but no change in actual red blood cell count after estrogen administration. This hemodilution effect is found in pregnancy and in the hyperstimulation syndrome seen following induction of ovulation. The authors speculate that the extravascular fluid as well as the intravascular fluid might be increased under estrogen domination. Such a finding might account for preovulatory and premenstrual edema.

Skin and Appendages. Estrogens oppose the effect of androgens on sebaceous glands and hair follicles in the sexual regions.

Mechanisms of Action

The current theory for the intracellular mechanism of estrogenic action is that of gene activation. Estrogen target cells contain specific loci, receptor proteins, which bind estrogens. These cytosol proteins have a sedimentation rate of approximately 8 S (S = Svedberg unit.) As the hormone is bound, the protein splits to form a hormone complex and a 4 S protein. The hormone receptor complex must then be activated in order for it to be translocated into the nucleus where it combines with an acceptor protein. This nuclear acceptor protein is not hormone specific. It will accept other molecules such as insulin, glucagon and aminopeptides. Once in the nucleus, the hormone acceptor complex can act as a gene derepressor by combining with a repressor protein on the surface of the gene; it removes the repressor and allows gene activation. This results in replication of RNA polymerase, which in turn increases ribosomal RNA and transfer RNA, thus setting into motion all of the necessary reactions for the synthesis of proteins (enzymes) which are characteristic of the target cell response to estrogen (Fig. 2.14).

Progesterone

Tissue Content and Metabolism

Progesterone has been isolated from ovarian corpora lutea, placental tissue, adrenal and testis.

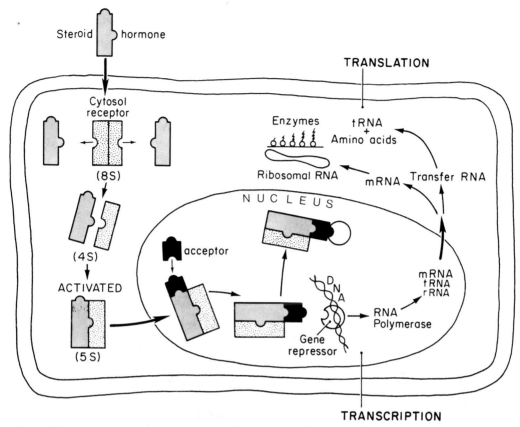

Figure 2.14.   Intracellular mechanisms of action of estrogen by gene activation.

Ovary

Human corpora lutea of different ages contain a measurable amount of progesterone on the first ovulatory day. This increases to a maximum by the 16th cycle day and remains elevated until the 24th cycle day. Appreciable amounts of progesterone are still present at the onset of menstruation, and traces are detectable in corpora of the previous cycle. Although two additional pregestational steroids have been isolated from human corpora (Table 2.6), there is some question as to the physiological activity of these compounds. The 20β-ol steroid is said to be inactive, and the activity of the α compound may depend upon the ability of the body to convert it to progesterone. Thus, although there are many naturally occurring estrogenic steroids, there seems to be only one naturally occurring steroid which has appreciable progestational activity.

Blood

Progesterone is transported in the blood by a specific binding protein. The low baseline serum progesterone level in the follicular phase of the menstrual cycle is compatible with adrenal function. Just prior to ovulation, a slight increase can be detected, apparently due to luteinization of the granulosa cells of the preovulatory follicle as the LH surge begins. Following ovulation, there is a gradual rise to a plateau between days 19 and 21 and a rather sharper decline to baseline values again at the time of menstruation (Fig. 2.15). The value of approximately 0.5 ng/ml in males and menopausal women is the same as that in the follicular phase of the cycle and represents the adrenal component.

The metabolic clearance rate of progesterone in males and ovariectomized females, is 2100 L/day. The rapid removal of progesterone from the blood and its equally rapid conversion to a biologically inactive steroid must be obviated for effective therapeutic administration of this hormone. This has been accomplished by frequent intramuscular administration, vaginal absorption, or synthetic chemical changes in the molecule which protect it from metabolism.

Table 2.6
Progestational Compounds Isolated from Human Corpora Lutea

Progesterone = Δ^4-3-ketopregnene-20α-one[a]
$\frac{1}{2}$–$\frac{1}{3}$ activity of progesterone = Δ^4-3-ketopregnene-20α-ol[b]
$\frac{1}{5}$–$\frac{1}{10}$ activity of progesterone = Δ^4-3-ketopregnene-20β-ol[b]

[a] Isolated by Corner and Allen (1929) and identified by Butenandt and Schmidt (1934).
[b] Isolated by Zander, Forbes, von Munstermann, and Neher (1958).

Urine

Little or no progesterone is excreted in the urine. Sodium pregnanediol glucuronide is the metabolic product of progesterone which is excreted in the urine throughout the menstrual cycle. Before ovulation, between 0.2 and 1 mg of pregnanediol per 24 hours are excreted. This amount presumably represents the contribution from the adrenal gland. After ovulation, the excretion rises to between 3 and 6 mg per 24 hours at the peak of the luteal phase and falls again before menstruation. When measured as free pregnanediol, this metabolite represents approximately 20% of injected progesterone. Although other metabolic products of progesterone have been isolated from human urine (Fig. 2.16), only one, pregnanolone, is of any clinical importance.

Bile and Feces

Sodium pregnanediol glucuronide has been identified in the blood and has also been isolated from bile. In the feces, however, pregnanediol is found in the free form, indicating that hydrolysis occurs in the gut.

Summary. In summary, progesterone is probably the only naturally occurring progestational hormone of any significance. Small amounts may be synthesized by the cells of the follicle in the preovulatory swelling phase; however, the major production is by the corpus luteum cells of the ovary during the luteal phase of the cycle. It is constantly produced in small amounts by the adrenal gland and by the testis, and it probably serves as the precursor for corticoids and androgens. It is transported in the blood by a specific binding protein and metabolized and conjugated in the liver into sodium pregnanediol glucuronide; pregnanolone represents a minor metabolic product. The pregnanediol excreted in

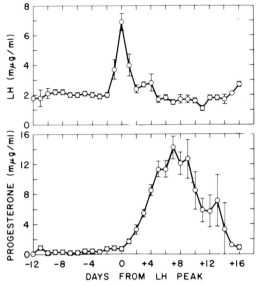

Figure 2.15. Serum progesterone during menstrual cycle. (From J. D. Neill et al.: *Journal of Clinical Endocrinology & Metabolism, 27:* 1167, 1967.)

the bile is enzymatically hydrolyzed by the gut, therefore, pregnanediol recovered in the feces is in the free form.

Functions

The major functions of progesterone are the preparation of the endometrium for implantation and the maintenance of pregnancy. Its physiologic effects, therefore, are almost entirely confined to the uterus. A peculiarity of progesterone activity is that usually an initial estrogenic stimulation is required prior to the progestational stimulation. This estrogen dependence may be due to the necessity for estrogen to induce the specific progesterone receptor protein.

Vagina

The vaginal epithelium following progesterone stimulation shows an increased number of precornified cells, mucus shreds, and aggregates of cells.

Uterus

Under progesterone dominance the cervical os is contracted, the mucus is scanty and thick. The endometrium shows the progestational changes classically described by Hitschmann and Adler and quantitated by Noyes et al. The normal menstrual flow occurs from such a progestational endometrium. The amount of progesterone necessary

PROGESTERONE METABOLITES

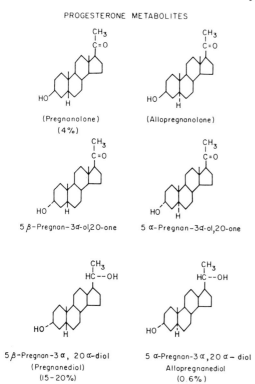

(Pregnanolone)
(4%)

(Allopregnanolone)

5 β-Pregnan-3α-ol,20-one

5 α-Pregnan-3α-ol,20-one

5 β-Pregnan-3 α, 20 α-diol
(Pregnanediol)
(15-20%)

5 α-Pregnan-3 α,20 α – diol
Allopregnanediol
(0.6%)

Figure 2.16. The metabolic products of progesterone isolated from human urine.

to produce these typical endometrial changes is influenced by the previous estrogenic stimulation as well as by the duration and the continuity of the progesterone dosage. In addition to deposition of glycogen in the endometrium under the influence of progesterone, the carbonic anhydrase is increased. Böving believes that it is this enzyme which, in conjunction with the carbonate from the blastocyst, disrupts the epithelial cement substance allowing the trophoblast to implant. A protein, blastokinin, specifically induced by progesterone without previous estrogen stimulation, has been described in the rabbit uterus and tentatively identified in the human. This protein seems to be one of the first manifestations of progesterone stimulation. It is apparently necessary for normal implantation of the rabbit blastocyst. If induction of this same type of protein can be substantiated in the human, this may well be the most important action of progesterone. The uterine musculature under the influence of progesterone becomes quiescent, thus allowing for the continued growth and development of the implanted trophoblast.

Fallopian Tubes

Like the uterine musculature, the fallopian tubes show a decreased motility under progesterone dominance.

Ovary

Reinitiation of meiosis in the oocyte just prior to ovulation has been suggested as progesterone-dependent.

Breasts

Development of acinar buds from the breast ducts is stimulated by progesterone administration.

Pituitary and Hypothalamus

As previously stated, the effects of steroids on pituitary function are at least partially mediated through the hypothalamus. Many of the synthetic progestational compounds used in oral contraception have a marked suppressive effect upon the cyclic secretion of LH, the LH surge. Progesterone per se, however, has very little gonadotropic suppression or stimulation activity.

General Systemic Effect

Thermogenic Effect. The ability of progesterone to induce a rise in the basal body temperature is conveniently used as an index of ovulation in the human. This effect is apparently mediated through the central nervous system.

Anesthetic Action. Selye noted that progesterone, given in massive doses, caused an anesthetic-like reaction in rats. Rothchild and Rapport confirmed this effect in the human.

Skin and Appendages

An antiandrogen effect of progesterone has been reported on the hair follicles and sebaceous glands. This is thought to operate through a competition for both the testosterone protein-binding carrier and the androgen cytosol receptor in the target cells.

Mechanisms of Action

Progesterone exerts its action as a gene activator in exactly the same way that estrogen does.

Wade and Jones showed that resynthesis of high energy phosphate in the electron transport chain is blocked by progesterone. In the process, the hormone is metabolized. The experiments indicated that one locus of the steroid inhibition, and perhaps metabolism, is between reduced diphosphopyridine nucleotide (DPNH) and cytochrome c in the electron transport chain. This effect would lead to energy storage rather than energy utilization and account for many of the known properties of progesterone such as the accumulation of glycogen in the endometrial cells, the inhibition of muscle contractility, and the anesthetic action which occurs when a massive dosage of progesterone is given, blocking all high energy phosphate regeneration.

Gonadotropic Hormones: FSH, LH, Prolactin

Chemistry, FSH, LH

The three pituitary hormones which are glycoproteins, follicle-stimulating hormone (FSH), luteinizing hormone (LH) and thyrotropic hormone (TSH), as well as the placental hormone, human chorionic gonadotropin (hCG), are water-soluble, heat-labile and orally inactive. They are composed of three basic units, an α-peptide chain and a β-peptide chain which are noncovalently bonded, and a carbohydrate moiety with a sialic acid component (Table 2.7). Biologic activity is dependent upon receptor recognition and presence of the two protein chains. However, the specificity of biologic activity is determined by the β-subunit. The α-subunit is interchangeable among the four hormones. There is evidence that the units are synthesized by the pituitary independently and secondarily combined. This might explain the extremely infrequent occurrence of gonadotropin or thyrotropin-secreting pituitary tumors and some apparently hormonally inert chromophobe adenomas. The sialic acid moiety protects the molecule from metabolic destruction by the liver, thus increasing the circulation time and enhancing biologic activity.

Some pituitary hormones including somatotropin and prolactin, are species specific. However, the gonadotropins are not. Although certain animal gonadotropins are physiologically active in the human, antigenicity makes these unsuitable for therapeutic agents.

Tissue Content and Metabolism

The pituitary gonadotropins, follitropin (FSH, follicle-stimulating hormone) and lu-

tropin (LH, luteinizing hormone) have been isolated from human pituitaries, serum and urine. Prolactin, perhaps to be regarded in the human as an antigonadotropin, has also been isolated from these sources.

Pituitary

The pituitary gonadotropic cells are small basophils, and are located in the anterior pituitary angles adjacent to the pars intermedia with additional clumps of cells in the central zone. These cells must be differentiated from a rather similar type of β cell which produces thyrotropic hormone (TSH). A compilation of the data seems to indicate that there are some cells which synthesize only FSH or LH while others synthesize both. The pituitary of menstruating women contains approximately 700 I.U. of LH and 200 I.U. of FSH. After the menopause, the LH is 1700 I.U. and the FSH approximately 450 I.U. The turnover rate of stored gonadotropins is calculated to be between 12 and 24 hours. The LH production rate in menopausal women is estimated to be between 3 and 4000 I.U./day. No detectable gonadotropin is found in the pituitary during pregnancy.

Blood

Serum gonadotropin levels are elevated in infancy. FSH values in female infants tend to be higher than LH values. These elevated levels gradually fall reaching the lowest level at about 2 years. A secondary rise then begins at about the age of 5 years and continues until adult levels are reached. The rise in LH values occurs approximately 2 years prior to puberty, at about 8 years, but the change is not really significant until the menarche at approximately the age of 12 years. Rhythmic pulsatile FSH patterns and an elevation during sleep are the first changes in the prepubertal gonadotropic function. A pulsatile LH pattern during sleep is seen next. Just prior to the menarche, no further sleep elevations occur. A pulsatile discharge is maintained during the entire 24 hours. At the menarche the cyclic changes associated with ovulation are manifest, the cyclic LH surge being the most dramatic (Chapter 4).

In cyclic women, the FSH shows a rise in the first part of the follicular phase which begins prior to menses at aproximately day 25 or 26 of the 28-day cycle and declines after day 7, reaching a nadir just prior to the

Table 2.7
Glycoprotein Hormones: Follicle-stimulating Hormone (FSH), Luteinizing Hormone (LH), Thyrotropic-stimulating Hormone (TSH), Human Chorionic Gonadotropin (hCG), Placental

		Structure	Function
Protein		(1) α-Subunit	+ β = Receptor recognition
		(2) β-Subunit	Biologic specificity
Carbohydrate		(1) Glucosides	Biologic activity
		(2) Sialic acid	Increased circulation time

ovulatory LH surge at day 13. With this surge, there is an associated but lesser FSH surge, the importance of which is not documented (Fig. 2.17). It is possibly related to preovulatory expansion of the cumulus (Eppig).

In the perimenopause, as the numbers of oocytes and follicles in the ovary decrease, in response to a decreased follicular *inhibin*, the FSH begins to rise. When the follicular estrogen values fall associated with failing ovulatory function, LH rises, and both gonadotropin levels remain elevated during the rest of the individual's life span. Thus, it is the change in FSH pattern which first signals a change in ovarian function at both extremes of menstrual life, the menarche and the menopause (Chapters 4 and 32).

As LH is released in a pulsatile manner, frequent sampling is necessary to assure a proper baseline value. Stimulation of the peptidergic LRH neurons by catecholamine neurons from extra-hypothalamic sources is thought to be the origin of this pulsatile discharge. The amplitude of the pulse, if calculated as percentage of the baseline LH, gives one an excellent idea of permeability of the pituitary gonadotropin cell membrane and the amount of LH accumulated in the cell prior to the pulse. Hopkins has shown that, in tissue cultures of dissociated pituitary cells, LRH releases, in 2 min, only 0.1% of the cell LH content. During the next 90 min a maximum of only 10% of the total cell LH content is released. In the normal male and in the female in the early follicular phase, when the estrogen exposure is low and the pituitary cell membrane is apparently stable, an LRH stimulation induces an average LH peak, height from the baseline, of approximately 3 times the baseline. This also applies for the menopausal patient even though the LH baseline is extremely high. However, in the midcycle

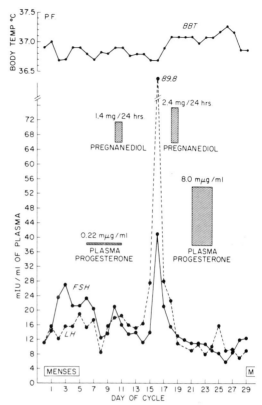

Figure 2.17. Plasma follicle-stimulating hormone (FSH) and luteinizing hormone (LH) values in an ovulatory cycle of a normal fertile woman in relation to clinical parameters of the basal body temperature (BBT), urinary pregnanediol excretion and plasma progesterone. (From C. M. Cargille, G. T. Ross, and T. Yoshimi: *Journal of Clinical Endocrinology & Metabolism, 29:* 13, 1969.)

after high estrogen exposure, the percent increase from the baseline may be 5 to 10 times that of the baseline. This increased LH response to LRH in relation to the LH baseline persists during the luteal phase of the cycle, while estrogen and progesterone remain elevated.

Urine

Fractionation of the gonadotropins into LH and FSH activity during a normal menstrual cycle indicates that the urinary pattern closely approximates that in serum. Total gonadotropins are elevated postmenopausally or in the castrate woman and tend to remain so for the duration of life. Christiansen's work indicates that although FSH rises slightly with age in the male, there is no significant rise in the LH.

The circulating half-life of FSH is estimated to be about 170 min, while that of LH is about 30 min. The renal clearance of FSH is 0.58 ml/min and LH is 0.14 ml/min, while hCG, a closely related placental glycoprotein, has a renal clearance of 0.95 ml/min.

Function

Follitropin, FSH

The function of FSH in the human female is to stimulate the ovarian granulosa cells to secrete (1) a high affinity estrogen binding-protein which allows concentration of estradiol in the follicle cells, and therefore replication of the granulosa cells; (2) to stimulate the secretion of mucopolysaccharides, the ground substances for the follicular fluid the basement membrane of the follicle and the zona pellucida of the oocyte; (3) to stimulate production of a protein hormone inhibin which regulates the FSH internal feedback; and (4) to stimulate the formation of LH receptors on both the granulosa and the theca cells. Thus, the initial FSH stimulation of the developing Graafian follicle must be adequate if there is to be a normal corpus luteum with a normal luteal span and function.

Lutropin, LH

In the human female, contrary to the male, LH action is dependent upon prior FSH stimulation. When FSH stimulation has induced LH receptors on theca and granulosa cells, steroidogenesis is activated by an LH stimulation. Estrogen is synthesized by theca cells. Estrogen triggers the LH surge, for luteinization of the granulosa cells, progesterone production and corpus luteum formation. The normalcy of luteal function is therefore dependent upon an adequate LH surge acting upon granulosa cells which have been adequately stimulated by FSH. The 14-day luteal span is maintained by a residual minimal LH stimulation.

In addition to the initiation and maintenance of progesterone production by the corpus luteum, the LH surge may also be important in oocyte maturation and resumption of meiosis. Following the initial stimulatory phase associated with the LH surge a "desensitization" of LH receptors occurs. This "down-regulation" results in a refractory stage, during which there is an absence of cyclic AMP accumulation and no steroidogenesis. It is associated with a decrease in both the numbers and the sensitivity of the LH receptors and is transcriptionally related

as it can be blocked by actinomycin D (Lamprecht).

As high cyclic AMP levels inhibit ovulation (LaMaire and Ryan and Coronel) by inhibition of prostaglandin (Challis et al.) this desensitization phase is necessary for ovulation and also explains the decreased estrogen synthesis following the LH surge. Decreased estrogen may also be important for ovulation as collagenase or plasminogen are inhibited by estrogens and these enzymes may be necessary to digest the basement membrane of the follicle, at the stigma, during ovulation.

Mechanisms of Action

The pituitary gonadotropins, FSH and LH, are protein hormones and exert their biologic effect by interacting with cyclic AMP, the so-called second messenger. These hormones have their receptor proteins on the outer cell membrane and never enter the cytoplasm. The hormone protein complex on the outer membrane reacts with adenylcyclase, an enzyme on the inner cell membrane which in turn catalyzes the conversion of adenosine triphosphate, ATP, to cyclic adenosine monophosphate, cAMP. cAMP, by activation of protein kinase, is then able to phosphorylate all enzymes necessary to induce the responses characteristic of the hormones. The release of calcium ions in the first step of conversion of ATP to cAMP is possibly a key reaction, as the free calcium ions increase cell membrane permeability and therefore allow access to the cell of extracellular elements necessary to generate the energy for protein or steroid synthesis. Calcium ions may also provide a mechanism for intracellular feedback which blocks the synthesis of cAMP. An additional intracellular control mechanism is the enzyme diphosphodiesterase which likewise inhibits the synthesis of cAMP (Fig. 2.18).

Prolactin Chemistry

Prolactin is not a glycoprotein but an alcohol soluble protein with a relatively low molecular weight of 22,000. There are 198 amino acids with 3 disulfide bonds in the hormone, the peptide sequence of which has been described.

Prolactin Tissue Content and Metabolism

Pituitary

The pituitary lactotrophic cells are localized in the lateral medial area of the pituitary

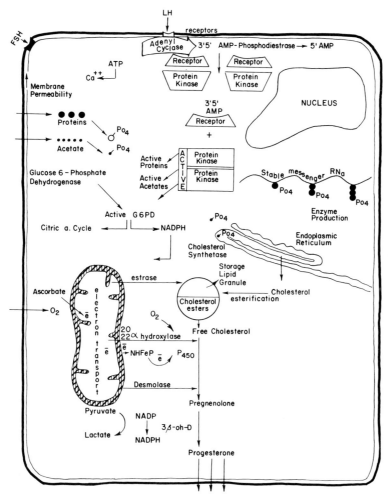

Figure 2.18. Intracellular mechanism of action of protein hormones by activation of "the second messenger" cyclic adenosine monophosphate, cAMP. (From S. J. Behrman and R. W. Kistner (eds.): *Progress in Infertility*, Ed. 2, Little Brown, Boston, 1975.)

and are acidophilic. This peripheral location makes the surgical approach to prolactinomas relatively feasible. Prolaction is closely related structurally to growth hormone and both are primitive hormones which may derive from a single anlagen.

The prolactin content of the pituitary, which is highest during pregnancy, remains high throughout pregnancy and falls during lactation. The fetal pituitary secretes relatively large amounts of prolactin as the dopamine content of the hypothalamus is relatively low, while the adult pituitary has a low prolactin content, apparently in relation to the hypothalamic dopamine. Prolactin, in addition to being produced by the pituitary, is synthesized in the decidualized endometrial stroma. Its function in this location is yet

unknown, but the release is not controlled by dopamine.

Prolactin secretion is pulsatile, augmented by sleep and probably autonomously regulated by an internal feedback on its own synthesis. The secretion is controlled by an hypothalamic inhibitory factor, probably dopamine. Thyrotropic-releasing hormone stimulates prolactin secretion, but no specific prolactin-releasing hormone has as yet been identified.

Many stimuli induce prolactin release through suppression of dopamine from the hypothalamus. Stress is perhaps one of the most important factors. ACTH and β-enkephalin, both of which are increased with stress, also are associated with elevated prolactin levels.

Drugs, estrogen and some progestogens stimulate prolactin secretion as do phenothiazide, dopamine antagonists.

Blood

Prolactin can be detected in the fetus by 20 weeks, and levels remain fairly high throughout fetal life. Just at the time of delivery a precipitous rise occurs, perhaps related to the stress of delivery. Elevations continue to be seen in the newborn for the first several days or week of life, and then fall to a low level where they remain throughout life in the male, and until puberty in the female (Table 2.8). There is no marked variation in prolactin throughout the menstrual cycle. Prolactin values, however, are increased in pregnancy, and specifically at lactation with suckling. As nursing continues, prolactin values return to normal menstrual levels, and rise only when the infant is put to breast. As prolactin is pulsatile and shows elevations at night, a single assay can give false impressions of the patient's prolactin exposure.

Prolactin Function

Prolactin has at least two functions in the human. It is necessary for lactation, and is an antigonadotropin. It has also been implicated as important in the control of osmolality, subcutaneous fat metabolism, calcium metabolism and steroidogenesis. This last function may be related to its antigonadotropin effect.

Steroidogenesis

Prolactin receptors have been identified in the adrenal as well as in the breast and, although much of prolactin research is handicapped by the failure to work with species specific hormone, in spite of this technical problem, it seems that prolactin stimulates the enzymes of the adrenal androgen pathway facilitating the conversion of pregnenolone to dihydroepiandrosterone (DHEA) and DHEA sulfate (DHEAS). In the testes, prolactin stimulates 3-β-ol dehydrogenase activity increasing testosterone production. Steroidogenesis in the ovary has also been shown to be affected by prolactin. In a normal individual, progesterone synthesis by the luteinized granulosa cell is decreased when the normal prolactin level is significantly **lowered** by bromocryptine. Paradoxically, however,

Table 2.8
Serum Prolactin Values[a]

Age	Mean Values (ng/ml)
Term (cord blood)	246
Day 1	278
6 Weeks	17
1 Year	10
2–12 Years	5
Adult	5
Adult	8
Follicular phase	6.7
Luteal phase	9.0
Menopause	5

[a] Modified from H. J. Guyda and H. C. Friesen: *Pediatric Research, 7:* 534, 1973.

elevated prolactin levels are also associated with lowered progesterone. Inhibition of steroidogenesis by an elevated prolactin could be explained on the basis of a defective neurotransmitter, dopamine, causing both hyperprolactinemia and a lowered LH surge. Under these circumstances, the steroidogenic changes in the ovary would be secondary to a hypothalamic-pituitary defect and could be normalized by a *dopamine agonist*, bromocryptine. Inhibition of steroidogenesis by deficient prolactin might be explained by a critical level of prolactin below which the ovarian 3-β-ol dehydrogenase is not activated. Under these circumstance, steroidogenesis is abnormal secondary to the ovarian enzyme defect and should be normalized by administration of prolactin or a *dopamine antagonist*.

Prolactin Mechanisms of Action

Although prolactin, like other pituitary hormones has a receptor on the cell membrane of its target endorgans, breast, adrenal, ovary, testis, kidney and liver, and exerts its action through the second messenger cyclic AMP, practically no specific enzyme effects can be cited. Thus, although prolactin is necessary for milk production, its exact intracellular function has not been described. In the adrenal, ovary and testis it is said to promote the LH action "on cholesterol utilization."

Hafiez et al. report that prolactin activates the 3β-ol dehydrogenase enzyme, and in the kidney Spanos et al. describe activation of the 2-hydroxylase enzyme which converts vitamin D precursor to its active form.

Hypothalamus

Anatomy

The hypothalamus is the rostral part of the midbrain, the diencephalon, forming the floor and the lower portion of the lateral walls of the third ventricle. It is just posterior to the optic chiasma, and anterior to the mamillary bodies. The pituitary lies immediately below it in the bony sella turcica. The posterior pituitary is anatomically continuous with the hypothalamus via the median eminence and the pituitary stalk, which passes through the sella diaphragm.

The blood supply is of key importance. It was the knowledge that the blood was carried in an hypophyseal portal system from the hypothalamus to the pituitary, rather than in the opposite direction, which first alerted Harris to the conclusion that substances from the brain might be contributing to the control of pituitary function. It is now realized from the work of Bergland and Page, and others, that there is also blood flow from the pituitary to the brain. This vascular connection would allow for behavior modification by pituitary hormones such as enkeflin and feedback modifications of the hypothalamic hormones by their pituitary target cell hormones.

Although the hypothalamus is composed mainly of nonmyelinated nerves there are also myelinated axons. Neurons of nonmyelinated nerves lie completely within the hypothalamus while the myelinated nerves have neurons outside of the hypothalamus, only axons being represented in the hypothalamus.

The nonmyelinated system is composed of peptidergic neurons synthesizing hypothalamic releasing hormones (Table 2.1). These neurons are loosely collected in areas called nuclei. Their unmyelinated axons terminate on the vessels of the hypothalamic portal system in the region of the median eminence. Oxytocin and vasopressin neurons, however, have axons which transverse the pituitary stalk and terminate in the posterior pituitary.

The myelinated axons are mainly norepinephrine and serotonin secreting, arising from neurons in the locus subceruleus and raphe nucleus, reaching the arcuate and suprachiasmatic nuclei by ascending and descending tracts mainly via the fornix, the striae terminalis, the reticular formation, the retinohypothalamic tract, and the medial forebrain bundle (Table 2.9). The norepinephrine stimulus is thought to increase, while serotonin decreases, secretion of the hypothalamic peptidergic neurons.

Function

The peptidergic neurons of the hypothalamus referred to in Table 2.1 control the vegetative nervous system regulating food intake, fluid balance, temperature, sleep, the respiratory and circulatory systems, growth and development, and reproductive functions. The hypothalamus also maintains body homeostasis and integrates physiologic hormonal changes with internal environment, external environment and behavorial functions. In reproductive physiology, this is particularly in relation to nutrition, sensory stimuli, steroids and stress.

In addition to the **hypothalamic pituitary hormones** mentioned above, two **hormone carrier peptides** have been identified: estrogen-sensitive neurophysin, which may carry LRH through the pituitary portal system, and nicotine-neurophysin, which is the carrier protein for oxytocin and vasopressin. A third group of **hypothalamic** peptides with less well understood functions are also produced in the **brain**, pituitary, gastrointestinal tract (including the pancreas), and the placenta, and have as their common functional characteristic amine precursor uptake and decarboxylation. They are therefore referred to as the **APUD series**. It is beyond the scope of this text to expand further on these peptides, but it is of interest that tumors from these cells are characterized by production of multiple (two or more) hormones.

Hypothalamic Hormones

Chemistry of Luliberin (Luteinizing Release Hormone, LRH, LH-RH or GnRH)

Luliberin, LRH, the hypothalamic luteinizing release hormone, sometimes referred to as GnRH, gonadotropic-releasing hormone, because both LH and FSH release are stimulated, is a decapeptide with the formula as illustrated (Fig. 2.19). It is not species specific, and is physiologically active by any mode of administration.

LRH Tissue Content and Metabolism

Blood

Like LH, LRH is released in a pulsatile manner and there is no evidence for a mid-

Table 2.9
Some CNS-Hypothalamic Pathways Important in Reproduction

A. Descending			
Neurons of Origin	Tracts	Hypothalamic Tracts	Hypothalamic Nuclei
Amygdala	Stria terminalis	Medial hypothalamic area	Anterior hypothalamic area, supraoptic nucleus
Retina	Retinohypothalamic	Optic chiasma	Suprachiasmatic nucleus
Olfactory tubercule	Medial forebrain bundle	Lateral hypothalamic area	? Premamillary nucleus
Hippocampal formation	Fornix	Medial corticohypothalamic tract	? Arcuate nucleus

B. Ascending				
Monoamine Neurons	Brainstem	Tract	Hypothalamic Tracts	Hypothalamic Nuclei
Norepinephrine	Locus ceruleus subceruleus	Reticular formation	Medial forebrain bundle	Preoptic and arcuate nucleus
Serotonin	Raphe nucleus	Ventral tegmental area	Medial forebrain bundle	Preoptic and arcuate nucleus

cycle LRH elevation to account for the midcycle LH surge.

Hypothalamus

The major site of LRH production is in neurons of the arcuate nucleus. An axonal regulatory mechanism of dopamine on LRH release is probable.

Metabolism of LRH

The half-life is between 2 and 4 min. Uptake and retention were measured in the rat. Although immediate uptake was highest in the kidney, the pituitary showed the greatest uptake by 90 min, and the activity was retained during the 360 min of the experiments. The liver showed some retention up to 120 min. Neither the cerebral cortex nor the hypothalamus concentrated LRH; 1% of the total dose was excreted in 4 hours.

Function

Luliberin (LRH)

LRH is associated with synthesis and release of both LH and FSH, albeit FSH is stimulated less consistently and to a lesser degree. The LRH release effect reaches a maximum at 30 min, and this rapidity of action, along with its obligatory link with calcium ions, indicates that it is a function of the gonadotropic cell membrane. Liu and Jackson have shown that LRH induces synthesis of the carbohydrate fractions of the gonadotropic glycoproteins, therefore stimulating glucide neogenesis rather than the protein synthesis. This synthetic function is tied to cyclic AMP accumulation and requires 2 to 8 hours for initiation and maximum response.

Steroid Modulation

The location of the steroid modulation of the pituitary gonadotropins is as yet undecided, and the intracellular mechanism which controls it is even less well understood. There are estrogen receptors in both the hypothalamic and pituitary cells. Thus, some estrogen modulation would be expected to occur at the pituitary level. The negative estrogen feedback, however, is usually thought to be in the hypothalamus, but the specific neurons on which it is located are undetermined. There are at least two general possibilities: the LRH neuron per se, or the neuron which controls the release of LRH.

The negative estrogen feedback, i.e. the lowering of basal LH by estrogen, can apparently be explained by the inhibition of synthesis or release of LRH. This inhibition is in a linear dose-related relationship. The positive estrogen feedback, although specifically due to increased release of LH at the membrane of the pituitary gonadotroph, may also be primarily due to a hypothalamic influence. At the present writing, it seems that substance P is an LRH inhibitor. This hypothalamic

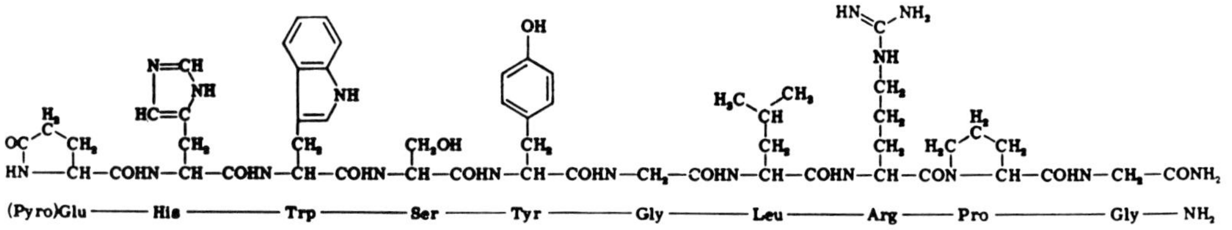

Figure 2.19. Hypothalamic luteotropic releasing hormone is a decapeptide. (From A. V. Schalley et al.: *Science, 179:* 341, 1973.)

peptide, by stabilizing the gonadotroph membrane, may inhibit LH release. If substance P production is inhibited by estrogen, the membrane would become permeable, and the LH flood occur. Thus, the "positive" estrogen feedback may be an inhibition of an inhibition. The positive feedback, however, unlike the negative feedback, does not exhibit a linear dose relationship, but is dependent upon a specific estrogen dose acting over a specific period of time.

Other steroids which possibly exert a feedback action on the hypothalamic neurons or the noradrenergic nervous system are testosterone and progesterone. Testosterone is a potent LH inhibitor, but a poor FSH inhibitor, and a testosterone level in the adult male range is necessary for this effect. Progesterone, per se, is not effective either as a stimulator for LH release or a tonic LH inhibitor in the human. If it is effective at all, it apparently requires a preliminary estrogen priming action.

Mechanisms of Action

The LRH receptor on the external cell membrane of the pituitary gonadotroph interdigitates with a specific adenyl cyclase system activating the conversion of ATP to cyclic AMP. **Calcium ions** which are released during this reaction, **facilitate the release** of LH and FSH by increasing the cell membrane permeability. The **cyclic AMP** activates a specific protein kinase which in turn allows transcription and translation of the enzymes **necessary to synthesize** the carbohydrate fractions of the pituitary gonadotropins, LH and FSH.

VASCULAR PHENOMENA OF MENSTRUATION

Menstruation is in the last analysis a vascular phenomenon; two groups of blood vessels supply the endometrium: (1) the straight arteries and (2) the coiled arteries. The straight vessels undergo no fundamental change during menstruation, supplying the basal third or so of the endometrium (Chapter 3).

Much more important are the coiled arterioles, which alone supply blood to the superficial third and most of the middle third of the endometrium. Throughout the earlier part of the cycle the endometrial vessels exhibit a rhythmic, alternating, vasoconstriction. As endometrial growth advances, the arterioles become more and more coiled because their length increases more rapidly than the endometrium thickens. This increased coiling is accentuated by a regression in endometrial growth beginning some days before the onset of menstrual bleeding and leading to a stasis, with or without vasodilatation. For this description we are indebted to Markee, who observed that, following this phase of slowed circulation, there occurs an intense vasoconstriction which is probably due to prostaglandin formation in relation to the decreased steroid milieu. This constriction causes anoxia with tissue and vessel damage. The dissolution of the endometrium releases acid hydrolases which have hitherto been confined in the cell lysosomes. These liberated enzymes are then able to disrupt the endometrial cell membranes further and thus complete the process of menstruation. The platelet clot which forms at the site of vessel damage is digested, further slough and endometrial digestion occurs, and the process is repeated until the entire functional endometrium is desquamated. It is important to realize that the usual hemostatic mechanism, **the filbrin clot**, does not occur.

Preovulation: Follicular Phase

The preovulatory estrogen peak stimulates the LH surge on approximately the 14th day of an ideal 28-day cycle, and ovulation occurs sometime within the 24-hour period thereafter. The most precise observations point to 28 hours after the beginning of the LH rise. Although ovulation is dependent upon the LH surge which is triggered by the estradiol surge, the specific process, characterized by follicle migration to the cortex, stigma formation and rupture, is probably initiated by prostaglandin and made possible by the vascular and stromal composition of the ovary.

Ovulation

The loose syncytial stromal arrangement in the ovarian medulla and the spiral arteries allow growth of the young antrum follicle. However, as the follicular size increases, it impinges on the cortex, stretching the straight arterioles and branching arcades (Fig. 2.20), which are unable to compensate. The ensuing impairment in the blood supply, perhaps in conjunction with vasoconstriction of prostaglandin, induces the stigma, an avascular area on the surface of the follicle through which ovulation will occur. However, the massive LH surge may also specifically contribute to ovulation by desensitization of the LH receptors. This desensitization causes temporary impairment of steroidogenesis and cyclic AMP accumulation. Decreased cyclic AMP allows prostaglandin activity, and decreased estrogen stimulus allows activation of collagenase, an enzyme necessary for dissolution of the stigma. At follicle rupture, the follicular fluid containing the oocyte collects in the cul-de-sac pool.

The extruded ovum is directed toward and into the fimbriated end of the tube by two forces, viz. (1) the ciliary current in the peritoneal fluid produced by the cilia of the epithelium of the fimbria ovarica and (2) the motility of the tube. The latter is apparently by far the most significant.

Postovulation: Luteal Phase

With the rupture of the follicle, blood vessels infiltrate, organization of the central blood clot occurs, and cells are rapidly luteinized. The stratum granulosa cells, hitherto functioning as nurse cells for the ova, producing the mucopolysaccharides of the follicular fluid, begin to show luteinization and lipid droplets, signifying progesterone production some 24 hours before ovulation and shortly after the beginning of the LH flood. Increased amounts of progesterone are secreted after reactivation or resynthesis of LH receptors. Estrogen is produced, perhaps by the same corpus luteum cells, but more probably by the stimulated theca interna cells. The peak steroid production by the corpus luteum of menstruation is between the 18th and 22nd day of an ideal 28-day cycle, or day 4 to 9 of the luteal phase. The fixed life span of the corpus luteum (in the absence of pregnancy), which usually averages between 14 and 16 days, may be determined by the inability of the cells to augment precursor substances laid down in the preovulatory phase, or by the inability of the minimal amount of LH available in the luteal phase of the cycle to stimulate steroid synthesis for a longer period of time. However, a luteolytic action, related to estrogen and/or its effect on the luteal synthesis of prostaglandin, may be responsible for the final demise of the corpus luteum.

Paralleling the corpus luteum phase in the ovary, the endometrium in the postovulatory

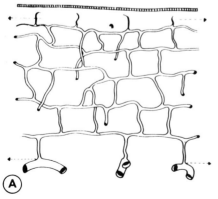
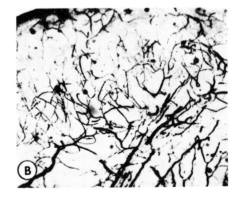

Figure 2.20. Demonstration of the relation of ovarian vascular pattern to follicular growth and ovulation. (From G. Reeves: *Obstetrics & Gynecology, 37:* 832, 1971.)

phase shows increasing evidence of the characteristic progesterone effects, such as increasing thickness and edema, increased tortuosity of the glands, steadily increasing secretory activity of the glandular epithelium, and decidual-like hypertrophy of the stromal cells. These histological changes are described in the chapter on cyclical changes in the endometrium (Chapter 3).

Menstruation: Menstrual Phase

The height of the progestational phase is reached, not at the beginning of the next menstrual bleeding, but probably 4 to 6 days before this, as regression of the corpus luteum begins. When this endocrine support is rather abruptly withdrawn, retrogression occurs in the previously built-up endometrium. Although estrogen deprivation can produce bleeding experimentally, the evidence indicates that in the usual ovulatory cycle the deprivation of progesterone plays a more important role than estrogen withdrawal. With the decline of corpus luteum function approximately 2 to 4 days before menstruation, the estrogen, and perhaps progesterone, inhibition of the pituitary gonadotropins is released and another crop of follicles starts to mature as the next cycle begins.

The endometrium, under the influence of progesterone, synthesizes prostaglandin and, as the endometrium breaks down with the withdrawal of ovarian estrogen and progesterone steroid support, prostaglandin is released causing vasoconstriction and increased endometrial disruption. Lysosomes, intracellular packets which contain acid hydrolase enzymes, are also increased under progesterone influence and, as the cell membranes are disrupted, these enzymes are released and cause further cellular dissolution and digestion. The hemostatic mechanism in the endometrium is via a platelet not a fibrin clot. Therefore, an intact fibrolytic system is not necessary.

ENDOCRINES IN PREGNANCY

If however, the egg is fertilized, the corpus luteum continues to produce increasing amounts of progesterone and the endometrium is not only not cast off but continues to develop further, becoming the decidua of early pregnancy. The decidua has been shown to be producing prolactin. The func-

tion of this hormone in the endometrium at the present time is unknown, but it is known that decidual prolactin is not controlled by a dopamine inhibition.

The corpus luteum of pregnancy probably continues to function for several months. However, progesterone secretion may be taken over by the placenta at a relatively early date. Thus, although corpus luteum activity usually continues through at least the first trimester, substantial placental takeover of progesterone production may occur prior to the second missed period.

Function of progesterone in pregnancy is manifold. It may stimulate maturation in the egg and reinitiation of meiosis. It may slow the tubal motility and allow sperm to ascend more easily, and the egg to rest after fertilization. It may cause quiescence of uterine motility preventing egg expulsion. It may stimulate a "blastokinin-like-protein" which promotes implantation. It may be important in inducing changes which allow for implantation. The function of the decidua and associated prolactin production is unknown. Siiteri et al. believe that progesterone may prevent rejection of the "foreign" embryonic tissue by inhibiting T-lymphocyte cell-mediated responses.

Placental Function

Chorionic Gonadotropin, hCG

The prolonged luteal function in pregnancy is caused by a third gonadotropin, chorionic gonadotropin (hCG) which is closely related both biologically and chemically to the pituitary hormone LH. The α-chain is interchangeable with that of pituitary FSH and LH. The β-chain is immunologically distinguishable from both FSH and LH, allowing for a specific radioimmunoassay. Plasma clearance of hCG is relatively slow; the half-life in human serum is estimated at 26 hours by radioimmunoassay (Midgley and Jaffe, 1968). The renal clearance is approximately 1 ml/min, considerably slower than the estimated 7 ml/min for LH. The function of hCG to prolong the corpus luteum life span in the early part of pregnancy is well documented. To this end, the amount of hormone produced increases rapidly from first detection at 5 to 6 days, prior to the first missed period to a peak at the 60th day (Fig. 2.21). Thereafter it falls somewhat less pre-

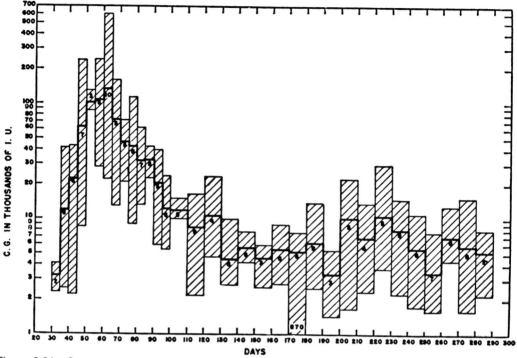

Figure 2.21. Serum chorionic gonadotropin throughout normal pregnancy in 24 women (Delfs method). Gonadotropin in international units (I.U.) is plotted against duration of pregnancy in days, counting from Day 1 of the last menstrual period. Heavy black line shows average gonadotropin level. Cross-hatched area indicates extreme variation for the period with the number of determinations in each. Plotted on semilogarithmic graph scale. (From G. E. S. Jones, E. Delfs, and H. M. Stran: *Bulletin of the Johns Hopkins Hospital,* 75: 359, 1944.)

cipitously until about 90 days, at which point it maintains a fairly stable level until delivery. Chorionic gonadotropin is the basis for most of the biological and immunological pregnancy tests. The values in the serum are slightly higher than those in the urine. The quantitative serum chorionic gonadotropin levels are helpful in the evaluation of the normalcy of fetal growth and development in the first trimester of pregnancy. Assays are also important in the diagnosis and follow-up examinations of patients who have had trophoblastic disease, hydatidiform moles or chorioepithelioma (Chapter 27). The thyroid stimulating activity sometimes seen in the presence of trophoblastic tumors, when hCG titers are high, is in fact hCG. It is responsible for the clinical hyperthyroidism sometimes seen in association with these conditions.

Chorionic Somatomammotropin, hCS

Another specific placental protein hormone is placental lactogen or placental human chorionic somatomammotropin (hCS). The values during pregnancy are shown (Fig.

2.22). The functions of this hormone are as yet undetermined. It can be used as a measure of placental competence after the first trimester.

Prolactin

As stated above, the maternal placenta, the decidua, has been shown to produce prolactin. This cell, however, is not controlled by a dopamine inhibition. As the pituitary also secretes increasing amounts of prolactin through pregnancy (Fig. 2.23), the contribution of the decidua to the second and third trimester prolactin values cannot be assessed.

Progesterone

The placenta is also responsible for steroid production and, as indicated, by 36 days may have assumed sufficient progesterone production to allow a pregnancy to progress following ablation of the corpus luteum. The placenta in the last trimester of pregnancy is able to secrete 250 mg of progesterone per 24 hours. About 2.5 to 3.9 μg of progesterone

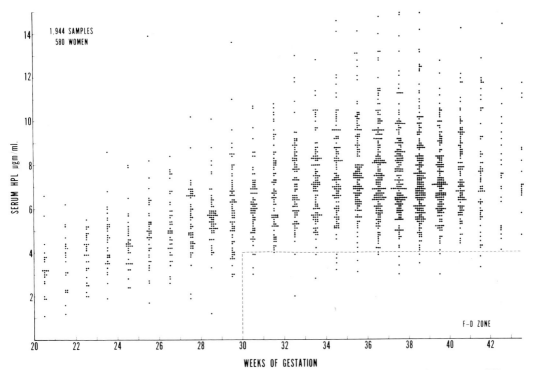

Figure 2.22. Serum somatomammotropin (placental lactogen) values throughout normal pregnancy. F-D zone indicates the area of concern for fetal danger. (From W. N. Spellacy and J. E. Cohn: *Obstetrics & Gynecology, 42:* 330, 1973.)

per gram of placenta. Blood levels of progesterone in pregnancy roughly approximate the rise in progesterone production previously indicated by studies of the urinary pregnanediol excretion (Fig. 2.24). It is assumed that the function of progesterone in pregnancy is to maintain the quiescence of the uterus. Serum progesterone or urinary pregnanediol after the third month, can serve as an index of placental competence.

Estrogen

Placental cells are also capable of synthesizing estrogens, and the rising urinary estrogen values for estrone, estradiol, and estriol (Fig. 2.25) in part reflect this function. The tremendous amounts of estriol which are found in urine during pregnancy have, however, been shown to be derived from the fetal adrenal steroid dehydroepiandrosterone. This is metabolized in the fetal liver to 16-hydroxydehydroepiandrosterone which is converted by the placenta to estriol. Therefore, urinary estriol is a sensitive measure of fetal well being, after the first trimester.

Measurement of these steroids in amniotic fluid has been accomplished, and the findings

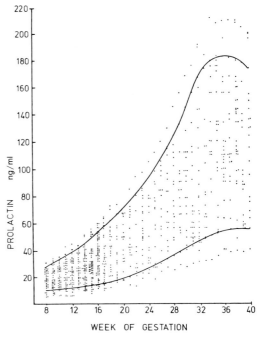

Figure 2.23. Serum prolactin values in normal pregnancies showing 90th and 10th centiles (From Biswass: *British Journal of Obstetrics & Gynaecology, 83:* 683, 1976.)

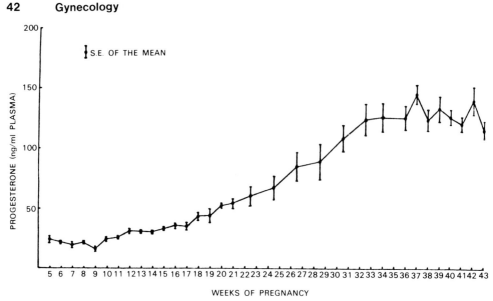

Figure 2.24. Plasma progesterone levels throughout normal pregnancy. (From E. D. B. Johansson: *Acta Endocrinologica, 61:* 692, 1969.)

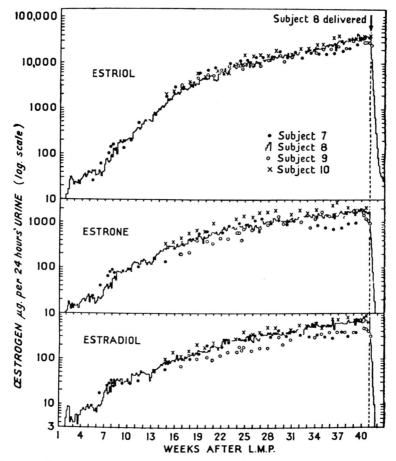

Figure 2.25. Excretion of estriol, estrone, and estradiol during pregnancy in the four subjects, and during the puerperium in Subject 8. L.M.P., last menstrual period. (From J. B. Brown: *Lancet, 1:* 704, 1956.)

are more closely related to the actual status of the fetus, as no consideration need be given to the maternal liver and kidney function. If 16α-hydroxydehydroepiandrosterone is measured, the factor of aromatization by the placenta is also eliminated, giving an even closer approximation of the actual fetal physiology (Schindler and Ratanasopa). The importance of evaluation of both urinary and serum estriol levels under specific circumstances is apparent.

Estetrol is the final product in the metabolic pathway for the peripheral inactivation of estrogens during pregnancy. Serum estradiol, estrone, estriol and estetrol values throughout normal pregnancy as reported by Levitz and Young are shown (Fig. 2.26). Values for conjugated and free estriol serum levels in late pregnancy were reported by Klooper et al.

Pregnancy Tests

Chorionic gonadotropin hormone in pregnancy urine or serum is the basis for the validity and accuracy of the biological and immunological pregnancy tests. The tests may be expected to be positive when the trophoblast is living and functioning, and when the hormone has access to the maternal circulation. Even if trophoblast is present, the test will be negative if the trophoblastic cells have degenerated and ceased to function or if the physiological level is too low to detect by the assay method used. Although the chorionic hormone is present throughout pregnancy, it reaches its greatest concentration between 50 and 90 days, following which there is a decline to a low level, which is maintained throughout pregnancy.

The biological urine pregnancy tests have been replaced by the immunological assays. The hCG-receptor assay is specifically equivalent to a biological assay. Barr reports a 97.4% accuracy rate, the disadvantage being that there were 2.3% false-positive reactions.

When the diagnosis is uncertain and true complications of pregnancy are suspected, such as a missed abortion or an hydatidiform mole, or when one wishes to evaluate the normalcy of the developing trophoblast, a specific quantitative serum test is indicated. Vaitukaitis et al. have described an immunoassay, based on an hCG β-subunit, which avoids reactivity with LH and thereby allows improved specificity. There are currently several such hCG β-subunit assays available.

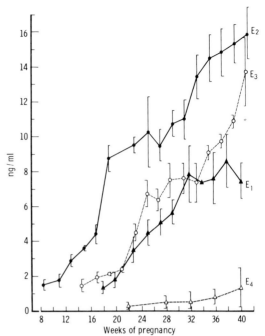

Figure 2.26. Serum values for estradiol (E_2), estriol (E_3), estrone (E_1) and estetrol (E_4) during weeks of pregnancy. (From M. Levitz and B. K. Young: *Vitamins and Hormones, 35:* 109, 1977.)

When trophoblastic disease, hydatid mole or chorioepithelioma is present, it is also desirable to have a bioassay, such as the Delfs assay, for comparison with the immunoassay. If an abnormal molecule is present, it may not react with the specific radioimmunoassay system, whereas a serum bioassay may detect such structurally abnormal hormones.

References and Additional Readings

Abraham, G. E.: Ovarian and adrenal contributions to peripheral androgens during the menstrual cycle. J. Clin. Endocrinol. Metab., *39:* 340, 1974.
Aksel, S., Schomberg, D. W., and Hammond, C. B.: Prostaglandin $F_{2\alpha}$ production by the human ovary. Obstet. Gynecol., *50:* 347, 1977.
Aksel, S., Schomberg, D. W., and Hammond, C. B.: Prostaglandin $F_{2\alpha}$ levels in human ovarian plasma in pregnancy in a case of Halban's disease. Obstet. Gynecol., *52:* 421, 1978.
Ambrus, C. M., Niswander, K. R., Courey, N. G., and Mink, I. B.: Effect of contraceptive drugs on blood coagulation system. Hematol. Rev., *2:* 163, 1951.
Barr, W. A.: A comparison of the Hogben pregnancy test with an immunological method. J. Obstet. Gynaecol. Br. Commonw. *70:* 551,1963.
Bergland R. M., and Page, R. B.: Pituitary-brain vascular relations: a new paradigm. *Science 204:* 18, 1979.
Bischoff, K., Bettendorf, G., and Steger, H. E.: Pituitary content of FSH and LH in accident victims. Arch. Gynecol. *208:* 44, 1968.
Borgeat, P., Garneau, P., and Labrie, F.: Calcium requirement for stimulation of cyclic AMP accumulation in anterior pituitary and LHRH. Mol. Cell. Endocrinol., *2:* 117, 1975.
Böving, B. G.: Implantation. Ann. N.Y. Acad. Sci., *75:* 700, 1958.
Cantarow, A., Rakoff, A. E., Paschikis, K. E., Hansen, L. P., and

Walkling, A. A.: Excretion of exogenous and endogenous estrogen in bile of dogs and humans. Proc. Soc. Exp. Biol. Med., *52:* 256, 1943.

Challis, J. R. G., Davies, I. J., and Ryan, K. F. The concentrations of progesterone, estrone and estradiol-17β in the plasma of pregnant rabbits. Endocrinology *93:* 971, 1973.

Chow, B. F., van Dyke, H. B., Greep, R. O., Rothen, A., and Shedlobsky, T.: Gonadotrophins of the swine pituitary. Endocrinology, *30:* 350, 1942.

Colburn, P., and Buonassisi, V.: Estrogen-binding sites in endothelial cell cultures. Science, *201:* 817, 1978.

Corner, G. W., and Allen, W. M.: Physiology of the corpus luteum; II. Production of a special uterine reaction (progestational proliferation) by extracts of the corpus luteum. Am. J. Physiol., *88:* 326, 1929.

Dawood, M. Y., and Ratnam, S. S.: Serum estradiol-17β in normal pregnancy measured by radioimmunoassay. Obstet. Gyencol., *44:* 194, 1974.

Flerko, B., and Szentagolhai, I.: Oestrogen sensitive nervous structures in the hypothalamus. Acta Endocrinol. (Kbh.), *26:* 121, 1957.

Funk, C., Chamelin, I. M., Wagreich, H., and Harrow, B.: Study of hormonal factors which influence production of insulin. Science, *94:* 260, 1941.

Gallagher, T. F., Peterson, D. H., Dorfman, R. I., Kenyon, A. T., and Koch, F. C.: Daily urinary secretion of estrogenic and androgenic substances in normal men and women. J. Clin. Invest., *16:* 695, 1937.

Gethmann, V., Ball, P., and Knuppen, R.: Effect of 2-hydroxyesterone in gonadotropin secretion in ovariectomized rat. Acta Endocrinol. (Kbh.) (Suppl.), *215:* 102, 1978.

Goldstein, J. L., and Brown, M. S.: The LDL pathway human fibroblasts: a receptor/mediated mechanism for the regulation of cholesterol metabolism. Curr. Top. Cell. Regul., *11:* 147, 1976.

Greep, R. O., van Dyke, H. B., and Chow, B. F.: Use of anterior lobe of prostate gland in assay of metakentrin. Proc. Soc. Exp. Biol. Med., *46:* 644, 1941.

Haafiez, A. A., et al.: The role of prolactin in the regulation of testis function: the effects of prolactin and luteinizing hormone on plasma. J. Endocrinol. *52:* 327, 1972.

Harris, G. W.: *The Neural Control of the Pituitary Gland.* Edward Arnold, London, 1955.

Hitschmann, F., and Adler, L.: Der Bau der Uterusschleimhaut des Geschlectesreifen Weibes mit besonderer Berücktigung der Menstruation. Monatsschr. Gerburtschilfe Gynaekol., *27:* 1, 1908.

Hopkins, C. R.: Short term kinetics of luteinizing hormone secretions studied in disassociated pituitary cells attached to manipulable substrates. J. Cell. Biol. *73:* 685, 1977.

Hunzicker-Dunn, M., Jungmann, R. A., and Birnbaumer, L.: Hormone action in ovarian Follicles: Adenylyl cyclase and protein kinase enzyme systems. In *Ovarian Follicular Development and Function*, edited by A. R. Midgley, Jr. and W. A. Sadler, p. 267. Raven Press, New York, 1979.

Kérdelhue, B., Valens, M., and Langlois, Y.: Stimulation de la sécrétion de la LH et de la FSH hypophysaires aprène, chex la ratte cyclique. C. R. Acad. Sci. (D) (Paris), *286:* 977, 1978.

Kirchick, H. J., Keyes, P. L., and Frye, B. E.: An explanation for anovulation in immature alloxan-diabetic rats treated with pregnant mare's serum gonadotropin; reduced pituitary response to gonadotropin-releasing hormone. Endocrinology, *105:* 1343, 1979.

Klooper, A., Strong, J. A., and Cook, L. R.: The excretion of pregnanediol and adrenocortical activity. J. Endocrinol., *15:* 180, 1957.

Kuhl, H., and Taubert, H. -D.: Short loop feedback mechanism of lutenizing hormone; LH stimulates hypothalamic L-cystine arylamidase to inactivate LH-RH in the rat hypothalamus. Acta Endocrinol., *78:* 649, 1975.

Laragh, J. L.: Oral contraceptive induced hypertension, nine years later. J. Obstet. Gynecol., *126:* 141, 1976.

LeMaire, W. J.: Hormone action in ovarian follicles. In *Ovarian Follicular Development and Function*, edited by A. R. Midgley, Jr. and W. A. Sadler, p. 305. Raven Press, New York, 1979.

Levitz, M., and Young, B. K.: Estrogens in pregnancy. Vitam. Horm., *35:* 109, 1977.

Liu, T., and Jackson, G. L.: Effect of in vitro treatment with estrogen on luteinizing hormone synthesis and release by rat pituitaries in vitro. Endocrinology, *100:* 1294, 1977.

Longcope, C., Layne, D. S., and Tait, J. F.: Metabolic clearance rates and interconversions of estrone and 17β-estradiol in normal males and females. J. Clin. Invest., *47:* 93, 1968.

Markee, J. E.: Menstruation in intraocular endometrial transplants in the rhesus monkey. Contrib. Embryol., *28:* 219, 1940.

Marsh, J. M., Yang, N. S. T., and LeMaire, W. J.: Prostaglandin synthesis in rabbit Graafian follicles in vitro. Effect of luteinizing hormone and cyclic AMP. Prostaglandins, *7:* 269, 1974.

McNeil, T. H., and Sladek, J. J.: Fluorescence immunocytochemistry. Simultaneous localization of catecholamines and gonadotrophin releasing hormone. Science, *200:* 72, 1978.

Merimee, T. J., Burgess, J. A., and Rabinowitz, D.: Sex-determined variation in serum insulin and growth hormone response to amino acid stimulation. J. Clin. Endocrinol., *26:* 791, 1966.

Midgley, A. R., Jr., and Jaffee, R. B.: Regulation of human gonadotropins; II. Disappearance of human chorionic gonadotropin following delivery. J. Clin. Endocrinol. Metab., *28:* 1712, 1968.

Miller, G. J., and Miller, N. E.: Plasma-high-density lipoprotein concentrations and development of ischemic heart disease. Lancet, *1:* 16, 1975.

Moore, R. Y.: Visual pathways to CNS control of diurnal rhythms, p. 537. *The Neurosciences, Third Study Program*, edited by F. O. Schmitt and F. G. Worden. MIT Press, Cambridge, Mass., 1979.

Morato, T. K., Raab, H. J., Brodie, M., Hyano, M., and Dorfman, R. I.: The mechanisms of estrogen biosynthesis. J. Am. Chem. Soc., *84:* 3764, 1962.

Myer, R.: Anovulatory cycle and menstruation. Am. J. Obstet. Gynecol., *51:* 39, 1946.

Naftolin, F., Morishita, H., Davies, I. J., Todd, R., Ryan, K. J., and Fishman, J.: 2-Hydroxyesterone induced rise in serum luteinizing hormone in the immature male rat. Biochem. Biophys. Res. Commun., *64:* 905, 1975.

Noyes, R. W., Hertig, A. T., and Rock, J.: Dating the endometrial biopsy. Fertil. Steril., *1:* 3, 1950.

O'Malley, B. W., and Means, A. R.: Female steroid hormones an target cell nuclei. Science *183:* 610, 1974.

Rothchild, J., and Rapport, R. S.: The thermogenic effort of progesterone and its relation to thyroid function. Endocrinology, *50:* 580, 1952.

Ruf, K. B.: How does the brain control the process of puberty? Z. Neurol., *204:* 95, 1973.

Ryan, W. L., and Coronel, D. M.: Adenosine 3',5'-monophosphate as an inhibitor of ovulation and reproduction. Am. J. Obstet. Gynecol., *105:* 121, 1969.

Santen, R. J., and Bardin, C. W.: Episodic luteinizing hormone secretion in man. J. Clin. Invest., *52:* 2617, 1973.

Schindler, A. E., and Ratanasopa, V.: Profile of steroids in amniotic fluid of normal and complicated pregnancies. Acta Endocrinol., *59:* 239, 1968.

Selye, H.: *Textbook of Endocrinology.* University of Montreal Press, Montreal, 1947.

Shinn, S. H., and Howitt, C.: Evidence for the existence of LHRH binding protein. Neuroendocrinology, *24:* 14, 1977.

Shutt, D. A., Clarke, A. H., Frasier, I. S., Goh, P., McMahan, G. R., Saunders, D. N., and Sherman, R. P.: Changes in concentration of prostaglandin F and steroids in human corpus luteum in relation to growth of corpus luteum and luteolysis. J. Endocrinol., *71:* 453, 1976.

Siebke, H., and Schuschania, P.: Ergebnisse von Mengenbestimmungen des Sexualhormons; Sexualhormon in Harn und Kot bei regelmassigem mensuellem Zyklus Zyklusstorungen und bei Hormontherapi. Zentralbl. Gynaekol., *54:* 1734, 1930.

Sinding, C., and Robinson, A. G.: A review of neurophysins. Metabolism, *26:* 1355, 1977.

Spanos, E., Pike, J. W., Haussler, M. R., Colston, K. W., Evans, I. M. A., Goldner, A. M., McCain, T. A., and MacIntyre, I.: Circulating l 25-digydroxy vitamin D in the chicken: enhancement by injection of prolactin and during egg laying. Life Sci. *19:* 1751, 1976.

Stone, R. T., Mauer, R. A., and Gorski, J.: Effect of estradiol-17β on preprolactin messenger ribonucleic acid activity in the rat pituitary gland. Biochemistry, *16:* 4915, 1977.

Strickland, S., and Beers, W. H.: Studies of the enzymic basis and hormonal cartel of ovulation. In *Ovarian Development and Function,* edited by A. R. Midgly and W. A. Sadler. Raven Press, New York, 1979.

Tulchinsky, D., Osathamonda, R., and Finn, A.: Dehydroepiandrosterone sulfate loading test in the diagnosis of complicated pregnancies. N. Engl. J. Med., *294:* 517, 1976.

Vaitukaitis, J. L., Graunstein, G. D., and Ross, G.T.: A radioimmunoassay which specifically measures human chorionic gonadotropin in the presence of human luteinizing hormone. Am. J. Obstet. Gynecol., *113:* 751, 1972.

Vijayan, E., and McCann, S. M.: In vivo and in vitro effects of substance P and neurotensis on gonadotropin and prolactin release. Endocrinology, *105:* 64, 1979.

Wade, R., and Jones, H. W.: Effect of progesterone on oxidative phosphorylation. J. Biol. Chem., *220:* 553, 1956.

Witten, C. L., and Bradbury, J. T.: Hemodilution as a result of estrogen therapy. Estrogenic effects in the human female. Proc. Soc. Exp. Biol. Med., *78:* 626, 1951.

Zander, J., Forbes, T. R., von Munstermann, A. M., and Neher, R.: Δ^4-3-Ketopregnane-20α-ol and Δ^4-3-ketopregnane-20β-ol, two naturally occurring metabolites of progesterone. J. Clin. Endocrinol., *18:* 337, 1958.

Zeleznik, A. J., Midgley, A. R., Jr., and Riechart, L. E., Jr.: Granulosa cell maturation in the rat. Increased binding of the human chorionic gonadotrophin following treatment with follicle stimulating hormone in vivo. Endocrinology, *95:* 818, 1974.

CHAPTER 3

Cyclical Cytology and Histology of the Genital Tract

CYCLIC CHANGES IN THE VAGINA AND CERVIX

While histologically the vagina and exocervix have only a subtle cyclicity with the menstrual cycle, these changes are quite identifiable by a study of the cells exfoliated from the cervix and vagina.

The Specimen

While the total thickness of the vaginal epithelium is affected by its endocrine milieu, cytohormonal evaluation depends upon the state of the epithelial cells lying upon the surface of the epithelium. *Natural* exfoliation therefrom or *gentle* scraping, therefore, yield a reproducibility which cannot be achieved when specimen depth artificially varies due to variations in scraping technique.

Lateral Vaginal Wall Scraping

This specimen obtains material directly from the organ of response (i.e., vaginal epithelium). Thus it does not have to accumulate in the vaginal pool reservoir and is most free of contaminating material from the cervix and endometrium. *Light uniform* scrapings from the midportion of the lateral vaginal wall is the most accurate and preferred specimen for cytohormonal evaluation.

Vaginal Pool Specimen

This is very satisfactory material for accurate cytohormonal evaluation *provided* that one evaluates *only* the *vaginal* wall portions of the pool, recognizing and entirely disregarding those portions coming from the cervix. When this is not possible (i.e., inexperi-

ence; severe cervicitis) lateral vaginal wall scraping should be utilized.

Vaginal pool material should be, and usually is, a part of a routine cancer detection specimen, either as a separate slide or a part of a combined single-slide specimen (i.e., Fast vaginopancervical). A cervical scraping by itself does *not* suffice for cancer detection, and is *un*reliable for hormonal evaluation.

In this way, therefore, accurate cytohormonal evaluation is available to all patients with routine cancer detection cellular examination if it includes vaginal pool material. A cytohormonal evaluation should be made on all such cancer detection material, and reported upon if abnormal.

Cervical Specimen

This material is *not* reliable for cytohormonal evaluation.

Serial Specimen

When serial evaluation is important (i.e., cycle, ovulation, drug response), *daily serial* smears are invaluable.

Staining by the classical Papanicolaou method is preferred for an accurate evaluation and permanent record, or the more rapid Shorr stain can be used. For an immediate clinical impression, it can be stained fresh by a rapid method (i.e., Rakoff's stain (Paschkis et al.)) and microscopically examined directly.

In *children* and the *aged*, great care must be exercised to obtain the specimen only from the vaginal vault. It must not be contaminated by touching either the labia, the vestibule, or the ungloved examiner's fingers. A nonabsorbent cotton swab, moistened with saline and introduced through a nasal speculum or drinking straw, gives an adequate vaginal smear for cytohormonal evaluation of a child.

Cellular Morphology Response

The most dependably valuable information is obtained from cellular morphology. Both the relationships of one cell to another *and* their individual state of cellular maturation are evaluated. The former includes their sticky behavior with clumping *versus* a tendency to remain separate as individual cells, and a tendency to lie flat *versus* a crinkling and retraction of the outer margins of the cytoplasm with a characteristic folding upon itself in a navicular fashion.

Numerous indices have been used to describe only the squamous cells, or squames. The percentage of squamous cells with nuclear pyknosis is referred to as the karyopyknotic index (K.I.). The percentage of squamous cells showing cytoplasmic acidophilia is termed the cornification index (C.I.), eosinophilic index (E.I.), or acidophilic index (A.I.).

The maturation index (M.I.) expresses most of the above information *plus* information regarding maturation only to the level of parabasal cell exfoliation as found in atrophy. The maturation value (M.V.) expresses most of the information of the latter index in one figure.

Maturation Index (M.I.)

The maturation index is a concise and objective method for gaining insight regarding the endocrine milieu. This expresses conveniently the level of cellular maturation attained at the time of exfoliation as a delicately changing ratio. A differential of the three major types of cells shed from the stratified squamous epithelium of the lateral vaginal wall, is expressed as percentages present of the parabasal, the intermediate, and the superficial cells *in that order* (Fig. 3.1). The nomenclature used for these three major types of cells shed from squamous epithelium, is the International Nomenclature which was informally agreed upon in 1958. Nomenclature used previously differs from this.

The M.I. of a patient exfoliating no parabasal cells, 55% intermediate cells, and 45% superficial cells is written 0/55/45 and accurately reflects their ratio on the surface of her vaginal epithelium. This order (parabasal/intermediate/superficial) of the M.I. is important to obviate confusion and mistake. It is analogous to the Arneth index in which the level of maturation of the neutrophils exfoliated from marrow into circulating blood is represented with the least mature cell on the left (i.e., band or stab cell) and the most mature cell on the right (i.e., segmented polymorphonuclear cells). Likewise, a shift to the left denotes less mature cells being released (exfoliated), whereas a shift to the right indicates more mature cells. Arrows written over the M.I. may be used to more clearly indicate the direction and degree of the maturation shift (i.e., $\overrightarrow{0}/55/\overleftarrow{45}$).

These three normal cells shed from the noncornified, stratified, squamous vaginal epithelium are usually easily told apart:

First, one determines the cytoplasmic thickness (Fig. 3.1). If it is *thick*, the cell is a *parabasal* regardless of the nuclear pattern or cytoplasmic color, size, or shape. If the cytoplasm is "wafer-thin" the cell is a squame of either intermediate or superficial type.

Second, if it is a squame, one then determines the nuclear size and chromatin pattern. If the nucleus of this squame is plump and vesicular with an intact chromatin pattern, the cell is termed an *intermediate* (Fig. 3.1); if it is pyknotic, shrunken below 6 μm, hyperchromatic, and lacks chromatin pattern, the cell is a *superficial*, regardless of cytoplasmic color.

A sharp distinction is usually obvious with a good nuclear stain, such as the Papanicolaou stain, on properly fixed material. In poor nuclear stains and in dried or poorly fixed cell preparations, a sharp differentiation may be difficult. Under phase contrast microscopy, pyknosis usually is accompanied by a very characteristic red sheen to the nucleus.

One must be very careful not to include *dyskaryotic* cells in the M.I. Such contaminating cells from cervical or vaginal atypias or from dermatological conditions must be recognized as *not* belonging in the *normal* squamous series and therefore must *not* be counted in the M.I. The cells of the dyskaryotic series have larger than normal nuclei. Frequently, the nucleus is hyperchromatic, the nuclear membrane is wavy, and the chromatin is granular and uniformly dispersed. In severe dysplasia, the cytoplasm of the dyskaryotic cell may be scanty and thick, so that

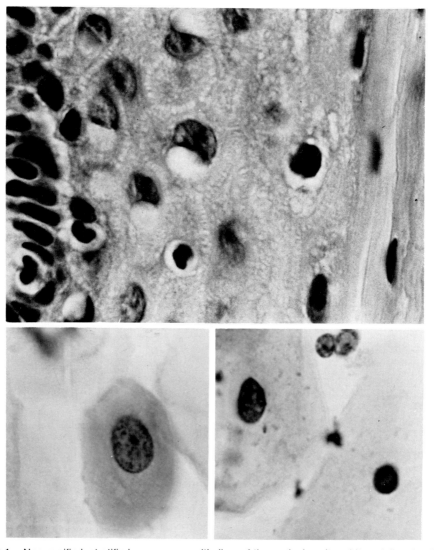

Figure 3.1. Noncornified, stratified, squamous epithelium of the vaginal vault and its exfoliated cells. *Upper section, from left to right*: basement membrane, true basal cells, parabasal cells, intermediate cells, superficial cells (×1100). *Lower left*, parabasal cell (exfoliated, in vaginal smear); cytoplasm is *thick* from nucleus to cell border (×1500). *Lower right*, intermediate cell (*left*) and superficial cell (exfoliated, in vaginal smear); cytoplasm of both is uniformly "wafer-thin" from nucleus to cell border. The intermediate cell nucleus is vesicular and retains chromatin pattern. The nucleus of the superficial cell is pyknotic, measuring less than 6 μ, hyperchromatic, and has lost chromatin pattern. For size reference, a neutrophil is in upper midfield (×1500).

the cell would seem to be a parabasal cell to the unwary who did not recognize the enlarged nucleus. This is the greatest cause for incorrectly identifying three cell types as being present in the vaginal smear at the same time, which is very rare. Dyskaryotic cells must *not* be included in the M.I.

It is obvious from the foregoing that the karyopyknotic index (K.I.), which expresses the percentage of squamous epithelial cells having pyknotic nuclei, and the acidophilic indices (A.I., C.I., E.I.), which express the percentage of cells having yellow, orange, or red cytoplasm usually will approximate closely the right hand figure of the maturation index. The K.I. is exactly the right hand figure, if there are no parabasal cells present (it is rare to have three cell types at the same time). The acidophilic indices, on the other hand, may differ significantly from the right hand cell of the M.I., due, in great part, to the artifacts of drying or inflammation and the variations of staining.

Normal Cytohormonal Patterns of the Endocrine Periods

Childhood Period

This period produces one of the most dependable and constant patterns, except for the very beginning and end of the period. *At birth* the vaginal epithelium of the female infant is thick and lush in response to circulating maternal hormones, including massive progesterones, estrogens, and adrenocortical compounds (Fig. 3.2). The surface cells are mainly of intermediate type, so that the M.I. of the cell spread is characteristic of pregnancy, $\overleftrightarrow{0/95/5}$. Desquamation rapidly takes place and within a few weeks it becomes the thin atrophic epithelium so characteristic of *childhood*, with the M.I. markedly shifted to the left (c. $\overrightarrow{100/0/0}$ or $\overrightarrow{70/30/0}$). The surface cell matures to the parabasal level at exfoliation, with only a few intermediates and with *no* superficials.

Perimenarchal Period

Around the age of 8 years, but with great individual variation, there begins a gradual increase of noticeable sex steroid activity until the reproductive level is reached at menarche, about the age of 14. This gradual increase is evidenced in the vaginal epithelium by thickening and proliferation, with increasing numbers of suface cells maturing to the intermediate and superficial types as sex hormone production increases. The vaginal smear mirrors this, with an increasing shift of the M.I. to the right, until the appearance of menses and the full-blown cellular endocrine pattern of the reproductive age.

Therefore, as this perimenarchal period is a continuing transition from childhood atrophy (M.I., c. $\overleftrightarrow{100/0/0}$ to $\overleftrightarrow{70/30/0}$) to the lush epithelium of the reproductive period, (M.I., c. $\overrightarrow{0/70/30}$ to $\overrightarrow{0/40/60}$), great variation can be encountered. Age is the major factor in evaluating endocrine status of this period.

Reproductive Period

During the childbearing age, from perimenarche to perimenopause, the endocrine

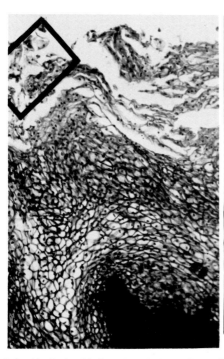 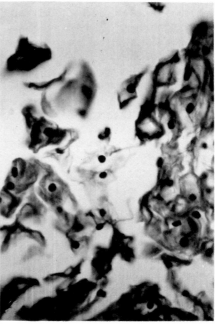

Figure 3.2. Vaginal epithelium, female fetus, 6-month gestation. *Left,* the lush epithelium so typical of both a female fetus en utero and a pregnant woman (H & E stain, ×40). *Right,* intermediate cells exfoliating from the surface of the same epithelium. Maturation index, 0/95/5 (H & E, × 160).

milieu shows great cyclic fluctuation. Following the initial period of endocrine adjustment in the establishment of menses and extending into the disruption of endocrine interplay of the perimenopausal period, the pattern is a series of menstrual cycles. Although the hormonal patterns vary widely between individuals, they are usually mirrored in repetition for a given individual. Their constancy is broken normally only by childbearing, so that the cellular patterns of the *menstrual cycle*, or *pregnancy*, and of the *postpartum period*, are characteristic.

Throughout the *menstrual cycle* with a normal ovulatory pattern, superficial cells and intermediate cells vary in exfoliation from 30 to 60% (M.I. from c. $\overleftarrow{0/40/60}$ around ovulation to c. $\overrightarrow{0/70/30}$ around menstruation) in response to estrogen and progestogen levels. At the time of ovulation, high and unopposed estrogen is present with a moderate shift of M.I. to the right (c. $\overrightarrow{0/40/60}$). With ovulation, circulating estrogen drops rapidly. Shortly thereafter estrogen rises again with the development of the corpus luteum during the secretory phase, but at this time it is accompanied by progestogens. Just before menstruation the progestogen opposition is at its highest and produces a moderate M.I. shift to the midzone (M.I., c. $\overrightarrow{0/70/30}$). During menstruation both estrogen and progestogen sharply drop. Soon, from the developing new follicle, estrogen again rises alone during the proliferative phase, shifting the M.I. to the right until the ovulatory pattern (M.I., c. $\overrightarrow{0/40/60}$) is once more reached, two weeks before menses.

Except postpartum, the parabasal type cell does not exfoliate normally until the later years of the reproductive period or in the perimenopausal period. In some patients, the parabasal cell may not exfoliate at any time during the reproductive and postmenopausal periods if at the latter time they go into intermediate cell atrophy $\overleftrightarrow{(0/100/0)}$ rather than parabasal cell atrophy ($\overleftarrow{100/0/0}$).

As with a single basal body temperature determination, a *single* vaginal smear evaluation gives only limited endocrine information. This is not only because of the great endocrine variations encountered during the menstrual cycle, but also because of the fact that many combinations of dynamic factors can produce similar static cytohormonal patterns *Daily* vaginal pool aspiration smears obtained and prepared by the patient along with her basal body temperature, are invaluable in detecting ovulation, anovulation, time in cycle, endocrinopathies, etc. Almost as valuable and easier to obtain, are the twice-a-week series taken every 3–4 days. Such complete cytohormonal evaluation yields valuable dynamic endocrine information.

In *pregnancy*, the cytohormonal pattern is characteristic and is "locked in" by massive levels of hormones. With conception the normal luteal phase M.I. shift toward the midzone, proceeds just as in the nonpregnant menstrual cycle; however, when the pattern reaches the menstrual M.I. (c. $\overrightarrow{0/70/30}$), it does not recede, but continues its midzone climb. Within a few weeks it has reached the pattern so characteristic of pregnancy, with the extreme M.I. midzone shift ($\overrightarrow{0/95/5}$) maintained throughout gestation. The levels of estrogens, progestogens, and cortical steroids are so massive in the normal pregnancy that this M.I. is not altered by usual doses of hormones. This forms the basis for Wied's test for menopausal amenorrhea versus pregnancy. Direct effect of infection upon the vaginal epithelium, however, will artificially alter even the hormonal pattern of pregnancy, with a characteristic inflammatory "spread" of the M.I. (e.g., from $\overline{0/95/5}$ toward c. $\overrightarrow{33/34/33}$).

In the absence of inflammation, therefore,

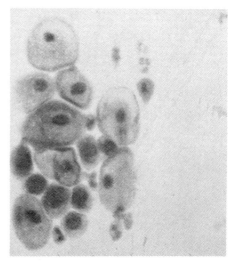

Figure 3.3. Postpartum or lactational pattern; maturation index, $\overleftarrow{100/0/0}$. This peculiarly teleatrophic pattern contains only parabasal cells. It occurs abruptly at the end of gestation and is a marked change from the lush intermediate cell exfoliation of pregnancy (×160).

it is significant when the usual pregnancy M.I. of 0/95/5 varies markedly either to the right or to the left. Hormonal change must be great indeed, to effect such an alteration in a pattern normally held to by massive levels of hormones. Abortions having an endocrine basis are heralded by a bizarre M.I. either to the right or to the left. If this threatened or impending abortion then leads to fetal death, it is signaled by a drastic shift of the M.I. to the left, similar to the postpartum pattern.

The *postpartum* pattern is striking (Fig. 3.3) Around the time of delivery another mammoth hormonal change takes place. The M.I., heavily shifted to the midzone throughout pregnancy, briefly shifts to the right in some patients and then, after delivery, shift to the left (from 0/95/5 to 100/0/0). This teleatrophic postpartum or lactational pattern (Fig. 3.3) is striking in a young woman. It can be altered by hormones administered for suppression of lactation. After varying lengths of time it gradually returns to the normal menstrual cyclic pattern.

Perimenopausal Period

For years, both before and after the actual cessation of menses, there are gradually progressive alterations and diminutions in the orderly cyclic endocrine patterns of the reproductive period. These are mirrored in the vaginal epithelium and its cytohormonal pattern. This process of alteration begins in the latter part of the reproductive period and continues through the menopause and for years thereafter, with the cyclic hormonal variations decreasing in intensity and varying in frequency. The onset of this perimenopausal period is gradual and varies greatly among individuals. If cessation of cycles does occur before death, it is insidious and without clinical fanfare.

Cytohormonally, perimenopausal patients appear to fall into two well defined categories, those developing intermediate cell atrophy (toward M.I., 0/100/0) with apparent lack of any estrogen effect, or *estratrophy*, and those developing parabasal cell atrophy or *teleatrophy* (towards M.I., 100/0/0) with total absence of evidence of any effect of vaginal maturation. The reasons for the differences are not clear. Adrenal cortical function may well play a larger role than generally appreciated, and probably accounts for the M.I. "midzone" shift of intermediate cell atrophy, even though small levels of estrogens have

also been implicated. Why all do not follow this pattern is not clear. Variations in hypophysial response to feedback may underlie these patterns, and at times adrenal androgens are suspected of playing a role.

In the development of intermediate cell atrophy throughout the perimenopausal period, there is an increasing number of intermediate cells exfoliated at the expense of superficials, without significant production of parabasals. This shift toward the midzone of the M.I. may be gradual, with 0/100/0 being reached years after actual cessation of menses. This is not an atrophic vaginal epithelium clinically, but is lush and resistant to infection; however, of great importance is the virtual absence of superficial cells (less than 10%). This total lack of apparent estrogen stimulation may reflect relatively high or unopposed cortisone levels.

In the development of the other frequent pattern, that of *teleatrophy*, there is a gradual increase in exfoliation of parabasal cells at the expense of superficial cells, and later of the intermediate cells. Finally complete atrophy, or teleatrophy, appears with total shift of the M.I. to the left (100/0/0). Clinically, vaginal atrophy is present and the epithelial resistance to infection is low. Senile vaginitis is frequent in this group.

Postmenopausal Period

Either of the two major patterns are assumed as the stormy perimenopausal phase passes into this relatively quiescent postmenopausal period, that of intermediate cell atrophy (M.I., 0/100/0) or of parabasal cell atrophy (M.I., 100/0/0) with variations in between. Cyclic fluctuations become less intense and frequent. Intermediate cell atrophy, in which the epithelial surface is completely covered with intermediate cells, is usually asymptomatic. This pattern predominates when inflammatory patterns are removed from consideration.

Teleatrophy, or parabasal cell atrophy, frequently becomes inflamed and infected, producing senile vaginitis. At times bizarre parabasal cell changes come about from irritation which, in morphology, can *approach* dysplasia or even closely resemble neoplasia. These problems are dissipated with small amounts of oral or vaginal estrogens, to which the epithelium is very sensitive, and reevaluating cytologically biweekly thereafter.

Without extrinsic estrogens and in the absence of inflammation, the presence of significant numbers of superficial cells is abnormal in this postmenopausal period. They rise in infection, chronic irritation (procidentia, etc.), leukoplakia, vaginal dermatoses, and estrogen administration. In the absence of those, however, a significant rise in superficial cells may indicate the presence of certain neoplasms (endometrial, ovarian, mammary, etc.), and hormonal abnormalities. Contamination of the vaginal specimen with vulvar cells must be ruled out.

Cervical Mucosa

The endocervix is of Müllerian origin, and it would seem quite certain that it must show some sort of cyclical response to the ovarian hormones. One of the most complete studies thus far made is that of Sjövall, who con-cluded that the cervical epithelium, under the influence of the ovarian estrogenic hormone, increases in height until after ovulation, becoming lower and increasingly secretory thereafter under the influence of the progesterone then operative. The glands become increasingly large and tortuous, but no evidence of menstrual desquamation is found. Topkins has not been impressed by cervical cyclic changes although cytopathological smears indicate that some type of cycle undoubtedly exists in the lower genital tract. Study of the cervical mucus is of importance in the study of infertility.

Pregnancy Changes in Cervix

It is apparent that the *endocervical glands increase strikingly in size and tortuosity* in pregnancy, producing a lacy adenomatous pattern of the thickened mucosa (Fig. 3.4).

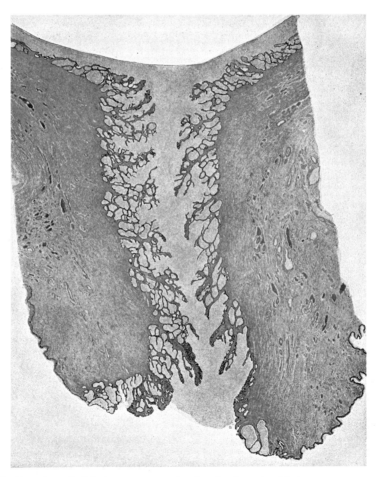

Figure 3.4.   Section of cervix late in pregnancy showing the hypertrophied, spongy mucosa. (From H. J. Stander (Ed.): *Williams' Obstetrics*, Appleton-Century, New York, 1941.)

Similar but more striking changes mimicking adenocarcinoma, although reversible, may be produced by contraceptive pills (Graham et al.) The changes induced by the oral contraceptives is referred to as *microcystic mucoid metaplasia.*

There have been numerous reports of *decidual changes* in the cervix, so that the occurrence is no longer considered rare. Estimates as to the frequency vary greatly, but Epperson and his co-workers, on the basis of a large series of cervical biopsies in pregnant women, found an incidence of 10.4%. Sometimes the decidual change occurs in the form of small patches, but often large fields of typical decidual cells are observed. The decidual change is limited to the stromal elements, so that it would be illogical to assume that the decidua is merely a pregnancy response of a preceding cervical endometriosis. For some reason the cervical stromal elements of such cervices show a sensitivity to the pregnancy hormones, as may connective tissue elements in the ovary and pelvic peritoneum in the fairly frequent instances of ectopic decidua, of which cervical deciduosis must be considered a form.

CYCLIC CHANGES IN THE ENDOMETRIUM

Thorough familiarity with the appearance of the endometrium at different stages of the cycle will permit the experienced pathologist to estimate the time of the menstrual cycle.

This can be done to within a 48-hour span (as day 18–19 or day 23–24). Our criteria are essentially those of Noyes et al. with slight modifications as noted in Table 3.1. Dating the endometrium prior to ovulation is of no practical importance.

The *endometrium*, under the immediate influence of the two ovarian hormones, estrogen and progesterone, exhibits certain characteristic cyclical changes, which may be most conveniently divided into four phases.

Postmenstrual Phase

The endometrium is thin, measuring ordinarily only 1 or 2 mm in thickness. The surface epithelium, as well as that lining the glands, is of cuboidal type. The glands are straight, narrow, and collapsed, whereas the stroma is dense and compact. This phase may arbitrarily be put as including the four or five days immediately following cessation of a period. There is some evidence to indicate that a period of *rest* may at times occur just after menstruation, but this applies chiefly to women with abnormally long cycles, with marked prolongation of the preovulatory phase.

Proliferative Phase

By a gradual transition the postmenstrual phase is followed by the interval stage, during which the continued action of estrogen brings about increased thickness of the uterine mucosa. The surface epithelium becomes taller and columnar, as does that of the glands, while mitotic figures are quite numerous, more so than in the immediately postmenstrual phase. Ciliated cells are a normal finding according to Fleming et al. and Schueler. The *early interval* phase antedates ovulation, and during this period no evidence of secretory activity is to be seen in the gland epithelium (Fig. 3.5), as the secretion of progesterone has not yet begun. This non-secretory portion of the cycle is usually spoken of as "proliferative" and is characterized primarily by growth.

Secretory or Progestational Phase

After ovulation, in the *late interval* or *secretory* phase, the evidence of secretory activity in the gland epithelium becomes more and more marked (Fig. 3.6). If differential staining for glycogen is carried out, granules of glycogen are demonstrable, at first only few in number and within the cytoplasm of the cells, but later more abundant in the cells and in increasing amount in the gland lumina. Subnuclear vacuoles (Figs. 3.7 and 3.8), which are believed to represent a prosecretion phase, begin to crowd the nuclei from the base of the cells toward the lumen. Despite some uncertainty, it is generally assumed that these prosecretion vacuoles represent the earliest stages of progesterone activity. The stroma is more abundant and more vascular than in the postmenstrual phase, particularly in the later stage of the interval, which extends to within a week of the next menstrual phase.

Premenstrual Phase

During this stage the secretory function of the now fully mature corpus luteum brings

Table 3.1

A. Endometrial Dating

Day	Criteria
16	Subnuclear vacuoles Pseudostratification Mitoses, glands and stroma
17	More or less orderly row of nuclei Cytoplasm above nuclei and subnuclear vacuoles below Gland and stromal mitoses Very minimal secretion
18	Vacuoles above and below nuclei Improved linear arrangement of nuclei Gland mitoses rare Stromal mitoses rare Bubbles of secretion seen at luminal border
19	A few vacuoles remain in cell; mainly active evacuation with intraluminal secretion No gland or stromal mitoses May look like day 16 but *NO* pseudostratification
20	Peak secretion with ''ragged'' luminal border Vacuoles are rare—all subnuclear vacuoles gone; inspissation may be beginning
21	Abrupt onset of stromal edema Gland secretion prominent (inspissated) ''Naked'' stromal nuclei begin to appear
22	Peak edema Marked appearance of ''naked'' stromal nuclei; stromal cells small and dense filamentous cytoplasm Active secretion, but subsiding Rare stromal mitoses
23	Prominent spiral arterioles Periarteriolar cuffing with enlargement (earliest predecidual change) of stromal cell nuclei and cytoplasm Stromal mitoses Glands with secretory ''exhaustion''—low columnar cells, luminal edges ragged
24	Definite predecidual cells around arterioles with early subepithelial changes Greater stromal mitoses Ragged cell borders; i.e., secretorily exhausted
25	Definite subcapsular predecidua Inspissated secretion noted to begin Early stromal infiltration with lymphocytes and occasional polymorphonuclear leukocytes
26	Generalized decidual reaction—decidual islands in stroma Polymorphonuclear leukocytic invasion (lymphocytes may accompany or precede)
27	Solid sheet of decidua Marked leukocytic infiltrate; polymorphonuclear leukocytes Inspissated secretion with variable intracellular secretory activity
28	Focal necrosis and hemorrhage Peak leukocytic infiltration; polymorphonuclear leukocytes prominent Cells may show secretory exhaustion or may show active secretion Beginning stromal clumping and fragmentation of glands *Menstruating* Disruption of capsular layer Stromal clumping Glandular breakup and hemorrhage Variable leukocyte infiltration Edema After 24 hours, metaplastic alterations on surface

Table 3.1—*continued*

B. Dating the Corpus Luteum

Day	Criteria
Proliferation (days 14–15)	Collapsed follicle Unluteinized granulosa Absence of blood vessels in granulosa Vascularized theca with ovoid or polyhedral cells No blood in lumen
Vascularization (16–17 days)	Invasion of granulosa by thin blood channels Blood in lumen next to granulosa Large polyhedral granulosa cells
Maturity (day 18)	Mitosis in granulosa ends in day 18 Broad lutein zone traversed by traveculae of theca interna with numerous blood vessels Presence of paralutein cells Fibrous layer lining lutein zone
Retrogression (begins about day 22–23)	Increase in lipids in and fibrosis of lutein zone Presence of "mulberry" cells (vascularized lutein cells) Theca cells smaller in size, resemble ordinary connective tissue Hyalinization occurring over several weeks, cicatrization and formation of corpus albicans over several months

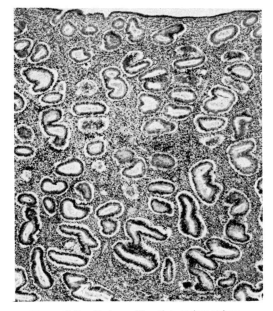

Figure 3.5.   Early proliferative endometrium.

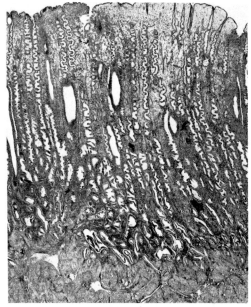

Figure 3.6.   Late interval endometrium showing definite secretory activity.

about a full-blown secretory response in the endometrium, which now is soft, velvety, and edematous, measuring from 4 or 5 mm to as much as 6 or 7 mm in thickness. Whereas the surface epithelium is still tall and cylindrical, that of the glands is now low, the nuclei having receded toward the base of the cells, and the cytoplasm appearing to melt into the lumen, so that the edge is apt to appear frayed.

The glands are wide and assume a characteristic corkscrew pattern, the convolutions producing tuftlike accumulations of epithelium on either longitudinal or cross section. The necks of the glands often remain rather

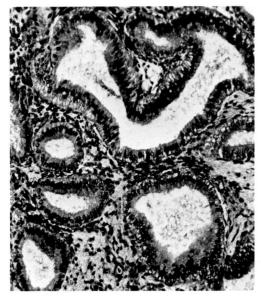

Figure 3.7. Early secretory pattern showing subnuclear vacuoles.

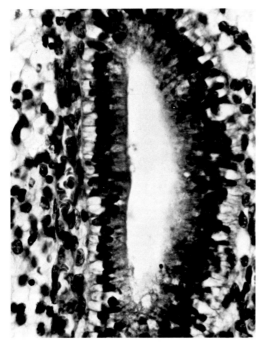

Figure 3.8. Subnuclear vacuoles, the earliest histological evidence of secretory activity (high power).

narrow and straight, the tortuosity involving chiefly the middle or spongy zone of the endometrium. The growing tips of the glands in the basalis, in immediate contact with the musculature, are lined by an immature type of epithelium which is apparently unrespon-

sive to progesterone, so that a secretory reaction is lacking (Fig. 3.9).

The stroma becomes edematous and loose textured, especially in its superficial layer, and the constituent cells undergo hypertrophy, with an increased amount of cytoplasm. This gives them an appearance suggesting decidual cells, and in many cases the resemblance is so striking that one might well suspect the existence of early gestation. Wienke et al. note that the stroma shows an increased ability to respond to hormonal stimuli as the cycle progresses.

In this phase one can distinguish the same three layers which one sees even more sharply delimited in the young decidua. The uppermost layer is compact in appearance, consisting of broad fields of hypertrophied stromal cells between the rather narrow necks of the glands. It is called the *stratum compactum.* The *stratum spongiosum* (middle zone) presents a lacy, labyrinthine appearance because of the preponderance of dilated and tortuous glands, with very little intervening stroma. Finally, the deepest layer (*basalis*) in contact with and often penetrating the muscularis for short distances is made up of the growing tips of the glands, with a dense, compact stroma surrounding them. Because it is composed of an immature refractory tissue it may exhibit only a proliferative pattern even in the premenstrual phase of the cycle, in as much as this undifferentiated endometrium has not acquired the ability to respond to progesterone.

The compacta and spongiosa together make up the portion of the endometrium chiefly participating in the cyclical phenomena of menstruation, so that together they comprise the so-called *functional zone.* The basalis, on the other hand, is the layer responsible for growth and regeneration of the endometrium.

It is not uncommon to find even large areas of unripe endometrium, often showing the Swiss cheese pattern of hyperplasia (see Chapter 14) in endometria which otherwise are typically secretory or progestational in character. It is apparent that curettings from such a uterus would show a mixture of secretory and unripe endometrium, constituting the so-called *mixed endometrium.* Such localized areas of unripe or hyperplastic endometrium seem to produce no such menstrual excess as is so often seen in association with

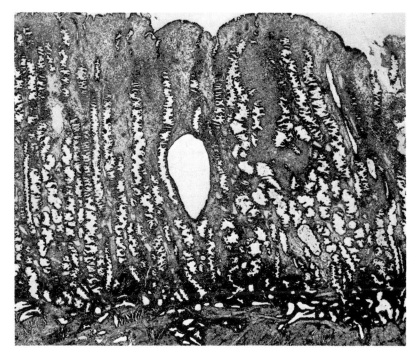

Figure 3.9. Premenstrual or progestational endometrium (25th day).

diffuse Swiss cheese hyperplasia of the endometrium.

Differential staining in the progestational phase reveals increasing quantities of *glycogen*, the first appearance of which, in the form of small intracellular granules, is noted about the time of ovulation, but which in the progestational phase are much more richly distributed, not only within the cells but also in the gland lumina. Quantitative studies on this point have been made by a number of investigators who conclude that *mucin* is also present but appears to be independent of hormonal influence and is found, not in the cells, but only in the gland lumina or in the uterine cavity.

The blood vessels of the endometrium are most conspicuous in the premenstrual phase, and this applies especially to the coiled or spiral arterioles, which are best seen in the lower and middle zones of the endometrium.

Degenerative changes make their appearance in the endometrium well before the onset of menstrual bleeding. The immediately premenstrual phase is characterized especially by a rather massive infiltration by polymorphonuclear and mononuclear leukocytes, producing a *pseudoinflammatory* appearance. The staining reaction of the upper layer be-

comes impaired, suggesting their impending dissolution (Fig. 3.10).

Menstrual or Bleeding Phase

On the first day of the period the tissue loss is quite patchy and only slight and fragmentary. The factor responsible for both the death of tissue and the bleeding is the ischemia produced by the prolonged and intense vasoconstriction of the coiled arterioles. Fibrinolytic activity is increased in the premenstrual and menstrual phases of the cycle and may be related to endometrial desquamation and the fluidity of menstrual blood.

The area supplied by each of these vessels exhibits its own individual degenerative and bleeding changes, and the sum total of many such localized phenomena produces the composite changes characterizing menstruation. Because of the constrictive occlusion of the arterioles, the blood from the endometrial veins backs up into the venules and capillaries, and many of these venous channels rupture, so that small lakes of blood are produced which often cause the appearance of subepithelial hematomas. Strips of tissue are cast off in scattered areas as the process advances, whereas bleeding increases not only as a re-

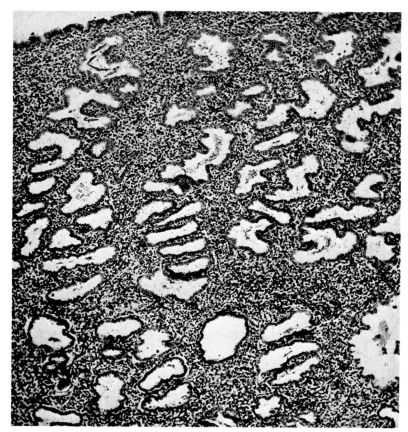

Figure 3.10. Endometrium from patient just about to menstruate showing marked infiltration with leukocytes and wandering cells.

sult of actual rupture of blood vessels but also from increased permeability of the blood vessel walls.

By the second day of bleeding the tissue loss is extensive, practically the entire surface being denuded. There is much individual difference in the amount of endometrium thrown off, but as a rule the entire compacta and a considerable portion of the spongiosa are lost, although the deeper portions of the latter are left behind.

Even while desquamation is still proceeding, evidences of *regeneration* of the surface are usually apparent. This takes place from the epithelium of the gland stumps in the basalis and the shrunken retracted portions of compacta which may remain. The surface is restored with amazing rapidity. Baggish et al. indicate that the superficial stromal cells may actually undergo metaplasia into epithelium. The regeneration of the endometrium is so rapid that if a uterus, removed immediately after the cessation of the flow, is examined, the surface is complete.

The Endometrium of Pregnancy (Decidua)

In the event of pregnancy the hypertrophic and secretory changes of the pregravid phase become even more marked, so that there is an insensible transition between the premenstrual picture in the nonpregnant and the very early decidua of the pregnant woman. In fact, it is not always easy to make the distinction in the laboratory unless embryonic elements, such as villi or trophoblast are present in the section. The *glands* of the decidua present marked sawtooth convolution and scalloping, and the *epithelium* is low, pale staining, and actively secretory. At a little later stage the tortuosity of the glands is much less and the epithelium becomes very flat, so that there may be difficulty in distinguishing the glands from lymphatics or venules.

The *stromal* cells become large and polygonal, with a wide zone of cytoplasm surrounding the nucleus. They now constitute the characteristic *decidual cells*, and are arranged in mosaic or tile-like fashion, occurring in large fields in the superficial or compact layer of the endometrium, where the gland elements are sparsest. In the middle or spongy zone (Fig. 3.11), on the other hand, the hypertrophy and convolution of the glands are most pronounced, and the interglandular septa are thin and delicate, so that an intricate lacy pattern is produced.

In certain cases of pregnancy, both intrauterine and extrauterine, the endometrium exhibits an intensely adenomatous, hypersecretory response with the cells lining the glands mimicking malignant cells by marked mitotic activity, hyperchromatic nuclei, and bizarre abnormal cell types. This *Arias-Stella* reaction is further described and depicted in Chapter 26. Finally, the basalis stands out in even sharper contrast with the upper layers of the endometrium than in the nonpregnant woman, the tips of the glands being lined by a cuboidal nonsecretory type of epithelium quite different from that in the upper reaches of the gland.

Progestational Therapy

In recent years there has ensued a widespread tendency to utilize various progestogens in treating bleeding problems, endometriosis, dysmenorrhea, etc., as well as provid-

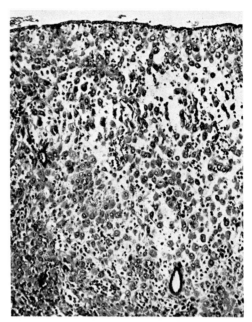

Figure 3.12. Full thickness of endometrium in patient treated by prolonged continuous progesterone. There is almost complete absence of glands along with marked edema of the decidualized stroma. Changes are less pronounced in the lower (basal) portion.

ing contraception. It is important to become familiar with the appearance of the endometrium that has been subjected to prolonged progestational therapy.

There is a striking conversion of the endometrial stroma into typical decidual cells (Fig. 3.12) with simultaneous suppression of the glandular components so that these undergo almost complete exhaustion. This "glandular atrophy" is much more striking with the combined than with sequential hormones. It is apparent that the progestational drugs affect only the functional zone of the endometrium, with the basal layer exhibiting only an estrogen response.

The Senile Endometrium

After the menopause the endometrium may undergo shrinkage, becoming thin and atrophic. This is what one would expect from the withdrawal of the estrogenic hormone which supplies the normal growth stimulus to the genital mucosa. The surface epithelium becomes lower, whereas the glands are narrow and sparsely distributed in the stroma, which with increasing years assumes a more and more fibrotic appearance (Fig. 3.13). The

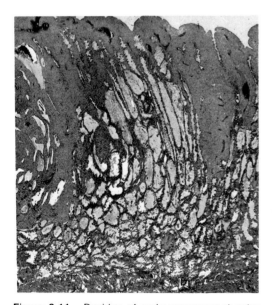

Figure 3.11. Decidua of early pregnancy showing the superficial compact zone in contrast with the spongy middle portion. The basalis is not well shown in this field.

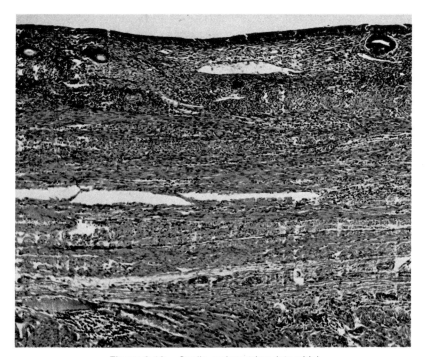

Figure 3.13.   Senile endometrium (atrophic).

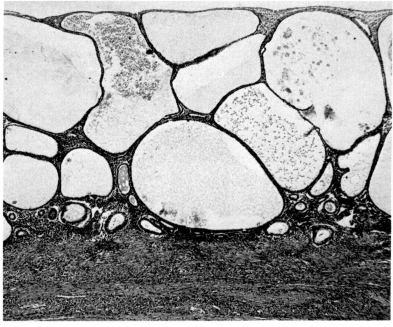

Figure 3.14.   Cystic enlargement of glands in senile endometrium (patient aged 57), a persistence of the Swiss cheese pattern of hyperplasia, but of inactive or retrogressive type.

thinned out atrophic mucosa is prone to superficial punctate ulceration and infection, resulting in the so-called *senile endometritis*, a not infrequent lesion which is of importance because it sometimes produces postmenopausal bleeding which calls for diagnostic differentiation from that produced by adenocarcinoma of the uterus. However, atrophic vaginitis rarely coexists with adenocarcinoma which is characterized by a well supported mucosa and a shift to the right in the maturation index (M.I.).

Although the atrophic changes described above are common, it must be remembered that for a considerable time after the last menstruation, the endometrium may show little atrophy and it may actually present a hyperplastic appearance (Fig. 3.14). In other words, the disappearance of an estrogen influence is not always abrupt, and we know now that even after complete cessation of menstrual function, estrogen may still be produced by some ovarian or extragenital source, most likely the adrenal cortex.

CYCLIC CHANGES IN THE OVARY

Following menstruation a number of follicles begin to mature in the ovary, but, with rare exceptions, only one of these undergoes full maturation, as evidenced by ovulation. The remainder of the follicles are blighted at various phases of development, through the process known as *atresia folliculi.* The process of maturation of the follicle from its early primordial phase (Fig. 3.15) to that of the full development which is attained just before ovulation is characterized by the following chief features.

1. The originally flat follicular epithelium or *membrana granulosa* becomes cuboidal, with later stratification and multiplication of cells, so that at maturity it consists of several layers. The *granulosa* possesses no blood vessels of its own, receiving its nutrition from the *theca interna*; after ovulation the thecal blood vessels grow into the granulosa layer.

2. The oocyte becomes embedded in a well marked peninsula of granulosa cells, the *cumulus oophorus* (see Fig. 3.17) or *discus proligerus.* Call-Exner bodies (small folliculoid areas resulting from cystic degeneration with a surrounding rosette of granulosa cells) are frequent, as they are in certain granulosa cell tumors (Chapter 24).

3. The follicle develops a central cavity or *antrum* filled with a clear fluid or *liquor folliculi.*

4. The *theca interna*, at first poorly developed, becomes a conspicuous zone, the cells of which, as maturity is approached, become large and polyhedral, with abundant lipoid content, presumably going to the nutrition of the nonvascular granulosal layer.

The fully mature follicle consists of the following layers, from without inward (Figs. 3.16 and 3.17).

1. The *theca externa*, a layer of condensed ovarian tissue merging imperceptibly with the stroma.

2. The *theca interna*, as above described: It has been established that these are the cells which are responsible for estrogen production, and the granulosa are more concerned with progesterone formation.

3. The *membrana granulosa.*

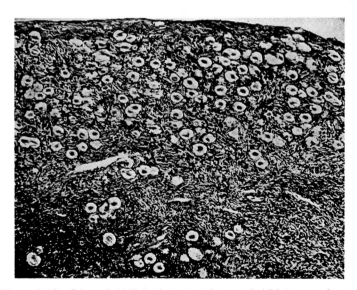

Figure 3.15. Primordial follicles in cortex of ovary of child 4 years of age.

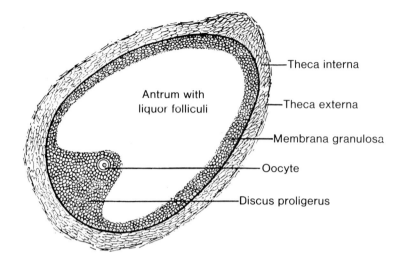

Figure 3.16. Diagram of chief constituent elements of mature follicle.

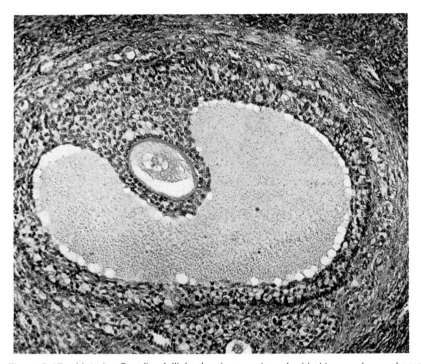

Figure 3.17. Maturing Graafian follicle showing oocyte embedded in cumulus oophorus.

4. The central cavity or *antrum*, filled with the liquor folliculi.

5. The *cumulus oophorus* or *discus proligerus*.

6. The *corona radiata*, the layer of cells of the discus immediately surrounding the egg, and arranged in radial fashion.

7. The *zona pellucida*, a thin, refractile, amorphous zone just within the corona radiata.

The rupture of the follicle is attended by extrusion of the egg and, with it, of the zona pellucida, corona radiata, and a considerable number of the cells of the cumulus. No one but a pathologist will understand the extreme difficulty in distinguishing between a mature follicle and an early corpus luteum, because the lutein changes in granulosa and theca cells are not abrupt but very gradual in their evolution. The collapse of the follicle (Fig.

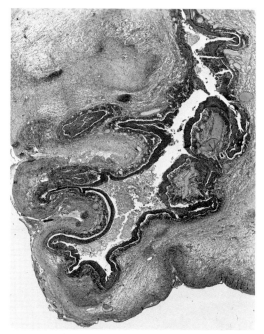

Figure 3.18. Freshly ruptured follicle showing crumbling of wall.

3.18) with the subsequent crumbled festooned pattern is probably the most reliable index of ovulation.

Strassman showed that the theca interna forms a wedgelike cone directed toward the surface of the ovary and thus plays an important mechanical role in ovulation. The cavity collapses with the escape of the follicular fluid, and the second or *corpus luteum phase* of development now begins, reaching its maximum several days before the onset of the next menstrual period. It should be stressed, however, that the corpus luteum is only a modified follicle, and an exact line of demarcation is histologically impossible. For purposes of description, its life cycle can be divided into the following stages, according to the plan originally suggested by Meyer.

1. The stage of *proliferation* immediately following rupture of the follicle: As might be expected, therefore, the wall of the corpus luteum in its earliest stage is identical with that of the fully mature follicle. The granulosal layer, however, soon shows evidence of

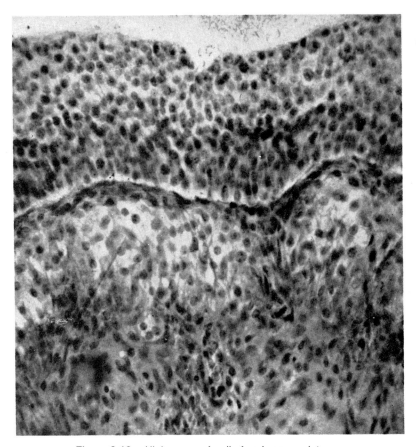

Figure 3.19. High power of wall of early corpus luteum.

beginning transformation into the large, poly-hedral, often vacuolated cells known as lutein cells (Fig. 3.19). Between the granulosa and theca there is a zone of blood vessels known as the perigranulosal vascular wreath.

Grossly the corpus luteum in this early stage is a very inconspicuous structure, its thin wall being crenated and folded on itself because of shrinkage of the cavity. There is no such festooning of the wall as is seen in later stages, and its color is a grayish yellow instead of the bright carroty yellow of late stages.

2. The stage of *vascularization* (Figs. 3.20–3.21): This phase is so designated because its chief characteristic is an invasion of the layer of now definite lutein cells by blood vessels from the theca. These channels extend to the very lumen, and hemorrhage into the latter is a normal feature of this phase. Characteristically it is of limited amount, the blood forming a zone along the luminal edge of the lutein zone. At times, however, the cavity may be distended with blood. The theca interna has undergone retrogressive changes, its cells having shrunken through disappearance of the rich lipoid content of the earlier phase.

Grossly, the corpus luteum is now a rather large structure of hemorrhagic appearance. It may measure 10 or 12 mm in diameter, and is usually recognizable on the surface of the ovary, where it often forms a slight mound. On section the bright yellow lutein zone is

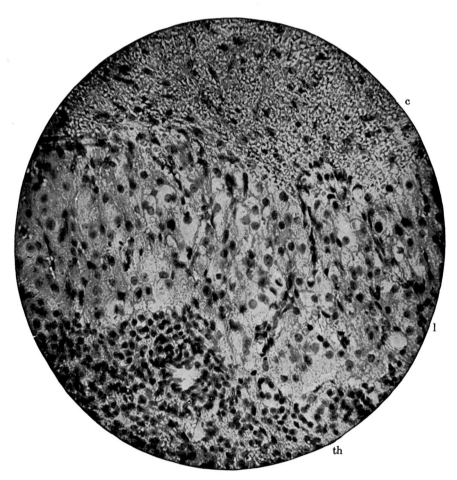

Figure 3.20.   Wall of corpus luteum in stage of early vascularization (16th day). Blood vessels from the theca are pushing into the granulosa layer (*l*) which now shows definite lutein characteristics. The theca cells (*th*) have undergone retrogression. The blood now in the cavity (*c*) is beginning to be invaded by endothelial cells. (From *Novak's Gynecologic and Obstetric Pathology*, Ed. 7, W. B. Saunders, Philadelphia, 1974.)

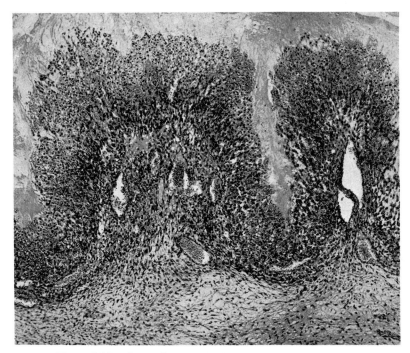

Figure 3.21. Corpus luteum in early stage of vascularization.

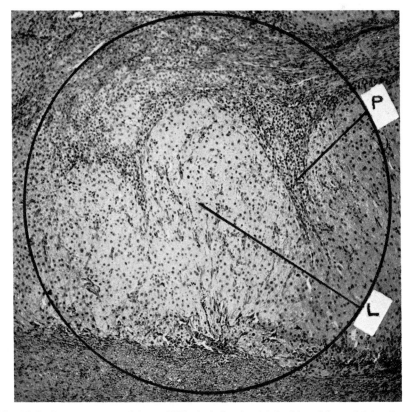

Figure 3.22. Wall of mature corpus luteum (27th day) showing lutein (*L*) and theca-lutein of paralutein (*P*) cells. The latter are not always so well marked.

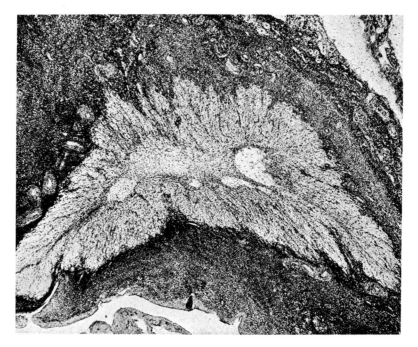

Figure 3.23. Retrogressive corpus luteum.

seen to be fairly wide and moderately festooned, its color contrasting sharply with the blood which is present in the lumen.

3. The stage of *maturity*, which parallels the progestational phase in the endometrium: The broad yellow lutein zone is thrown into festoon-like bunting, the color being due to the presence of the pigment carotene. The theca pushes down into the lutein zone in wedgelike septa which divide the lutein into broad folds and alveoli. The cells of the theca themselves often show luteinization, constituting the theca lutein or paralutein cells (Fig. 3.22), although these are always much smaller than the granulosa lutein cell. Along the inner edge of the lutein zone a layer of fibroblastic tissue appears to shut off the lutein cells from the cavity. The latter contains a varying amount of fluid, including usually unresorbed blood elements from the preceding stage.

The gross appearance of a mature corpus luteum is not always the same, nor is its size, which varies from 10 to 20 mm in diameter. Its yellowish color can often be seen shimmering through the surface of the ovary, above which it may project as a more or less conspicuous mound, at times actually polypoid. In other cases the corpus may seem to lie

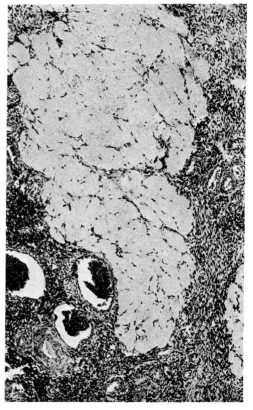

Figure 3.24. Corpus albicans.

beneath the surface, being revealed only by cutting into the ovary. The cavity may be small, with only a scant amount of fluid, or it may be very large and distended with a yellowish liquid.

4. The stage of *retrogression* (Fig. 3.23): The maximal development of the corpus luteum is attained on about the 4th to the 6th day before the appearance of menstrual bleeding. The retrogression of the corpus is marked by fatty degeneration, fibrosis, and later by hyalinization of the lutein zone, with increase of the cicatricial tissue within the cavity. The yellowish color may persist for a long time, even several months, but ultimately it disappears.

The end product is the *corpus albicans* (Fig. 3.24) appearing as a whitish, hyalinized, convoluted structure which slowly decreases in size. Its morphology has been discussed by Joel and Foraker. It is not difficult to "date" the corpus luteum of the present cycle; to ascertain whether it is 2 or 6 months old may be more of a problem.

Corpus Luteum of Pregnancy

In the event of fertilization of the egg, the corpus luteum does not undergo retrogression, but continues to develop, becoming considerably larger than the corpus luteum of menstruation, and comprising sometimes one-third or even one-half of the ovarian volume. The large size is often due to cystic distention, but there is considerable variation in this respect, some corpora lutea of pregnancy being of rather solid structure. The lutein cells are large and tilelike in appearance, and paralutein cells are often conspicuous (Fig. 3.25). The maximum of histological development is reached at about 10–12 weeks.

Csapo and Pulkkinen have reviewed the role of the corpus luteum in human pregnancy and demonstrated that progesterone was indispensable and the corpus luteum likewise as long as it was the major source of progesterone. It can be removed after the placenta is producing adequate progesterone.

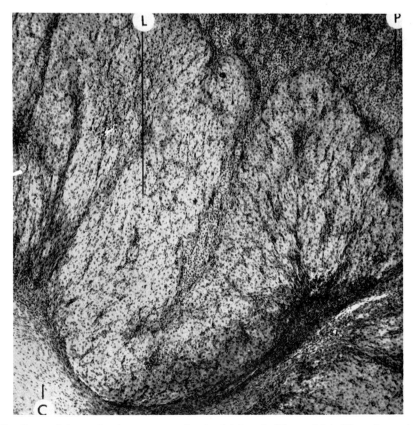

Figure 3.25. Corpus luteum of early pregnancy showing lutein cells (*L*), paralutein (*P*), and organization along inner wall of lutein layer (*C*).

There is some variation in this point from patient to patient.

References and Additional Readings

Baggish, M. S., Pauerstein, C. J., and Woodruff, J. D.: Role of stroma in the regeneration of the endometrial epithelium. Am. J. Obstet. Gynecol., 98: 459, 1967.

Csapo, A. I., and Pulkkinen, M.: Indispensability of the human corpus luteum in the maintenance of early pregnancy; luteectomy evidence. Obstet. Gynecol. Survey, 33: 69, 1978.

Epperson, J. W. W., Hellman, L. M., Galvin, G. A., and Busby, T.: Morphologic changes in cervix during pregnancy, including intraepithelial carcinoma. Am. J. Obstet. Gynecol., 61: 50, 1951.

Fleming, S., Tweedale, D. N., and Roddick, J. W.: Ciliated endometrial cells. Am. J. Obstet. Gynecol., 102: 186, 1968.

Fraenkel, L.: Die Funktion des Corpus luteum. Arch. Gynaekol., 68: 438, 1903.

Garcia, J., Jones, G. S., and Wentz, A. C.: The use of clomiphene citrate. Fertil. Steril., 28: 707, 1977.

Govan, A. D. T.: The human ovary in early pregnancy. J. Endocrinol., 40: 421, 1968.

Graham, J., Graham, R., and Hirabyashi, K.: Reversible "cancer" and the contraceptive pill. Obstet. Gynecol., 31: 190, 1968.

Joel, R. V., and Foraker, A. G.: Fate of the corpus albicans: a morphologic approach. Am. J. Obstet. Gynecol., 80: 314, 1960.

Markee, J. E.: Menstruation in intraocular endometrial transplants in the rhesus monkey. Contrib. Embryol., 28: 219, 1940.

Meyer, R.: Über Corpous Luteumbildung beim Menschen. Zentralbl. Gynaekol., 46: 1206, 1911.

Noyes, R. W., Hertig, A. T., and Rock, J.: Dating the endometrial biopsy. Fertil. Steril., 1: 3, 1950.

Papanicolaou, G. N., Traut, H. F., and Manchetti, A. A.: Epithelia of Woman's Reproductive Organs: A Corrrelative Study of Cyclic Changes. Commonwealth Fund, New York, 1948.

Paschkis, K. E., Rakoff, A. E., Cantarow, A., and Rupp, J. J.: Clinical Endocrinology, Ed. 3, Hoeber Medical Division, Harper & Row, New York, 1967.

Schueler, E. F.: Ciliated epithelium of the human uterine mucosa. Obstet. Gynecol., 31: 215, 1968.

Sjövall, A.: Untersuchungen uver die Schliemhaut der cervix uteri. Acta Obstet. Gynecol. Scand. (Suppl. 4), 18: 4, 1938.

Strassman, E. O.: Theca interna cone and its role in ovulation. Surg. Gynecol. Obstet., 67: 299, 1938.

Topkins, P.: Histologic appearance of endocervix during menstrual cycle. Am. J. Obstet. Gynecol., 58: 654, 1949.

White, A. J., and Buchsbaum, H. J.: Scanning electron microscopy in the human endometrium; I. Normal. Gynecol. Oncol., 1: 330, 1973.

Wied, G. L.: Climacteric amenorrhea; a cytohormonal test for differential diagnosis. Obstet. Gynecol., 9: 646, 1957.

Wienke, E. C., Jr., Cavazos, F., Hall, D. G., and Lucas, F. V.: Ultrastructure of the human endometrial stroma cell during the menstrual cycle. Am. J. Obstet. Gynecol., 102: 65, 1968.

CHAPTER 4

Pubertal Development and Menstruation

NORMAL PUBERTAL DEVELOPMENT

Introduction

Puberty is the term applied to the period of sexual maturation during which the child becomes capable of reproductive function. Dynamic changes occurring in the hypothalamic-pituitary-ovarian axis are mirrored by changes in body habitus and appearance. These outwardly observed manifestations include the growth spurt, development of secondary sexual characteristics, and the occurrence of menstruation. Dynamic emotional, psychological, and behavioral changes also occur during this period and must be taken into consideration in the evaluation of abnormalities of puberty and in the understanding of the total developmental picture.

Since puberty is an ongoing process, it is worthwhile to recapitulate briefly the endocrinology of the fetus, the newborn, and the child, as these hormonal foundations provide the basis for later development and one period merges indistinguishably into the next.

Endocrinology of the Fetus

Development of the Fetal Ovary

Until the 12-mm stage, approximately 42 days of gestation, the embryonic gonads of both males and females are indistinguishable. The absence of a Y chromosome dictates the formation of an ovary; a gene or set of genes on the short arms of the Y chromosome causes the indifferent gonad to develop into a testis.

The primordial germ cells originate in the endoderm of the yolk sac from which they migrate during the 4th and 5th week of gestation through the dorsal mesentery to reach the urogenital ridge, the site of the undifferentiated gonad. Some 300–1300 germ cells reach this area, and increase in number through *mitotic* division. In the embryonic ovary, at 77–84 days, long after differentiation of the testis in the male fetus, ovarian differentiation begins as primordial germ cells divide to form millions of oogonia; this process of germ cell multiplication then ceases before birth. At the 11th and 12th week, some oogonia begin to enter meiotic prophase, characterizing the transition of oogonia into oocytes, which become enveloped by a single layer of flattened granulosa cells to form the first primordial follicles. This development coincides with the appearance of follicle stimulating hormone (FSH) and luteinizing hormone (LH) in the fetal circulation, and is maximal by 20–25 weeks, at which time some of the primordial follicles have developed into primary follicles, and the morphologic features of the ovary can be clearly recognized.

Fetal Hormonal Secretion

FSH and LH have been detected as early as 9 weeks gestational age in human fetuses delivered by hysterotomy. Prior to 12 weeks of fetal age, pituitary, serum and amniotic fluid concentrations of LH and FSH are low or unmeasurable but increase beginning at approximately 12 weeks gestational age. An unequivocal sex difference in fetal serum FSH levels has been consistently observed, with FSH concentrations higher in female than in male fetuses. The finding of relatively high serum FSH levels in the female fetus in the presence of serum estradiol concentrations as high or higher than those in the male and as high as those seen in the maternal circulation, suggests that the fetal pituitary is not suppressed by an estrogen-mediated feedback system. The high FSH levels in female fetuses may play a role in fetal ovarian differentiation, since they coincide with the stage of follicular development (Reyes; Clements et al.).

To determine whether or not fetal pituitary hormones are essential for the normal development of the fetal gonad, hypophysectomy has been performed by Gulyas at various ages in the Rhesus monkey. The Rhesus is an animal model of particular efficiency in the discrimination between fetal, placental, and maternal endocrine secretion. Chorionic gonadotropin is not detectable in serum, urine, or placental extract beyond the 6th week of pregnancy, leaving the fetal and maternal pituitaries as the only apparent potential sources of gonadotropins. Ablation of either the fetal or maternal pituitary permits study of the dependence of fetal gonads on the secretion of the fetal or maternal pituitary. Ablation of the fetal pituitary leads to a marked hypoplasia of the fetal gonads at birth, and the orderly progression of oogenesis is disrupted in the ovary. On the other hand, maternal hypophysectomy performed between 56 and 71 days of gestation has no discernible effects on fetal gonad development. The fetal gonads are therefore dependent upon the secretions of the fetal pituitary during development, especially in mid- and late gestation. Depriving the fetus of its own pituitary secretions leads to striking retardation of normal gonadal growth and differentiation, reducing survival of germ cells at birth.

Fetal ovarian function, however, is not well understood. The steroidogenic potential of the fetal ovary has been investigated only to a limited degree. Estrogen formation by the fetal ovary has been recorded in some species, but significant estrogen synthesis may be prevented by the apparent absence of enzymes capable of removing the side chain of C-21 steroids to form C-19 steroids. Embryonic ovaries from humans and monkeys have been incubated with a variety of potential radioactive precursors, but estrogen synthesis has been difficult to demonstrate. Ovaries of 12–22 week fetuses, cultured in the presence of FSH/LH, human chorionic gonadotropin (hCG), or cyclic-AMP can produce progesterone, estrone, estradiol, androstenedione, testosterone, 17-hydroxypregnenolone, and dehydroepiandrosterone (DHEA) depending entirely on the precursors provided. The fetal ovary is capable of aromatization and spontaneous steroidogenesis, and stimulation can increase both steroid synthesis and release. The ovary, compared to the testis, is less able to synthesize testosterone; Wilson and Jawad suggest that the fetal ovary is deficient in both 17-oxidoreductase and 3β-ol-dehydrogenase activity, although active in aromatization. Therefore, the ovary is steroidogenically capable in utero, but with reduced activity compared to that of fetal testis because of enzyme deficiencies, an absence of precursors, and a deficiency of LH-like gonadotropin binding.

The stage of fetal development at which inhibitory feedback mechanisms of sex-hormones mature is not specifically known. Steroidogenic activity in the fetal testes can be demonstrated from the 6th week of gestation, and testosterone production occurs at the age of 12 weeks. The steroid synthesis of the human fetal ovary is practically negligible, but estrone, estradiol, and estriol are present in the fetal circulation around the 12th–15th week of gestation with increasing levels at the age of 20 weeks. This increase in fetal sex hormones correlates with a fall of both pituitary content and serum concentrations of LH and FSH. This might indicate the development of the sex hormone-hypothalamic-pituitary negative feedback mechanism at this time.

During the remainder of fetal development in utero, the concentration of fetal serum LH and FSH rises to peak levels by midgestation, and then decreases, possibly due to maturation of hypothalamic receptors sensitive to feedback inhibition by extremely high levels of circulating placental estrogens. From the 7th fetal month on, ovarian development continues to be a dynamic process, with maturation of cohorts of primordial follicles, and prominent atresia. Granulosa cells proliferate, the theca differentiates into an internal and external layer, and antral fluid accumulates to form a typical Graafian follicle. Even ovarian cyst formation has been reported in the fetal ovary. The process of atresia results in a decline in the ovarian germ cell population to approximately two million at birth. Following birth, there is a further fall to a few hundred thousand oocytes by the time of the first ovulation at puberty.

In late fetal life, the high estrogen production from the placenta appears to suppress fetal gonadotropin output, suggesting that a negative feedback can occur before birth. At delivery, estradiol levels drop rapidly, resulting in a compensatory increase in FSH and LH output, with FSH levels approaching those observed in the postmenopausal female. These elevated gonadotropin levels in early life can cause follicular development and the output of measurable estradiol. This may cause a small degree of breast development in early infancy, which then regresses by age 2–3 when gonadotropin levels are low and estradiol stimulation is minimal.

Endocrinology of Early Childhood

Following delivery, FSH levels are markedly elevated in the female, and LH levels remain relatively low. Estradiol output peaks at about the 2nd month, suggestive of an insensitivity of the hypothalamic-pituitary centers to negative feedback signals. By 4 years of age, FSH levels have reached a nadir, although some evidence of early response to negative feedback is shown by agonadal patients whose FSH levels are always higher than those in normal children.

During childhood, the period from 4–8 years, gonadotropin levels remain low and ovarian stimulation is minimal, although waves of follicular development in the ovary have been observed. Also, in the prepubertal period, cyclic gonadotropin output with increased estradiol production has been identified in young girls. During childhood, a gradual rise in the secretion of dehydroepiandrosterone (DHEA) and dehydroepiandrosterone sulfate (DHEAS) occurs, presumably by adrenal secretion, but not due to increasing adrenocorticotropic hormone (ACTH) stimulation or to a direct effect of gonadotropins upon the adrenal cortex. The beginnings of maturation of the androgenic zone of the adrenal cortex can be seen by about age 7 in girls, and represents the "adrenarche" phase of pubertal maturation. Other endocrine changes, including an increased LH output during sleep, became more pronounced as puberty approaches.

Gradually, increasing FSH levels are seen and, almost imperceptibly, pubertal development has begun.

Theories of Pubertal Initiation

The onset of puberty is determined by a process of central nervous system (CNS) maturation leading to increased pituitary secretion of FSH and LH, increased ovarian follicular maturation, increased circulating estrogens and androgens, and increased secondary sexual development culminating in the development of an individual capable of reproduction. The specific mechanisms involved in the timing of puberty are not completely understood and are quite complex. Among those aspects to be considered in any discussion of the initiation of pubertal development are the following:

1. Critical weight and body mass relationships
2. A change in the setting of the "gonadostat," involving decreased sensitivity to sex steroids, and a decreased negative feedback of estradiol on pituitary function
3. Onset of adrenal activity as the trigger of puberty, as reflected by increased DHEA and DHEAS
4. The possible involvement of prolactin
5. Mechanisms involving hormonal changes during sleep
6. Pineal input to maturation processes, due either to output of melatonin or to storage of LH-RH
7. Physical maturation of the central nervous system, as reflected by increased arborization of CNS neurons, resulting in increased neurotransmitter output, increasing LH-RH stimulation particularly during sleep, resulting in pulsatile sleep-associated LH secretion, and increased activation of the hypothalamic-pituitary-gonadal axis.

Although other factors probably are involved in initiating puberty, for example genetic determinants, these factors appear to be the most important.

Critical Weight and Body Mass Relationships

In 1970, Frisch and Revelle proposed that menarche in normal Caucasian girls in the United States is closely correlated with the attainment of a critical body weight, specifically 47.8 ± 0.5 kg. This hypothesis promoted considerable criticism and controversy, and was revised in 1974, when the percentage of body fat was thought to be of greater importance than the critical weight. The minimal weight for height at menarche is indicated by the 10th percentile of fractional body water at menarche, 59.8%, which is equivalent to about 17% fat of body weight. Between the age of menarche and 18 years, some 4.5 kg of fat are gained: at age 16, mean fat is 15.7 kg or 27% of body weight and, at age 18, mean fat is 16.0 kg or 28% of the mean body weight of 57.1 kg. Reflecting this increase in fatness, the total water/body weight percentage decreases from 55.1% at menarche, to 52.1% at age 18 years.

Frisch and McArthur postulated that mean body fatness is important in both the establishment and the continuation of normal reproductive function. The sequence of events would be: altered body composition and weight, altered metabolic rate, and diminished hypothalamic sensitivity followed by an increase in gonadotropin secretion and estrogen production leading to pubertal development and menarche.

In contrast, Crawford and Osler concluded that menarche is not necessarily triggered by achievement of a critical body weight: girls with tall stature significantly exceeded the "critical" weight of 47.8 kg before achieving menarche but had onset of menses in accordance with the body composition hypothesis;

hypothyroid girls without adolescent development had a body composition similar to age-matched controls; obese girls under age 8 years had an even greater percentage of body fat than normal menarcheal girls, but showed no signs of puberty; patients with gonadal dysgenesis, whose gonadotropins are moderately elevated from infancy to the end of the first decade, had a further increase at approximately the same time that their normal counterparts were entering puberty, obviously in the absence of any estrogen exposure. Crawford and Osler reported that neither the fall in fractional body water nor the accumulation of fat are direct determinants of the adolescent gonadotropin rise; they suggested that pituitary gonadotropins may play a role in determining body composition at menarche, rather than vice versa.

If fatness is important in initiating puberty, then obesity and early menarche should be correlated. Estrogen is metabolized mainly by 16α-hydroxylation to estriol and by 2-hydroxylation leading to the synthesis of 2-hydroxyestrone and 2-hydroxyestradiol, the catechol estrogens (Fig. 4.1). Fishman and colleagues have indicated that patients with anorexia nervosa and with obesity metabolize estrogens differently. Obese patients have an increased production of biologically active

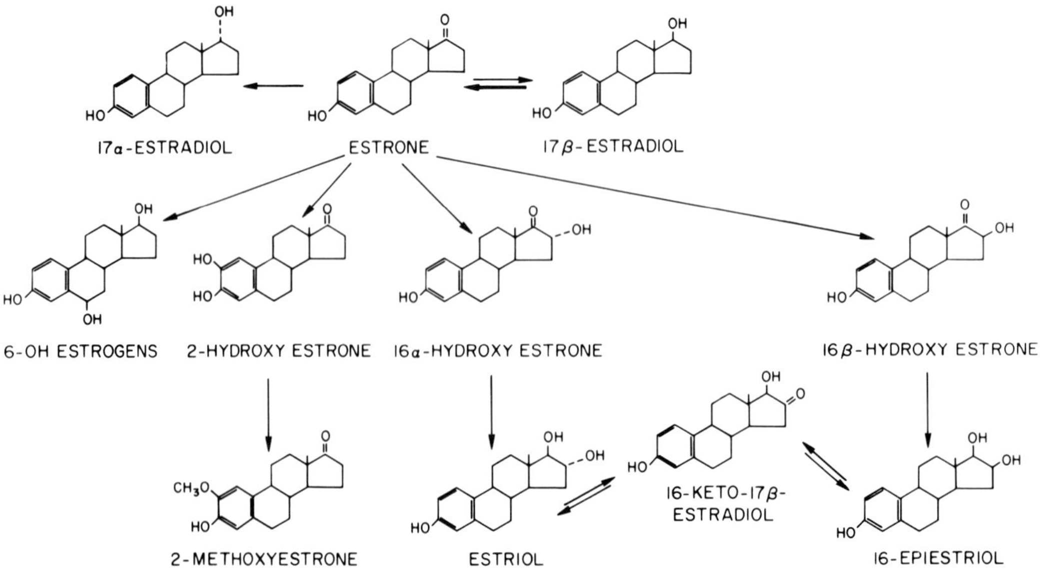

Figure 4.1 Metabolism of estrogen occurs predominantly via 16α-hydroxylation leading to estriol, or through 2-hydroxylation with formation of the catecholestrogens. Obese patients tend to metabolize estrogen via the 16α- and 6-hydroxylation pathways; patients with anorexia nervosa have an increased catecholestrogen metabolism.

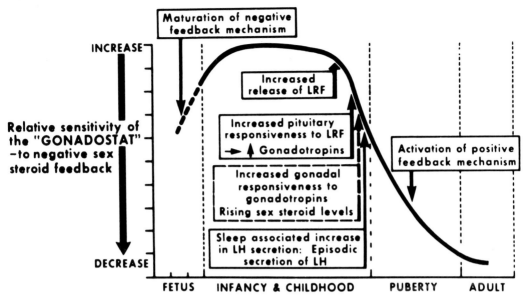

Figure 4.2   The change in set point of the hypothalamic "gonadostat" (denoted by the *dashed* and *solid* lines) and the maturation of the negative and positive feedback mechanisms from fetal life to adulthood in relation to the normal changes of puberty. (Reproduced with permission from M. M. Grumbach et al., *Control of the Onset of Puberty*, edited by M. M. Grumbach, G. D. Grave, and F. D. Mayer, Ch. 6, p. 115. John Wiley & Sons, Inc., New York, 1974.)

estrogens, via both 16α- and 6-hydroxylation, and obesity could be associated with an earlier increase in circulating estrogen in early puberty. Also, obesity is a stress, inducing increased adrenal activity in both adults and children, reflected by increased urinary excretion of 17-ketosteroids and 17-hydroxycorticoids, increased cortisol production and secretion rates, and a reduction in the half-life of exogenous tritiated cortisol. However, in obese prepubertal girls, fatness was not associated with early estradiol output: pregnenolone and DHEA levels were as high as in adult women; progesterone, androstenedione and prolactin levels were elevated and cortisol, testosterone, LH, and thyroxine were normal for puberty. Estradiol levels were markedly *depressed* in obese girls, and FSH levels were higher. Maturation of adrenal gland function is therefore enhanced, whereas gonadal secretion of estradiol is impaired in prepubertal obesity (Genazzani and colleagues).

The prolactin (PRL) elevation in the obese individuals suggests a possible association with increased endorphin production. Alternatively, another hormone of pituitary origin other than ACTH and prolactin, which might be responsible for the development and

growth of the cells of the adrenal zona reticularis, has variably been named adrenal androgen-stimulating hormone (AASH) (Grumbach et al.), or cortical androgen-stimulating hormone (CASH) (Parker and Odell). Overproduction of or hypersensitivity to this or these factors could be responsible for the enhanced adrenal function in obese prepubertal girls.

To summarize, body weight and body fat are involved in normal pubertal development and obesity or malnutrition may change the timing of pubertal onset. However, there are other important considerations in determining what initiates puberty.

The "Resetting the Gonadostat" Theory

Over the years, Grumbach, Kaplan, and their numerous associates have developed and refined the concept of the "gonadostat" (Fig. 4.2). The present hypothesis of neuroendocrine regulation of gonadal maturation requires a functionally intact hypothalamic-pituitary-gonadal axis. Release of LH-RH into the portal system results in synthesis and release of pituitary FSH and LH which, in turn, stimulate ovarian follicular development. Output of sex steroids, particularly estradiol, inhibits the release of both hypothalamic and pituitary hormones, so that, by negative feedback, a type of equilibrium is reached. Pubertal development is initiated as the sensitivity of this feedback setting changes with age. Thus, hormonal changes occurring in puberty are but part of a continuum of endocrine changes which start in the fetus and end with mature ovulatory reproductive function.

Crucial to the theory are two points: firstly, the CNS and not the pituitary gland or gonad restrains activation of the hypothalamic-pituitary-ovarian (H-P-O) axis; and secondly, a separate pituitary hormone, AASH, may be secreted to stimulate adrenal activation and puberty.

The inhibitory effect of the CNS appears to be mediated by the hypothalamus via the neurosecretory neurons that synthesize and secrete LH-RH. The hypothalamic-pituitary-gonadotropin unit is not solely influenced by sex steroids and inhibin; other complex neural mechanisms integrate a variety of intrinsic and extrinsic stimuli.

The neural control of puberty includes two major aspects: the *timing* of puberty, which is poorly understood but strongly influenced by genetic factors and inheritance, and modified by a variety of environmental factors; and changes in *feedback sensitivity* which control the transition from prepuberty to complete sexual maturation.

The negative feedback mechanism is at maximal sensitivity at about 4 years of age, when estrogen levels are very low, yet inhibit gonadotropin output effectively. At this time, exogenous administration of very small amounts of estrogen cause a greater-than-expected suppression of FSH and clomiphene citrate, ordinarily an antiestrogen, functions as an estrogen and can also lower gonadotropin levels.

In prepuberty, before secondary sexual development is noted, the sensitivity of the negative feedback mechanism begins to change. The sensitivity of CNS mechanisms to circulating sex steroids decreases, there is less restraint on gonadotropin secretion, and FSH begins to rise. With increasing gonadotropins increasing ovarian stimulation, gonadal steroid secretion rises. Waves of follicular development occur in the juvenile ovary and the increased estradiol levels are reflected in the onset of secondary sexual development. Through puberty, the negative feedback sensitivity continues to decrease until an adult equilibrium is reached. At mid-to-late puberty, the positive feedback effect of estradiol resulting in an LH surge-like output becomes mature and exogenous estrogen administration can induce LH release.

Thus, in theory, the maturation of the H-P-O axis involves decreased negative feedback sensitivity of the CNS to sex steroids leading to increased LH-RH release and increased serum gonadotropin output. With a change in the feedback setting, there is less suppression of FSH and LH output, and more ovarian stimulation. With increased gonadal secretion of estradiol comes increased pituitary sensitivity and ultimately the development of a positive feedback inducing the LH surge. The "resetting of the gonadostat" is not visualized as an abrupt phenomenon; it is a useful integrating concept, but does not address itself to the mechanism of initiation of these events nor to the determining factors.

Onset of Adrenal Activity

The role of the adrenal has been intensely investigated, yet controversy as to its triggering or initiating involvement remains.

DHEA elevations are observed prior to the first signs of puberty, including any increase in FSH levels, suggesting a role for the adrenal androgen DHEA in the maturation of the H-P-O axis (Sizonenko and Paunier; Hopper and Yen). Girls reach a higher DHEA concentration at a similar bone age than boys, possibly because adrenal maturation occurs at an earlier bone age in girls than boys. Gonadotropin concentrations do not have a triggering effect on adrenal maturation, as human luteinizing hormone (hLH) given to patients with gonadal dysgenesis produces no alteration in serum DHEA, DHEAS, estrone, or testosterone (Lee and colleagues); the addition of estrogen also produced no change, leading to the conclusion that gonadotropin and/or estrogen concentrations do not trigger or determine maturation of the adrenal.

DHEAS and DHEA are produced in increasing amounts at the time of puberty, and are probably responsible for the physical changes of adrenarche. However, there has been no conclusive evidence that the increase in DHEAS output is the initiating feature of pubertal development. ACTH stimulation of the adrenal does not increase at puberty and 17α-hydroxyprogesterone and cortisol do not rise at this time. Also, children with chronic adrenal insufficiency have a normal adolescent growth spurt, suggesting that adrenal steroids, although important in the entire picture, probably do not play a role in the initiation of pubertal development.

Prolactin Mechanisms

Animal studies reveal that the adrenal has specific prolactin receptors, that prolactin is capable of stimulating Δ^4 androgen production by an increase in 3β-ol dehydrogenase activity, that prolactin injections advance the time of female sexual maturation in rats, and that prolactin acts synergistically with ACTH in rats to augment adrenal androgen production or effects. In humans, however, some studies have shown no significant change in prolactin levels from years 2 to 12, producing doubt that prolactin could be a primary or permissive stimulus for adrenal steroidogenesis in childhood (Parker et al.). Others have shown a slow progressive increase of prolactin through childhood, correlated with rising estrogen levels. In premature thelarche the mean basal prolactin level and the TRH-stimulated response are not significantly different from those of control individuals, so prolactin is not thought to play a major role in isolated prepubertal breast development (Caufriez and colleagues). Prolactin levels are higher in girls than boys in Stage III of pubertal development; serum estradiol correlates with prolactin, and a prolactin elevation was not documented prior to the onset of significant pubertal development (Thorner et al.). Polleri et al. have definitively shown that prolactin levels are elevated at night throughout prepuberty, childhood, and puberty with no significant increase during early puberty. Thus, prolactin does not seem to be the trigger for pubertal development.

Sleep Mechanisms

A number of polypeptide pituitary hormones are secreted in close relationship to various phases of the sleep-waking cycle, frequently with a distinctive episodic or pulsatile pattern.

Prolactin levels are related to sleep, with concentrations increasing episodically following onset of sleep, becoming progressively higher as sleep proceeds, with the highest concentrations during the early morning hours. TSH has a similar pattern, with a peak at about 3 A.M.

There is, however, a striking sleep-related augmentation of LH during puberty in both males and females, which increases as puberty progresses, and which appears to correlate with the physical (Tanner) stage of development.

Sleep-associated hormone secretory events have been studied in an attempt to gain insight into basic neuroendocrine mechanisms that govern pituitary hormone secretory activity. REM sleep, or desynchronization, results from neural activity in the nucleus locus ceruleus and requires a serotoninergic mechanism for its initiation, and noradrenergic and cholinergic mechanisms for its maintenance. These studies provide a rationale for suggesting that neurotransmitters involved in the synthesis and release of hypothalamic releasing and inhibiting hormones may also be important in the initiation and maintenance of the REM-non-REM sleep cycle.

Prolactin secretion is increased 60–90 minutes after onset of sleep, and achieves maximal levels in the early morning about 5 A.M. Studies using antiserotonin agents suggest that serotonin has a stimulatory effect on prolactin secretion during sleep but, as with growth hormone, the area is still controversial.

Children have an increase in LH output during sleep compared to waking hours, but this is maximized in puberty. An increase in pulsatile LH secretion occurs with sleep onset, with a seeming relationship to the number of sleep cycles. As puberty progresses, the pulsatile activity can be observed through the 24-hour day. In pubertal boys, there is a simultaneous augmentation of testosterone secretion. In females, the sex steroid augmentation is not correlated with sleep, but estradiol levels are increased during the early afternoon after the sleep-associated LH increase. The lag in the rise of plasma estradiol is interesting, and may result from the requirement of two coordinated cellular systems needed in the ovary to synthesize estrogen.

Much needs to be learned about neurotransmitter function during sleep, as stimulation and suppression of reproductive function seems to change both with age as well as sleep-stage.

Receptors Regulating Gonadal Responsiveness

The human ovary contains receptors for estrogen at an early stage. At the ovarian level, FSH stimulates synthesis of its own receptor, an effect that occurs (although less efficiently) without estrogen. This suggests that rising levels of FSH in early puberty can increase FSH receptors resulting in an increase in ovarian responsiveness to FSH. FSH also stimulates the synthesis of LH receptors, a process which is enhanced in the presence of estrogen. Receptors for gonadotropins must exist in intrauterine life, and certainly are present in early childhood when waves of follicular development have been documented. Although the ovary is responsive to variations in gonadotropin output at all stages, the induction of LH receptors by FSH may be a modulating mechanism controlling ovarian function.

The gonad, however, may be unnecessary for the change in negative feedback sensitivity to occur. Winter and Faiman (1972, 1973) postulated that if the low serum gonadotropin levels of childhood are the result of feedback inhibition by gonadal secretions, then absence of the gonad during childhood should be accompanied by elevations of serum FSH and LH to levels similar to those found in castrate adults. Conversely, if the prepubertal gonad is nonfunctional in a negative feedback fashion, then elevations of serum gonadotropins should not be found in agonadal individuals until after the normal age of puberty; such an elevation at this time would imply the operation of some stimulus to gonadotropin secretion or the removal of some inhibiting influence exclusive to the gonad. Serum FSH concentrations in agonadal patients are always elevated above the age-specific normal range, and serum LH levels are usually higher. However, after the normal age of puberty, a further increment in serum gonadotropin concentrations occurs in agonadal subjects, suggesting that the hypothalamic "gonadostat" resets in the absence of a functional gonad. Presumptively then, the stimulus is a central one.

Maturation of the Central Nervous System

The mechanism by which a change in feedback sensitivity might occur at central levels has recently surfaced in work by Ruf, and by Knobil and colleagues, in the Rhesus monkey. Ruf has postulated that the resetting of the hypothalamic "gonadostat" is caused by the growth and functional maturation of steroid-sensitive adrenergic systems. Two anatomically distinct systems may be involved, the tubero-infundibular tract, which originates entirely within the basal hypothalamus and which is predominantly dopaminergic; and another system of noradrenergic neurons whose cell bodies lie outside the basal hypothalamus and whose axons probably travel within the medial forebrain bundle entering the median eminence from a lateral and anterior direction. In adult animals, brain catecholamines promote the discharge of gonadotropin-releasing neurohormones into the hypophysial portal system, while certain indoleamines inhibit the activation of the hypothalamic-pituitary-gonadal axis. In particular, norepinephrine appears to be stimulatory to LH release, whereas dopamine is inhibitory, except in the circumstance of an increased estrogen milieu as in the midcycle, when dopamine may become stimulatory.

Ruf has postulated that growth and functional maturation of steroid-sensitive adrenergic nervous systems results in an increased gonadotropin secretion. To explain the increased hypothalamic drive necessary for the activation of the pituitary-gonadal axis, Ruf suggests a plasticity of the central nervous system, with a continued increase in the physical number of nerve endings throughout childhood and into puberty. This continued arborization results in increased brain catecholamines, promoting the discharge of increased gonadotropin-releasing neurohormone (LH-RH) into the portal system, resulting in increased gonadotropin release. Because the increased physical number of nerve endings are more responsive to circulating sex steroids, a mechanism is developed for positive and negative feedback function. This working hypothesis brings together several separately proposed theories for the initiation of pubertal development.

An interesting observation, reported by Ruf, is that the aminergic fiber system shows a remarkable capacity for regenerative sprouting and growth when injured, or when given access to areas previously innervated by other fiber projections. The resetting of the "gonadostat" during puberty may result from an increase in the terminal arborization of adrenergic neurons, possibly associated with an increase in their number, synapsing directly or indirectly with neurons elaborating gonadotropin-releasing factors. The consequence of this process is an increase in the hypothalamic drive to activate the pituitary-gonadal axis. Thus, the decrease in neuronal steroid-sensitivity is only apparent and, due to the fact that a rise in gonadal steroid output is compensated for by an increase in the respective distribution volume in the body. Therefore, steroid concentrations at neuronal receptor sites do not necessarily rise with gonadal output and may even decrease. In any case, this theory can explain why pubertal development is slow but progressive, why gonadotropin-releasing factors are present in the hypothalamus long before adult reproductive function is established, and why the prepubertal pituitary readily discharges gonadotropins in response to releasing hormone stimulation. It allows an explanation for the growth spurt accompanying puberty, since the release of growth hormones is likewise under adrenergic control. It provides an explanation for the synchronization of LH release with sleep, in which catecholamines play a regulatory role. Additionally, since increased arborization is stimulated by injury, it provides an explanation for precocious puberty caused by brain lesions, tumors, and other pathology.

Fitting with this hypothesis is the work of Knobil, done primarily in the Rhesus monkey. Searching for the site and mechanism of the negative and positive feedback control, Knobil began to explore the pulsatile LH output. Knobil observed in the Rhesus (as have Ehara, Yen, and Siler; Boyar et al.; and others, in the human) that the secretion of LH in the adult is always pulsatile or episodic, occurring about every 2 hours. Measurable gonadotropin output patterns reflect the stage of pubertal development, and an increase in LH synchronized with sleep is one of the earlier signs of developing puberty. Presumptively, FSH is also released in a pulsatile manner, but its half-life is longer than that of LH, which prevents the detection of the pulsatile episodic release pattern. The tonic or basal pituitary secretion of gonadotropins is dependent upon the frequency and amplitude of the pulsatile output. Estrogen (E_2) induces an increase in pituitary response of LH to LH-RH stimulation, so that rising E_2 levels induce a higher pulsatile amplitude of LH secretion; this evolves into an LH-surge-like output, the positive feedback. The tonic or basal secretion of FSH is regulated mainly by negative or inhibitory feedback influences exerted by estradiol and also by inhibin, a protein component probably synthesized by the granulosa cell. The cyclic secretion of LH is induced by positive feedback in which an increment in circulating estradiol, reaching a critical level for a particular duration, will cause a surge-like output of LH. A synchronous release of FSH occurs, and the FSH surge-like output may share a role with LH in inducing the physical act of ovulation.

During these investigations, Knobil found that radiofrequency or chemical lesions, or knife-cut isolation experiments leaving islands of intact hypothalamus, or even aspiration of virtually the entire brain, did not destroy positive and negative feedback control of LH output as long as hypothalamic-pituitary connections, a source of rising estrogens and the *arcuate* nucleus in the mediobasal hypothalamus were present. Knobil showed that an LH surge from the pituitary could be induced by estrogen if the arcuate nucleus were destroyed as long as LH-RH was administered in pulsatile hourly fashion to the animal. Thus, the arcuate nucleus plays a permissive role and serves as an LH-RH pump; but estrogen levels at the pituitary determine LH and FSH output.

Importantly, Knobil studied prepubertal Rhesus monkeys in the same way. An immature animal, when given intermittent hourly pulsatile LH-RH injections, shortly develops both a positive feedback to its own endogenous ovarian estrogen output, as well as an LH surge; ovulation occurs in these monkeys. When the pulsatile LH-RH stimulation is stopped, the animals revert to immaturity. Thus, the immature or prepubertal monkey is like an arcuate-lesioned adult. All that is needed to induce maturity is the pulsatile, episodic LH-RH output, signals for which appear to originate in the arcuate nucleus. Ruf has provided some evidence for the mechanism, possibly increased numbers of synapses due to increased arborization. In summary, a triggering event initiating puberty is not needed; pubertal H-P-O maturation appears to be an on-going multisystem event.

Physical Changes in Puberty

Physical changes in puberty include the development of breasts and pubic hair growth, and the adolescent growth spurt. Less obvious is the stimulation occurring in the target organs of the sex steroids; the vaginal mucosa becomes thickened and rugated, the uterine fundus enlarges more so than the cervix, the cervical glands are stimulated to produce a copious mucus, secretory glands of the vagina become active, and the labia minora and majora enlarge. Changes in body fat distribution and bodily contour occur. Body odor changes with development of glands of the skin, and acne and comedones may form.

The Tanner classification (Table 4.1) describes the stages of pubertal development. It is preferable to consider breast development, (Fig. 4.3), under estrogen influence primarily, separately from pubic hair growth (Fig. 4.4), which is controlled by adrenal androgen output; however, despite the different influencing hormones, there is only slight variation and development is remarkably parallel.

The first physical sign of puberty is ordinarily breast budding, which usually precedes pubic hair growth, which occurs earlier than axillary hair growth. The adolescent growth spurt, observed in retrospect, can be divided into three stages, the minimum growth velocity, peak height velocity (PHV), and the stage of decreased velocity with cessation of growth at epiphyseal fusion. PHV occurs about a year after the onset of breast development,

and about a year and a half before menarche. Girls grow approximately 25 cm between growth take-off and cessation, and reach PHV before menarche so that there is limited growth potential in a postmenarcheal girl. Age at menarche and PHV are not good

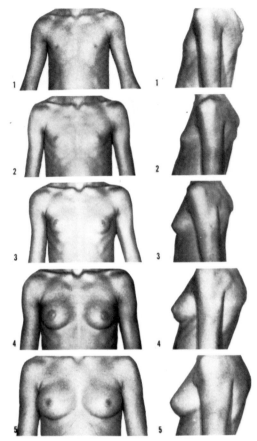

Figure 4.3 Standards for evaluating breast development. (Reproduced with permission from J. M. Tanner, *Growth at Adolescence*, p. 152. Blackwell Scientific Publishing Co., Oxford, 1962.)

Table 4.1
Tanner Classification[a] of Pubertal Development

Stage	Pubic Hair	Breasts
1	None	Elevation of the papilla only
2	Sparse growth, labia majora only	Breast budding and areolar enlargement with mound-like elevation of breast and papilla
3	Coarse curled hair sparsely over mons	Continued enlargement of breast and areola without separation of contours
4	Adult in character but not in distribution	Areola and papilla project above breast contour
5	Adult hair spread to medial aspects of thighs	Adult, with areola recessed to contour of the breasts

[a] The classification does not consider breast size and inherent shape, which are determined by genetic and nutritional factors.

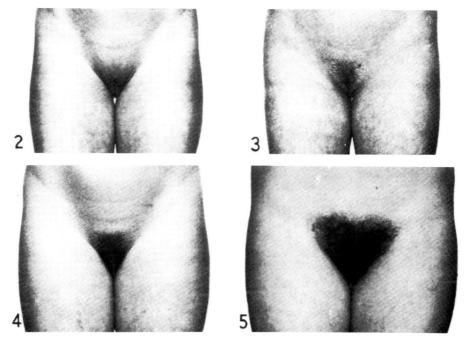

Figure 4.4 Standards for evaluating pubic hair growth. (Reproduced with permission from J. M. Tanner, *Growth at Adolescence*, p. 152. Blackwell Scientific Publishing Co., Oxford, 1962.)

predictors of adult height, nor does the age of PHV or the age of initiation of pubertal signs correlate well with duration of pubertal development. Accumulation of body fat continues until, at age 16, girls have twice as much fat as boys. There is an increase in fatness between menarche, and Tanner Stage V complete physical maturation.

Importantly, some variation does occur in the pattern of pubertal development. One fifth of girls have pubic hair as the earliest secondary sexual characteristic, and PHV occurs before the development of pubic hair in some 25% of girls. In another 25%, the initial stages of breast development occur first. Menarche ordinarily occurs within 2½ years of the onset of breast budding.

Bone age is an index of physiologic maturation and closely correlates with menarche; bone age is far more useful than chronological age in determining the onset of secondary sexual development and in evaluating possible delayed puberty.

Hormonal Changes at Puberty

Gonadotropins FSH and LH

During childhood, the rise in FSH precedes that in LH, when these hormones are measured over time. In the patient with ovarian failure or gonadal dysgenesis, an elevated FSH can be observed as early as age 6. Ordinarily, the beginning increase of FSH is observed in the normally developing female at about age 8.

One of the first definite signs of impending puberty is an increased LH output associated with REM sleep, a time of norepinephrine output. The pattern of LH secretion is episodic and pulsatile, with hourly increases; as puberty advances, the amplitude increases.

In late puberty, the adult pattern gradually begins to appear. This does not have a sleep-associated LH increase, but has an episodic pulsatile LH output that occurs throughout the 24-hour day, which is modulated by the sex steroid milieu.

Estrogens

Estradiol, the major estrogen secreted by the follicle, rises steadily through puberty, reaching adult levels at about the time of Tanner Stage IV, when menarche ordinarily occurs. Waves of follicular development have been documented to occur throughout puberty; even before the first period, cyclic gonadotropin output associated with increasing, and then waning, estradiol levels have been documented.

When correlated with the sleep-associated

LH increase, estradiol is not elevated; consistently, the estradiol increase is seen early the next afternoon and is maximal at about 2 P.M.

Androgens

Androgens, particularly testosterone and androstenedione output, are not as important in females as in males. However, testosterone increases gradually throughout puberty. In males, a testosterone elevation is closely correlated with the sleep-associated LH increase.

Progesterone

Progesterone levels are ordinarily very low in the pubertal female. The first menstrual period is usually anovulatory, and progesterone is not increased following an LH surge which may be observed in middle to late puberty. A low progesterone output reflects inadequate corpus luteum development in the year after the first period but, with time, normal progesterone output and duration of the luteal phase is achieved.

Adrenal Androgens

Plasma DHEAS and DHEA begin to increase in girls by approximately 8 years of age, and continue to increase until about age 13–15. DHEA has a diurnal rhythm similar to that of cortisol, but DHEAS does not. It is unclear whether this increase in adrenal androgens is associated with the initiation of pubertal development, but certainly adrenarche, growth of pubic and axillary hair, is a result of adrenal androgen output.

Prolactin

Prolactin has not been shown to be responsible for the initiation of pubertal development. Ordinarily, circulating prolactin levels are correlated with levels of estradiol, and prolactin, therefore, gradually increases throughout puberty. At all ages, prolactin is increased during sleep.

Behavioral Development at Puberty

The somatic changes in sexual maturation are accompanied by the important process of psychic maturation. Menarche provides a landmark in physical female development, but adolescent psychology is characterized by contradictions in actions and words.

In dealing with pubertal and adolescent patients in the office, the adolescent should initially be seen alone, without the presence of parents. The basis of confidentiality should be stated early and adhered to, and a relaxed, open, flexible, and unhurried approach is essential. The adolescent should be spoken with on her own level, not as to a younger child. It is helpful to observe the parent-adolescent relationship, which is easily done at the end of the interview, when the patient may be asked if she wishes to have certain facts explained to her parents in her presence. The questions of the adolescent should be answered honestly, simply, and completely, with factual information provided. The adolescent's point of view should be respected, and explanation provided for any disagreement.

DELAYED PUBERTAL DEVELOPMENT

Introduction and Definitions

Delayed puberty, a common cause of primary amenorrhea, is primarily a diagnosis of exclusion. Primary amenorrhea, discussed in "Amenorrhea," Chapter 30, is ordinarily defined as failure of menarche by age 16. However, menarche is the culmination of pubertal maturation, which includes development of the breasts, growth of axillary and pubic hair, and the appearance of an estrogenic vaginal smear, and of accelerated linear skeletal growth. It is more important to think in terms of maturational delay and abnormality than whether or not menstruation has begun. Yet, the complaint of "no periods" is more commonly heard than worry over delayed secondary development.

It is useful to establish criteria for deciding which children deserve evaluation. Puberty is considered delayed in girls if secondary sexual development has not occurred by the age 14; menarche is considered delayed if bleeding has not occurred by the age 16. Additionally, if height and/or weight are significantly retarded for age, or if two years have elapsed from the onset of breast growth (thelarche) without the occurrence of menses, then evaluation of the child is indicated. Finally, if the child or her parents are unduly concerned about her lack of development at an even younger age, then potentially some investigation should be undertaken.

The differential diagnosis of delayed puberty is shown in Table 4.2. The goals of the evaluation of an individual with delayed pu-

Table 4.2
Etiologic Classification of Delayed Puberty

I. Lesions of central origin
  A. Functional and organic brain disease
    1. Traumatic, toxic, and infectious lesions
      a. Encephalitis, epilepsy, hypothalamic tumors
    2. Neuroendocrinologic dysfunction
      a. Neurotransmitter excess or deficiency
      b. Releasing hormone
      c. Feedback defects
    3. Ahumada-del-Castillo syndrome
    4. Isolated releasing hormone deficiencies
      a. Hypothalamic hypogonadism
    5. Kallmann's syndrome—hypogonadotropic hypogonadism with anosmia
  B. Psychogenic amenorrhea
    1. Major and minor psychosis, emotional shock
    2. Anorexia nervosa
  C. Pituitary disturbances
    1. Tumors
      a. Nonfunctioning
      b. Functioning: prolactin, hCG, ACTH, TSH
    2. Congenital defects
      a. Isolated gonadotropin deficiency (pituitary hypogonadism)
    3. Empty sella syndrome
II. Lesions of intermediate origin
  A. Chronic illness
    1. Rheumatic fever, tuberculosis, childhood leukemia
  B. Metabolic diseases
    1. Thyroid
    2. Diabetes mellitus (juvenile)
    3. Adrenal
      a. Congenital adrenal hyperplasia
      b. Cushing's syndrome
      c. Virilizing tumor
  C. Nutritional disturbances
    1. Malnutrition
    2. Exogenous obesity
III. Lesions of peripheral origin
  A. Ovarian causes of delayed puberty
    1. Congenital developmental defects
      a. Ovarian dysgenesis
      b. True hermaphroditism
      c. Virlizing or feminizing male hermaphroditism
    2. Tumors
      a. Virilizing and feminizing tumors
    3. Insensitive ovary syndrome (Savage syndrome)
  B. Vaginal and uterine defects
    1. Congenital defects
      a. Imperforate hymen, transverse vaginal septum
      b. Congenital absence of the vagina and uterus
      c. Congenital malformation of the uterus
    2. Traumatic and infectious lesions
      a. Stenosis of vagina or cervix
      b. Asherman's disease—endometrial sclerosis
IV. Physiologic amenorrhea—pregnancy

berty are to distinguish those patients who will undergo spontaneous puberty from those who have disorders that lead to sexual infantilism and require treatment.

Evaluation

A careful history includes details of the general physical health, analysis of previous records of height and weight, and a history of the timing of the onset of puberty in other family members. One needs to know of any chronic or intermittent illnesses, accidents and injuries, and all details pertaining to growth and development. Disorders of pregnancy, abnormalities of labor and development, or birth trauma might suggest a congenital or neonatal event related to the delay in puberty. Neonatal and childhood linear growth and nutrition status are important as these may reflect long-standing abnormalities of development. Growth charts should be reviewed. A history of consanguinity is important in the detection of chromosomal recessive disorders.

The family history may reveal a delayed onset of menarche in family members. Isolated gonadotropin deficiency may occur in families, and Kallmann's syndrome, characterized by anosmia or hyposmia due to agenesis or hypoplasia of the olfactory bulbs, is associated with LH-RH deficiency and delayed puberty. Autosomal dominant, autosomal recessive, and X-linked inheritance have all been suspected.

The physical examination must include body measurements, precise staging of any secondary sexual changes, and a careful neurologic examination including vision fields, funduscopy, and assessment of sense of smell. Signs suggesting hypothyroidism, gonadal dysgenesis, hypopituitarism, or chronic illness, should be noted. When puberty begins normally but menses are delayed, the possibility exists of an abnormality of the vagina, including vaginal atresia or aplasia, Mullerian agenesis, or imperforate hymen. The uterus is likely to be absent if the vagina is absent. In complete testicular feminization the amenorrheic, androgen-resistant patient shows feminine external genitalia and habitus, normal breast development, sparse pubic and axillary hair, no uterus, bilateral inguinal or abdominal testes, and a 46XY karyotype.

The laboratory evaluation of the patient with pubertal delay involves the determination of karyotype, circulating gonadotropin levels, and bone age. Under certain circumstances, a skull film or x-ray of the sella turcica is needed to rule out an intracranial process, but the necessity for other tests and studies depends upon what has been suggested from history and physical examination. A buccal smear is of limited value because of its inability to differentiate most mosaic patterns.

Further evaluation might involve the use of an LH-RH stimulation to assess the response of the pituitary to provocative testing. During pubertal development, FSH first increases, and an increase in the FSH response to LH-RH is observed in early puberty. As pubertal development progresses, baseline LH rises and later the peak response following LH-RH stimulation also increases (Fig. 4.5). The LH-RH induced gonadotropin output is correlated to some extent with the degree of secondary sexual development, and is only of limited value in establishing a diagnosis and prognosis in pubertal delay.

Clomiphene citrate, an antiestrogen with weak estrogenic properties, decreases gonadotropin levels in prepubertal patients, but increases gonadotropin output in later pubertal individuals and in adults. The response to clomiphene correlates with the degree of secondary sexual development, and thus, the administration of clomiphene alone is of limited usefulness.

Estrogen provocation testing is also of interest, but of limited help in assessing which individual will continue to progress in puberty. It is not always possible to differentiate the late bloomer from the individual with a congenital deficiency, causing hypogonadotropic hypogonadism (HH). Patients with delayed puberty are usually shorter than their peers, although growth spurt and height velocity are usually appropriate for bone age. A positive family history for delayed menarche is often obtained and, in general, these individuals seem to be consistently slow in achieving developmental landmarks and are physically less mature throughout childhood. Bone age has a much better correlation with the onset of and progression through puberty than chronologic age. The earliest signs of sexual maturation begin at a bone age between 11 and 13 for girls.

It is important to distinguish between delayed and arrested patterns of growth. In both, the bone age is retarded, but the distinguishing feature is growth velocity. If the growth rate of a short girl with retarded bone age is normal, somewhere between 1.5 and 2 inches/year, then the patient probably has a delayed growth pattern. If the growth rate is less than 1 inch/year, the patient has an arrested growth pattern and almost certainly

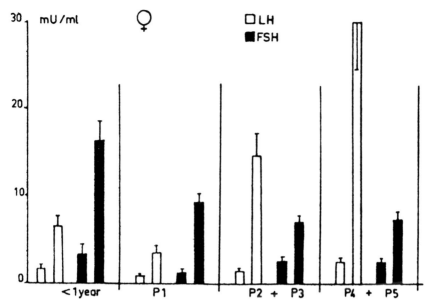

Figure 4.5   LH-RH test (0.1 mg/m²) in normal girls with different developmental stages. Mean ± SEM basal and peak levels of luteinizing hormone (*LH*) and follicle stimulating hormone (*FSH*). The possible utility of the LH-RH stimulation test is illustrated as the expected response can be compared to that observed, with an assessment of the normality of pubertal maturation. (Reproduced with permission from Job et al., *Hormone Research, 8:* 171, 1977.)

something is wrong. Differential diagnosis of an arrested growth pattern includes the lack of growth hormone, thyroid hormone and/or sex hormones, excess glucocorticoids, certain disorders such as rickets and uremia, and systemic disease. Regional enteritis may be completely silent, suggested only by an arrested growth pattern, although a low albumin and high sedimentation rate can be measured.

In cases where the distinction between delayed puberty and hypothalamic hypogonadism is unclear, a period of watchful waiting for approximately 6 months is in order before therapy is instituted. Patients with delayed puberty will show, in 6 months, some progression of secondary sexual development, or an increase in baseline gonadotropins, or a change in the gonadotropin response to LH-RH administration.

PRECOCIOUS PUBERTAL DEVELOPMENT

Definition

Precocious puberty is defined as a premature initiation of either sexual development and/or menstrual bleeding before the age of 8 years in the female. Such development can occur at any time after birth.

Classification

Precocious puberty is divided into two major categories:

1. True, complete precocious puberty, indicative of premature maturation of the hypothalamic-pituitary-ovarian axis resulting in total ovarian function with ovulation
2. Incomplete pseudoprecocious puberty, in which either gonadotropin output or sex steroid secretion occurs with stimulation of secondary sexual characteristics only, without evidence of ovulation

True, complete precocious puberty, the most common form of sexual precocity, is defined as the premature initiation of the normal physiologic and endocrinologic processes of puberty before the age of 8 years. Premature activation of the hypothalamic-pituitary-ovarian mechanism occurs without a demonstrable organic lesion of the central nervous system, and in the absence of gonadotropin secreting tumors, and adrenal or gonadal disorders. Children with complete precocity are able to conceive and suitable precautions must be taken.

Incomplete isosexual pseudoprecocious puberty is development appropriate to the sex in the presence of any of several lesions. Oocyte maturation does not occur, and development of secondary sexual characteristics may be isolated; premature thelarche, breast development, may occur in the absence of pubarche, pubic hair development, or vice versa.

Heterosexual precocious puberty is the development of pubertal maturational changes inappropriate for the sex of the individual. Virilization in the female or feminization in the male may occur when enzyme disorders or tumors allow production of sex hormones inappropriate to gender.

Precocious puberty is associated with accelerated growth; accelerated osseous maturation also occurs resulting in ultimate short stature, although the sexually precocious individual may be the tallest and largest of his or her peer group. Some 50% of sexually precocious girls do not attain an adult height of 5 feet. Interruption and treatment at an early age allows these individuals to gain more adult height. Prior to epiphyseal closure, such children are always larger than their peers, but the intellectual and psycho-sexual development is appropriate for their chronologic age.

The differential diagnosis of precocious puberty is shown in Table 4.3. The sex distribution among the various subdivisions is interesting: precocious puberty of the idiopathic type is three to four times more common in girls; precocious puberty due to neurogenic causes is almost evenly divided between the sexes; pineal tumors and ectopic hCG-producing hamartomas are far more common in males. In contrast, McCune-Albright syndrome is virtually limited to females, but the cause of sexual precocity is unexplained. This syndrome, characterized by areas of increased skin pigmentation, a sclerotic overgrowth of the base of the skull, and disseminated areas of osseous rarefaction has no reported genetic component. The sequence of pubertal change is frequently deranged, and vaginal bleeding may precede other signs of maturation by several years. The precocious development may occur as a result of pressure on the hypothalamus due to sclerosis of the base of the skull; the endocrine manifestations, including hypothyroidism, may represent a widespread failure of catecholamine neuroendocrine control, with inappropriate secretion of one or more of the releasing factors.

The sexual precocity that occasionally ac-

Table 4.3
Differential Diagnosis of Precocious Puberty

   I. Complete, true precocious puberty
     A. Idiopathic or constitutional
     B. Neurogenic, cerebral lesions
        1. Tumors of hypothalamus, pineal, or cortex: hamartoma, craniopharyngioma, glioma
        2. Infections: toxoplasmosis, encephalitis, meningitis
        3. Neurocutaneous syndromes: neurofibromatosis
        4. Developmental defects: tuberous sclerosis, microcephaly, aqueduct stenosis, craniostenosis
        5. Trauma
        6. Miscellaneous: Sturge-Weber syndrome, diffuse encephalopathy, idiopathic epilepsy
     C. McCune-Albright syndrome
     D. Juvenile primary hypothyroidism
     E. Silver syndrome (cranial facial disproportion, small stature, retarded bone age, increased gonadotropin levels)
  II. Incomplete or pseudoprecocious puberty
     A. Premature pubarche
     B. Premature thelarche
     C. Adrenal lesions: congenital adrenal hyperplasia, Cushing's syndrome, tumors
     D. Ovarian tumors: estrogen-producing (granulosa-theca cell, luteoma)
     E. Iatrogenic: androgen or estrogen administration, geriatric vitamins, oral contraceptives
 III. Extrapituitary gonadotropin production
     A. Gonadotropin-secreting tumors (choriocarcinoma, teratoma, hepatoblastoma, dysgerminoma)
     B. Exogenous gonadotropin administration

---

companies hypothyroidism in the prepubertal child has been called the "hormonal overlap syndrome." In this syndrome, there is dissociation of the pubertal changes, with breast development and a milky galactorrhea, but with delayed and scanty sexual hair growth. Hypothyroidism associated with precocious puberty and lactation is rare. The etiology of this syndrome depends upon the cross-reactivity of LH with TSH and the response of prolactin to the stimulation of TRH. These children have severe hypothyroidism, no negative feedback from T_3 and T_4 at the pituitary level and, therefore, a marked elevation of pituitary TSH and hypothalamic TRH. The excessive TSH gives an LH-like biologic effect stimulating ovarian estrogen secretion. The estrogen, however, is unable to turn off TSH; therefore, precocious puberty and occasionally dysfunctional anovulatory uterine bleeding ensue. The TRH stimulates excessive prolactin production and galactorrhea. The treatment of this condition is obviously thyroid replacement.

Since 90% of the cases fall in the idiopathic category, it follows that precocious puberty in general is frequently seen in females. A constant concern is that a small neoplastic lesion of the hypothalamus, or a scar in the connecting tracts may be the real etiologic factor. The theory of Ruf as to the initiating factor of puberty suggests that the inherent plasticity of the adrenergic nervous system allows injury or trauma to cause excessive sprouting of nerve endings. This arborization then results in increased catecholamine neurotransmittor function, resulting in increased stimulation to the pituitary and ultimately to premature ovarian function. The initiating factor then may be infectious, traumatic, developmental, or inherited, but the worry of neoplasia is real.

Neoplastic processes can produce virilization, feminization, and precocious sexual development. The pathophysiology of these changes varies with the cell-type and location of the tumor, and the clinical syndromes produced vary with the host, the age and sex, and also with the hormones produced. The primary concern of any physician presented with a patient complaining of altered or accelerated sexual development is whether or not a tumor is involved. An understanding of the ways in which neoplasms cause these changes, coupled with rapidly improving laboratory technology, should make the task relatively simple.

Incomplete precocious puberty does not involve activation of the hypothalamic-pituitary axis, and therefore the development observed may be partial. Breast development or sexual hair growth may occur independently, and again the worry is of a steroid-producing tumor. Granulosa-theca cell tumors are the most common ovarian tumor causing sexual development, but other tumors such as thecomas and rarely teratomas have been seen. Autonomous ovarian cysts, with cessation of sexual precocity following resection, have been reported; Wieland et al. described a follicular cyst in a 4-year-old girl which caused premature vaginal bleeding; its removal rapidly decreased levels of circulating estradiol, caused regression of the breasts, normalized the gonadotropin levels, and halted sexual development. Although usually unnecessary, endocrine assays can be used to differentiate idiopathic precocious puberty from that caused by steroid-producing tumors. With a sensitive radioimmunoassay, it is now possible to demonstrate increased FSH and LH levels compatible with the stage of sexual development, not chronological age, in children with precocious puberty of idiopathic origin. Patients with precocious thelarche may have an elevation of LH only. Patients with tumors have some elevation of the serum estrogen levels and low or undetectable serum FSH and LH levels. However, perhaps the most clinically applicable hormone assay in precocious puberty is the pregnancy test. This should be obtained in every case as it is such a simple assay. If positive, the diagnosis of tumor, probably chorionepithelioma or teratoma, is assured.

Premature Thelarche

Unilateral or bilateral breast development without other signs of sexual maturation (for instance appearance of sexual hair or growth of the labia minora and uterus) is not uncommon in infancy and childhood. It is usually seen before 2 years of age, and may be due to the relative increase in gonadotropin output observed during this time, which can stimulate a responsive ovary to produce estradiol.

Premature thelarche is rarely observed after the age of four; its appearance in the older child may be the first sign of impending (precocious) puberty. Plasma estrogens may be slightly elevated for age, but are usually quite low. Nipple development is ordinarily absent, and the estrogenic dulling of the vaginal mucosa is uncommon. Ordinarily, the breast enlargement regresses after a few months; transient episodes of estrogen secretion, or possibly even estrogen contained in follicular fluid of an ovarian cyst, can be responsible. Premature thelarche is by definition benign, and progressive sexual development and accelerated growth and bone maturation do not occur.

Premature Pubarche or Precocious Adrenarche

Premature pubarche refers to the isolated appearance of pubic hair (and rarely axillary hair) before the age of 8 with no other manifestations of sexual maturation or virilization. It is more common in older but still prepubertal children, although it may occur in infancy. Pubarche is the first sign of adolescent development in 20% of normal girls over age 8; differentiating normal from premature pubarche is difficult. Circulating levels of adrenal androgens are increased for age, but appropriate for the stage of sexual hair growth. Premature adrenarche is a nonprogressive disorder compatible with normal secondary sexual maturation at a later age.

Iatrogenic Sexual Precocity

Prepubertal children are exquisitely sensitive to exogenous sex steroids, and unusual sources of androgens or estrogens may induce a remarkable response. Some sex hormones have been found in vitamin preparations, tonic lotions or cremes, and these used to be a common cause of sexual precocity when these agents were more readily available. However, precocious sexual development due to the ingestion of the mother's oral contraceptives still happens.

Heterosexual Precocious Puberty

Virilization in a girl usually indicates significant organic disease, the most common of which is congenital adrenal hyperplasia due to a 21-hydroxylase or an 11β-hydroxylase deficiency; clitoromegaly, short stature, hirsutism, and acne are manifiested. Rarely, an ovarian or adrenal androgen-producing tumor can cause virilization. Heterosexual precocious puberty in the female requires a diligent search for androgen secretion from a virilizing tumor, or that due to congenital adrenal hyperplasia.

Diagnosis of Sexual Precocity

The first priority in the investigation of a child with precocious sexual development is to identify potential life-threatening disorders: neoplasm of the central nervous system, ovary, or adrenal or ectopic chorionic tissue. Ordinarily, no serious cause of the precocious puberty is discovered. The next priority is to determine if, over time, the pubertal changes are progressive or whether the process is self-limited.

The first step involves taking a detailed history that may reveal symptoms suggesting intercurrent disease, perinatal abnormalities or injuries, previous infections, ingestion of sex steroids, or the presence of similar conditions in family members. Specific information is needed regarding headache or other neurologic symptoms, exposure to medications, and the occurrence of vaginal bleeding. The history of the previous development of the individual is important, including measurements which can be plotted on a growth chart to determine the onset of increase in height velocity, and the degree of correlation between height and weight measurements.

The physical examination should detail the degree and synchrony of the secondary sexual development, and the appearance of acne, facial, and body hair, axillary glandular development, body odor, muscular development, and galactorrhea. Neurologic examination is essential with assessment of visual fields and optic discs. Attention should be paid to note the skin lesions of McCune-Albright syndrome and of neurofibromatosis. Examination should be made for abdominal, gonadal, or adnexal masses, and for coexisting endocrine disease.

Another important examination is that of the internal genitalia to assess the appearance and normality of the uterine cervix; the rectal examination should ascertain uterine size and absence of adnexal or ovarian masses. Vaginal lesions or foreign bodies which could result in external bleeding should be detected. Examination under anesthesia may be necessary in a resistant child, but a great deal of information can be obtained from the simple observation of vaginal mucosa, labia minora, the appearance of vaginal cells in the wet mount, and rectal examination. An important observation is whether estrogenization has occurred.

If a proper diagnostic survey is made, it is seldom necessary to resort to an exploratory laparotomy. Such a survey should include an examination of the vagina with a small cystoscope to exclude a foreign body, especially when vaginal bleeding is the sole manifestation of precocity, ultrasonography, and possibly an examination under anesthesia to eliminate the possibility of an ovarian tumor (however, by the time the precocity is recognized, the tumors are usually of sufficient size to be palpated abdominally). An enlargement of one ovary may represent only a follicle cyst. No operative procedure is indicated if regular ovulatory bleeding occurs even in the presence of such an ovarian enlargement. Documentation of ovulation can be made by basal body temperature chart kept by the mother, and serial vaginal or urinary sediment smears. If an incomplete precocity exists and a tumor is diagnosed, a pregnancy test should be done to diagnose a chorionepithelioma. A careful neurological and ophthalmological examination are important to detect an intracranial lesion. Finally, a thyroid study is indicated if any signs of hypothyroidism are present.

Radiological examination is important both to rule out intracranial disease by a skull film or by tomography or a computed axial tomography (CAT) scan as well as to assess bone age, taken usually from a left-hand film. Sex steroids accelerate osseous maturation. Additionally, intracranial calcification, signs of raised intracranial pressure, or the basal sclerosis characteristic of the McCune-Albright syndrome may be observed. Serial bone-age determinations may be helpful as a guide to the rate of progression of the pubertal process. Pneumoencephalography or carotid arteriography should be carried out only if there is other evidence of central nervous system lesions. A pneumoencephalogram, however, is usually not indicated as a rapidly growing intracranial tumor will usually cause death within 5–7 months, or by the time precocity is established, whereas a hamartoma may be impossible to diagnose even with this diagnostic aid. CAT scans may be useful in the diagnosis of small tumors in, or adjacent to, the hypothalamus.

Further laboratory evaluation includes the assessment of circulating FSH and LH values, testosterone, estradiol, and other measurements as indicated by history and/or physical examination. The measurement of DHEAS and/or DHEA may be valuable or a 17α-hydroxyprogesterone measurement may indicate the presence of congenital adrenal hyperplasia. Thyroid function tests and a prolactin assay may be important to rule out primary hypothyroidism. Ordinarily, in true precocious puberty, those parameters measured agree with the bone age and not the chronologic age of the individual. However, in sexual precocity due to tumor steroid production, gonadotropin levels usually will be depressed by the sex steroid.

Treatment of Precocious Puberty

Diagnosis is the key to management of precocious puberty if a reason explaining the premature development can be found. However, as isosexual idiopathic precocious puberty is most common, usually attempts must be made to suppress the gonadotropin secretion. The treatment of precocious puberty has as its objective two major purposes: (1) suppression of menstruation, ovulation, and fertility; and (2) prevention of excessively short stature.

Treatment with progestational agents, preferably those without androgen or estrogen activity, will successfully accomplish the first objective. The goal of ideal sex steroid treatment includes stopping the progression of puberty, and rapid intervention is indicated if menarche has occurred, or if the child is at risk for significant psychologic trauma. Equally important is the attempted reversion to pubertal growth rates, with deceleration of skeletal maturation, resulting in comparable changes of height and bone age resulting in attainment in the expected adult height. At discontinuation of the ideal sex steroid treatment, normal reproductive and hormonal function should resume, and there must be a lack of significant side effects, specifically due to glucocorticoid or androgenic properties of the agent. Unfortunately, treatment effective in the suppression of menses and secondary sexual development has been successfully developed, but does very little to increase the ultimate height of the child.

Medroxyprogesterone acetate (MPA; Depo-Provera), in doses of 100–200 mg I.M. weekly or biweekly, is the treatment of choice; menses and further breast enlargement will cease but there is no useful effect upon the rate of growth and bone maturation, so patients are likely to be short. The drug has side effects, including suppression of adrenal cortical function, weight gain, possible acceleration of the onset of diabetes mellitus in predisposed individuals and mild blood pressure elevation. MPA does not prevent skeletal maturation but remains the drug of choice.

Cyproterone acetate is an antiandrogenic drug which also inhibits gonadotropin release. Used orally in a dosage of 50–200 mg/meter^2/day, or I.M at a dosage of 100–250/m^2 every 2–4 weeks, it effectively suppresses ovarian function, stops menstruation, and may have a mildly beneficial effect upon ultimate adult height. Side effects include suppression of adrenal cortical function, and low-grade hyperprolactinemia.

Danazol, a 2,3-isoxasol derivative of 17α-ethinyltestosterone, is an impeded androgen with some progestational effects. Although effective in stopping menses and inhibiting further breast development, Danazol does not appear to exert a beneficial effect upon ultimate height and can cause virilization. An advantage is good suppression of gonadotropin secretion, and suppression of steroidogenesis at the level of the gonad. The oral dosage is 150–300 mg/m^2/day, which effectively causes inhibition of sexual development and suppression of sex steroid secretion, but has no beneficial effect on growth rate. With all current forms of therapy, the ultimate adult height in patients with precocious puberty is approximately five feet.

Finally, and importantly, children with precocious puberty have a physical appearance that outstrips their psychosexual and psychosocial maturation. Thus, many have severe psychologic disturbances, are shy and withdrawn, and counseling may be a helpful component of therapy. Although these individuals tend to seek the company of children closer to their size and strength, their social skills are not equivalently advanced, and problems can occur. Advanced school placement should be considered for those with appropriate intellectual development, and sexual education may be of importance.

MENSTRUATION

Introduction

Menstruation may be defined as a bloody, vaginal discharge which is spontaneous, periodic, and has as its source the uterine mucous membrane. Histologic evaluation of endometrial tissue reveals two major patterns, that from endometrium under the stimulation of unopposed estrogen and that from endometrium having a secretory pattern induced by ovarian progesterone. "Bleeding endometrium" is defined as endometrium shed from a proliferative pattern, implying unopposed estrogen activity in the absence of ovulation. "Menstruating endometrium" is diagnosed when a secretory pattern induced by progesterone implies that ovulation has occurred.

The menstrual cycle is judged as normal by the duration, amount, and periodicity of the menstrual flow. Characteristic of normal ovulatory menstruation are certain symptoms including cramping pain with menses, breast tenderness and recurrent cyclic manifestations, which are to be regarded as within normal limits or otherwise, depending upon the ability of the individual to function normally.

Characteristics of Normal Menstruation

Interval and Duration of Bleeding

Although the traditional menstrual interval, counting cycle day 1 as the first day of bleeding, is about 28 days, there are wide variations from this rule both in different women and in the individual. Ross and colleagues found the average cycle length to be 29.1 ± 0.6 days, and an extensive study of some 20,655 cycles in 2,316 women indicated a variation between 24 and 30 days with less than one-sixth of the cycles being the lunar 28 days.

The duration of normal ovulatory menses is usually between 3 and 7 days and, in any one woman, the duration of the flow is usually uniform.

Menstrual cycles are less regular in duration and interval at both extremes of menstrual life. Dewhurst and colleagues documented irregular and increased cycle length most often in postmenarcheal females and next in perimenopausal women. Concern about menstrual irregularities during the first 2 years of menstrual life are ordinarily unnecessary, and irregular periods can be thought of as a usual childhood disease. However, in the perimenopausal era, menstrual irregularities may signal more serious lesions of the endometrium.

Amount of Blood Loss

Hallberg and co-workers, in a study of 476 randomly selected Swedish women, reported a mean value of 33.2 ± 1.6 ml for blood loss during the menstrual period. The younger age women, less than 20 years of age, showed less loss while the 30-year-old group had higher losses: the top normal values varied between 60 and 80 ml. Seventy-eight percent of all menstrual blood loss occurred during the first 2 days and 91% during the first 3 days of menses.

The circulating hemoglobin concentration varies with the measured menstrual blood loss. A decrease in hemoglobin is usually evident when blood loss exceeds 80 ml, but may be seen at 60 ml. Beaton and associates calculated that the average iron intake is 12.4 mg/day and the menstrual iron loss averages 0.4 mg/day. Menstrual loss may not be compensated, and iron depletion may result if the iron intake is below 11 mg/day.

A rough estimate of blood loss can be made from the number of pads soiled or tampons used and from the hematocrit taken immediately before and immediately after the flow. Subjectively, it is difficult to quantitate menstrual blood loss, as women who state that they are "hemorrhaging," may have completely normal blood counts.

Composition of Menstrual Blood

Menstrual discharge is characteristically a dark reddish color like that of venous blood. The offensiveness of the discharge is due not only to decomposition of the blood elements but also to the admixture of the secretions of the vulvar sebaceous glands. When menstrual bleeding is profuse, the discharge is often a brighter red color. The menstrual blood does not coagulate and contains no fibrinogen. It is characteristically dark red, containing red blood cells, endometrial tissue, cervical mucus, cervical and vaginal cells, bacteria and enzymes. Among those identified are alkaline and acid phosphatases, high levels of β-glucuronidase, acid cathepsin-D, plasminogen and fibrinolysins.

Recent work on the exfoliative cytology of menstrual blood has revealed that different types of endometrial cells are shed. These include columnar as well as short fusiform cells, stratified squamous epithelium, histiocytes, endometrial stroma, spindle-shaped mast cells, and epithelial debris as well as cornified and noncornified cells of the navicular type. Cells containing squamous metaplasia are seen, parabasal cells can be isolated, and large clusters of adequately preserved endometrial cells suggest a convenient, noninvasive technique which could be used in conjunction with current methods of endometrial cellular collection (aspiration, lavage or scraping) to detect abnormal endometrial cells.

The fluidity in menstrual blood, and the lack of gross clot formation within the uterus, may be explained by the rapid activation of intrauterine fibrolytic systems, as evidenced by the lack of fibrinogen and the large amounts of fibrinolysis breakdown products in the menstruum. Occasional small clots are passed, and this is thoroughly within normal limits. Intrauterine clotting does occur, but is a limited process in which fibrin formation does not go beyond the monomer stage. Rapid bleeding can cause expulsion of clotted blood from the uterine cavity before liquefaction has occurred. Although the lack of fibrinogen in the menstrual discharge is well documented, clot formation in the vagina is not infrequent. Beller demonstrated that the vaginal clots are not composed of fibrin; they are red cell aggregations to mucoid substances, mucoproteins and/or glycogen, rather than the end product of the coagulation scheme. Clots associated with dysfunctional bleeding and heavy blood loss are also free from fibrin and indistinguishable from normal menstrual clots on both histological and histopathological examination. Fibrin clots, however, do occur following curettage.

Mechanisms Involved in Menstruation

The morphologic sequences of endometrial desquamation and regeneration are still somewhat controversial. The endometrium and its vessels are extremely sensitive to the sex steroids estrogen and progesterone, and under the influence of the former, the Golgi apparatus in the epithelial cells becomes progressively more complex. The numbers of lysosomes and other vesicles containing acid hydrolytic enzymes increase. In the postovulatory phase of the cycle, under the influence of both estrogen and progesterone, these changes are accentuated and become most marked in the late secretory phase. Failure of implantation of the fertilized oocyte results in involution of the corpus luteum and a fall in the sex steroid levels; a series of reactions is initiated which then leads to endometrial desquamation. Firstly, a 30–50% regression of the endometrium above the basalis occurs, which causes the elongated spiral arterioles which have grown to the tip of the surface of the epithelium to coil and to become compressed. Protracted contractions of these spiral arteries associated with the hormone deprivation causes a decreased endometrial blood supply, resulting in hypoxia of the vessels, stasis, and more vasoconstriction. Fragility of the lysosomal membranes increases, allowing a gradual release of the destructive hydrolytic enzymes and accumulation of catabolic materials leading to tissue destruction. The destructive hydrolytic enzymes further digest cellular membranes causing endothelial breakdown of the small arterioles. Depolymerization of the acid mucopolysaccharides and digestion of the endometrium continues, red cells are released from breaks in the capillaries and from defects in the arterioles and venules, and bleeding and sloughing of the tissue through the compact and spongy layers occurs. Plasminogen activators from the lysosomes convert plasminogen into plasmin which digests fibrin, and perhaps fibrinogen, prior to fibrin polymerization. The fibrinolytic system activated by cellular necrosis, together with the lysosomal acid hydrolytic enzymes, cause a consumption of plasma clotting factors, leading to a decreased concentration of Factors II, VII, and X in menstrual blood, an absence of fibrin, and increased fibrinogen degradation products.

The endometrial prostaglandin content which is low during the proliferative phase increases following ovulation. The highest concentrations of the $F_2\alpha$, E_1 and E_2 prostaglandins are found in the menstrual flow. These concentrations should, and apparently do, result in vasoconstriction causing slowing of the blood flow in the venous lacunae of the endometrium and permitting increased aggregation of platelets at the points of vascular rupture. This prevents too rapid blood loss and allows the process of tissue digestion which ensures orderly desquamation of the endometrium. Thus, the platelet plug is reinforced by small amounts of monomer fibrin formed probably both by tissue and blood thromboplastin. Plasmin digests the fibrin clot, thrombin is lysed, blood again flows from the endometrial vessels, the platelet plug is again formed, and the process is repeated.

The resulting fibrinolytic activity contributes to the complete breakdown of fibrinogen and fibrin before blood leaves the uterine cavity. This clotting and fibrinolysis which continue side by side allows the endometrium to be gradually desquamated. If the fibrinolytic activity, which is apparently dependent upon the plasminogen activators and acid hydrolytic enzymes from the lysosomes, is inadequate and fibrin is deposited in the stroma and not completely redigested, abnormal bleeding associated with incomplete endometrial shedding may occur.

Desquamation of the endometrium takes place predominately in the superficial areas of the endometrium, and comprises the compacta and varying amounts of the spongiosa only. Epithelialization is first observed at 36 hours, with regenerating epithelium appearing first from glandular stumps, which become joined in a form of bridge between glands; denuded areas are almost completely covered by regenerating epithelium by 48 hours. By 60 hours, most of the desquamation has taken place and regeneration is almost complete. The amount of desquamation varies as, in some areas, only minimal shedding of the compacta occurs and, in others, shedding progresses irregularly to the muscularis. Desquamation does not necessarily occur in a uniform manner in the uterus, and the depth of necrosis is not related to a specific area of the uterine cavity. Neither are the compacta and spongiosa completely shed, nor is the so-called basalis left bare. Flowers and Wilborn further contributed the documentation that regression rather than cell death is the chief event of menstruation, with the vast majority of the cells of the spongiosa remaining viable and undergoing remodeling to participate in the new cycle. The regression involves autophagocytosis, heterophagocytosis and the release of enzymes from the leaky or damaged cells. These events are set into motion when conception does not occur, and are designed to save as much of the endometrium as possible and to prepare it for another attempt at reproduction. Individually and collectively, all of the processes contribute to the orderly regression and survival of the endometrium.

Menstruation in Hematologic Disorders

Normal mechanisms involved in hemostasis are usually only evoked in response to injury, and require *blood platelets* which maintain normal capillary resistance and *blood coagulation*, the result of a complex enzymatic conversion of fibrinogen to fibrin, requiring the presence of multiple clotting factors. Disturbances of those factors related to fibrin clot formation are usually unassociated with menstrual bleeding problems, while those related to vessel fragility or platelet insufficiency are associated with abnormal uterine bleeding.

Abnormalities of menstrual flow can therefore be predicted in particular situations. For instance, patients anticoagulated with coumadin or heparin may have serious problems with hematuria, epistaxis and bleeding into muscles but usually have normal menses. Patients with congenital afibrinogenemia (I), hypoprothrombinemia (II), or deficiencies of Factors III, IV, VI, VIII, IX, and possibly XII have no problems with menstruation. On the other hand, patients with deficiencies of Factors V, VII (proconvertin) and X, factors concerned with hemostasis rather than coagulation, may have menorrhagia. Patients with Von Willebrand's disease, an hereditary bleeding disorder in which a prolonged bleeding time is the only demonstrable disorder, have severe menorrhagia. Excessive blood loss at menstruation is also seen with all illnesses causing platelet deficiency. Acute leukemia, lupus erythematosus and, infrequently, pernicious anemia may be present with menorrhagia because of associated thrombocytopenic purpura.

References and Additional Readings

Apter, D., and Vihko, R.: Serum pregnenolone, progesterone, 17-hydroxyprogesterone, testosterone and 5α-dehydrotestosterone during female puberty. J. Clin. Endocrinol. Metab. *44:* 1039, 1977.

Beaton, G. H., Thein, M., Milne, H., and Veen, M. J.: Iron requirements of menstruating women. Am. J. Clin. Nutr. *23:* 275, 1970.

Beller, F. K.: Observations on the clotting of menstrual blood and clot formation. Am. J. Obstet. Gynecol. *111:* 535, 1971.

Bidlingmaier, F., Butenandt, O., and Knorr, D.: Plasma gonadotropins and estrogens in girls with idiopathic precocious puberty. Pediatr. Res. *11:* 91, 1977.

Boyar, R. M., Finkelstein, J. W., David, R., Roffwarg, H., Kapen, S., Weitzman, E. D., and Hellman, L.: Twenty-four hour patterns of plasma luteinizing hormone and follicle-stimulating hormone in sexual precocity. N. Engl. J. Med. *289:* 282, 1973.

Boyar, R. M., Wu, R. H. K., Roffwarg, H., Kapen, S., Weitzman, E. D., Hellman, L., and Finkelstein, J. W.: Human puberty: 24-hour estradiol patterns in pubertal girls. J. Clin. Endocrinol. Metab. *43:* 1418, 1976.

Caufriez, A., Wolter, R., Govaerts, M., L'Hermite, M., and Robyn, C.: Gonadotropins and prolactin pituitary reserve in premature thelarche. J. Pediatr. *91:* 751, 1977.

Clements, J. A., Reyes, F. I., Winter, J. S. D., and Faiman, C.: Studies on human sexual development. III. Fetal pituitary and serum, and amniotic fluid concentrations of LH, CG, and FSH. J. Clin. Endocrinol. Metab. *42:* 9, 1976.

Couture, M. L., Freund, M., and Sedlis, A.: The normal exfoliative cytology of menstrual blood. Acta Cytol. *23:* 85, 1979.

Crawford, J. E., and Osler, D. C.: Body composition at menarche: the Frisch-Revelle hypothesis revisited. Pediatr. *56:* 449, 1975.

Davie, R., Hopwood, D., and Levison, D. A.: Intercellular spaces and cell junctions in endometrial glands: their possible role in menstruation. Br. J. Obstet. Gynaecol. *84:* 467, 1977.

Dewhurst, C. J., Cowell, C. A., and Barrie, L. A.: The regularity of early menstrual cycles. J. Obstet. Gynaec. Br. Commonw., *78:* 1093, 1971.

Ducharme, J. R., Catin-Savoie, S., Tache, Y., Bourel, B., and Collu, R.: Sequential hormonal changes and activation of the hypothalamic-pituitary-gonadal axis. J. Steroid Biochem. *11:* 563, 1979.

Ehara, U., Yen, S. S. C., and Siler, T. M.: Serum prolactin levels during puberty. Am. J. Obstet. Gynecol. *121:* 995, 1975.

Fishman, J., Boyar, R. M., and Hellman, L.: Influence of body weight on estradiol metabolism in young women. J. Clin. Endocrinol. Metab. *41:* 989, 1975.

Flowers, C. E., and Wilborn, W. H.: New observations on the physiology of menstruation. Obstet. Gynecol. *51:* 16, 1978.

Frisch, R. E., and McArthur, J. W.: Menstrual cycles: fatness as a determinant of minimum weight for height necessary for their maintenance or onset. Science *185:* 949, 1974.

Frisch, R. E., and Revelle, R.: Height and weight at menarche and a hypothesis of critical body weights and adolescent events. Science *169:* 397, 1970.

Genazzani, A. R., Pintor, C., Facchinetti, F., Carboni, G., Pelosi, U., and Corda, R.: Adrenal and gonadal steroids in girls during sexual maturation. Clin. Endocrinol. *8:* 15, 1978.

Genazzani, A. R., Pintor, C., and Corda, R.: Plasma levels of gonadotropins, prolactin, thyroxine, and adrenal and gonadal steroids in obese prepubertal girls. J. Clin. Endocrinol. Metab. *47:* 974, 1978.

Greenstein, B. D.: The role of hormone receptors in development and puberty. J. Reprod. Fertil. *52:* 419, 1978.

Grumbach, M. M., Roth, J. C., Kaplan, S. L., and Kelch, R. P.: Hypothalamic-pituitary regulation of puberty in man: evidence and concepts derived from clinical research. *In Control of the Onset of Puberty,* M. M. Grumbach, G. D., Grave, and F. D. Mayer, Ch. 6, p. 115. John Wiley & Sons, Inc., New York, 1974.

Gulyas, B. J., Tullner, W. W., and Hodgen, G. D.: Fetal or material hypophysectomy in Rhesus monkeys (*Macaca mulatta*): effects on the development of testes and other endocrine organs. Biol. Reprod. *17:* 650, 1977.

Hallberg, L., Hogdahl, A. M., Nilsson, L., and Rybo, G.: Menstrual blood loss — a population study. Acta Obstet. Gynecol. Scand. *45:* 320, 1966.

Hansen, J. W., Hoffman, H. J., and Ross, G. T.: Monthly gonadotropin cycles in premenarcheal girls. Science *190:* 161, 1975.

Hopper, B. R., and Yen, S. S. C.: Concentrations of dehydroepiandrosterone and dehydroepiandrosterone sulfate during puberty. J. Clin. Endocrinol. Metab. *40:* 458, 1975.

Job, J. C., Chaussain, J. L., and Carnier, P. E.: The use of luteinizing hormone-releasing hormone in pediatric patients. Horm. Res. *8:* 171, 1977.

Kauli, R., Prager-Lewin, R., Keret, R., and Laron, Z.: The LH and FSH responses to LH-releasing hormone (LH-RH) in girls with true precocious puberty treated with cyproterone acetate. Eur. J. Pediatr. *125:* 205, 1977.

Knobil, E., and Plant, T. M.: The hypothalamic regulation of LH and FSH secretion in the Rhesus monkey. In *The Hypothalamus,* edited by S. Reichlin, R. J. Baldessarini, and J. B. Martin, p. 359. Raven Press, New York, 1978.

Knobil, E., Plant, T. M., Wildt, L., Belchetz, P. E., and Marshall, G.: Control of the Rhesus monkey menstrual cycle: permissive role of hypothalamic gonadotropin-releasing hormone. Science *207:* 1371, 1980.

Lee, P. A., Kowarski, A., Migeon, C. J., and Blizzard, R. M.: Lack of correlation between gonadotropin and adrenal androgen levels in agonadal children. J. Clin. Endocrinol. Metab. *49:* 664, 1975.

Lightner, E. S., Penny, R., and Frasier, S. D.: Growth hormone excess and sexual precocity in polyostotic fibrous dysplasia (McCune-Albright syndrome): evidence for abnormal hypothalamic function. J. Pediatr. *87:* 922, 1975.

Marshall, W. A., and Tanner, J. M.: Variations in pattern of pubertal changes in girls. Arch. Dis. Child. *44:* 291, 1969.

Norman, R. L., and Spies, H. G.: Effect of luteinizing hormone-releasing hormone on the pituitary-gonadal axis in fetal and infant Rhesus monkeys. Endocrinology *105:* 655, 1979.

Parker, L. N., and Odell, W. D.: Evidence for existence of cortical androgen-stimulating hormone. Am. J. Physiol. *236:* E616, 1979.

Parker, I. N., Chang. S., and Odell, W. D.: Adrenal androgens in patients with chronic marked elevations of prolactin. Clin. Endocrinol. *8:* 1, 1978.

Payne, A. H., Jaffe, R. W.: Androgen formation from pregnenolone sulfate by the human fetal ovary. J. Clin. Endocrinol. Metab. *39:* 300, 1974.

Polleri, A., Masturzo, P., Viguola, G., Barreca, T., and Gallamini, A.: Sleep-wake differences in serum prolactin levels in children. J. Endocrinol. Invest. *1:* 347, 1978.

Reyes, F. I., Boroditsky, R. S., Winter, J. S. D., and Faiman, C.: Studies on human sexual development. II. Fetal and maternal serum gonadotropin and sex steroid concentration. J. Clin. Endocrinol. Metab. *38:* 612, 1974.

Ross, G. T., Cargille, C. M., Lipsett, N. B., Rayford, P. L., Marshall, J. R., Strott, C. A., and Rodbard, D.: Pituitary and gonadal hormones in women during spontaneous and induced ovulatory cycles. Recent Prog. Horm. Res. *26:* 1, 1970.

Ruf, K. B.: How does the brain control the process of puberty. Z. Neurol. *204:* 95, 1973.

Rybo, G.: Menstrual blood loss in relation to parity and menstrual pattern. Acta Obstet. Gynecol. Scand. 45, Suppl. 7, 1966.

Shaw, S. T.: On quantifying menstrual blood loss. Contraception *16:* 283, 1977.

Sizonenko, P., and Paunier, L.: Hormonal changes in puberty III: Correlation of plasma dehydroepiandrosterone, testosterone, FSH, and LH with stages of puberty and bone age in normal boys and girls and in patients with Addison's disease or hypogonadism or with premature or late adrenarche. J. Clin. Endocrinol. Metab. *41:* 894, 1975.

Tanner, J. M.: *Growth at Adolescence*, p. 152. Blackwell Scientific Publishing Co., Oxford, 1962.

Thorner, M. O., Round, J., Fahmy, A. J. D., Groom, G. V., Butcher, S., and Thompson, K.: Serum prolactin and oestradiol levels at different stages of puberty. Clin Endocrinol. *7:* 463, 1977.

Weitzman, E. D., Boyar, R. M., Kapen, S., and Hellman: The relationship of sleep and sleep stages to neuro-endocrine secretion and biological rhythms in man. Recent Prog. Horm. Res. *31:* 399, 1975.

Widholm, O., Vartiainen, E., and Tenhunen, T.: On iron requirement in menstruating teen-age girls. Acta Obstet. Gynecol. Scand. 46, Suppl. 1, 1967.

Wieland, R. G., Bendezu, R., Hallberg, M. C., Tang, P., and Webster, K.: Hormonal evaluation of premature menarche produced by a follicular cyst. Am. J. Obstet. Gynecol. *126:* 731, 1976.

Wilson, E. A., and Jawad, M. J.: The effect of trophic agents on fetal ovarian steroidogenesis in organ culture. Fertil. Steril. *32:* 73, 1979.

Winter, J. S. D., and Faiman, C.: Serum gonadotropin concentrations in agonadal children and adults. J. Clin. Endocrinol. Metab. *35:* 561, 1972.

Winter, J. S. D., and Faiman, C.: The development of cyclic pituitary-gonadal function in adolescent females. J. Clin. Endocrinol. Metab. *37:* 714, 1973.

Winter, J. S. D., Faiman, C., Hobson, W. C., Prasad, A. V., and Reyes, F. I.: Pituitary-gonadal relations in infancy. I. Patterns of serum gonadotropin concentrations from birth to four years of age in man and chimpanzee. J. Clin. Endocrinol. Metab. *49:* 545, 1975.

Zipf, W. B., Kelch, R. P., Hopwood, N. J., Spencer, M. L., and Bacon, G. E.: Suppressed responsiveness to gonadotropin-releasing hormone in girls with unsustained isosexual precocity. J. Pediatr. *95:* 38, 1979.

CHAPTER 5

Gynecological History, Examination, and Operations

GYNECOLOGICAL HISTORY

The aim of each history should be to obtain a complete picture of the patient and her illness at the time of her examination. Indeed, a strongly presumptive diagnosis can frequently be made from the history alone, before examination.

Patient's Complaint

The general nature of the patient's complaint should be ascertained at the beginning of the consultation and should be stated as nearly as possible in the patient's own language. This may not always be very precise, or even literate, but it will at least be authentic and will often point the way to later questioning.

Family History

Special attention should be directed to the pedigree if a heritable disease is suspected (see Chapter 7). Certain families have a predilection for ovarian and breast cancer. In congenital defects the history of the mother's pregnancy may be revealing, e.g., maternal diethylstilbestrol (DES) ingestion causes vaginal adenosis.

History

A record of the patient's previous illnesses and, especially, of any operations is of obvious importance. It is remarkable how little many women know as to the nature of previous surgery.

Menstrual History

Since menstrual symptoms are of more significance than any other in gynecological patients, a complete menstrual history should be obtained in every case. Countless women today are taking contraceptive pills, which may modify the periods. The history should note any forms of contraception and include the following data.

Age at Onset. An unusually early menarche, especially when accompanied by general developmental changes, may be indicative of certain endocrinopathies, whereas others are characterized by the late appearance of puberty.

Interval. Although the traditional menstrual interval is 28 days, there are wide individual variations even in normal women. Departures from the woman's norm, however, are frequently produced by either functional or anatomical abnormalities.

Duration. The same general statement may be made concerning the duration of the flow. Most frequently this parallels the quantity, a prolonged flow being usually an excessive one, and a very short period being scanty, but a 2- to 7-day flow represents normal variation.

Amount. Although variations in the amount of blood lost at menstruation by different women are wide, a marked diminution is suggestive of an endocrine or constitutional abnormality of some sort, whereas menstrual excess is produced by either functional or structural lesions, often the latter. A rough idea as to the amount of menstrual flow may be obtained by inquiry as to the number of pads or tampons required daily.

Character of Menstrual Discharge. The menstrual blood is characteristically of dark venous appearance and normally is unclotted. When menstruation is excessive, however, the blood may be bright red with clots.

It is not unusual to find some clotting even with normal menstruation but when clots are numerous and large, dysmenorrhea is usually a complaint.

Menstrual Pain. Pain with menstruation is one of the most common gynecological symptoms, and many factors may be responsible. These need not necessarily be of anatomical or structural character, for often constitutional, psychogenic, and other general factors may be concerned. In questioning patients, it is wise to inquire as to the character of the pain, which is usually of either a bearing down or colicky character, and also as to the time of its onset and its duration. For example, in the common type of primary dysmenorrhea, it most characteristically begins a day or two before the onset of the period and disappears after menstruation has been well established. In other cases, it may persist throughout the flow or even beyond. Any increased dysmenorrhea should require further elucidation.

Intermenstrual Bleeding. It is important to ascertain whether or not there is bleeding between the menstrual periods, and whether this is apt to occur after coitus or other contact. Bleeding of this type is the most characteristic symptom of early cervical cancer, although it is also common with such innocuous lesions as cervical polyp or erosion.

The Date of the Last Menstrual Period. When this is inquired for, the physician will often find the patient's memory very hazy, and this item in the history is sure to be inaccurate in many cases. Yet it is often of great importance, as in cases of possible early gestation, intra- or extrauterine. When possible, it is desirable also to secure the menstrual data preceding the last period, as well as information as to the normalcy of the period, subsequent spotting, etc.

Vaginal Discharge

Leukorrhea is such a common gynecological symptom that it merits a special heading. The duration of the leukorrhea, the character, color, possible odor, and possible irritativeness of the discharge are among the items of inquiry. The budding physician will soon learn that certain fastidious women will complain bitterly about a minor discharge. Others are seemingly oblivious to a copious leukorrhea (see Chapter 28.).

Obstetrical History

Whether the patient is single or married is less important than duration of sexual exposure with or without contraception. Even more so is the history of the pregnancies and labors, with especial reference to their number, character, and possible complications. Other important items concern miscarriages or abortions, either spontaneous or induced. On the other hand, a history of infertility, when there has been no contraception, may be of significance.

Urinary Symptoms

The great frequency of urinary symptoms among women, not only in association with urinary tract disease but also with various gynecological disorders, makes it important to inquire as to such items as increased frequency, pain, incontinence, nocturia, and hematuria. A history of previous urinary tract disease, such as cystitis or pyelonephritis may, likewise, be of much value in the interpretation of existing urinary symptoms.

Gastrointestinal Symptoms

Anorexia, bloating, belching, and discomfort after eating may be secondary to gynecological disease, or they may suggest functional or organic abnormalities of the abdominal viscera. The same statement may be made concerning nausea and vomiting. The latter symptoms, when associated with amenorrhea, would naturally make the physician think of the possibility of pregnancy, to give only one illustration of their possible significance. Constipation is especially common in gynecological patients but may be a rather direct result of certain pelvic lesions associated with pressure or rectal pain.

Present Illness

Last and perhaps most important comes the most comprehensive heading, that of the history of the present illness, which constitutes a summation of those previously mentioned. Chronological appearance of all gynecological symptoms is particularly desirable with brief mention only of the many irrelevant problems that many women include. Evaluation of the sexual habits are of particular importance in infertility problems.

GYNECOLOGICAL EXAMINATION

Although the gynecologist's examination will naturally be directed chiefly toward the pelvic and abdominal organs, it must include a general survey of the entire physical make-up.

General

Among the general items to be included are the height, weight, and general build of the patient, and, in the case of obese patients, the regional distribution of the adipose tissue, as well as any abnormalities of hair distribution. The thyroid should be examined, and at least a superficial examination of the heart and lungs made. The blood pressure should be taken, and the urine examined for protein and sugar, with, usually, a microscopic examination.

Examination of the Breast

Certain gynecological textbooks have attempted to include sections on the diagnosis and treatment of this most common type of female malignancy. Benign and malignant breast disease is so complex and so highly specialized that it warrants not a chapter but a textbook of its own. In most areas of the United States breast surgery is the domain of the general surgeon or the breast surgeon; in many areas it falls within the realm of the gynecologist and, indeed, operative surgery on the breast is fully sanctioned by the American Board of Obstetrics and Gynecology. Whether he performs breast surgery himself, or refers it to a fellow surgeon, careful history, inspection, and palpation of the breast by the gynecologist is mandatory as part of a gynecological "checkup," for breast cancer is more common than any other form of carcinoma which the female may acquire. Palpation of the breast should be done bimanually with the patient in the sitting position and with the flat of the fingers with the patient in the lying position.

Mammography

Low-dose mammography or xeromammography is a most important diagnostic aid in the early detection and diagnosis of small breast cancers. The benefits far exceed the risks when mammography is used wisely and within accepted guidelines. In routine gynecological examinations it should be used cautiously in young women who may or may not be pregnant. In older women it could allow us "to see today with the eyes of tomorrow."

Mammography should be considered of value for the following patients: (1) All women with signs or symptoms of breast cancer, regardless of age. (2) Asymptomatic women between 40 and 50 years of age with high-risk factors (strong family history, cancer of one breast, nulliparity, late menopause, late pregnancy, and recurrent fibrocystic disease) should have a mammogram every 3 years, depending on the individual factors in each patient. (3) Asymptomatic women with or without high-risk factors after the age of 50 should have a routine mammogram every 1 to 3 years, depending on physical signs and risk factors. (4) Women with signs and symptoms of fibrocystic disease after the age of 50 should have a mammogram every 1 to 2 years supplemented by a careful breast examination. (5) Periodic screening by mammography for asymptomatic low-risk younger women under the age of 40 is not routinely recommended. It should be used only occasionally but may be helpful in searching for an occult primary lesion.

Sonography and thermography are of limited clinical value in breast examinations, but computerized tomography (CT) scanning is a new and interesting innovation which may be used with or without contrast media enhancement. All women should be encouraged to practice breast self-examination once a month, preferably after their menstrual period.

Differential Diagnosis

A careful breast examination by the gynecologist doing a routine pelvic examination is essential to assist in the differential diagnosis between benign breast disease and breast cancer. About 30% of all adult women will have mild to moderate symptomatic benign breast disease; this includes fibroadenomata in young women, fibrocystic disease, sclerosing adenosis or chronic cystic mastitis in midlife, and intraductal hyperplasia, papillomatosis, and ductal ectasia in later life. Premenstrual mastodynia associated with thickening, multiple areas of nodularity, and bilateral shottiness are quite characteristic of these all too common conditions. The upper and outer quadrant or axillary tail of Spence seems to be involved most often, but any discrete, solitary, or dominant tumor mass which has a firm or hard consistency, with or without the classic signs of retraction or a positive plateau test, must be considered suspect and further study or biopsy recommended. Aspiration, needle biopsy, or excisional biopsy can be done under either local or general anesthesia. Cost containment makes it advisable to consider biopsy on an ambulatory basis unless the clinical diagnosis of breast cancer seems likely.

Breast cancer is the most common site of malignancy in women and is the leading cause of cancer deaths in American females. About 27% of all cancers in females occur in the breast, and 6% of all women will develop this malignant disease. About 106,000 new cases of breast cancer occur annually in the United States. The peak incidence occurs between the ages of 50 to 55, and the upper and outer quadrant of the breast is the most likely site. The malignant lump in the breast is usually of firm or hard consistency, often attached to the surrounding tissue, and frequently fixed to Cooper's suspensory ligaments, giving a positive retraction sign or plateau test. The axillary and supraclavicular nodes should be carefully examined. Minimal breast cancer can be diagnosed fortuitously by routine mammography and consists of very early breast cancer, which is highly curable. It consists of (1) lobular carcinoma in situ, (2) intraductal carcinoma in situ, and (3) minimally invasive carcinoma.

"Beware of the ample bosom" is a wise admonition based on bitter experience. Nipple secretion should be studied by cytological examination, even though it is often unrewarding. Bloody secretion may be associated with intraductal papillomatosis or cancer, and a clear or turbid secretion may result from many conditions including the taking of phenothiazine tranquilizers or chronic cystic mastitis.

Weight reduction, salt and fluid restriction, diuretics, or discontinuing hormones or the birth control pill will often relieve breast pain and cause premenstrual thickening and nodularity to decrease. These women are to be carefully *rechecked* following their next menstrual period. Women in the high-risk group—including women with a strong family history of breast cancer, extensive recurrent benign breast disease (the "busy bosom syndrome"), or cancer of one breast—should be discouraged from the prolonged use of estrogens.

Palpation of the regional nodes including the axillary and supraclavicular areas should be included in the routine breast examination. Despite some difference of opinion, the majority of scientific studies indicate that proliferative fibrocystic disease predisposes to the later development of breast cancer.

The surgical treatment of benign breast disease may vary from local excision to bilateral subcutaneous mastectomy with silastic implants, depending on the severity of the disease, the age of the patient, and the risk factors involved.

Adjuvant Chemotherapy

Adjuvant chemotherapy, using combined drugs in addition to primary surgery and/or radiotherapy, has resulted in a notable improvement in the survival rate of premenopausal patients with positive axillary nodes. Patients with negative axillary nodes are not treated with adjuvant chemotherapy. Improved survival rates in postmenopausal patients have not been quite as impressive with the use of adjuvant chemotherapy. The use of antiestrogen therapy in patients with positive estrogen receptor assays has been most helpful both in the specific treatment of advanced or metastatic disease as well as in combined drug adjuvant treatment for the primary disease.

Hormone Receptor Assays

The discovery that the positive binding of estrogen and progesterone to cytosol receptors in breast cancer tissue is associated with a favorable response to endocrine therapy in patients with advanced or metastatic breast cancer is a very important medical advance. These assays should be done on all patients with breast cancer where tumor tissue is available. About 50 to 65% of primary breast cancers are estrogen receptor positive (ER+), depending on the level selected as the criterion. Positive estrogen receptor assays also have been correlated with a more favorable prognosis and a prolonged disease-free interval. This prognostic index is independent of axillary node metastases, tumor size, or menopausal status of the patient. Whether or not hormone receptor assays will also serve to predict a response to chemotherapy is still uncertain. Those patients with a high level of both estrogen and progesterone receptor activity in tumor tissue have the most favorable prognosis.

The Relation of the Ovary to Breast Cancer

Like the uterus, the breast is a target end organ insofar as stimulation by the ovarian hormone is concerned. It has been pointed out by Randall and Harkins that a significant number of women continue to show evidence of estrogen effect on the vaginal mucosa for many years after the cessation of the menses, and there is general agreement with this observation. It has been well documented that in certain animals, even of the male sex, breast cancer can be produced by protracted doses of estrogen. Gynecomastia can be caused by hormonal stimulation in men receiving estrogens for cancer of the prostate or other medical reasons. Enlargement of the male breast has been observed in stilbestrol factory workers, as well as in men with estrogen-producing tumors. Therefore, it seems quite obvious that both endogenous and exogenous hormones—particularly estrogens—can affect the breast and thus may be important in the etiology of breast cancer. It has likewise been noted that women with breast cancer who are subjected to oophorectomy reveal a considerable degree of so-called "ovarian stromal hyperplasia," and thus such gonads seem to harbor cells morphologically akin to the theca cells which normally secrete estrogen. It would, therefore, seem highly rational, as noted by Rosenberg and Uhlmann, to advocate *routine castration in the menstruating woman* to avoid further stimulation of an already proved malignant end organ. Patterson and Russell suggest ovarian irradiation as an effective and simple method of ablating ovarian functions.

The study of Feinleib would suggest that early castration for gynecological problems in the woman *less than* 40 markedly decreases the expected incidence of subsequent breast cancer. *After* 40 years the difference is less striking, and it is suggested that removal of the cyclic stimulation of the functioning ovary may be of importance.

Unfortunately, the problem is not nearly so simple, for it is well established that the adrenal gland is quite capable of estrogen secretion. Review by Brown, Falconer, and Strong indicates that *castrated* patients treated with adrenocorticotrophin (ACTH) have a large measurable amount of urinary estrogen, almost certainly of adrenal origin. For this reason, certain gynecologists, surgeons, and endocrinologists have adopted a policy of oophorectomy for the young menstruating patient and adrenalectomy or hypophesectomy for the older patient, when the estrogen receptor assay is positive and when there has been evidence of metastatic disease. That this approach is not entirely satisfactory is suggested by a series of articles by Bulbrook and Greenwood.

Prophylactic versus Therapeutic Castration in the Total Treatment of Breast Cancer

Modern studies have shown that bilateral oophorectomy performed in premenopausal women for pelvic disease unrelated to the breast resulted in a lowered incidence of breast cancer. Feinleib of Boston has shown that women who undergo an artificial menopause early in life by the removal of their ovaries have a reduced risk of developing breast cancer by about 75%. MacMahon et al. reported that those women with first births after the age of 35 had three times the risk of breast cancer as did those with first births before the age of 18. Statistical studies both here and abroad have noted a definite break or "hook" in the incidence of breast cancer during the age range of the menopause. This has been attributed to hormonal changes within the body occurring at this time of life.

In several comprehensive reviews, Lewison has pointed out that for many years the rival merits of prophylactic versus therapeutic castration have been enthusiastically endorsed (mainly on empirical grounds) by those clinicians concerned with the total treatment of breast cancer. In premenopausal patients with operable breast cancer, is it wise to perform prophylactic castration as an adjunct to surgery or is it wiser to reserve this procedure for the palliative treatment of recurrent or metastatic disease? This is, indeed, the doctor's dilemma! As long as the practice of medicine remained a "science of uncertainty and an art of probability" doctors were destined to be impaled upon the horns of this dilemma. However, today, fortunately, we are on the threshold of a new and exciting era in science—a new generation of radioisotope tests called endocrine receptor assays. The results of these steroid hormone receptor assays can be a very specific and selective cytoplasmic binder for tumor tissue. When these results are combined with sophisticated nuclear scans and data gleaned from biochemical tumor markers, this information may provide us with new and valuable guidelines for the resolution of this clinical dilemma, namely which patients will be most likely to respond favorably to castration, endocrine ablation or hormone therapy. Additional tests of hormone dependence currently under study may be even more valuable in the future.

Therapeutic castration performed either by surgery or radiotherapy in premenopausal patients with advanced or metastatic breast cancer will result in a favorable therapeutic response in about 30% of all patients. However, by selecting those patients with a positive estrogen receptor assay (or even better those patients with a *high* estrogen and progesterone receptor assay) one can expect a favorable objective regression in about 60 to 75% of these patients. The addition of antiestrogen therapy may enhance the benefits of therapeutic castration.

Prophylactic castration in patient with operable breast cancer has been recommended in premenopausal women for the following reasons: (1) castration will prevent future pregnancy, which may be harmful; (2) castration decreases the ovarian source of estrogenic activity, which may help control micrometastases present systemically.

In a large clinical trial reported by Ravdin et al., premenopausal patients with operable breast cancer were treated by radical mastectomy and then randomized to receive prophylactic surgical castration in one-half of the series. Recurrence and survival rates in 357 patients were determined every 6 months for 3 years. No significant difference either in survival rate or recurrence rate was noted between those patients receiving surgical castration prophylactically and the controls. Estrogen receptor assays were not being done at the time of this study.

In patients with breast cancer, the following conclusions can be drawn regarding castration:

1. Prophylactic castration is not recommended in premenopausal patients with localized Stage I operable ($T_1N_0M_0$) breast cancer.

2. Prophylactic castration may be recommended in premenopausal patients with extensive axillary involvement in Stage II operable ($T_2N_1M_0$) breast cancer, particularly if the estrogen assay is positive. "Prophylactic" castration in these patients is probably early "therapeutic" castration because of micrometastases and occult systemic dissemination.

3. Therapeutic castration is recommended in premenopausal patients with advanced, recurrent, or metastatic breast cancer who have a positive estrogen receptor assay. Chemotherapy and/or radiation therapy is to be used if the estrogen receptor assay is negative.

4. Therapeutic castration plus antiestrogen therapy is recommended in the early postmenopausal patient with advanced or metastatic disease with either the primary tumor or the metastasis being estrogen receptor positive.

5. Pregnancy is to be avoided for 3 to 5 years postoperatively in patients who have had breast cancer.

6. Exogenous estrogens are to be avoided in patients with breast cancer.

Castration and antiestrogen therapy are important therapeutic measures in premenopausal patients with advanced or metastatic breast cancer in whom the estrogen receptor assay is positive. The stronger the positive assay, the better the result of treatment.

Abdominal Examination

Simple inspection will reveal such abnormalities as undue prominence or asymmetrical contour, as well as variations in abdominal and pubic hair distribution. Any masses or tenderness should be carefully noted. Previous surgical scars should be noted.

If an abnormal mass of any kind is felt, its position and its relation to any abdominal or pelvic organ or region should be noted, together with its size, shape, contour, consistency, movability, and tenderness or lack of tenderness. Percussion is of special value in the case of certain large tumors, such as ovarian cysts, which must be distinguished from ascites. Shifting dullness suggests ascites.

Pelvic Examination

It is in the examination of the pelvic organs proper that the special training of the gynecologist comes into play. The more experienced, thorough, and methodical he is, the more he will learn from the examination.

Preparation and Position of the Patient. The clothing having been removed, the patient lies in the dorsal recumbent position, with flexed thighs and knees, the feet resting on the stirrups of the examining table, and the limbs and lower abdomen being draped with a sheet. The presence of a nurse, or of a female relative or friend, should be looked upon as essential, for obvious reasons. It is of great importance that the patient's bladder be emptied just before the examination.

The examining hand is covered with a rubber or "throw-away" plastic glove, for the protection of the physician perhaps even more than of the patient, and the index finger is well lubricated. The traditional examining hand of the gynecologist is the left, and the expert gynecologist soon learns to feel both sides of the pelvis equally well with the left hand. A reason for use of the left hand is that the more useful right hand is free to handle the instruments which are at times called for during the examination.

Careful inspection of the external genitalia is the first step of the pelvic examination. This will take cognizance of the presence of any anatomical or pathological abnormalities, the presence of any skin lesions or of any inflammation or irritation of the vulvovaginal mucosa and urethra, the presence or absence of the hymen, the size of the clitoris, etc.

Before proceeding with the vaginal examination, the presence of urethral or Bartholin's gland disease should be excluded. Urethral caruncle or erosion will usually be evident on inspection, but the distal portion of the urethra should be gently stripped to ascertain whether a purulent exudate can be milked from either the urethra, the subjacent Skene's ducts, or a suburethral diverticulum infection.

Speculum examination of the cervix is performed before pelvic examination, because any type of lubricant will make evaluation of a cytopathological smear more difficult. Smear should be performed where indicated; in addition visualization of the cervix may provide certain information. The presence of polyps, eversion, or retention cysts must be looked for, and the character, amount, and probable source of any discharge noted. The vaginal mucosa should likewise be inspected.

The gonococcus may be sought for and cultured from the secretion from the cervical canal or urethra, whereas the trichomonas can be found in the exudate obtained from the speculum in the posterior fornix. This technique for these various tests is described in the appropriate chapters.

The examination of the cervix with a speculum is an essential part of the work-up. Although the later stages of cancer are ordinarily unmistakable, the early lesions are not characteristic and present no specific appearance. One must suspect any cervical lesion and settle the question definitely, as it can practically always be settled, by smear, colposcopy, and if necessary, biopsy. These and other special diagnostic methods are discussed in Chapters 12 and 15.

One or more well-lubricated fingers are then introduced into the vagina, and as the fingers pass into the vagina one can note the degree of relaxation if any is present. Ordinarily the patient is asked to bear down for a moment, as this will indicate the degree of any cystocele, rectocele, or uterine descensus which may be present.

In the case of patients in whom an intact hymen would render digital examination of the vagina impossible or very painful, the examination of the pelvic organs should be made *per rectum*. Occasionally examination under anesthesia is desirable, especially in the case of young girls.

The examination of the internal genitalia begins with careful *palpation of the cervix*, making note of such data as its size and shape, the direction in which the cervix points, whether or not there is any laceration or hypertrophy, and whether such digital contact with the cervix causes bleeding, as it so commonly does with certain lesions (polyp, cancer).

The examining fingers now seek to determine the size, shape, and position of the uterus; the external hand is called into play, and the real *bimanual procedure* begins. The purpose is to map out the organs between the internal fingers and the hand externally, and the cooperation of the patient is indispensable for good results. When the abdominal wall is very thick and obese, one can scarcely expect to be able to outline the organs as clearly and sharply as in the case of women with thin and flabby abdominal walls (Fig. 5.1).

A common complaint of beginners is that

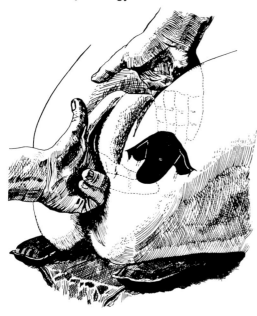

Figure 5.1. Bimanual palpation of pelvic viscera.

the fingers are too short to permit satisfactory outlining of the internal genital organs. During the examination the fingers should hug the posterior rather than the anterior wall, for pressure against the urethra may cause much discomfort. On the other hand, the perineum can be pressed backward toward the rectum quite freely and painlessly. By passing the finger along the front of the cervix one comes to the anterior surface of the uterine body, which can be felt through the anterior vaginal fornix, especially if the external hand gently presses the uterus down toward the internal. Between the two the fundus can then be clearly felt, and one can determine its size, contour, and movability quite accurately. An irregular, knobby outline, combined with enlargement of the uterus, for example, makes it quite certain that the uterus contains myomatous tumors. The posterior wall can likewise be readily palpated in most cases.

When, on the other hand, the fundus cannot be felt anteriorly, the finger passed upward along the posterior surface of the uterus encounters the firm uterine body posteriorly, so that *retroposition* can be easily diagnosed.

The idea, in other words, is simply to play one hand against the other, groping gently about to outline the various normal or abnormal pelvic contents. In palpating behind the cervix one incidentally notes any tenderness or thickening in the uterosacral region.

This is sometimes due to nodules of endometriosis or to inflammatory thickening of the ligaments themselves, but it is often due to the presence of prolapsed, inflamed, and adherent adnexa.

The sides of the pelvis are then carefully and gently explored by the external hand in an effort to feel the lateral organs between the two hands. In most cases the normal ovaries are readily palpable and are tender to palpation. Any enlargement is noted, as well as the movability or fixation of the organ. Although the normal tube cannot be felt, any noteworthy enlargement, as with pyosalpinx, leads to a definite, usually fixed and adherent mass of varying size, inseparable from the ovary.

Examination of the Rectum

Finally, examination of the rectum is of importance, especially in those cases in which rectal symptoms, especially bleeding or pain, have been complained of. External hemorrhoids, fissures, and fistulous openings are readily seen, but other abnormalities require digital or proctoscopic examination. Many rectal carcinomas are low enough to be felt by the examining finger. Frequently, combined examination, with one finger in the vagina and one in the rectum, will be informative.

AUXILIARY METHODS OF EXAMINATION

Even with a careful history and physical examination, it is often not possible to be satisfied that a precise diagnosis can be made. Under these circumstances, help from various auxiliary methods of examination involving specialized equipment and technique is often possible. These include various forms of roentgenography, ultrasonography, computerized axial tomography, and, finally, diagnostic laparoscopy, colposcopy, or hysteroscopy.

Roentgenography

A "plain film" of the abdomen sometimes referred to as a K.U.B. (kidneys, ureters, and bladder) may reveal calcifications or other abnormalities that furnish a key to a diagnosis.

Fibromyomata, particularly if they have been present for a prolonged period, become

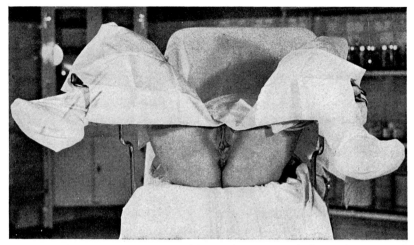

Figure 5.2. Dorsal lithotomy position used for most vaginal operations.

calcified and visible by roentgenography. So-called psammoma bodies are microscopically calcified areas that are sometimes found in tumors of the ovary, particularly epithelial tumors of the serous variety. These may be visible by roentgenography. A tooth or other calcified structures may be seen in a plain x-ray film of a dermoid cyst.

An intravenous pyelogram (I.V.P.) may be useful in gynecological diagnosis by revealing obstruction or distortion of the urinary tract by pressure from tumors of the generative tract.

A hysterosalpingogram, obtained by injection of radiopaque material through the cervix, is useful in visualizing the endometrial cavity and ascertaining patency and contour of the fallopian tubes.

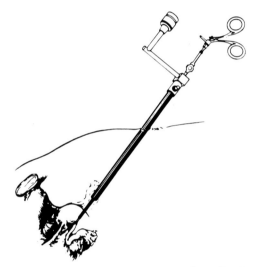

Figure 5.3. Single incision laparoscopic sterilization.

Ultrasonography

Ultrasonography has come into widespread use in gynecological diagnosis. Although at times it may be misleading, it is useful in locating pelvic masses and can usually ascertain if they are solid or cystic. The method has many other uses. For example, an intrauterine device may be located or an ectopic pregnancy sometimes identified.

Computerized Axial Tomography

Computerized axial tomography (CAT) has potential in identifying very small subtle space-occupying lesions. At the time of writing, its application to gynecological problems is not clearly established because of the accessibility of the pelvic organs to other meth-

ods of examination. Theoretically, CAT scanning should be able to identify very small lesions. The method is presently quite useful in identifying enlargements of gynecological interest and significance in areas not available to other easy methods of examination, for example, the adrenal.

Endoscopy

Laparoscopy

This diagnostic method is considered under "Gynecological Operations" in this chapter, as it has important therapeutic functions as well as diagnostic capability.

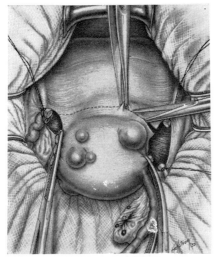

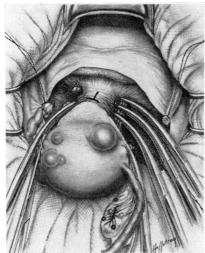

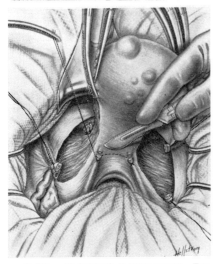

Colposcopy

In patients who have a cervix which appears more or less normal to the naked eye but whose smear is either equivocal or even positive, colposcopy is a necessary procedure to help to identify any abnormality. A colposcope is nothing more than a low-power microscope mounted with a suitable light source to allow a magnified view of the cervix. This procedure and its potential will be discussed in greater detail in Chapter 12 on carcinoma of the cervix.

Hysteroscopy

The hysteroscope is very useful in examining the endometrial cavity for polyps, submucous myomas, adhesions, and other lesions of importance. Except for the treatment of adhesions by the operative hysteroscope, the therapeutic use of this instrument is somewhat limited. Sigler and Kemmann have reviewed the contemporary control of the hysteroscope in gynecology and obstetrics.

GYNECOLOGICAL OPERATIONS

A textbook on clinical gynecology cannot satisfactorily include adequate coverage of operative gynecology. Attempts to achieve this have invariably resulted in rather obvious shortcomings in discussion of the surgical methods or of such aspects as pathology or endocrinology—which are more important to the student or general practitioner than is operative technique. However, it seems advisable to describe a few gynecological operations which, with certain variations, comprise probably 90% of most standard surgical procedures. This attempt should in no way be construed as a half-hearted portrayal of operative technique, but only as a realistic effort to illustrate and explain a few methods which are referred to repeatedly throughout this text.

Dilatation and Curettage

This is one of the most common operations performed by the gynecologist, for it is standard procedure to investigate *any unexplained atypical or irregular bleeding* by simply

Figure 5.4A. Abdominal hysterectomy. *Top,* left tube, uteroovarian and round ligaments divided and doubly ligated; bladder peritoneum mobilized. *Middle,* uterine vessels doubly ligated. *Bottom,* division of uterosacral ligaments and posterior peritoneum; an inverted T-incision has been utilized anteriorly to push the pubocervical fascia laterally along with the ureter (as per Richardson).

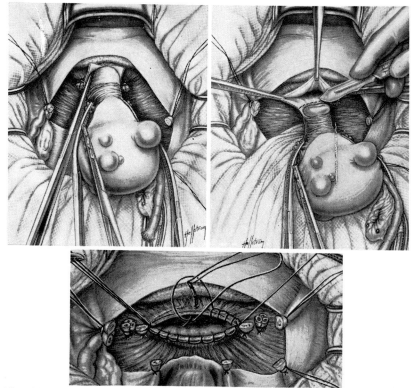

Figure 5.4B. Abdominal hysterectomy (*continued*). *Top left*, cardinal ligaments clamped, staying within the fascia reflected by the T-incision. *Top right*, cervix excised, clamp at both angles as well as anterior and posterior, according to individual technique. *Bottom*, lock, or some kind of hemastatic suture, of vaginal cuff.

"scraping out" the lining endometrium when no cause for bleeding has been found in preliminary office examination.

Curettage may yield many ancillary benefits. It is our custom to perform routine preoperative *examination under anesthesia*, because a much more accurate assessment of the female organs is afforded in the completely relaxed patient. In most instances it is logical to perform certain minor operative procedures as curettage on an outpatient basis.

The technique of curettage is simple. With the patient in the dorsal lithotomy position (Fig. 5.2), after preliminary examination under anesthesia a vaginal retractor is inserted, and the cervix is grasped with a tenaculum clamp. The uterine cavity is then measured by a sound, after which the cervix is dilated by various methods. Thorough curettage is then accomplished, after which the cavity is probed by certain types of "*polyp forceps.*" Pregnancy and acute infections are obvious contraindications to curettage. Where early therapeutic abortion is performed, curettage is preceded by suction.

Laparoscopy

The use of the laparoscope for diagnostic and therapeutic measures has become increasingly popular. Either the two-incision techniques, in which the laparoscope and probe or other instrument are utilized through separate incision, or the one-incision technique, with the fiber-optic operating laparoscope with an electric coagulation forceps, may be used (Fig. 5.3).

The abdomen is insufflated with carbon dioxide, after which a trocar is introduced through the lower portion of the umbilicus. The laparoscope is then inserted, and the pelvic organs can be visualized. Previous surgery or obesity can make visualization difficult, but the well trained operator can generally overcome these. It is our clinic policy to handle these women as outpatients, allowing them to go home in the late afternoon. However, various medical complications may dictate overnight admission.

Perhaps the most widespread use of the laparoscope is as a method of providing sterilization of the patient by the application of bands or clips or by coagulation of the tubes. In our area this is done on an outpatient basis and is colloquially referred to as "band aid" surgery, because the patient leaves the same afternoon with a simple dressing over the umbilicus.

Laparoscopy is not without complication, even when performed by a skilled operator. Bleeding may be a problem; it is generally controlled by coagulation or application of a band, but on occasion laparotomy may be necessitated. Uterine perforation may occur if the intrauterine cannula, which is utilized to mobilize the uterus, is manipulated too briskly. Burn at the trocar site may occur, as may infection or cardiac arrhythmia. Far and away the most serious complication, however, is damage to the bowel, which is generally in the nature of a burn, leading to subsequent bowel perforation and peritonitis. Although the exact mechanism of this is uncertain, it has happened in at least half a dozen cases in this community, and unfortunately this is the type of problem that leads to medicolegal intervention.

Hysterectomy for Benign Disease

The most common major gynecological operation is removal of the uterus for benign disease by either the *abdominal* or *vaginal* route. Each approach has various indications and contraindications.

Abdominal Hysterectomy (Fig. 5.4, *A*, *B*, and *C*). In past years there was considerable debate as to the relative desirability of total or subtotal hysterectomy (preservation of the cervix). Today no one will question preference for the total operation as a prophylaxis against cervical stump cancer as well as persistent leukorrhea. *Panhysterectomy* refers to removal of the corpus and cervix and implies nothing with regard to the removal of the adnexa. In many instances preliminary subtotal hysterectomy with removal of a bulky myomatous tumor or large adnexal masses will improve exposure and facilitate removal of the cervix. Amirikia and Evans indicate that the mortality of total hysterectomy is 0.23%.

The abdominal approach is favored for large myomatous tumors, ovarian lesions, and for certain conditions in which the uterus is apt to be fixed, as in endometriosis, inflammatory disease, certain types of previous surgery, etc. Desire to repair a ventral hernia,

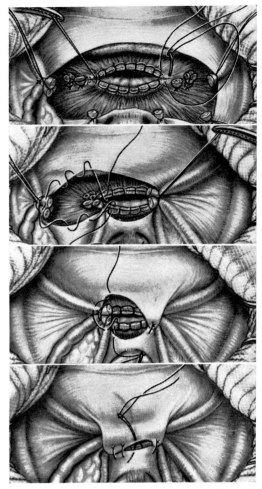

Figure 5.4 C. Abdominal hysterectomy (*continued*). *Top*, attachment of uterosacral and cardinal ligaments to angles. *Second from top*, round ligaments, tubes, and uteroovarian ligaments attached to angles. *Third from top* and *bottom*, complete peritonealization. (From L. A. Gray: *American Journal of Obstetrics & Gynecology, 75:* 33, 1958.)

remove the appendix, or explore for pain are indications for laparotomy when hysterectomy seems indicated.

Oophorectomy with Benign Disease? Although it is generally accepted that complete removal of all pelvic organs is the preferred treatment in most cases of pelvic malignancies (with such exceptions as certain ovarian tumors or intraepithelial cervical cancer in the youthful woman), there is the greatest difference of opinion as to removal of the gonads prior to the expected time of menopause in a woman who is having abdominal

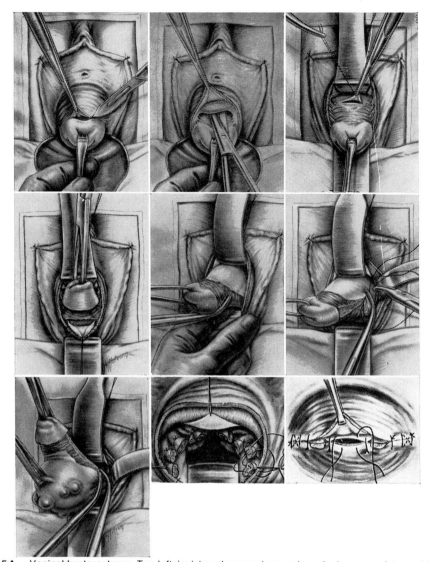

Figure 5.5A. Vaginal hysterectomy. *Top left*, incision above and around cervix, low enough to avoid damage to bladder. *Top middle*, separation of bladder from cervix up to peritoneal reflection; note bladder pillars with ureters in close proximity. *Top right*, peritoneal cavity entered anteriorly so that long Heaney retractor may be inserted beneath bladder. *Center left*, entry into posterior cul-de-sac (this is frequently preferable initially, because early division of the uterosacral ligaments will increase mobility of uterus). *Center middle*, division and suture of uterosacral ligaments. *Center right*, ligation of uterine vessels, preferably double. *Bottom left*, fundus delivered, either posteriorly or anteriorly, with suture of tubes, uteroovarian and round ligaments. *Bottom middle*, suture of ligaments to provide support for vagina. Heaney method utilizes peritoneum, tube, uteroovarian and round ligaments to respective anterior vaginal apex. Mayo-Simpson suspension interposes ligaments from both sides in midline under bladder. In either plication of uterosacral ligaments with posterior vagina is utilized to prevent enterocele (illustrated before approximation of ligaments). *Bottom right*, suture of mucosa, if no repair.

hysterectomy for a benign disease such as myomata, recurrent bleeding, etc.

One can find no set criteria for removal or preservation of the adnexa, and although Randall has presented all of the questions pertinent to the removal or conservation of the gonads, he has unfortunately not provided any certain formula for the harassed gynecologist to follow.

The problem revolves around several

points. (1) Although it is generally accepted that ovarian cancer will afflict less than 1 of every 100 40-plus-year-old women, it is nevertheless an extremely insidious and usually fatal disease. (2) The importance of the aging gonad is not fully understood, especially its possible role in preventing skeletal, cardiovascular, and other changes. One may find the greatest difference of opinion, Parrish et al. emphasizing that castration 10 years before the usual menopausal age of 50 years is attended by a high incidence of atherosclerosis. On the other hand, Plotz et al., and Novak and Williams, are not impressed by such an association. Actually today it might appear that protracted exposure to estrogen is associated with increased cardiovascular problems. (3) A not infrequent occurrence is an enlarged cystic ovary, generally func-

tional, but not always, which is extremely worrisome to the conscientious gynecologist who will be aware of the fact that 5 to 10% of all ovarian cancers will develop in the posthysterectomy female. Grogan has always stressed the frequency of posthysterectomy functional cysts of the ovary, but we regard them as infrequent.

Although we will propose no inviolable routine, preferring to individualize according to the patient's psyche, familial history for cancer, etc., our inclination is toward the radical approach, namely removal of the gonads if the patient is over about 40 years of age. Where vasomotor symptoms appear, these are generally controlled by various oral hormones with minimal complications if the uterus is out. Although *not* advocating replacement therapy for every aging female, we

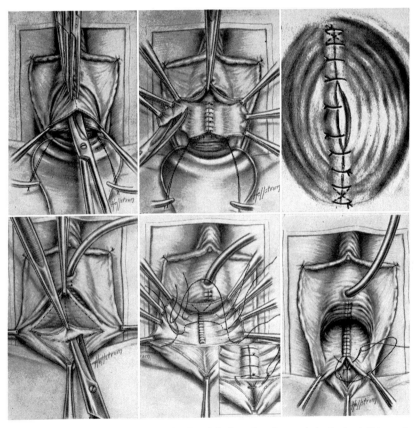

Figure 5.5B. Vaginal hysterectomy (*continued*). *Top left*, if cystocele repair is desired, it is performed after suspension of the vagina; note separation of mucosa from bladder and fascia. *Top middle*, excision of redundant mucosa after approximation of pubocervical fascia (plication of sphincter where necessary). *Top right*, closure of vault with excision of redundant vaginal mucosa. *Bottom left*, posterior repair begun by elevating mucosa. *Bottom middle*, approximation of levator ani (repair of perirectal fascia is often desirable). *Bottom right*, running lock suture of posterior vaginal wall. (From L. A. Gray: *Vaginal Hysterectomy.* Charles C Thomas, Springfield, Ill., 1955.)

are certainly more inclined to utilize it *when necessary* if the uterus is absent.

Vaginal Hysterectomy (Fig. 5.5, *A* and *B*). This procedure has enjoyed a tremendous surge of popularity in the last 30 years and has considerable to recommend it. Postoperative discomfort is minimal and mortality is low, although morbidity is not uncommon, particularly when cystocele repair is also carried out. Pratt has recently compiled the complications, dividing them into vascular, urinary, and pyogenic varieties, as well as indicating that morbidity is increased in the woman less than 35 years old (because of pelvic vascularity) and more than 60 years old (due to the problems associated with increasing age).

Specific indications for a vaginal approach are prolapse and outlet relaxation, with associated rectocele, enterocele, and urinary incontinence. Appropriate reparative procedures are then combined with hysterectomy. However, cases of recurrent functional bleeding, painful retropositions, and small myomas are also amenable to surgery by the vaginal route. Lack of descensus or even nulliparity is not a contraindication, but large tumors (especially ovarian), endometriosis, or inflammatory disease should suggest laparotomy. A previous lower midline scar is not in itself a contraindication (as noted by Coulam and Pratt) but dictates sober discretion. Such procedures as ventrofixation and other types of suspension can make subsequent vaginal hysterectomy of considerable difficulty. One of the nicest features of the vaginal approach to hysterectomy is that it spares the surgeon the decision as to how to handle the ovaries. These are rarely removed during the course of the average vaginal operation, although this would often technically be easy. Vaginal hysterectomy (with or without adnexectomy) is occasionally expedient in treating endometrial adenocarcinoma as noted by Pratt, Symmonds, and Welch.

References and Additional Readings

Allen, J. L., Rampone, J. F., and Wheeless, C. R.: Antibodies in gynecological operations. Obstet. Gynecol., *39:* 218, 1972.

Amirikia, H., and Evans, T. N.: Ten year review of hysterectomies: trends, indications and risks. Am. J. Obstet. Gynecol., *134:* 431, 1979.

Beatson, G. T.: On the treatment of inoperable cases of carcinoma of the mamae; suggestions for a new method of treatment. Lancet, *2:* 104, 1896.

Brown, J. B., Falconer, C. W. A., and Strong, J. A.: Urinary estrogens of adrenal origin in women with breast cancer. J. Endocrinol., *19:* 52, 1959.

Bulbrook, R. D., and Greenwood, F. C.: Persistence of urinary estrogen excretion after oophorectomy and adrenalectomy. Br. Med. J., *1:* 662, 1957.

Coulam, C. B., and Pratt, J. H.: Vaginal hysterectomy—is previous operation contraindicated. Am. J. Obst. Gynecol. *15:* 252, 1973.

Ellsworth, H. S., et al.: Prolapse of the tube following vaginal hysterectomy. J.A.M.A., *224:* 891, 1973.

Feinleib, M.: Breast cancer and artificial menopause: a cohort study. J. Natl. Cancer Inst., *41:* 315, 1968.

Gray, L. A.: *Vaginal Hysterectomy.* Charles C Thomas, Springfield, Ill., 1955.

Gray, L. A.: Techniques of abdominal total hysterectomy. Am. J. Obstet. Gynecol., *75:* 334, 1958.

Gray, L. A.: The place of vaginal hysterectomy in gynecological surgery. West. J. Surg., *67:* 153, 1959.

Grogan, R. H.: Reappraisal of residue ovaries. Am. J. Obstet. Gynecol., *97:* 124, 1967.

Hebert, L. A., and Lemann, H. Jr.: Operative risk: clinical evaluation and management of disorders of water and electrolyte balance. Clin. Obstet. Gynecol., *16:* 195, 1973.

Lewison, E. F.: Prophylactic versus therapeutic castration in the total treatment of breast cancer: a collective review. Obstet. Gynecol. Surv., *17:* 769, 1962.

Lewison, E. F.: Prophylactic versus therapeutic castration in the total treatment of breast cancer: Current concepts in cancer. Int. J. Radiat. Oncol. Biol. Phys., *4:* 477, 1978.

MacMahon, B., Cole, P., and Brown, J.: Etiology of human breast cancer: a review. J. Natl. Cancer Inst., *50:* 21, 1973.

Mattingly, R. F., and Wilkinson, E. J.: Thromboembolism in pelvic surgery. Clin. Obstet. Gynecol., *16:* 162, 1973.

Novak, E. R., and Williams, T. J.: Autopsy comparison of cardiovascular changes in castrated and normal women. Am. J. Obstet. Gynecol., *80:* 863, 1960.

Parrish, H. M., Carr, C. A., Hall, D. G., and King, T. M.: Time interval from castration to development of excessive coronary arteriosclerosis. Am. J. Obstet. Gynecol., *99:* 155, 1967.

Patterson, R., and Russel, M. H.: Clinical trials in malignant disease. II. Breast cancer; value of irradiation of the ovaries. J. Fac. Radiol., *10:* 130, 1959.

Plotz, E. J., Wiener, M., Stein, A. A., and Hahn, B. D.: Enzymatic activities related to steroidogenesis in postmenopausal ovaries in patients with and without endometrial carcinoma. Am. J. Obstet. Gynecol., *99:* 182, 1967.

Pratt, J. H.: Operative and postoperative difficulties of vaginal hysterectomy. Obstet. Gynecol., *21:* 220, 1963.

Pratt, J. H.: Wound healing—evisceration. Clin. Obstet. Gynecol., *16:* 126, 1973.

Pratt, J. H., and Galloway, J. R.: Vaginal hysterectomy in patients less than 30 or more than 60 years of age. Am. J. Obstet. Gynecol., *93:* 812, 1965.

Pratt, J. H., Symmonds, R. E., and Welch, J. S.: Vaginal hysterectomy for carcinoma of the fundus. Am. J. Obstet. Gynecol., *88:* 1063, 1964.

Radman, H. M., and Korman, W.: Uterine perforation during dilatation and curettage. Obstet. Gynecol., *21:* 210, 1963.

Randall, C. L.: Ovarian conservation. Obstet. Gynecol., *20:* 880, 1962.

Randall, C. L.: The risk of gynecological malignancies in older women. Clin. Obstet. Gynecol., *7:* 545, 1964.

Randall, C. L., and Harkins, J. L.: Ovarian function after the menopause. Am. J. Obstet. Gynecol., *74:* 719, 1957.

Ravdin, R. G., Lewison, E. F., Slack, N. H., Dao, T. L., Gardner, B., State, D., and Fisher, B.: Results of a clinical trial concerning the worth of prophylactic oophorectomy for breast carcinoma. Surg. Gynecol. Obstet., *131:* 1055, 1970.

Rosenberg, N. F., and Uhlmann, E. M.: Prophylactic castration in carcinoma of the breast. Arch. Surg., *78:* 376, 1959.

Sapon, I. P., and Solberg, N. S.: Prolapse of the uterine tube after hysterectomy. Obstet. Gynecol., *42:* 26, 1973.

Schinziger, A.: Verh. Dtsch. Ges. Chir., *18:* 28, 1889.

Sigler, A. M., and Kemmann, E.: Hysteroscopy. Obstet. Gynecol. Surv., *30:* 567, 1975.

Twombly, G. H.: Hemorrhage in gynecological surgery. Clin. Obstet. Gynecol., *16:* 135, 1973.

Williams, E. A.: Vaginal hysterectomy, J. Obstet. Gynaecol. Br. Commonw., *69:* 590, 1962.

CHAPTER 6

Embryology

DEVELOPMENT OF THE OVARY

The Indifferent Stage

The first gonadal structures are recognizable in human embryos when they measure about 5 mm crown rump length (approximately 4 weeks). It is not possible to assign a specific sex to this first gonadal primordium, and the so-called indifferent stage lasts until the embryo has reached about 15 mm (between 6 and 7 weeks) when, according to Gillman, testicular differentiation begins.

The germ cells have an extragonadal origin. McKay et al. were able to observe the migration of the germ cells from early stages by their high alkaline phosphatase activity. These cells can first be identified in the endodermic wall of the primitive gut from which they migrate to the gonadal site. Germ cells never persist outside of the genital ridge.

By examination of a section through the gonadal structure of a 7.4 mm embryo (approximately 5 weeks) (Fig. 6.1), several different components may be recognized: (1) germinal epithelium, a well established name but misleading in that it apparently does not have the capacity to produce germ cells; (2) underlying loose embryonic connective tissue; and (3) germ cells which have wandered in from the outside as previously described and which seem to accumulate beneath the germinal epithelium.

The derivation and subsequent development of the structures referred to above have been the subject of considerable difficulty and controversy. According to earlier studies, for example, that of Witschi, during the indifferent stage of gonadogenesis, cellular condensations lying more or less at right angles to the celomic epithelium could be distinguished. These were referred to as medullary cords. More contemporary studies, such as those reviewed by Baker and by other authors do not describe these cords, which were probably artifactual in earlier work due to the thicker sections necessarily in use in former times.

Differentiation of the Testis

According to Gillman the differentiation of the testis first becomes recognizable in an embryo with a crown rump length of 14 to 16 mm (6 to 7 weeks). Condensations of mesenchymal cells (formerly called medullary cords) which become the seminiferous tubules of the testis acquire a prominence. During this same time the germ cells disappear from the mesenchymal areas, the cells of the outer epithelium flatten, and a connective tissue layer develops between the sex cords and the covering epithelium. In a male fetus the sex gland of a 27 mm embryo (about 8 weeks) is a typical testis.

According to Gillman's studies, the interstitial cells show their first signs of specialization in a fetus of about 31 mm crown rump length (about 10 weeks). By the time the fetus reaches 50 mm (about 11 weeks), they begin to increase enormously and the tubules, now properly called seminiferous tubules, are separated by large areas of hypertrophied cells with abundant cytoplasm. This increase continues until the fetus reaches a length of 160 or 190 mm (5 to 6 lunar months), when the interstitial cells suddenly shrink or degenerate. The possible functional significance of these with respect to the development of the sex ducts should be kept in mind.

Differentiation of the Ovary

After the embryo reaches 14 to 16 mm (6 to 7 weeks), the conversion of the gonad into

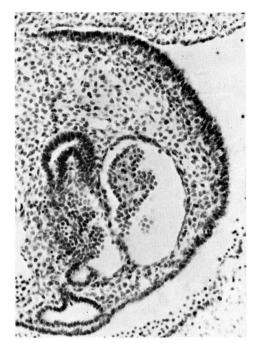

Figure 6.1. Human embryo 7.4 mm. Cross section through left urogenital fold at indifferent gonad stage. The cortex consists of the much thickened celomic epithelium and contains several germ cells. The medulla is composed of a nucleus of blastema cells. (Reprinted by permission from H. W. Jones, Jr., and W. W. Scott: *Hermaphroditism, Genital Anomalies and Related Endocrine Disorders,* Ed. 2. Williams & Wilkins, Baltimore, 1971.)

an ovary is not so prominent as its conversion into a testis. The young ovary seems to remain in the indifferent stage for a longer period of time. Finally, the germinal epithelium becomes thicker and more prominent. In places, massive clumps of sex cells are visible. The first follicles, constituted of oocytes surrounded by recognizable layers of granulosa cells, appear initially in the central part of the ovary when the fetus measures about 150 mm crown rump length (slightly younger than 5 lunar months).

As described above, the primitive germ cells have an extragonadal origin and migrate to the indifferent gonad. After arrival in the gonad of the female, the germ cells may be called oogonia. They are noted as early as the fifth week, although the gonad cannot be identified as an ovary at that time. According to Baker, whose account is followed, oogonia may be found through the seventh month of fetal life. They undergo mitotic division with great frequency, and their maximal number is at the fifth month, when their estimated number is about 2.6 million.

The oogonium is said to become an oocyte when it enters the first of its two meiotic divisions. The first oocyte may be recognized at about 8 weeks, and their maximum number is likewise at about 5 months, when their number approximates 4.2 million. At birth, no oogonia remain, and the oocytes have been reduced to 2.0 million. By the seventh postnatal year, there remain only about 300,000.

The primary oocyte remains in a kind of hibernation in the prophase of the first meiotic division for many years. Completion of the first meiotic division is simultaneous with preovulatory follicular maturation and ovulation. The second meiotic division usually occurs after ovulation and is completed only if there is sperm penetration.

Considerations of Ovarian Development

The descriptive account of the development of the ovary given above is purely in morphological terms and gives no understanding of the mechanisms involved or their causes. Understandably, there are no data on experimental studies of human embryos, but there is an enormous amount of animal work which shows that the normal development of the gonad can be altered in important ways by suitable experiments. The application of these data to the human is, of course, only speculative, but, from a theoretical point of view, it does shed some light on certain clinical situations.

It seems clear that the genetic sex factors are responsible for the sexual differentiation of the gonads, but the exact mechanism by which this is translated into an ovary or a testis, as the case may be, remains obscure. However, for reasons which will be given later, it is likely that this determination is the only specific duty of the sex determining genes.

Among the many experiments bearing upon this subject, the data on amphibians reviewed by Jost may be cited as an example. In amphibian larvae, which are either united in heterosexual parabiosis or receive heterosexual gonadal grafts from other individuals, the sex inductor of the genetic male usually predominates and inhibits the ovarian development of the females. Depending upon the stage of development, the ovary may become quite reduced or even undergo a complete sex reversal if the male component is able to develop.

In placental mammals, gonadal reversal studies have met with limited success. By transplanting fetal ovaries and testes of rats under the kidney capsule of a castrate host, MacIntyre, Baker, and Wykoff demonstrated that the testes could suppress ovarian development and vice versa, depending upon the relative age of the transplants. Somewhat similar studies by Turner and Asakawa in mice showed that an ovotestis could be produced in this way. The germ cells in the ovarian portion exhibited the morphological characteristics of oocytes, while the germ cells in the testicular portion exhibited the characteristics of spermatocytes. These experiments confirmed in the placental mammal the findings in lower animals that the germ cells assume the role of the germ cell of the organ in which they develop, while retaining their original genotype.

In 1974, it was noted by Wachtell et al. that male, but not female, mammals were positive for a cell surface histocompatability antigen called the H-Y antigen. This led Ohno and others to suggest that the H-Y antigen was *the* Y-linked testis determining gene product. Although H-Y antigen positivity correlates well in a variety of normal mammals, Jones et al. noted certain discrepancies in patients with abnormal sexual development so that the precise role of the H-Y antigen in testicular development must be regarded as unsettled.

DEVELOPMENT OF INTERNAL AND EXTERNAL GENITALIA

The Morphological Differentiation of the Fallopian Tubes and Uterus

The genital tract appears later than the sex glands. At about the time when differentiation of the indifferent gonads begins (between 14 and 16 mm at 6 to 7 weeks), the various structures which ultimately contribute to the internal genitalia are recognizable. At this time the mesonephros is the functioning kidney. The mesonephric urinary duct, generally known as the Wolffian duct, opens at its posterior end into the urogenital sinus, a specialized part of the cloaca formed when the

urorectal septum divides the cloaca into rectum and urogenital sinus.

About this same time a second pair of ducts, the Müllerian ducts, are developing anterior and external to the mesonephros. Cranially they appear as a funnel of the celomic epithelium, and later this funnel will become the ostium of the fallopian tube. The blind end of this funnel proliferates posteriorly and pushes a cord of cells lateral to the Wolffian duct. The Müllerian ducts reach the urogenital sinus at about 32 mm crown rump length (about 10 weeks). At this stage, the fetus may be considered to be provided with both Müllerian and Wolffian structures and is sexually undifferentiated and bisexual with respect to the gonaducts. Near the cloaca the two urogenital ridges approach medially and fuse into the so-called genital cord. At this level the Müllerian ducts, originally lateral in position in the cephalic area as described, are medial to the mesonephric ducts and brought side to side in the midline where they fuse and end blindly at the Müllerian tubercle. This tubercle is a median protuberance into the dorsal wall of the urogenital sinus but at this time contains no lumen or opening into the sinus (Fig. 6.2).

In the female, when somatic sex differentiation begins somewhere around the 10th week, the Wolffian ducts retrogress, perhaps due to failure of androgen support. In the adult female these structures are sometimes represented as tiny tubules near the ovaries, called the epoophoron. On the contrary, the Müllerian ducts persist and differentiate into tubes and uterus. The fallopian tubes are derived from those portions of the Müllerian ducts which remain unfused, and the uterus is derived from the fused caudal portion of the Müllerian ducts.

The Morphological Differentiation of the Vagina

It should be recalled that when the posterior ends of the Müllerian ducts reach the urogenital sinus they make contact with the epithelium of the sinus at the level where the Wolffian ducts open into the sinus. This point of contact with the dorsal wall of the sinus is known as the Müllerian tubercle. At the time and place of contact, the two Müllerian ducts have fused into a genital canal and end blindly against the sinus, as already noted. Progressively, this united blind core of cells,

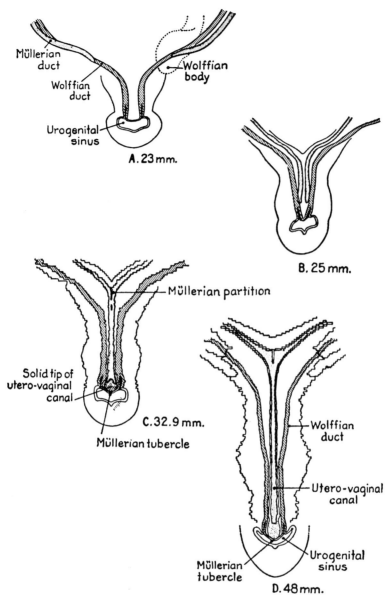

Müllerian
duct

Wolffian
duct

Wolffian
body

Urogenital
sinus

A. 23 mm.

B. 25 mm.

Müllerian partition

Solid tip of
utero-vaginal
canal

C. 32.9 mm.

Müllerian tubercle

Wolffian
duct

Utero-vaginal
canal

Müllerian
tubercle

Urogenital
sinus

D. 48 mm.

Figure 6.2.   The relations between the Müllerian and the Wolffian ducts at various phases of early embryonic development. (From A. K. Koff: *Contributions to Embryology*, No. 140, 1933.)

which now might be called the vaginal cord or the vaginal plate, lengthens and becomes the vagina when a lumen appears in it.

There has been considerable debate about the origin of the cells comprising the vaginal cord. The description here will largely follow that of Vilas which was confirmed by Meyer and which fits in well with what would be expected from the comparative study of the development of the vagina.

As has been said, the Wolffian ducts open into the sinus, whereas the Müllerian ducts are only in contact with the urogenital sinus. As development proceeds, the epithelium from the urogenital sinus progressively extends around the posterior part of the Wolffian ducts and between the Wolffian and the Müllerian ducts. Therefore, the ends of the degenerating Wolffian ducts are embedded in a mass of cells coming from the sinus. There has been special dissonance about the participation of the Wolffian epithelium in the vaginal plate. Several earlier workers thought so, and Forsberg, who has made an extensive study of vaginogenesis in several species including the human, favors the view that the adult human vaginal epithelium is derived through the vaginal plate from Wolffian epithelium, although agreeing that its origin from sinus epithelium cannot be excluded. Cunha has emphasized the role of the perivaginal connective tissue in the differentiation of the adult epithelium.

As mentioned, this description favors the view that the adult epithelium is of urogenital sinus origin. As development progresses, the Müllerian ducts which contain a lumen end against the solid cord of cells constituting the vaginal plate, which in turn ends against the urogenital sinus which progressively becomes smaller as development continues. The vaginal plate acquires a lumen first at the end nearest the urogenital sinus at the stage of about 150 mm (slightly less than 5 months). The fornices and a continuous lumen all through the canal appear at about the stage of 200 mm.

From this course of events, it is clear that there has been a junction between the epithelium of the urogenital sinus and that of the Müllerian ducts. The exact site of this junction has been the subject of considerable discussion. Vilas, and Meyer, have held that the junction is marked in the adult by the squamocolumnar junction in the cervix. Both Vilas and Meyer felt that they had demonstrated that the sinus epithelium actually invaded the cervical canal, but that these squamous elements were forced out by the proliferating endocervical cells which descended from the uterine cavity. On the other hand, Koff concluded from his studies that the junction was in the upper third of the vagina. Fluhmann reviewed the previous evidence and presented some of his own which he believed showed that the junction was in the internal os where the endocervical and endometrial mucosa joined.

The Morphological Differentiation of the External Genitalia

Like the other portions of the genital tract, the external genitalia pass through a bisexual period before specialized differentiation appears at about 50 mm (2 months) (Fig. 6.3).

At early stages the external genitalia are constituted by (1) a genital tubercle or phal-

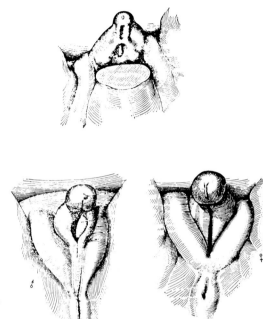

Figure 6.3. Development of the human external genitalia. *Upper,* undifferentiated external genitalia of an embryo 16.8 mm. long. *Lower,* external genitalia during the period of sexual differentiation. *Lower left,* male embryo (45 mm long.); *lower right,* female embryo (49 mm long). (Reprinted by permission H. W. Jones, Jr., and W. W. Scott: *Hermaphroditism, Genital Anomalies and Related Endrocrine Disorders,* Ed. 2. Williams & Wilkins, Baltimore, 1971.)

lus, (2) the urethral groove which is limited laterally by the two urethral folds, and (3) the genital swellings (scrotolabial swellings) which appear on either side of the phallus.

The urogenital sinus opens into the urethral groove. The under surface of the phallus is composed of a urethral plate, which is a proliferation of sinus epithelium.

Sex differences become recognizable when the fetus measures about 50 mm (2 months). In males the urethral folds fuse first in the pelvic region, progressively bringing the urogenital ostium onto the phallus toward the glans penis. The fusion of the folds results in the formation of a perineal raphe which extends from the anus to the urogenital ostium. The genital swellings, which may now be called scrotal swellings, have migrated toward the anus and no longer flank the base of the phallus.

In female embryos the urethral groove remains open and becomes the vestibule. The urethral folds do not fuse but form the labia minora. The genital swellings, which may now be called labial swellings, become elongated and flank the base of the clitoris. The external genitalia are definitely female in character in a 3-month fetus.

Experimental Considerations in the Development of the Internal and External Genitalia

As was mentioned in discussing the experimental data on gonadal development, the genetic determination of sex may be confined to its influence in controlling the sex of the gonad. For various reasons which will now be elaborated, sexual differentiation of the ducts and external genitalia is greatly influenced by and normally seems to depend upon the proper hormonal environment at a specific time in embryonic life. This hormonal theory of sexual differentiation has been firmly established by a large number of investigators working primarily on convenient laboratory animals. It is, of course, not at all sure that such data apply to the human, but clinical data are such that it seems very likely that sexual differentiation in the human is hormonally controlled in a manner similar to other mammals.

Effect of Castration on the Differentiation of the Genitalia. Alfred Jost, in a series of brilliant experiments, elucidated the role of the developing gonads in the differentiation of the sex ducts in the rabbit. It was found possible to open the uterus of the pregnant doe, to surgically castrate fetuses at various stages of pregnancy, and to replace them in the uterus until near term, when they were delivered by cesarean section. Castration did not interfere with feminine differentiation of female rabbit fetuses; ovariectomized females developed a complete feminine genital tract. Thus, feminine organogenesis does not depend upon the presence of the ovaries. In the earliest castrated females the Müllerian ducts were somewhat reduced in size, indicating that some growth-contributing influence might arise from the ovaries.

Castration of male fetuses, on the contrary, showed the primordial import of the testis as a body sex differentiator, and in fetuses castrated before initiation of somatic sexual differentiation (day 19), no male characteristic developed and the whole genital tract became feminine, similar to that observed in castrated female fetuses. In other words, in the absence of the testis, the Wolffian ducts disappeared, and the Müllerian ducts were retained, and differentiated into fallopian tubes, uterine horns, and Müllerian vagina. The urogenital sinus and the external genitalia became feminine.

From such experiments arose the following concept about somatic sexual differentiation of the mammalian fetus. The neutral or gonadless type which develops in the absence of any sex gland (or in the presence of ovaries) is feminine. The testis prevents male embryos from acquiring a female body by suppressing very early the Müllerian ducts and by stimulating masculine organogenesis of the other parts of the genital tract. The Wolffian ducts are taken into the sexual sphere, and all masculine structures are stimulated to grow.

It might be conjectured whether feminine organogenesis of the genital tract in the absence of the testis is not imposed by maternal or extratesticular hormones. In vitro experiments (Jost, 1950), showing that isolated pieces of embryonic genital tract of rats also differentiate as in females, seem to rule out such a surmise.

Chemical Nature of Testicular Morphogenetic Secretion. It seems quite clear that the fetal testis produces morphogenetic secretions responsible for two effects during sexual differentiation: (1) suppression of Müllerian ducts which, in the absence of the testes, would otherwise persist, and (2) stimulation of the development of male structures.

The Müllerian inhibiting factor has been diligently studied by Natalie Josso and her associates. She has called it the anti-Müllerian hormone and demonstrated that it is a polypeptide produced by the Sertoli cells of the testes.

The substance which stimulates the developing male structures is probably testosterone itself. However, study of human cases of male hermaphroditism due to 5-α-reductase deficiency by Imperato-McGinley et al. has shown that testosterone is responsible for masculinization of the Wolffian duct derivatives, that is, the epididymis, vas deferens, and seminal vesicles. However, dihydrotestosterone is the derivative substance which masculinizes derivatives of the urogenital sinus, that is, the prostate and the urethra. Testicular production of testosterone, however, is necessary for this type of masculinization, for dihydrotestosterone is produced in the target end organ by conversion of testosterone by 5-α-reductase.

References and Additional Readings

Baker, T. G.: A quantitative and cytological study of germ cells in human ovaries. Proc. R. Soc. (Biol.), *158:* 417, 1963.

Baker, T. G.: Oogenesis and ovarian development. In *Reproductive Biology*, edited by H. Balin and S. Glasser, Vol. 7, p. 398. Excerpta Medica Foundation, Amsterdam, 1972.

Cunha, G. R.: Epithelial-stromal interactions in development of the urogenital tract. Int. Rev. Cytol., *47:* 137, 1976.

Cunha, G. R., and Lung, B.: The importance of stroma in morphogenesis and functional activity of urogenital epithelium. In Vitro, *15:* 50, 1979.

Fluhmann, C. F.: The developmental anatomy of the cervix uteri. Obstet. Gynecol. *15:* 62, 1960.

Forbes, T. R.: On the fate of medullary cords of the human ovary. Contrib. Embryol., *30:* 9, 1942.

Forsberg, J. G.: Development of the human vaginal epithelium. In *The Human Vagina*. Elsevier/North-Holland Biomedical Press, Amsterdam, 1978.

Gillman, J.: The development of the gonads in man, with a consideration of the role of fetal endocrines and the histogenesis of ovarian tumors. Contrib. Embryol., *32:* 81, 1948.

Imperato-McGinley, J., Guerrero, L., Gautier, T., and Peterson, R. E.: Steroid 5-α-reductase deficiency in man. An inherited form of male hermaphroditism. Science, *186:* 1213, 1974.

Jones, H. W., Jr., Rary, J. M., Rock, J. A., and Cummings, D.: The role of the H-Y antigen in human sexual development. Johns Hopkins Med. J., *145:* 33, 1979.

Josso, N., Tran, D. and Meusy-Dessolle, N.: Anti-Müllerian hormone is a functional marker of fetal Sertoli cells. Nature, *269:* 411, 1977.

Jost, A.: Sur le role des gonades foetales dans la differenciation sexuelle somatique de l'embryon de Lapin. C. R. Assoc. Anat., *34:* 255, 1947.

Jost, A.: Recherches sur la differenciation sexuelle de l'embryon de Lapin. II. Action des androgenes de synthese sur l'histogenese genitale. Arch. Anat. Microsc. Morphol. Exp., *36:* 242, 1947.

Jost, A.: Le controle hormonal de la differentiation du sexe. Biol. Rev., *23:* 201, 1948.

Jost, A.: Sur le controle hormonal de la differenciation sexuelle du Lapin. Arch. Anat. Microsc. Morphol. Exp., *39:* 577, 1950.

Jost, A.: A new look at the mechanisms controlling sex differentiation in mammals. Johns Hopkins Med. J., *130:* 38, 1972.

Koff, A. K.: Development of the vagina in the human fetus. Contrib. Embryol., *24:* 59, 1953.

MacIntyre, M. N., Baker, L., Jr., and Wykoff, T. W.: Effect of the ovary on testicular differentiation in heterosexual embryonic rat gonad transplants. Arch. Anat. Microsc. Morphol. Exp., *48:* 141, 1956.

McKay, D. G., Hertig, A. T., Adams, E. C., and Danziger, S.: Histochemical observations on the germ cells of human embryos. Anat. Rec., *117:* 201, 1953.

Meyer, R.: Zur Frage der Entwicklung der menschlichen Vagina, Teil IV. Arch. Gynaekol., *165:* 504, 1938.

Ohno, S.: Major regulatory genes for mammalian sexual development. Cell, *7:* 315, 1976.

Turner, C. D., and Asakawa, H.: Experimental reversal of germ cells in ovaries of fetal mice. Science, *143:* 1344, 1964.

Vilas, E.: Uber die Entwicklung der Menschlichen Scheide. Z. Anat. Entwicklungsgesch., *98:* 263, 1932.

Wachtell, S. S., Koo, G. C., Zuckerman, E. E., Hamerling, U., Schied, M. P., and Boyse, E. A.: Serological cross reactivity between H-Y (male) antigens of mouse and man. Proc. Natl. Acad. Sci. U.S.A., *71:* 1215, 1974.

Witschi, E.: Embryogenesis of the adrenal and the reproductive glands. Recent Progr. Hormone Res., *6:* 1, 1951.

CHAPTER 7

Genetics and Cytogenetics

THE CHROMOSOMES

The hereditary message of man is carried by the deoxyribonucleic acid (DNA) of the 46 chromosomes. A haploid set of 23 chromosomes, consisting of 22 autosomes and one sex chromosome, is contributed by each parent. Each of the 22 autosomes has a homologous partner, and each gene locus in the diploid set of autosomes is duplicated by an allelic gene for the given paired characteristic and located on the homologous chromosome.

The sex chromosomes represent a special situation in this regard. The basic facts of sex determination and the inactivation of the X chromosome in the female with the genetic consequences according to the hypothesis of Lyon have been discussed in Chapter 6 on Embryology. At this point it is only necessary to mention that the result of this inactivation is the reduction in the amount of active genetic material in female cells to approximately the amount of active genetic material in male cells. This has been referred to as *dosage compensation.* There are genetic reasons, which will be discussed in the appropriate sections, to believe that the inactivation of the X chromosome in man is not complete. Furthermore, cytological studies of meiosis in the human male indicate end to end pairing of the X and Y chromosomes (Fig. 7.1). Therefore, it is currently believed that there are pairs of allelic genes on at least parts of the X and Y chromosome. Although recombination of genes may occur during meiosis from these parts of the sex chromosomes, it is obvious that no recombination can occur between the sex-determining genes of the X and Y chromosomes, or else sex determination would not be precise. Thus, the X and Y chromosomes in part have genes which are unpaired and nonallelic and to which the term hemizygosity may be applied.

The chromosomes may be seen by the light microscope best during mitosis. When first visible in prophase but when better seen in metaphase, they consist of two identical chromatids attached only at the centromere. At anaphase the centromere will split to form two daughter chromosomes.

Three types of human chromosomes have been described according to the location of the centromere and the relative arm lengths: (1) the metacentric chromosome, where the centromere is approximately near the center; (2) the submetacentric, where the centromere is nearer one end than the other; and (3) the acrocentric, where the centromere is very near the extremity so that one arm of each chromosome is very short.

Chromosomes may be conveniently cultured from the peripheral blood for most clinical observations but can be obtained from other tissues. After fixation, staining, and photography, the chromosomes of an individual cell may be arranged in a karyotype in seven groups in order of descending length according to a standard arrangement (Fig. 7.2).

MENDELIAN INHERITANCE

From a clinical view, the identification of the type of Mendelian inheritance is made by an examination of the pedigree pattern. There are three principal types: autosomal dominant, autosomal recessive, and X linked.

At the time of the publication of the 5th edition of McKusick's *Mendelian Inheritance in Man* in 1978, there were 2,811 disorders which were considered to be genetic in origin and which were identifiable as inherited by

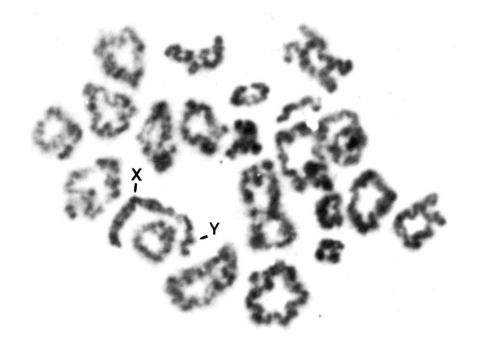

Figure 7.1. Photomicrograph of primary human spermatocyte at diakinesis. Clearly shown are 23 bivalents, the pairing in the autosomes being longitudinal and the pairing in the XY bivalent clearly shown to be end to end. The centromeres of the X and Y chromosomes are indicated by appropriate letters. (Courtesy of Dr. Malcolm Ferguson-Smith.)

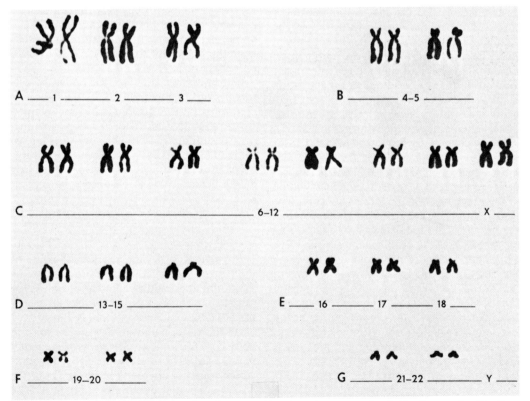

Figure 7.2. Chromosomes from a female cell arranged in a karyotype according to the Denver classification.

one of the three modes of inheritance. Of these, 1,364 were considered to have a particular mode of inheritance as quite certain. The remaining 1,447 composed a group for which the mode of inheritance was considered to be somewhat uncertain.

The Language of Pedigree Patterns

There is more or less general agreement on the method of representing the family of the individual who is affected with the particular disorder. The index person is often referred to as the propositus (female: proposita) (Fig. 7.3).

AUTOSOMAL DOMINANT INHERITANCE

Although McKusick lists 1,489 conditions transmitted as dominant, there are relatively few conditions which directly affect the female genitourinary tract and which are inherited by autosomal dominance.

However, one frequently seen condition which has been suspected of being transmitted by autosomal dominant inheritance is the Stein-Leventhal syndrome. Cooper et al.

(1968) suggested an autosomal dominant mode of inheritance on the basis of high frequency of hirsutism in the fathers, high frequency of hirsutism and oligomenorrhea in female sibs, the culdoscopic identification of ovaries which appeared to be affected by the Stein-Leventhal syndrome in 8 of 12 sibs, and elevated 17-ketosteroids in other related individuals. Although this may be so, as is often the situation in the human, it requires an assumption of considerable variation in the expressivity of the gene to account for the data. A representative pedigree pattern from Cooper indicates the type of information with which it is necessary to work in many areas of human genetics (Fig. 7.4).

A more clear cut dominantly inherited condition with important obstetrical implications is achondroplasia.

As a rule of thumb, autosomal dominant conditions are not sex related and have their source in but a single parent. If there is but one affected heterozygous parent, one-half the children will be affected heterozygotes and the other half will be normal. A thrice-married achondroplastic patient illustrates the mode of inheritance (Fig. 7.5).

The mutation rates of various genes can be

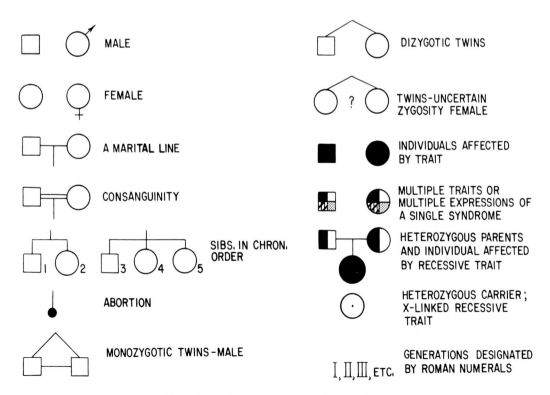

Figure 7.3. The language of pedigree patterns.

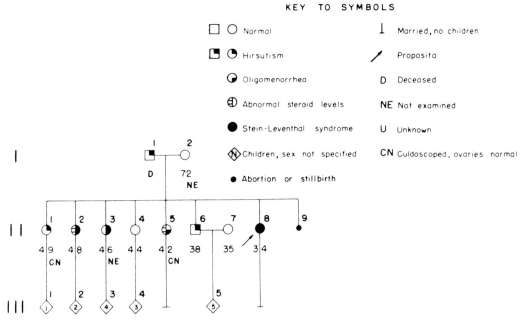

KEY TO SYMBOLS

□ ○ Normal   ⊥ Married, no children

◨ ◖ Hirsutism   ╱ Proposita

◔ Oligomenorrhea   D Deceased

⊕ Abnormal steroid levels   NE Not examined

● Stein-Leventhal syndrome   U Unknown

⬦ Children, sex not specified   CN Culdoscoped, ovaries normal

• Abortion or stillbirth

Figure 7.4. A pedigree pattern which indicates the mode of inheritance of patients with the Stein-Leventhal syndrome. (From H. E. Cooper et al: *American Journal of Obstetrics & Gynecology, 100*: 361, 1968.)

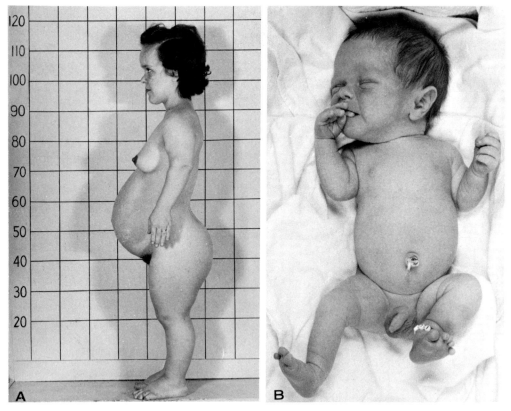

Figure 7.5 A and B. *A*, Photograph of pregnant patient with achondroplasia. (See *7.5C.*) *B*, photograph of unaffected child of achondroplastic patient.

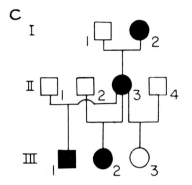

Figure 7.5 C. Pedigree pattern of thrice-married achondroplastic patient shown in *A*. The patient is II-3. (Courtesy of Dr. V. A. McKusick.)

accurately estimated if the mutation produces a dominant phenotype. In that case every affected child born to normal parents represents a fresh mutation. Thus, for achondroplasia it has been estimated that the percent fresh mutation rate is approximately 80%. At the other end of the scale, adult polycystic kidney disease, which is also an autosomal dominant, seems to have only about 1% fresh mutations.

AUTOSOMAL RECESSIVE INHERITANCE

Autosomal recessive traits occur without reference to sex and are inherited from both mother and father, both of whom are of necessity heterozygous. Consanguinity predisposes to this type of inheritance.

McKusick lists well over 1,000 disorders which seem to be transmitted as autosomal recessive difficulties. Of these, about half have firm data on their mode of transmission, whereas there are some uncertainties for the other half.

In general, diseases caused by enzyme defects are inherited as autosomal recessive disorders. This includes all classical so-called inborn errors of metabolism of the Garrodian type. Consanguinity is often found in the family history of affected homozygotes.

A general knowledge of autosomal recessive inheritance is very desirable for the obstetrician/gynecologist because of the possibility of prenatal diagnosis by amniocentesis for a substantial number of these disorders. At the time of writing these amount to approximately 100, or only about one-fifth of those difficulties for which autosomal reces-

sive inheritance seems sure. Tay-Sachs disease, the thalassemias, and the various glycogen storage diseases—such as Niemann-Pick disease, Gaucher's disease, Krabbe's disease, Pompe's disease—are among the better known disorders which are diagnosable by prenatal amniocentesis. For a complete list, a specialized reference work is necessary, as for example that of Milunsky, although new disorders are constantly being added to the list of diagnostic possibilities.

In addition, there are a number of autosomally transmitted diseases which cause malformations or malfunctions of the generative tract.

Among these are hydrometrocolpos and possibly agenesis of the Müllerian ducts (Rokitansky's disease). Many forms of male intersexuality are inherited as autosomal recessive disorders. For example, probably all enzyme deficiencies in the biosynthetic pathway of testosterone resulting in feminine or ambiguous genitalia are so inherited. In addition, the 5-α-reductase deficiency syndrome, which causes ambiguous genitalia because of peripheral failure of the urogenital sinus to convert testosterone to dihydrotestosterone, is an autosomal recessive disorder. Some forms of true hermaphroditism seem to be so inherited. There are also several endocrine disorders affecting female reproduction which belong in this group. For example, the ovarian insensitivity syndrome and various forms of central nervous system defects such as anosmic hypogonadism (Kallmann's syndrome) fall into this group.

Congenital, virilizing, adrenal hyperplasia is a classic example of an autosomally recessive trait which is of great familiarity to the gynecologist. It should be noted that the various forms of the disorder, e.g., 21-hydroxylase deficiency or 11-hydroxylase deficiency, etc., seem to behave genetically as distinct entities.

As mentioned, a very rare disorder, which seems to be transmitted in a recessive manner, is that of transverse vaginal septum (Fig. 7.6).

According to Mendelian principles, one-fourth of all offspring of heterozygous parents are affected homozygotes, one-half will be carriers, and one-fourth will be unaffected homozygotes. This information is exceedingly useful in counseling patients with virilizing adrenal hyperplasia or other such disorders, and it is important to know that, if an affected homozygote marries a normal mate,

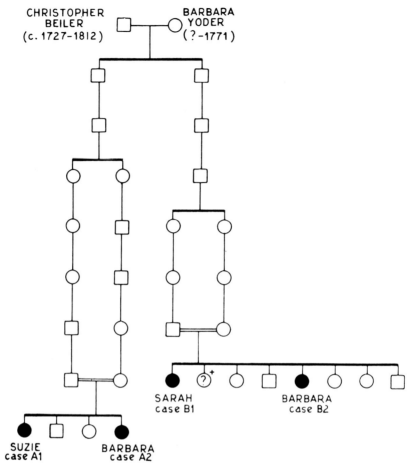

Figure 7.6. Pedigree pattern suggesting female limited autosomal recessive inheritance for patients with transverse vaginal septum. Drawing of the patient Barbara in the above pedigree pattern (from V. A. McKusick: *189:* 813, 1964) is shown in Figure 8.11 (next chapter).

none of their children will be affected but all will be carriers. If an affected homozygote, who is treated, happens to marry a heterozygote, one-half of their children will be affected and the other half will be carriers. The practicality of such information can be seen when it is realized that the gene for congenital virilizing adrenal hyperplasia seems to occur in the frequency of about 1 in 100 in Caucasians.

X-Linked Inheritance

The genes on the X chromosome may be expressed in either a dominant or a recessive manner. However, this is true only in the female. In the male, who is hemizygous for the major part of the X chromosome, all genes of the hemizygous portion are expressed, irrespective of their action in the female.

The number of known hereditary disorders attributable to X-linked inheritance is naturally far fewer than those linked to the autosomes. There are probably in excess of 200 such disorders. Slightly more than 100 of these have been firmly identified as transmitted in this manner, and the loci from many of these have been mapped.

No X-linked dominant condition with disorders of the genitourinary tract of special interest to the gynecologist has been described.

Hemophilia is a very well known example of an X-linked recessive trait. Although it does not specifically affect those organs normally dealt with by the gynecologist, he is very much concerned in caring for patients affected by hemophilia and is particularly concerned with the possibility of the intrauterine diagnosis of this condition.

Another disorder of special interest to the gynecologist is the androgen insensitivity syndrome or testicular feminization. As in all X-linked conditions, the inheritance is always through the mother and there is no male to male transmission. In the androgen insensitivity syndrome, there is a second reason for no male to male transmission in that affected males are incapable of reproduction. The children in such a family may be affected male, normal male, carrier female, or normal female (Fig. 7.7).

Another disorder of interest is the X-linked 46,XY familial form of streak gonads.

CHROMOSOMAL DISORDERS

A large number of chromosomal disorders have been described. In the monumental atlas of deGrouchy and Turleau, almost 50 specific syndromes were described due to numerical or structural anomalies of the autosomes. In addition, 20 or more disorders due to structural or numerical aberrations of the sex chromosomes have been recorded.

Furthermore, Borgaonkar and Lillard were able to describe over 200 different structural chromosomal variants among the autosomes and the sex chromosomes. The discrepancy between this number and the smaller number of specific syndromes catalogued by De-Grouchy and Turleau is perhaps understandable, as minor chromosomal variants seem to result in essentially the same syndrome, at least as identified by present methods of examination.

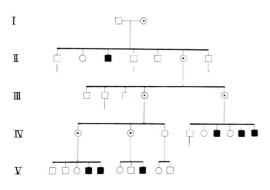

■ Testicular feminization

Figure 7.7. Pedigree pattern of family showing several members in several generations affected with testicular feminization.

The phenotype of the X chromosome anomalies is even more complex and is influenced not only by the loci on the X chromosome but by the Lyon phenomenon and by virtue of the failure of ovarian development in the event of most X chromosomal abnormalities.

The etiology of chromosomal diseases is not generally well understood. However, some disorders occur under special circumstances; thus, the 21-trisomy syndrome is known to occur more frequently with advancing maternal age.

In some circumstances, Mendelian-type inheritance is observed in chromosomal disorders. For example, a phenotypically normal mother might carry a balanced translocation, e.g., when all or essentially all of the long arm of the 21 chromosome is attached to the short arm of the 14 chromosome (14q21q). As this compound chromosome, which seems to behave in miosis as a number 14, piggybacks the number 21 chromosome, there are four possible gametes with respect to the 14 and 21 chromosomes: (1) the translocated chromosome plus a normal 21, (2) the translocated chromosome and no additional 21, (3) the normal 14 plus a normal 21, and (4) the normal and no 21. As fertilization of (4) would result in an autosomal monosomy, essentially all of which are lethal, only the first three combinations can result in embryogenesis. Fertilization by a normal sperm of gamete (1), (2), or (3) would result in (1) a translocation 21 trisomy, (2) a phenotypically normal balanced translocation carrier, or (3) a genotypically and phenotypically normal individual. Thus, theoretically, there is one chance in three of an abnormal child in the translocation situation and for female carriers this is close to the practical experience, as shown in the collected series of Lejeune.

Interestingly enough, if the father is the 14-21 carrier, although he has the same theoretical chance of one in three of an affected child, Lejuene's data show that only about 2% of children of such matings are affected. The discrepancy is apparently due to a disadvantage suffered by the spermatozoa burdened by the extra genetic material.

It is beyond the scope of this work to discuss in further detail the consequences of specific autosomal disorders, most of which result in abnormalities of only peripheral interest to the obstetrician/gynecologist. However, it should be mentioned that balanced translocation carriers may be responsible for repeated miscarriages. In fact, it is the rule rather than the exception for gametes with translocated chromosomes to be aborted. In several series of repeated miscarriage, the cause in about 5% of couples so affected has been found to be a translocation carrier in one or another parent, but mostly in the female and probably for the same reason as described above for the discrepancy in transmissal of translocation Down syndromes from mother and father. In 100 consecutively studied unpublished cases from Johns Hopkins, 7% were found to fall into this category.

INTRAUTERINE DIAGNOSIS

As physician to the fetus, the obstetrician has an obligation to attempt to make a diagnosis of genetic disease in the unborn child in high-risk pregnancies.

At the present time, the only therapy which can be offered to the pregnant patient with a genetically affected child is therapeutic abortion. As 2 or 3 weeks or longer may be required to make a suitable determination after obtaining material by amniocentesis and as a range of 20–26 weeks' gestation has been established by law in most states for considering therapeutic abortion, it is important that diagnostic procedures of this type be carried out as soon as possible. It is difficult to obtain sufficient amniotic fluid before about 16 weeks.

About 30 ml of amniotic fluid may usually be obtained from about the 16th week of pregnancy up to the 20th week without disturbing the course of the pregnancy. Using the supernatant fluid, it is possible that assays for enzyme defects or steroid disorders might be useful in diagnosing fetal disease. However, up to the moment, investigation of the supernatant fluid has produced very little of practical value except for α-fetoprotein.

The cells obtained by amniocentesis can be used for a variety of purposes. They may be used to determine the sex of the fetus by examination for the X- and Y-chromatin. This is of obvious importance in a variety of X-linked conditions. For example, a known hemophilia carrier may wish to be aborted if she carries a male child, half of whom could be expected to be affected.

The cells may also be cultured to determine the chromosome complement of the fetus. The principal usefulness here is when Down syndrome is suspected, from a previously affected child, or as a screening procedure in women above the age of about 35.

Several other types of chromosomal disorders have been diagnosed by this technique.

In addition to the chromosomal disorders, a number of inborn errors of metabolism can be diagnosed by a determination of the specific activity of the enzyme, the deficiency of which is responsible for the syndrome in question. If the heterozygous carrier state is determinable, as in the Tay-Sachs disease, the mating of two carriers is a clear indication for a prenatal assay of the first pregnancy. In situations where heterozygosity is not determinable, the need for amniocentesis is not evident except after the birth of an affected child.

Curiously enough, there is no autosomal dominant condition for which there exists a suitable test which lends itself to prenatal diagnosis.

Several series have now been published. An example from a very large series reported from the University of California at San Francisco by Golbus et al. is shown in the accompanying table (Table 7.1).

GENETIC COUNSELING

Genetic counseling in all its ramifications requires information far beyond that outlined in this chapter. Nevertheless, a discussion of the principles involved and the citing of a few examples may be worthwhile.

First and foremost, to provide intelligent counseling, a precise and accurate diagnosis of the alleged genetic condition is an absolute necessity. To this end, in the event there is a child, parent, prospective parent, or other relative with an alleged genetic defect, sophisticated cooperation from the appropriate pediatrician or internist or other consultant will most often be required. In the event the patient is pregnant, amniocentesis may be desirable to secure cytological or biochemical information about the unborn child.

The task of the counselor has been rendered infinitely more simple by *Mendelian Inheritance in Man*, a catalogue of autosomal dominant, autosomal recessive, and X-linked phenotypes compiled and frequently revised by McKusick and published by the Johns

Table 7.1
Indications and Results of Amniocentesis (3,000 Cases)*

Indication	No. of Pregnancies	Abnormalities Found
Chromosomal indications (total of 2,730):		
Maternal age 35–39 yr	1,843	17 trisomy 21 (1 mosaic); 5 other autosomal aneuploidy (4 mosaic); 9 translocations (3 unbalanced); 6 sex chromosome aneuploidy (4 mosaic); 1 anencephaly
Maternal age ≥40 yr	561	19 trisomy 21; 5 other autosomal aneuploidy (2 mosaic); 1 balanced translocation; 3 sex chromosome aneuploidy; 1 anencephaly
Previous trisomy 21	240	1 trisomy 21; 1 46,XX,7p+; 1 45,X
Previous trisomy 13 or 18	17	
Translocation carrier	14	8 translocation carriers
Miscellaneous	55	2 trisomy 18; 2 trisomy 21; 1 69,XXY
Sex determination (total of 49):		
Duchenne's muscular dystrophy	24	12 males (3 with normal fetal creatine phosphokinase carried)
Hemophilia A	7	3 males (1 not aborted)
Hemophilia B	4	3 males (2 not aborted)
Optic albinism	3	1 male
Renpenning syndrome	4	2 males
Lesch-Nyhan syndrome	1	1 male (unaffected)
Fabry's disease	1	
Newborn asphyxia	2	1 male
Lenz syndrome	2	
Wiskott-Aldrich syndrome	1	
Biochemical (total of 97):		
β-Thalassemia	46	7 affected
Sickle cell anemia	4	2 affected
α-Thalassemia	3	1 affected; 1 hemoglobin H disease
Tay-Sachs disease	7	1 affected
Niemann-Pick disease	5	2 affected
Gaucher's disease	3	1 affected
Krabbe's disease	2	2 affected
Pompe's disease	2	
Galactosemia	2	1 affected
Maple syrup urine disease	3	1 affected
Cystinosis	2	
Metachromatic leukodystrophy	1	
Arginosuccinic aciduria	1	1 affected (not diagnosed)
Hunter's syndrome	4	
Conradi's disease	1	
Achondrogenesis	1	1 affected
Acute intermittent porphyria	1	
T-cell disease	1	
Congenital osteogenesis imperfecta	2	1 mistakenly diagnosed as affected
Congenital adrenal hyperplasia	3	
Fetal blood typing	1	
Hypophosphatasia	1	
Morquio's syndrome	1	
α-Fetoprotein (total of 124):		
Previous neural tube defect	116	3 affected
Meckel-Gruber syndrome	4	
Pevious omphalocele	2	
Mother had spina bifida	2	

* From Golbus, M.D., et al.: N. Engl. J. Med., *300:* 157, 1979.

Hopkins University Press. This is a thumbnail sketch of almost 3,000 conditions with their type of inheritance and pertinent references to the literature. With an accurate diagnosis and by the use of this magnificent compendium, a knowledge of the basic principles of Mendelian inheritance, and an estimate of the frequency of the gene, it is often possible to formulate the probabilities of inheritance of a given trait.

A single example will suffice. The older sister of a patient who was treated for congenital adrenal hyperplasia is married and contemplates pregnancy. Recalling the difficulties of her sister as a child, she wishes to know what chance she has of producing an affected child. The counselor knows that this is an autosomal recessive disorder and that there are two chances out of three that unaffected sibs of such affected individuals are carriers. He also knows that one child out of four of two carrier parents is an affected homozygote. He also knows that in round figures, among Caucasians, the gene for congenital virilizing adrenal hyperplasia has a frequency of about 1 in 100. Therefore, the probabilities that the normal sister will produce an affected offspring are $\frac{2}{3} \times \frac{1}{4} \times \frac{1}{100}$ or 1 in 600.

Much more troublesome are problems involving congenital anomalies such as anencephaly, cleft palate, hare lip and the like, or mental retardation where genetic advice is very frequently sought. Such diseases are apparently multifactorial and are not inherited in a strict Mendelian fashion, although it is recognized that familial occurrence is above mere chance. So-called empirical risk figures for the disease in question must be used to predict the probabilities of trouble.

It has already been stated that chromosomal disorders are not inherited in the Mendelian sense except in special circumstances. However, Down syndrome has been much studied and certain risk factors are known. For example, Hook and Fabia have reported the frequency of Down syndrome by single year maternal age intervals and have shown

that the rate begins to increase rapidly in the early thirties. By age 40 the rate per 1,000 live births is 10 and by 45 is 30. However, in the translocation variety, Mendelian transmission does occur as referred to above for the D-G type. With a G/G translocation where the translocation is apparently 21/22 with either the father or the mother as the carrier, interestingly enough Lejeune's figures show that there is an exceedingly low probability of a mongoloid infant. On the other hand, where there is a 21/21 translocation, there is 100% probability of a mongoloid.

Although the diagnosis of genetic defects may require the skill of a variety of physicians, and while there is constant improvement in the treatment of patients with congenital defects—as for example, the control of adrenal hyperplasia with cortisone or the use of a suitable diet for phenylketonuria—it is nevertheless true that the gynecologist is often the critical physician in handling genetic defects in that it is he who advises about the intelligent selection of methods of pregnancy prevention, must make an intrauterine diagnosis, and must carry out the therapeutic abortion, if this seems indicated. For these and other reasons, the gynecologist must be well informed about genetics.

References and Additional Readings

Borgaonkar, D. S., and Lillard, D. R.: *Repository of Chromosomal Variants and Anomalies in Man*, Ed. 5. North Texas State University Press, Denton, 1978.

Cooper, H. E., Spellacy, W. N., Prem, K. A., and Cohen, W. D.: Heredity factors in the Stein-Leventhal syndrome. Am. J. Obstet. Gynecol., *100:* 371, 1968.

deGrouchy, J., and Turleau, C.: *Atlas des Maladies Chromosomiques.* Expansion Scientific Frances, Paris, 1977.

Golbus, M. S., Loughman, W. D., Epstein, C. J., Halbasch, G., Stephens, J. D., and Hall, B. D.: Prenatal genetic diagnosis in 3000 amniocenteses. N. Engl. J. Med., *300:* 157, 1979.

Hook, E. B., and Fabia, J. J.: Frequency of Down syndrome in live births by single year maternal age interval: results of the Massachusetts study. Teratology, *17:* 223, 1978.

Lejeune, J.: The 21 trisomy-current stage of chromosomal research. Progr. Med. Genet., *3:* 144, 1964.

McKusick, V.: *Mendelian Inheritance in Man*, Ed. 5. Johns Hopkins University Press, Baltimore, 1978.

Milunsky, A.: *The Prenatal Diagnosis of Hereditary Disorders.* Charles C Thomas, Springfield, Ill., 1973.

Rary, J. M., Park, I. J., Heller, R. H., Jones, H. W., Jr., and Baramki, T. A.: Prenatal cytogenetic analysis of women with high risk for genetic disorders. J. Hered., *65:* 209, 1974.

CHAPTER 8

Congenital Anomalies and Disorders of Sexual Development

EXTERNAL GENITALIA

Agglutination of the Labia

Properly speaking, agglutination of the labia is not a congenital anomaly of the external genitalia, but it is so often confused with an anomaly that it is properly considered at this point. The labia minora and the labia majora may be held together in the midline by such precise adhesions that at first glance one seems to be viewing the median raphe of a male perineum. Occasionally this fusion is so complete as to prevent normal voiding. The labia are adherent because of a mild childhood inflammatory process which has been insufficient to attract attention. Treatment consists of separation of the labia and the use of petroleum jelly or an estrogenic ointment to prevent the recurrence of the adhesions.

Masculinization of the External Genitalia

This subject is covered later in this chapter and will not be further considered at this point.

Imperforate Hymen

The hymen is the area where the embryonic vagina buds from the urogenital sinus. It is not to be confused with the so-called transverse vaginal septum. The hymenal area is entirely of urogenital sinus origin. If a lumen fails to develop at the point where the budding vagina arises from the urogenital sinus, the result is an imperforate hymen, a relatively rare condition.

It is unusual for an imperforate hymen to be discovered before the onset of puberty. If the condition is discovered before the onset of the menarche, the hymen should nevertheless be incised. At that time the vagina may be found to contain a clear, mucoid fluid which is apparently accumulated cervical secretion. On occasion the mucocolpos may reach considerable proportions. If the condition is not discovered until after the onset of puberty, symptoms arise from the accumulation of menstrual blood. Although cyclic lower abdominal pain is the common symptom, it is sometimes remarkable that a large amount of blood can accumulate in the vagina, uterus, and tubes and cause relatively little discomfort.

The treatment of this condition consists of simple incision of the hymen with excision of a triangular flap.

VAGINA

Congenital Absence of Vagina

Patients with congenital absence of the vagina usually also have absence of the uterus. Therefore, a more accurate term might be partial aplasia or dysplasia of the Müllerian ducts, for it is the absence of the Müllerian portion of the vagina that we are here concerned with. However, by common usage the term "congenital absence of the vagina" is used to describe the condition. The disorder is sometimes referred to as the Rokitansky-Küster-Hauser syndrome.

Such patients may have a normally developed lower vagina, which is derived from the urogenital sinus. However, the usual lesion includes absence of the middle and upper vagina, the uterus, and rarely the fallopian tubes. The ovaries are normal, anatomically and functionally. Such patients seek the physician after puberty because of the failure of the onset of menstruation. The external genitalia are normal except that the vaginal opening is absent or there may be a very shallow vagina.

In such instances the ovaries appear grossly normal as do the fallopian tubes. There seems to be a failure of fusion and development of the Müllerian ducts, and at the proximal end of each tube there are muscular thickenings which join in the midline by palpable and visible strands, suggesting a diminutive and undeveloped double uterus. On rare occasions there may be enough endometrial tissue in one of the rudimentary uteri to accumulate menstrual blood. When this occurs, cyclic lower abdominal pain will be encountered

and the rudimentary horn must be surgically removed. (Fig. 8.1).

Absence of uterus and vagina is associated with anomalies of the urinary tract in a significant number of cases. All patients with genital anomalies should have intravenous pyelograms.

Bony anomalies of the spine seem to be unduly common.

In addition to being associated with bony and kidney abnormalities, congenital absence of the uterus and vagina is associated with at least one specific syndrome. Park et al. described patients with shortness of stature, inlateral web neck, and deafness, with typical findings of the Rokitansky syndrome in the pelvis. Interestingly enough, deafness was due to bony defects of the small bones of the inner ear.

A few patients have been described who have normal ovarian development and normal development of the upper part of the Müllerian system consisting of bilateral fallopian tubes and only the corpus of the uterus. There is failure of development of the cervix and of the vagina. Such patients have endometrium which is functional; therefore,

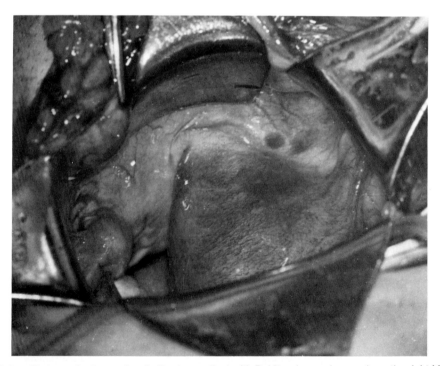

Figure 8.1.   Photograph of operative finding in a patient with Rokitansky syndrome where the right Müllerian anlage had enough functioning endometrium to cause an hematometra which required excision. On the left side may be seen the characteristic Müllerian rudiment usually associated with this syndrome.

soon after the onset of puberty blood will collect in the small endometrial cavity. This causes cyclic abdominal pain and very often by the time such patients seek medical help there has already been reflux of blood through the fallopian tubes causing ovarian hematomas and considerable internal endometriosis. When such a diagnosis is clearly established, hysterectomy can be recommended. This is unsatisfactory, but nevertheless a solution to a difficult problem (Fig. 8.2).

A small but special group of patients is encountered with congenital absence of most of the vagina but with normal development of the uterus and most often with a very small part of the upper vagina. Such patients may be looked upon as having an extraordinarily long transverse vaginal septum (see below). After the menarche they accumulate retained menstrual blood. A special technique for handling this situation was described by Jones and Wheeless.

Transverse Vaginal Septum

A patient with a transverse vaginal septum can easily be mistaken for a patient with congenital absence of the vagina and uterus if the examiner misinterprets the septum as the vaginal apex. This is a rather rare condition, and there are only a few pertinent reports in the literature. Bowman and Scott recorded four patients with this abnormality and briefly reviewed the literature.

The symptoms will depend entirely on whether the septum is imperforate or has a small opening. In the latter case, menstruation may be apparently normal and no difficulty is suspected until vaginal obstruction is encountered at marriage, or, as in a case reported by Bowman and Scott, until pregnancy occurs. If the septum is imperforate, external menstrual bleeding is, of course, impossible and symptoms will arise soon after the menarche because of retention of the blood.

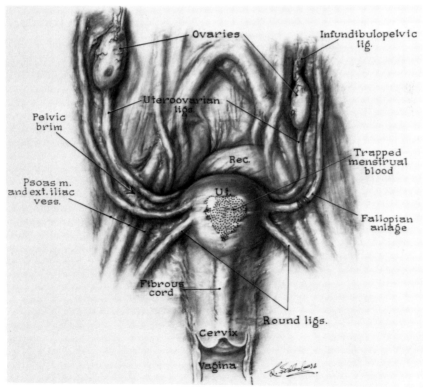

Figure 8.2. Drawing of patient with congenital absence of the cervix. There was sufficient development of the endometrial cavity to cause painful hematometra. The Müllerian anlage which was supposed to precede the fallopian tubes never developed a lumen. In this patient, the ovaries were unusually high and the one on the *right side* was just at the lower pole of the kidney.

Either manual dilatation or surgical excision of the septum is necessary and usually not difficult.

Double or Septate Vagina

A double vagina may occur with an entirely normal uterus and tubes. On the other hand, a complete double uterus and vagina are sometimes encountered. It is not uncommon to have a double vagina and double cervix and a single corpus. The septum, which is longitudinal and anterior-posterior, may be only partial or it may extend almost to the vaginal outlet. Both sides are usually patent but, in rare instances, the septum may deviate from the center and be fused with the lateral vaginal wall in such a way that one side of the vagina and uterus are obstructed and distended by retention of menstrual blood (Fig. 8.3).

The vaginal septum without obstruction is generally asymptomatic and undiscovered

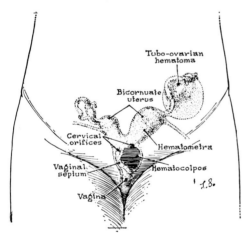

Figure 8.3. Sketch of situation in a patient with double uterus and double vagina with obstruction of the left half of vagina.

until marriage when it may be found to be a cause of dyspareunia. In other instances it may not be discovered until labor. Most obstetricians can relate cases they have seen or heard about in which a breech has straddled a septate cervix or vagina. If one side of the vagina is obstructed, symptoms from the retention of the menstrual blood will obviously occur.

Excision of the vaginal septum is usually rather simple but sometimes bloody. If the septum causes obstruction, dyspareunia, or dystocia it should be removed.

UTERUS AND TUBES

Absence of Uterus

In an otherwise normal female, absence of the uterus but with a vagina of normal length is almost unheard of. For the most part such individuals also have greater or lesser degrees of absence of the vagina, and this condition is essentially that of congenital absence of the vagina which has been previously discussed.

Unicornuate Uterus

If the development of one Müllerian duct is completely arrested, the uterus and fallopian tube may be formed entirely from the other. This so-called uterus unicornus or unicorn uterus seldom causes any clinical abnormality (Fig. 8.4, *left*).

Rudimentary Uterine Horn

When the development of one Müllerian duct is normal and the other very imperfect, various degrees of rudimentary uterine horns are produced. Most rudimentary horns are noncommunicating and are connected to the opposite unicornuate uterus by fibrous bands (Fig. 8.4, *right*). In some instances the endometrium is nonfunctional, so that no clinical

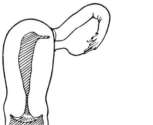
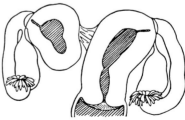

Figure 8.4. *Left,* sketch of uterus unicornus; *right,* sketch of a uterus with a rudimentary horn.

symptoms are present. A clinical situation may arise from the retention of menstrual blood in a rudimentary horn which does not communicate and where the endometrium is functional.

As with all examples of maldevelopment of the Müllerian ducts, anomalies of the urinary tract may be present. With rudimentary horns this is especially common. The anomaly of the urinary tract is, as a rule, on the same side as the most serious underdevelopment of the Müllerian duct. Although the kidney may be malrotated, low lying, or actually within the bony pelvis, complete agenesis is not uncommon.

Blind Uterine Horn

If the two Müllerian ducts develop about equally well but one fails to communicate, either with the other or exteriorly, the condition of a blind uterine horn results. The usual history is that of increasing dysmenorrhea with the development of a mass which presents in the lower abdomen and vagina lateral to the cervix. Pelvic endometriosis is a not uncommon accompaniment. Under this circumstance it is often possible to anastomose the blind horn with the opposite half of the uterus. Anomalies of the urinary tract are also common in this disorder.

Symmetrical Double Uterus

When the two Müllerian ducts develop side by side without communicating with each other, there is produced a so-called double uterus. Each duct forms one cervix and one uterine body with one fallopian tube attached to each. The duplication may continue down into the vagina in that part of the vagina formed by the Müllerian ducts. Such complete duplication may be referred to as the *uterus didelphys* (Fig. 8.5, *left*). However, most reduplicated uteri are not so complete, and the fusion may be only in the upper portion so that there will be a double uterus with a single cervix and a single vagina. If the two horns of such a partially fused uterus are recognizable, the uterus is designated as a *bicornuate uterus* (Figs. 8.5, *right*, to 8.7, inclusive). Sometimes, however, the external configuration of the uterus is relatively normal and the malfusion is represented only by a septum within the uterus. In that case the uterus may be referred to as a *septate uterus* (Fig. 8.8). If the condition is minimal, an *arcuate uterus* occurs.

These various degrees of reduplication of the uterus may be associated with reproductive failure. However, it should be emphasized that an anomalous uterus may be compatible with a normal reproductive history.

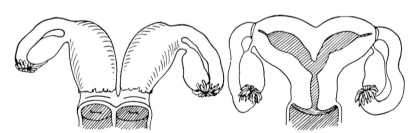

Figure 8.5. *Left*, sketch of uterus didelphys; *right*, sketch of a mild form of bicornuate uterus.

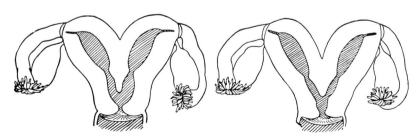

Figure 8.6. *Left*, sketch of a moderate form of bicornuate uterus; *right*, sketch of a more severe form of a bicornuate uterus.

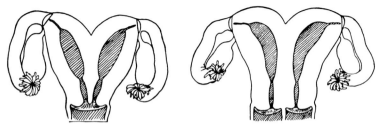

Figure 8.7.   Sketch of a bicornuate uterus. *Left*, with a double cervix but a single vagina; *right*, with a double cervix and a double vagina.

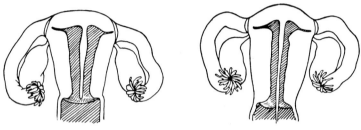

Figure 8.8.   Sketch of a septate uterus. *Left*, with a double cervix; *right*, with a double cervix and a double vagina.

Only about one-fourth of all women with this anomaly have reproductive problems. If it can be demonstrated by suitable tests that the double uterus is, in fact, responsible for the reproductive problem, surgical reconstruction of the uterus to form a single uterine cavity is entirely feasible. Various other factors which might lead to abortion should first be investigated by suitable studies. It is interesting that a septate uterus is more apt to cause difficulty than a true bicornuate uterus, although reproductive failure may be associated with either. Rock and Jones reported the problems encountered and the results of treatment in patients with double uterus. In properly selected cases, the results of treatment for reproductive failure are quite good.

OVARIES

Ovarian Aplasia

The subject of congenital absence of the ovaries, or ovarian aplasia or gonadal aplasia, is essentially a problem in sexual development and is considered later in this chapter.

Supernumerary and Accessory Ovaries

Ectopic ovarian tissue is an extremely rare condition. Wharton has thoroughly reviewed this subject. *Supernumerary ovaries* include those cases in which one or more normal extra ovaries are entirely separate from the normally placed ovaries. They would seem to arise through an embryological process accessory to that which was responsible for the normally placed ovaries. According to Wharton there are only four such acceptable cases in the literature.

Accessory ovaries include those cases in which excess ovarian tissue is situated near the normally placed ovary, may be connected with it, and seems to have developed from it. Such accessory tissue is invariably located near the normally placed ovary. Generally speaking, these accessory ovaries are small and almost always less than 1 cm in diameter. Most frequently they have been found attached to the broad ligament near the normal ovary. They have been described near the cornu of the uterus and between the leaves of the broad ligament. These small bits of tissue have usually been grossly mistaken for lymph nodes, and their true nature has been revealed only by microscopic examination. For the most part they have been solitary, but a few cases of two and even of three such accessory ovaries have been reported. They have universally been an incidental finding, although we have recently seen a granulosal thecal tumor arising from aberrant gonadal tissue well removed from the normal ovary.

In addition to supernumerary and accessory ovaries, there are other examples of heterotopic ovarian tissue. Very rarely, an ovary will be located at a position higher than normal, e.g., at the lower pole of the kidney.

Absence of One Tube and Corresponding Ovary

In addition to cases in which the heterotopic ovarian tissue seems to be the result of an embryonic aberration, ectopic ovaries might be the result of mechanical causes. An ovary is occasionally encountered which is parasitic to the omentum or other intraabdominal structure and is completely separate from its normal attachments. This condition is caused by torsion of the ovarian pedicle. At times, the parasitic ovary is represented only by a small calcified nodule in the omentum. At first glance in such a condition, there seems to be congenital absence of the tube and ovary. However, a small stump of tube and a tiny omental nodule indicates the true condition.

DISORDERS OF SEXUAL DEVELOPMENT

Criteria for Identification of Sex

Sex identification may be described in terms of at least seven characteristics. The first five of these are organic and the last two psychological: (1) Sex chromatin and the sex chromosomes; (2) gonadal structure; (3) morphology of the external genitalia; (4) morphology of the internal genitalia; (5) hormonal status; (6) sex of rearing; (7) gender role. The definition of all these is self-evident except perhaps for gender role, by which is meant the sex which the individual considers himself or herself to be.

Definition and Classification of Hermaphroditism (Intersexuality)

Although any of the several criteria of sex might be the basis of a classification of ambisexual individuals, the well established classification of Klebs is based upon the microscopic character of the gonad. Thus, any individual with testicular formation with contradiction of any of the anatomical criteria of sex (criteria 1–4 above) may be considered to be a male hermaphrodite or a male intersex. These terms are interchangeable. Please note

that this definition does not consider the hormonal status, sex of rearing, or gender role. Conversely, any individual with an ovary and a contradiction of one of the anatomical criteria of sex can be considered to be a female intersex, and any individual who has both testicular and ovarian formation is considered to be a true hermaphrodite.

Male Hermaphroditism

Classification

Normal male development depends upon the normal production during embryogenesis of testosterone and Müllerian-inhibiting hormone. These details are covered in Chapter 6 and should be reviewed.

Most male hermaphrodites have been found to have some problem with the biosynthesis or action of testosterone or some problem with either the production or expression of the Müllerian-inhibiting hormone. It is not always possible to pinpoint the precise nature of the defect, but a large number of abnormalities have been discovered, so it is convenient to classify patients into four general groups:

I. Male hermaphroditism due to defect in the central nervous system
II. Male hermaphroditism due to defect in the gonad
III. Male hermaphroditism due to defect in the end organ
IV. Male hermaphroditism due to defect in the Y chromosome (Table 8.1)

Group IV presents difficulties in classification, because patients with apparently similar chromosomal defects in some instances have streak gonads and in other instances have immature testicular formation. Therefore, it is moot whether such patients are considered under the rubric of hermaphroditism due to Y chromosomal defect (Group IV above) or under the rubric of streak gonads due to Y chromosomal abnormalities (see below). Under a strict definition of male hermaphroditism, they should be included with the hermaphrodite group because they do have testicular formation.

Etiology

Since 1970, rapid progress has been made in the pathogenesis of male intersexuality. In each of the subcategories in Group I, II, and III above, it can be stated with various de-

Table 8.1
Classification of Male Hermaphroditism

I. Male hermaphroditism due to a central nervous
   system defect
   A. Abnormal pituitary gonadotropin secretion
   B. No gonadotropin secretion

II. Male hermaphroditism due to a primary gonadal
    defect.
    A. Identifiable defect in biosynthesis of
       testosterone
       1. Pregnenolone synthesis defect
          (lipoid adrenal hyperplasia)
       2. 3β-hydroxysteroid dehydrogenase
          deficiency
       3. 17α-hydroxylase deficiency
       4. 17–20 desmolase deficiency
       5. 17β-ketosteroid reductase deficiency
    B. Unidentified defect in androgen effect
    C. Defect in Müllerian duct regression
    D. Familial gonadal destruction
    E. Leydig cell agenesis
    F. Bilateral testicular dysgenesis

III. Male hermaphroditism due to peripheral end
     organ defect
     A. Androgen-binding protein deficiency
     B. 5α-reductase deficiency
     C. Unidentified abnormality of peripheral
        androgen effect

IV. Male hermaphroditism due to Y chromosome
    defect
    A. Y chromosome mosaicism (asymmetrical
       gonadal differentiation)
    B. Structurally abnormal Y chromosome
    C. No identifiable Y chromosome

grees of confidence that the disorder is due to a genetic disorder of the Mendelian point mutation variety. Thus, all patients in these three groups have a normal 46, XY karyotype. Group IV, however, is characterized by a recognizable chromosome defect or discrepancy. As mentioned above, it presents a problem in classification in that all such patients have testicular development, whereas some patients with similar chromosome defects have streak gonads and are considered below in appropriate sections.

Among the Mendelian disorders of Groups I, II, and III, autosomal recessive transmission is clear in most categories, although the limited number of pedigree studies make this conclusion less than binding in all instances. However, in the androgen insensitive syndrome, inheritance is clearly X limited.

Male Hermaphroditism Due to a Defect in the Central Nervous System

Park et al. (1976) reported a patient who had a counterfeit gonadotrophin not recognized by the developing testis. The result of this was failure of testosterone production so that the external genitalia were not exposed to testosterone at any time during embryonic life and were therefore more female than male. However, the testis was competent with respect to its production of Müllerian-inhibiting factor and the Müllerian ducts were therefore suppressed.

Male Hermaphroditism Due to Defect in the Gonad

A large number of defects have been described in the biosynthesis of testosterone. An enzyme deficiency of each of the steps from pregnenolone to testosterone has been described (Fig. 8.9). Most of these are not complete, so that partial male development of the external genitalia does occur (Fig. 8.10).

In not all instances of low testosterone is it possible to pinpoint any enzymatic defect. It seems possible that a certain number of these cases are due to mistiming of the appearance of testosterone in embryonic life, so that the external genitalia which are responsive to androgen only at certain periods are not responsive when testosterone appears.

Other patients in this group of gonadal defects are considered in the hermaphroditic rubric by virtue of the fact that they have normal male external genitalia but also have well developed Müllerian ducts due to failure of the testis to produce or of the end organs to recognize the Müllerian-inhibiting factor. Elaboration of other categories may be found in the summary of Park et al. (1975).

Male Hermaphroditism Due to Defect in the End Organ

In this group are those patients who have normal production of testosterone by the testis but who are rendered hermaphroditic by virtue of the fact that the target organ fails to recognize and respond to testosterone. There are two principal categories in this group of patients. The first of these is the so-called *testicular feminization syndrome*, or perhaps more accurately the *androgen insensitivity syndrome*. A large number of these patients have absence of cytosol androgen-binding protein,

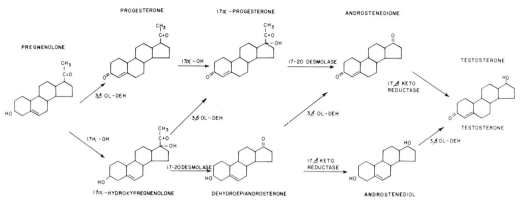

Figure 8.9.   Diagram of alternate pathways in the synthesis of testosterone from pregnenolone. (From I. J. Park, et al.: *American Journal of Obstetrics & Gynecology, 123:* 505, 1975.)

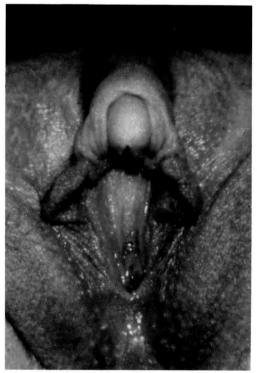

Figure 8.10.   Photograph of external genitalia of a patient with male intersexuality.

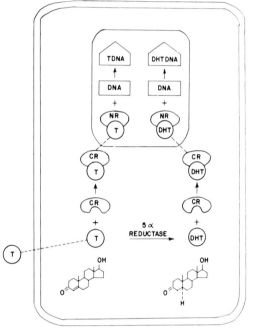

Figure 8.11.   Diagram of a target cell for testosterone action. *CR*, cytosol receptor; *DHT*, dihydrotestosterone; *DNA*, deoxyribonucleic acid; *NR*, nuclear receptor; *T*, testosterone. In the androgen insensitivity syndrome, in many cases, but not all, the deficiency is due to inaction of the cytosol receptor.

although Amrhein et al. described some families in which the cytosol androgen binding seemed to be normal. The testis is perfectly competent to suppress the Müllerian ducts, but the pedigree of such patients clearly indicates an X-limited mode of inheritance so that the disorder is invariably transmitted through the mother. There is no phenotypic expression of the mutant gene in the female.

A second category of patients with ambi-guity of the external genitalia is that due to 5-α-reductase deficiency (Fig. 8.11). In the normal formation of the external genitalia, testosterone is converted to dihydrotestosterone by 5-α-reductase, and it is dihydrotestosterone which is necessary for the masculinization of the external genitalia. This steroid masculinizes those structures which are derived from the urogenital sinus.

In both of the above disorders, a large number of patients have been described who seemed to have partial defects, so the clinical manifestation was modified accordingly.

Male Hermaphroditism Due to Defect in the Y Chromosome

A large number of cases have been described where there is testicular formation, ambiguity of the external genitalia with or without Müllerian duct development and some structural anomaly of the sex chromosomes.

A special situation exists when mosaicism of 45,X/46,XY occurs and where testicular formation occurs on one side and a streak gonad on the other. These cases have been described under the rubric of mixed gonadal dysgenesis or asymmetrical gonadal differentiation. Such patients are often short.

Treatment of Male Hermaphroditism

Approximately 80% of all male hermaphrodites have genitalia which are more feminine than masculine. In view of the fact that such patients generally are incapable of reproducing as a male, their interests are best served by female rearing. Therefore, treatment consists of surgical reconstruction of the external genitalia to make them cosmetically and functionally entirely female. This is best carried out in infancy and certainly before the child is 18 months of age so that therapy is complete before the development of memory. In addition, contradictory gonadal structures should be removed to prevent masculinization at puberty and to prevent the development of tumors which in retained testes are an increasing threat with age.

In addition, such patients will need to have exogenous estrogen started at the age of puberty or a little before in order to assure adequate secondary sex development.

Female Hermaphroditism

Classification

By far, the largest majority of patients with female hermaphroditism are affected by one or another of the types of congenital virilizing adrenal hyperplasia (Table 8.2).

Virilizing Congenital Adrenal Hyperplasia

Virilizing congenital adrenal hyperplasia may be due to a defect in any of the enzymic

Table 8.2
Classification of Female Hermaphroditism

I. Congenital virilizing adrenal hyperplasia
   A. 21-hydroxylase deficiency
   B. 11β-hydroxylase deficiency
   C. 17α-hydroxylase deficiency
   D. 3β-ol dehydrogenase deficiency

II. Maternal androgen
   A. Ovarian androgenic tumor
   B. Luteoma of pregnancy
   C. Adrenal androgenic tumor

III. Special or nonspecific

IV. Idiopathic

steps in the biosynthesis of cortisol (Fig. 8.12). However, more than 95% of these individuals have a failure of a 21-hydroxylation which prevents the conversion of 17α-hydroxyprogesterone to 11-deoxycortisol (Compound S). The disease is an autosomal recessive defect. The karyotype is 46,XX.

These individuals are hermaphroditic by virtue of masculinization of the external genitalia, but the Müllerian ducts and other internal genitalia are quite normal. Because of the failure of cortisol production, ACTH is greatly elevated and this stimulates the adrenal to produce abnormal amounts of estrogens and androgens, the latter of which are biologically dominant; therefore, the external genitalia exhibit various degrees of masculinization at birth (Fig. 8.13). In addition to the anatomical difficulty, if these individuals are untreated they will be subject to large amounts of virilizing hormone in infancy. As a result, bone growth will be abnormally rapid and epiphyseal fusion will occur at a very early date, so that as adults they will be extraordinarily short. Furthermore, the elevated steroids prevent puberty, and no secondary sexual development occurs. Primary amenorrhea is the rule (Figs. 8.14 and 8.15). The urinary 17-ketosteroids are elevated, and in infancy any confirmed value above 1.0 mg is significant. An elevated serum 17-hydroxyprogesterone is diagnostic. Salt loss occurs in the severe form of the disease, and low serum sodium and elevated potassium may be fatal.

It was discovered by Wilkins et al. that these undesirable metabolic disturbances could be overcome by the use of cortisone. Therefore, these individuals should be recognized at birth and treated promptly to pre-

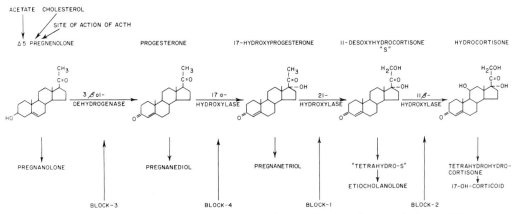

Figure 8.12. Enzymatic steps in cortisol synthesis—localization of defects in congenital adrenal hyperplasia.

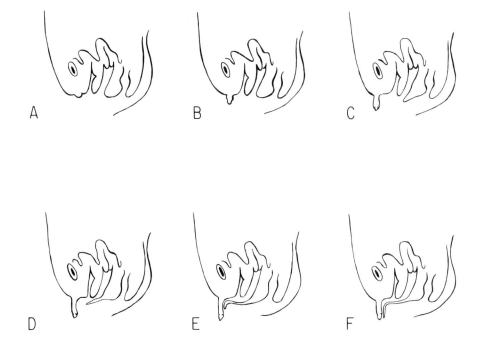

Figure 8.13. Diagram of degrees of abnormal development of the external genitalia in the adrenogenital syndrome. *A*, normal; *B, C, D,* and *E*, increasing degrees of fusion of the external genitalia; *F*, complete fusion with a phallic urethra.

vent the undesirable consequences as mentioned above. For the salt-losing form, deoxycorticosterone (DOC) may also be required. In addition to correcting the metabolic difficulty with cortisone and DOC, if necessary, surgical reconstruction of the external genitalia to provide cosmetic and functional female genitalia is necessary. This should be carried out at a very early age and certainly before the age of 18 months.

As noted in Chapter 30 on amenorrhea, there are various degrees of 21-hydroxylase deficiency. As a result, some individuals have little or no defect of the external genitalia, and have puberty which is not unusual, but, as adults, they suffer from oligomenorrhea and infertility. No surgical therapy is necessary in this group of patients, but menstrual periods are rendered regular and normal ovulation and pregnancy may occur by the use of appropriate doses of cortisol or one of its derivatives. Other details of the problem of 21-hydroxylase deficiency may be found in the summary by Jones (1979).

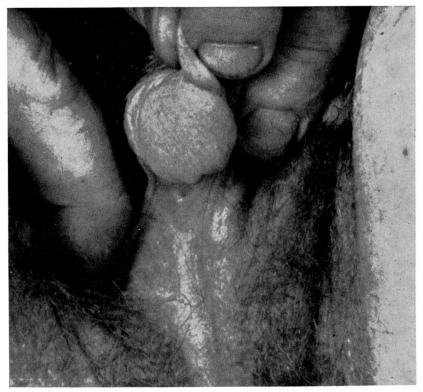

Figure 8.14. Characteristic genitalia of patient with congenital adrenal hyperplasia. (From H. W. Jones, Jr., and W. W. Scott: *Hermaphroditism, Genital Anomalies and Related Endocrine Disorders*, Ed. 2, Williams & Wilkins, Baltimore, 1971.)

Other Types of Female Hermaphroditism

Virilizing congenital adrenal hyperplasia is by all odds the most common cause of female intersexuality among genetic females. Nevertheless, fetal masculinization of the external genitalia does occur in otherwise normal females who have been subject to some virilizing influence during intrauterine life. Such patients, contrary to those with the adrenogenital syndrome, do not have postnatal elevations of androgenic substances, and, as they grow older, they do not show precocious development nor are they subject to the metabolic difficulties associated with the adrenal disorder. On the contrary, at the expected time of puberty, the nonadrenal patients will feminize normally and ovulate and have menstruation, except perhaps among the subgroup in whom there are associated anomalies of the Müllerian ducts where menstruation is precluded because of a uterine anomaly.

The diagnosis of female hermaphroditism not due to adrenal hyperplasia depends upon ambiguity of the external genitalia, the demonstration of a normal female karyotype, and the absence of an adrenal disorder. The relationship of the vaginal orifice and the female urethral meatus to the persistent urogenital sinus is essentially the same in the nonadrenal type of disorder as in the difficulty caused by adrenal hyperplasia. The differential diagnosis among the various conditions causing female pseudohermaphroditism is usually self-evident, but the differentiation of such patients from those with true hermaphroditism may be exceedingly difficult and in some circumstances actually require exploratory laparotomy in order to make the diagnosis with certainty.

True Hermaphroditism

Some individuals have gonads which are composed of various proportions of ovary and testis. Sometimes one gonad is entirely

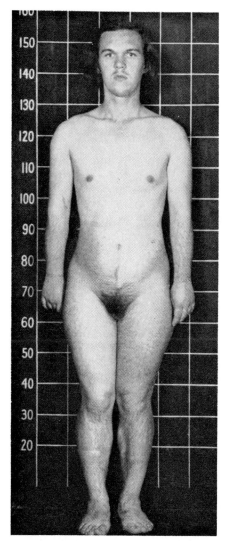

Figure 8.15. Photograph of patient with congenital adrenal hyperplasia. Note the rather characteristic stature of short arms and short legs. Also note the absence of breast development and the growth of hair on the face and body. This patient was 16 years old when the photograph was taken. She had been untreated and had not menstruated. (From H. W. Jones, Jr., and W. W. Scott: *Hermaphroditism, Genital Anomalies and Related Endocrine Disorders*, Ed. 2, Williams & Wilkins, Baltimore, 1971.)

testicular and the opposite one entirely ovarian, but most often one or the other of the gonads is an ovotestis. Most often the Müllerian ducts are reasonably well developed, and, if such patients are untreated, they will have female secondary sex development and menstruation. All of these individuals have various degrees of ambiguity of the external genitalia, so the diagnosis can and should be made in infancy. Approximately half of all these individuals have a 46,XX karyotype, but various types of mosaicism also occur. A small number of patients are true chimeras with two cell lines, one of which is 46,XX and the other of which is 46,XY. Interestingly enough, Jones et al. and others have shown that some but not all patients who have no apparent Y chromosome are positive for the H-Y antigen. It is possible in this group of patients that loci from the Y were translocated to the X during abnormalities of meiosis in the testis of the father. Exploratory laparotomy is usually necessary to confirm the diagnosis, which can be suspected in any patient with ambiguous genitalia and a normal 46,XX karyotype without any other obvious cause for the abnormality.

Treatment consists of surgical reconstruction of the external genitalia and removal of the contradictory gonadal tissue, which in most instances will require removal of the testicular portion of the gonad, because the ambiguity of the external genitalia is such that the sex of rearing can and should be female in most instances. There have been a few examples of reproduction in 46,XX true hermaphrodites. Van Niekerk has a very complete review of this problem.

X Chromosome Anomalies

Introduction

As of June, 1979 more than 300 loci had been mapped on the autosomes and the sex chromosomes. It is interesting that approximately one-third of these loci had been identified on the X chromosome. Interestingly enough, but a single locus (the H-Y antigen) had been definitely assigned to the Y chromosome. Mapping of the X chromosome is easier than mapping the autosomes because autosomal loci are available in double dose, so that a single mutant gene, as in a heterozygous carrier, is obscured by the normal allelic gene. On the other hand, due to lyonization, i.e., genetic inactivation of one of the two X chromosomes in normal women, the genes on the X chromosome are available in but a single dose. Thus, when there is a mutant gene on the active X chromosome, its presence is expressed and may be identifiable.

It is interesting to point out that of the more than 100 genes that have been mapped with confidence on the X chromosome, very few of them are associated with sexual development. Conversely, competence at loci on the autosomes is required for normal sexual differentiation; for example, 5-α-reductase is clearly an autosomal gene and yet, unless such a gene is available, male hermaphroditism will result because of failure to convert testosterone (T), to dihydrotestosterone (DHT), thereby causing failure of fusion of the urogenital sinus derivatives in the embryo. On the other hand, in female sexual development, even with two normal X chromosomes, masculinization of the external genitalia will occur if there is any difficulty with 21-hydroxylation by a gene which has been localized on chromosome 6. Thus, the separation of chromosomes into sex chromosomes and autosomes is at best only a rough estimation.

It is interesting that, although two normal X chromosomes are required for normal female development, there do not seem to be specific loci on the X chromosomes which code for ovarian development. Normal ovarian development seems to occur in the genital ridge by the mere presence of oogonia, and later oocytes, and it is competence of the two normal X chromosomes that is necessary for the development of these germ cells. Conversely, in the absence of germ cells, streak gonads are the consequence.

X-Inactivation

In the normal human female embryo one of the X chromosomes contracts, is thereby rendered genetically inactive, and is visible in somatic cells as the X-chromatin. This seems to occur at random in any given cell, so that approximately 50% of cells with maternally derived X's and 50% of cells with paternally derived X's are involved in this inactivation process. This process is initiated in the morula at about 16 days of embryonic life. Additionally all progeny cells of any given cell will always inactivate the same X, i.e., maternal or paternal, as in the parent cell. Reference has already been made to the general genetic consequences of this phenomenon.

It has been repeatedly observed that, when one X is structurally abnormal, it is the structurally abnormal X which is inactivated. Thus, random inactivation seems to be overridden in this situation. However, cells with inactivation of the normal X would be genetically unbalanced. Thus, it is very likely that random inactivation did in fact occur at the normal time but that the unbalanced disadvantaged cells were eliminated early in embryonic life, so that the remaining cells formed a normal embryo, all cells of which exhibited inactivation of the abnormal X.

There is evidence to indicate that the inactivation of the X chromosome arises from a center which is located very near the centromere on the long arm.

The above remarks about inactivation of one of the X chromosomes apply only when the autosomes are normal, which is the situation most of the time.

However, if there is an autosomal abnormality, such as a translocation of part of one autosome to an X chromosome, a special situation exists. If the autosome or portion of the autosome is translocated to the long arm of the X chromosome, this translocated portion will be involved in the inactivation process during lyonization. This would cause a partial autosomal deficiency in approximately one-half of all cells if random inactivation of the X took place. However, several case observations have indicated that under this circumstance it is the normal X which is inactivated, thus maintaining genetic balance. This apparently results from the elimination of the disadvantaged cells very early in embryonic life.

Classification of X Chromosome Anomalies

In addition to Mendelian problems, X chromosome anomalies may be divided into phenotypic discrepancy (streaks), monosomy (45,X), structural anomalies (isochromosomes, deletions, rings, etc.), translocations (X-autosome, XX, XY), polysomy (47,XXX; 48,XXXX, 49,XXXXX), and phenotypic anomalies (46,XX males; 46,XX true hermaphrodites).

It should be pointed out that, although 45,X is considered to be an X chromosome anomaly, it is perfectly obvious that the nature of the missing chromosome is not known.

As will become clear, the streak gonads, which most of these anomalies share in common, are the result of the absence of two normal X chromosomes. There are some minor exceptions to this, as will be noted. On the other hand, the somatic manifestations of the chromosomal abnormality are very much related to the presence or absence of the two short arms of the X chromosomes. When both short arms are present, there are no somatic abnormalities. On the other hand, with monosomy of the short arm, as in 45,X, shortness of stature and many other somatic abnormalities can be noted. These considerations can be used as genetic evidence that, even with genetic inactivation of one of the X chromosomes and the formation of the X-chromatin, not all of the X chromosome is inactivated.

Phenotypic Discrepancies—Streaks

Some patients who have no somatic anomalies, nevertheless have primary amenorrhea and failure of secondary sex development due to streak gonads, in spite of having a normal 46, XX karyotype. Thus, there is a clear discrepancy between the karyotype and the gonadal phenotype. The cause of this is quite unknown. However, on theoretical grounds, any noxious agent—a viral infection, drugs, etc.—which destroyed the germ cells early in embryonic life could cause streak gonads. As with essentially all patients with streak gonads, development of the uterus, fallopian tubes, and vagina is quite normal, and the external genitalia are female.

It is inappropriate to refer to such patients as having Turner's syndrome. (See below under 45,X.) It is permissible to refer to such patients as having *pure gonadal dysgenesis*, meaning that they are essentially normal except for gonadal maldevelopment. In this connection, it needs to be mentioned that patients with other karyotypes, such as 46,XY, may also have *pure gonadal dysgenesis*. In order to be absolutely specific, such patients may be referred to with a descriptive designation, for example, a patient with normal body type with streak gonads and a 46,XX karyotype.

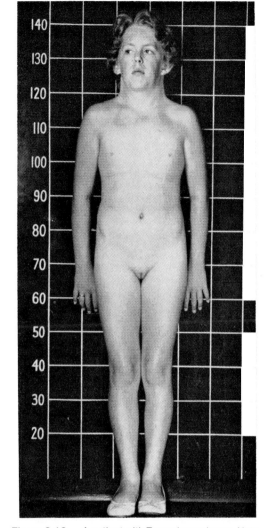

Figure 8.16.   A patient with Turner's syndrome. Note the short stature, webbed neck, and sexual infantilism in spite of the fact that the patient was 17 years of age. The karyotype was 45,X. (From H. W. Jones, Jr., and W. W. Scott: *Hermaphroditism, Genital Anomalies and Related Endocrine Disorders*, Ed. 2, Williams & Wilkins, Baltimore, 1971.)

45,X

The short stature, web neck, cubitus valgus, and other somatic abnormalities characteristic of the Turner phenotype are well known (Fig. 8.16). The failure of sexual development is associated with streak gonads which, as noted above, occur because of the absence of oogonia and oocytes. The characteristic body type (Turner phenotype) together with the streak gonads is Turner's syndrome. The de-

velopment of the Müllerian ducts (Fig. 8.17) are entirely female. This might be predicted from Jost's experiments in the rabbit which showed that Müllerian and Wolffian duct development, as well as the external genitalia (Fig. 8.18), was entirely dependent on the function of the gonad. In the absence of gonadal development, the duct development of the external genitalia was always female, regardless of the genetics of the individual.

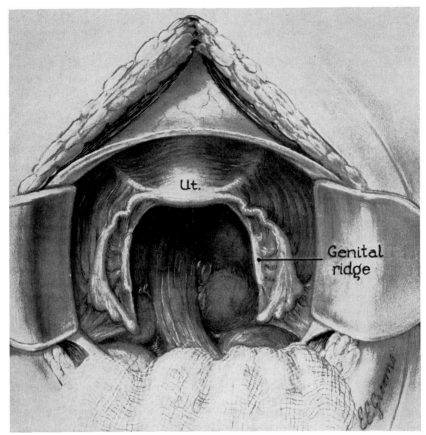

Figure 8.17. Internal genitalia of a patient with 45,X. Note that the uterus (*Ut.*), fallopian tubes, and round ligaments are normally formed but relatively undeveloped. The gonads are represented by thickenings or streaks.

Histological examination of the streaks reveals whirls of fibrous tissue that is indistinguishable from the stroma of the ovary, or for that matter of the testes. It shows rete tubules and, if examined after the time for the onset of puberty, invariably shows hilus cells. In addition, in the mesentery can always be found remnants of the Wolffian ducts. Not to be found are oocytes or those things which are induced by oocytes, namely the follicular apparatus. Thus, a streak gonad has all the components of a normal ovary except for oocytes and follicles (Fig. 8.19).

Endocrinologically, such patients have essentially no estrogen production. The gonadotropins are elevated even during infancy and childhood and after the age of puberty reach menopausal levels. The finding of elevated gonadotropins in addition to the phenotype is diagnostic.

Some individuals require no treatment except for counseling with regard to their somatic abnormalities and substitution therapy with estrogen for the development of secondary sexual characteristics. Exploratory laparotomy or even laparoscopy is not required for confirmation of the diagnosis, and no internal structures need to be removed. This is in contrast to individuals who have streak gonads associated with a Y chromosome where tumor formation is a concern.

As 45,X individuals are always short and as their epiphyses are not closed, it is usually desirable to gain some height by initiating treatment with relatively small doses of estrogen to prevent sudden closure of the epiphyses. Thus, initial therapy using no more than 0.6 mg of conjugated estrogen or its equivalent, beginning at about 11 or 12 years of age, will sometimes secure 1 or 2 inches of growth before the epiphyses close. After epiphyseal closure, larger doses of estrogen can be used to secure adequate breast development. This may amount to up to 2½ mg of conjugated estrogen a day for a period not to exceed 9 to 12 months. At the end of that time when

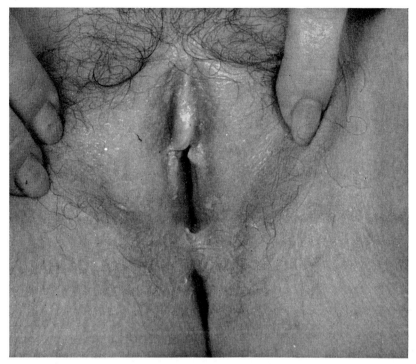

Figure 8.18.   External genitalia of patient with 45,X. The buccal smear of this patient was negative. (From H. W. Jones, Jr., and W. W. Scott: *Hermaphroditism, Genital Anomalies and Related Endocrine Disorders*, Ed. 2, Williams & Wilkins, Baltimore, 1971.)

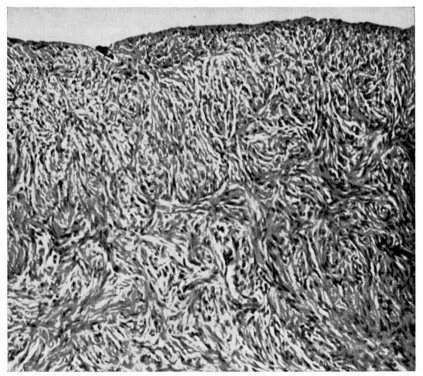

Figure 8.19.   Microscopic section through the genital ridge of a patient with streak gonads. Note that there is abundant stroma resembling ovarian stroma but no evidence of structures which would allow identification of either an ovary or a testicle.

secondary sex development is complete, it is important to reduce the dose to a maintenance figure of perhaps 0.6 mg a day or less or its equivalent in order to avoid the predisposition to endometrial cancer, which otherwise might be caused by unopposed high-dose prolonged estrogen action. Routine follow-up vaginal smears and endometrial sampling on a biannual basis are necessary to identify any early carcinoma of the endometrium.

Isochromosome X

As noted above, an isochromosome for the short arm of the X has probably not been well documented. On the other hand, many cases of isochromosome of the long arm of the X have been described, 46,X,i (Xq). These individuals have basically the Turner phenotype, as they are monosomic for the short arm of the X. The streak gonads of these patients are indistinguishable from the streak gonads of the 45,X patients both grossly and microscopically.

The treatment of these patients is identical with the treatment of patients with 45,X.

Ring X

Patients with Ring X are generally short, and in this respect they are very similar somatically to patients with 45,X. On the other hand, it is not at all unusual for patients with a Ring X chromosome to have a certain amount of spontaneous secondary sexual development and indeed to menstraute. A Ring chromosome implies there is some damage and probably loss of the tips of both the short arm and the long arm to enable healing to occur in a ring manner. It is the loss of the tip of the short arm which is responsible for the somatic expression. On the other hand, the loss of this small amount of genetic material does not always result in streak gonads, so that it is presumed that meiosis can take place at least for a sufficient number of cells to provide a certain amount of ovarian function. The ovaries of such a patient may be smaller than normal, but a biopsy of these ovaries does show oocytes which, through the light microscope, are no different from normal oocytes.

Pregnancy of a patient with a Ring chromosome has apparently not been reported.

Deletion of the Long Arm of the X Chromosome

Patients with deletion of the long arm of the X chromosome do not exhibit any somatic abnormalities. Thus, they are normally tall in contrast to patients who have loss of short arm material. However, because they do not have two normal X chromosomes, they do have streak gonads with the accompanying symptoms of high gonadotropins, failure of secondary sex development, and the like.

The treatment of these patients endocrinologically is the same as patients with streak gonads due to other chromosomal difficulties. No surgical treatment is required.

Other Structural X Anomalies

In addition to the anomalies already covered, various other anomalies of the X have been described (Table 8.4). Such patients have streak gonads and somatic anomalies in accordance with the presence or absence of the short arm of the abnormal chromosome.

Mosaicism

The karyotype-phenotype correlations recorded above apply only when mosaicism does not exist. In approximately 40% of individuals with streak gonads, mosaicism can be identified. In this circumstance, the karyotype-phenotype correlation is extremely difficult and apparently depends on the areas of the body occupied by one or another of the cell strains in the mosaic pattern. Most patients who have short stature and other somatic manifestations of Turner's syndrome, but who, nevertheless, have secondary sex development, menstruate and reproduce, are examples of a mosaic pattern. Although some patients with the Turner phenotype with menstruation and reproduction have not been found to be mosaic pattern, it needs to be remembered that the elimination of mosaicism by current methods of chromosome determination is almost impossible.

Polysomy X

The karyotype 47,XXX was described for the first time in 1959 by Jacobs, et al., under the name of "Super Female." However, it soon became apparent that this term was inappropriate, and it is seldom used. The disorder has a frequency of about 0.8 per

1,000 females. It is not associated with a recognizable syndrome at birth. According to the study of Robinson and his associates, it is characterized by birth weights that tend to be low but within normal limits. There is a higher than normal incidence of parents 35 years of age and older, and there is an increased incidence of clinodactyly. Full-scale IQ's are significantly lower in a portion of these individuals. It is often stated that approximately one-third of individuals have relatively normal or high IQ's, one-third have very average IQ's of approximately 100, and one-third have seriously depressed IQ's. This is consistent with the fact that the extra X chromosome undoubtedly has some active segments on the short arm which seem to interfere with mentation.

Secondary amenorrhea and premature menopause are common accompaniments, but there is no difficulty with puberty or secondary sex development. It is uncertain whether the menstrual difficulties are associated with the karyotype or associated with the psychogenic factors. Such patients can reproduce, and, for the most part, if they do reproduce, there is no chromosomal abnormality in their children.

The first description of a patient with 48,XXXX was in 1961 by Carr and his associates.

This disorder is quite rare and always associated with very serious mental retardation. In addition, various dysmorphias of the craniofacial area, thorax, and abdomen are common.

Secondary sexual development and menstruation are often normal, but amenorrhea or oligomennorhea is common. One woman with 48,XXXX gave birth to two children, each of whom had trisomy-21.

Patients with 49,XXXXX are quite rare, severely mentally handicapped, and have craniofacial and other dysmorphias.

Reproduction among such patients has apparently not been reported.

Y Chromosome Anomalies

Gynecologists encounter Y chromosome anomalies among the oligospermic or azoospermic husbands of infertile patients or in phenotypic females with amenorrhea where streak gonads may occasionally occur with a morphologically normal Y chromosome, but also when there is a structural abnormality of the Y chromosome.

Classification of Y Chromosome Anomalies

Y chromosome anomalies include patients with 46,XY in whom streaks have developed instead of testes. Such patients will have a female body type.

A second type of Y chromosome includes structural anomalies. Most frequently, because of the few bands on the Y chromosomes, the exact anomaly cannot be identified; such chromosomes are described as markers, but pericentric inversions, isochromosomes and deletions have been described.

A third group includes patients in whom there has been a translocation involving either the autosomes or the X chromosome with the Y.

Finally, polysomy (which includes 47,XYY, 48,XXYY, and 49,XYYYY) and Klinefelter's syndrome (which is typically 47,XXY but includes a variety of other karyotypes) are seen.

Phenotypic Discrepancies

Patients with a female body type with a karyotype 46,XY have been found to have streak gonads. These streaks on microscopic examination differ in no way from the streaks associated with other karyotypes. Individuals with 46,XY have no recognizable somatic abnormalities. They should not be labeled with the designation of Turner's syndrome, which implies shortness of stature and other characteristics of the Turner phenotype. Such patients have sometimes been referred to as having *pure gonadal dysgenesis*. Patients with other karyotypes also have pure gonadal dysgenesis, for example, patients with streak gonads and a female body type with a 46,XX karyotype.

These patients, of course, have no spontaneous secondary sex development or menstruation. They have female external genitalia, normal vaginas, and normal but infantile uteri. Their gonadotropins are at menopausal levels after the expected time of puberty. A number of such patients have been found to be normally positive for the H-Y antigen.

A special situation exists with the familial

type of XY streak gonads. A family studied by Ghosh et al. and another by Jones et al. (1979) showed that these patients were H-Y antigen negative. The mechanism of this is unclear. The pedigree of such patients clearly indicates that the disorder is an X-limited problem, and further study of this interesting phenonomen is obviously necessary.

Special mention should be made of the syndrome of normal female body type and 46,XY karyotype with spontaneous breast development. No such patient has apparently been reported with vaginal bleeding. Several such patients have been found to have gonadoblastomas in the streaks. In some instances, the gonadoblastoma has given rise to a dysgerminoma. It is thought that the presence of the tumor in the streaks stimulates the surrounding stroma to develop thecal estrogen production under the influence of the elevated gonadotropins. Presented with such a clinical situation, an x-ray of the lower abdomen will often reveal calcification in the gonadoblastoma.

Structural Anomalies

Because of the absence of a large number of bands on the Y chromosomes, it is often very difficult to determine precisely which part of a Y chromosome is missing. Therefore, there is a large literature on so-called marker chromosomes of the Y. Usually, these patients present with a female body type, streak gonads, and shortness of stature if the short arm of the Y chromosome is missing.

These patients have been particularly interesting to study for the H-Y antigen. The study of several patients with structural abnormalities of the Y chromosome seems to show rather conclusively that the locus which expresses the H-Y antigen is on the short arm of the Y, probably near the centromere. It is of interest that tumors of the streak can occur in patients with a negative H-Y antigen, so the H-Y antigen is of no clinical usefulness in ascertaining those patients with structural anomalies of the Y chromosome who are at high risk for tumor formation. This is perhaps not surprising, because the tumors which occur in these patients apparently arise from dysgenetic germ cells, and the H-Y antigen has been associated with testicular structure exclusive of germ cells.

As with all patients with Y chromosomes, removal of the streaks to prevent malignant tumor formation is recommended. Such patients who have a female body type will obviously need estrogen replacement therapy.

Translocations

A portion of the Y chromosome may be translocated either to an autosome or to an X chromosome. In such circumstances a female body type usually exists, and, in one patient reported by Park et al. (1974), the tumor formation in the streak caused sufficient estrogen not only for secondary sex development but for uterine bleeding, which was mistaken for normal menstruation.

As with all patients with a Y chromosome or a fragment of a Y chromosome, removal of the streaks is desirable to prevent serious tumor formation. Such patients must have substitution estrogen therapy.

Polysomy

Multiple Y Syndromes

The 47,XYY patient and others with even three or four Y's to one X chromosome are sometimes encountered as the oligospermic or azoospermic husband of an infertile patient. Originally, these patients were identified in screening mental and penal institutions, so it was thought that individuals with multiple Y chromosomes exhibited an aggressive tendency and were taller than expected. Further studies have tended to cast some doubt on this conclusion, and the matter has not been finally resolved. In reviewing the matter, Robinson and associates felt that no XYY syndrome could be identified, except for a possible skew to the lower levels in IQ scores. They felt that a longer period of follow-up was necessary before any final conclusions could be reached about the significance of the XYY karyotype.

As indicated above, oligospermia and azoospermia are not uncommon, although some such patients have apparently sired children.

Klinefelter's Syndrome

Patients with Klinefelter's syndrome typically have a karyotype of 47,XXY but might have a variety of other karyotypes with multiple X's and multiple Y's. These individuals are encountered as the azoospermic husbands of infertile patients. There are a number of somatic abnormalities described with this group of patients. According to Robinson et al., approximately 18% of such individuals have cleft palate, inguinal hernia, unilateral agenesis, and other somatic difficulties. A wide spread of full-scale IQ's has been described, but about one-third of patients have significantly depressed IQ's (below 90).

The testes are small, gynecomastia is common, and hyalinization or atrophy of the seminiferous tubules is characteristic. Germ cells are generally absent, and reproduction is not to be anticipated in this group of patients.

References and Additional Readings

Amrhein, M. A., Meyer, W. M., III, Jones, H. W., Jr., and Jones, G. S.: Methyltestosterone treatment of infertility associated with pelvic endometriosis. Proc. Natl. Acad. Sci. U.S.A., *73:* 891, 1976.

Bowman, J. A., Jr., and Scott, R. B.: Transverse vaginal septum. Obstet. Gynecol., *3:* 441, 1954.

Carr, D. H., Barr, M. L., and Plunkett, E. R.: An XXXX sex chromosome complex in two mentally defective females. Can. Med. Assoc. J. *84:* 131, 1961.

Garcia, J., and Jones, H. W., Jr.: The split thickness graft technique for vaginal agenesis. Am. J. Obstet. Gynecol., *49:* 328, 1977.

Ghosh, S. N., Shah, P. N., Rharpere, H. M., and Atherya, U.: H-Y antigen in human intersexuality. Clin. Genet., *14:* 31, 1978.

Jacobs, P. A., Baikie, A. G., Court-Brown, W. N., MacGregor, T. N., MacLean, N., and Harnden, D. G.: Evidence for the existence of the human superfemale. Lancet, *2:* 423, 1959.

Jones, H. W., Jr.: A long look at the adrenogenital syndrome. Johns Hopkins Med. J., *145:* 143, 1979.

Jones, H. W., Jr., Ferguson-Smith, M. A., and Heller, R. H.: Pathology and cytogenetics of gonadal agenesis. Am. J. Obstet. Gynecol., *87:* 578, 1963.

Jones, H. W., Jr., Rary, J. M., Rock, J. A., and Cummings, D.: The role of the H-Y antigen in human sexual development. Johns Hopkins Med. J., *145:* 33, 1979.

Jones, H. W., Jr., and Scott, W. W.: *Hermaphroditism, Genital Anomalies and Related Endocrine Disorders,* Ed. 2. Williams & Wilkins, Baltimore, 1971.

Jones, H. W., Jr., Turner, H. H., and Ferguson-Smith, M. A.: Turner's syndrome and phenotype. Lancet, *1:* 1155, 1966.

Jones, H. W., Jr., and Wheeless, C. R.: The salvage of the reproductive potential of women with anomalous development of the mullerian ducts: 1869–1968–2068. Am. J. Obstet. Gynecol., *104:* 348, 1969.

Klinefelter, H. F., Reinfenstein, E. C., and Albright, F.: Syndrome characterized by gynecomastia, aspermatogenesis, without aleydigism and increased excretion of follicle stimulating hormone. J. Clin. Endocrinol., *2:* 615, 1942.

Manuel, M., Katayama, K. P., and Jones, H. W., Jr.: The age of occurrence of gonadal tumors in intersex patients with a Y chromosome. Am. J. Obstet. Gynecol., *124:* 300, 1976.

McIndoe, A.: Discussion on treatment of congenital absence of vagina with emphasis on long term results. Proc. R. Soc. Med., *52:* 952, 1959.

McKusick, V. A., Bauer, L., Koap, C. E., and Scott, B.: Hydrometrocolpos as a simply inherited malformation. J.A.M.A., *189:* 813, 1964.

Milet, R. G., Plunkett, E. R., and Carr, D. H.: Gonadal dysgenesis with XX-isochromosome constitution and abnormal thyroid patterns. Acta Endocrinol., *54:* 609, 1967.

Park, I. J., Heller, R. H., Jones, H. W., Jr., and Woodruff, J. D. Apparent pseudo-puberty in a phenotype female with a gondal tumor. Am. J. Obstet. Gynecol., *119:* 661, 1974.

Park, I. J., Aïmakhu, V. E., and Jones, H. W., Jr.: An etiologic and pathogenetic classification of male hermaphroditism. Am. J. Obstet. Gynecol., *123:* 505, 1975.

Park, I. J., Burnett, L. S., Jones, H. W., Jr., Migeon, C. J., and Blizzard, R. M.: A case of male pseudohermaphroditism associated with elevated LH, normal FSH and low testosterone possible due to the secretion of an abnormal LH molecule. Acta Endocrinol., *83:* 173, 1976.

Park, I. J., Jones, H. W., Jr., Nager, G. T., Chen, S. C. A., and Hussels, I. E.: A new syndrome in two unrelated females: Klippel-Feil deformity, conductive deafness and absent vagina. Birth Defects, *8:* 311, 1971.

Robinson, A., Lubs, H. A., Nielsen, J., and Sorensen, K.: Summary of clinical findings: Profiles of children with 47,XXY, 47,XXX and 47,XYY karyotypes. Birth Defects, *15:* 261, 1979.

Rock, J. A., and Jones, H. W., Jr.: The clinical management of the double uterus. Fertil. Steril., *28:* 798, 1977.

van Niekerk, W. A.: *True Hermaphroditism.* Harper and Row, Hagerstown, Md., 1974.

Wharton, L. R.: Two cases of supernumerary ovary and one of accessory ovary with an analysis of previously recorded cases. Am. J. Obstet. Gynecol., *78:* 1101, 1959.

Wilkins, L., Lewis, R., Klein, R., and Rosemberg, E.: The suppression of androgen secretion by cortisone in a case of congenital adrenal hyperplasia. Bull Johns Hopkins Hosp., *86:* 249, 1950.

CHAPTER 9

Diseases of the Vulva

INFLAMMATORY DISEASE

The vulvar skin, of ectodermal origin, may be the site of any and all of the common dermatologic diseases. Furthermore, it is subjected to a great variety of local irritants—vaginal discharges, menstrual fluids, urine, and feces, as well as the secretion from the skin glands. As a final insult, these secretions are retained by tight, synthetic underwear, girdles, panty hose, and "slacks." Consequently, in the treatment of any vulvar irritation it is imperative to instruct the patient carefully as to local measures that should be instigated, regardless of the basic pathologic process. These include the use of loose cotton underclothing; the removal of undergarments that retain secretions in the anogenital area; the employment of drying agents (nonperfumed powder); the elimination of potentially irritating local agents (e.g., hygiene sprays, topical anesthetic agents, perfumed soaps, etc.) to which the tender vulvar skin may be sensitive; and a careful perineal toilet.

Intertrigo is common in the interlabial and crural folds, as in any area where moist folds of integument are constantly opposed. Treatment consists of drying powders, elimination of tight undergarments, and fluorinated hydrocortisone preparations for the elimination of the pruritus.

Seborrhea and Seborrheic Dermatitis. As with intertrigo, the excessive secretion of the sebaceous glands onto both labial folds produces an irritation which in the later stages demonstrates crushing and scaling of the skin.

Neurodermatitis has become a "waste basket," because any chronic irritative condition which does not seem to fall into a specific category may be labeled "neurodermatitis" since the patient is "nervous." In many instances, a careful history and examination will reveal the precipitating feature, and a diagnosis of "reactive dermatitis" would not only be more realistic but would assist the patient in preventing recurrences. The use of topical anesthetic agents, hygiene sprays, perfumed soaps or powders, strong detergents, and a host of other local irritants may be uncovered with a careful history.

Psoriasis is uncommon on the vulva. Nevertheless, vulvar psoriasis often does not appear as the classic lesion noted above but may be quite nonspecific. Correct diagnosis will lead to more appropriate therapy.

Moniliasis is currently the most common of the vulvar infections. It most frequently appears as a vulvovaginitis and is associated with severe pruritus. These mycotic infections may be associated with diabetes and its characteristic "beefy-red" vulva. The recognition of the combined etiologies depends obviously on careful urinalysis and blood sugar evaluations and on the demonstration of the offending organisms in vaginal smears. It should be appreciated that these infections not uncommonly follow the use of systemic antibiotics (See Chapter 10.) Therapy with one of the currently available fungicides such as Monastat, Mycostatin, or Lotrimin is usually satisfactory. Treatment should be continued daily for 7 to 10 days and the agent then used for 2 to 3 days pre- and postmenstrually for 3 months. Recurrences may be treated in the office by the use of 1% aqueous gentian violet. The cervix, vagina, and vulva should be painted thoroughly with the agent. Follow-up treatment with one of the above agents for 7 days is recommended.

Trichomonas and other vaginitides may cause minor pruritus, but these are reaction rather than direct infections.

DISEASES OF THE VESTIBULAR GLANDS

Since Bartholin's gland is commonly classed as one of the constituent structures of the vulva, a discussion of its diseases and those associated with the minor vestibular glands is properly included in this chapter. The lesions of these glands are either inflammatory or neoplastic, the former extremely common, the latter very rare.

Inflammation (Bartholin Adenitis)

Historically, in the majority of cases the causative organism has been the Gonococcus. There is no question, however, that other organisms may at times be the primary agents.

In the acute stage the major and most prominent gland becomes turgid, swollen, and painful, and a purulent exudate can be expressed from the duct by gentle pressure or may issue from it spontaneously. Abscess is a common sequel, manifesting itself by fluctuation and the associated edema may produce enormous swelling of the entire labium (Fig. 9.1).

Treatment. The treatment should consist of bed rest, sufficient analgesics to relieve the pain, local thermotherapy (ice pack or hot sitz baths), and antibacterial therapy. When abscess formation is evident, incision with drainage affords immediate relief. Marsupialization of the sac in the recurrent case may be attempted but is usually not successful in the acute stage due to the associated induration and edema.

Chronic Bartholin Adenitis

Chronic Bartholin adenitis may persist for many years. The only clinical evidence of the disease is the presence of a small nodular swelling, palpable deep beneath the posterior portion of the labium majus. The course of chronic bartholinitis may be punctuated by acute exacerbations, and, in the chronic cases, as a result of occlusion of either the main duct or one of its subdivisions, cysts of Bartholin's duct commonly develop and may undergo suppuration with abscess formation.

The pathological changes in chronic Bartholin adenitis are those characteristic of any chronic inflammation. Normally the main duct is lined by transitional epithelium, whereas a single layer of flattened cells lines

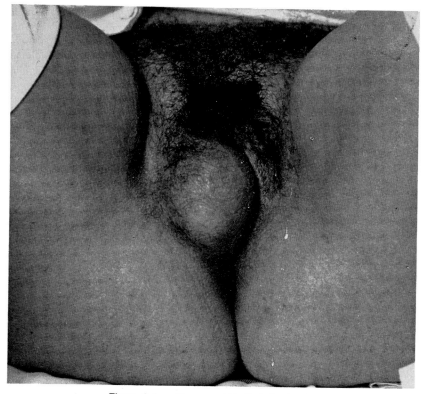

Figure 9.1. Abscess of Bartholin's gland.

the smaller branches. Severe inflammation may destroy all epithelium; however, the mucus-secreting acini are almost always demonstrable in the deeper tissues.

Treatment. No therapy is necessary for the asymptomatic chronically infected Bartholin gland or cyst. Simple marsupialization is quite efficacious for the uncomplicated cysts and may be an office procedure with the use of the "Word" catheter. However, when recurrent infection has been the problem, it is necessary to remove not only the cyst but the entire infected gland.

In addition to this major vestibular or Bartholin gland, it must be appreciated that the introitus contains many minor vestibular glands which may be the site of inflammation. The latter pose two problems. Often the patient complains of irritation, particularly with coitus, and small erythematous areas are noted at the outlet. These are difficult to eradicate, and biopsy of the foci may be taken. Often these are misinterpreted histologically because the duct is lined by transitional epithelium which may be interpreted as atypical due to the absence of "stratification."

HIDRADENITIS

Special consideration should be given to the infections which involve the apocrine system since they are unique to the areas which contain these specialized glands. The disease so commonly seen in the axilla and associated with local irritations is replicated in the vulva. This may lead to extensive tissue destruction, draining sinuses, and lymphedema, thus, simulating lymphopathia. In the mild case of recurrent pustule formation, the disease process may be modified by the use of oral contraceptives, which reduce the secretion of these specialized, cyclically functioning glands. Similarly the intense pruritus associated with focal dilatation of the glands, known as *Fox-Fordyce disease*, may be reduced strikingly with the use of such agents. In the later, the vulva is dotted with fine, slightly elevated papules.

Finally, in the patient with extensive suppurative disease, it may be necessary to perform wide, debriding surgery in an effort to stem the destructive process which has, on occasion, led to total vulvectomy and skin grafting.

ULCERATIVE LESIONS

Nonspecific Factitious and Aphthous Ulcers, Behçet's Disease and Crohn's Disease

Nonspecific conditions, previously designated as the acute ulcer of Lipschutz, may affect either the vulva or the lower vagina, the latter being more frequent. They appear as shallow, rounded, or oval lesions (Fig. 9.2) which produce only slight local discomfort and which are readily amenable to simple antiseptic treatment. The causative agent has been said to be *Bacillus crassus*, a normal inhabitant of the vagina; however, this is patently untrue. Such lesions may be due to local trauma (aphthous) and are evanescent. They may be self-inflicted (factitious) in the patient who is attempting to avoid coitus, or due to systemic disease such as lupus.

Behçet's "triple symptom syndrome" classically presents as recurrent ulcerations on vulvar and buccal mucous surfaces with irits or iridocyclitis. The latter may result in involvement of the central nervous system and death. Considered generally to be an autoimmune disease, cortisone is the currently accepted therapy, although recurrences are common.

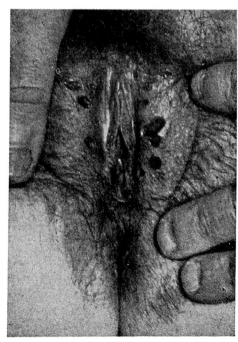

Figure 9.2.   Ulcus vulvae acutum; Lipschutz ulcer.

Crohn's disease may appear on the vulva as a diffuse ulcerative process. More commonly fistulae or draining sinuses develop in the perineum. The resultant rectovaginal fistula or destruction of the sphincter cannot be treated surgically without pre- and postoperative cortisone therapy.

CLASSIC VENEREAL DISEASES (SEXUALLY TRANSMITTED)

Chancroid (Soft Chancre, Ulcus Molle)

This lesion belongs to the group of venereal infections transmitted by coitus. The etiological agent is *Haemophilus ducreyi* which can be demonstrated in scrapings made from the base of the shallow ulcerations. The initial lesion presents as a small papule or pustule which appears within 2 or 3 days of exposure and progresses to ulceration but little induration. Characteristically, this ulcerative lesion is painful at the onset, thus differing from the majority of the other so-called "venereal diseases." Inguinal adenitis is frequent.

Diagnosis. The diagnosis of chancroid is based on the history of exposure, the short latent period of usually 2 to 4 days, the clinical characteristics of the ulcer as described above, especially the painful nature of the primary lesion, the usual absence of induration, and the demonstration of the Ducrey bacillus in smears or scrapings from the ulcer.

Treatment. The treatment of chancroid is meticulous cleanliness and the use of local antiseptics and sulfonamides, together with chloromycetin, achromycin, or other antibiotics.

Syphilis

(1) Chancre. This, the initial lesion of syphilis, is observed less commonly in women than in men. Chancre is recognized much more frequently on the vulva than in the vagina or cervix because the vaginal and cervical lesions are rarely visible or definitive. The lesion does not appear until 3 or 4 weeks after exposure. In many cases the initial lesion undoubtedly is overlooked due to its transient nature and minimal symptomatology.

The vulvar chancre presents as a rounded or ovoid ulcer with raised, indurated edges and a depressed center (Plate 9.4). It appears usually on the labium majus, in which case there may be considerable surrounding edema. There is marked associated inguinal lymphadenitis. The initial lesion usually regresses spontaneously in 4 to 6 weeks.

It must be emphasized that any ulcerative lesion, regardless of its apparent noncharacteristic appearance, must be suspect and thoroughly studied prior to any therapy.

Diagnosis. The diagnosis of syphilis in this primary stage is dependent upon the demonstration of the spirochete in the lesion. By firmly squeezing the lesion, droplets of lymph may be made to exude, and, if positive, examination of this transudate by the dark-field technique will reveal the characteristic spirochetes recognized by the corkscrew-like activity that is particularly well demonstrated by the fluorescent technique.

(2) Secondary Lesions—Condyloma Latum. The typical secondary lesion observed in the vulvar area is the condyloma latum, which often occurs simultaneously with the cutaneous macules or papules. The typical syphilitic condylomas are slightly raised, round or oval, plateau-like lesions of various sizes. The edges are slightly indurated, and the surface is moist, covered with a grayish necrotic exudate. The condylomas not only cover the vulva but extend to the surrounding perineum, the inner side of the upper thighs, and the buttocks. Again there is marked lymphadenitis.

The microscopic examination is made by the same technique as described for the initial lesion. In this stage, corroborative evidence for the existence of syphilis can be obtained from blood tests, which by this time are routinely positive.

The common treatment is 7 to 8 million units of penicillin given over a period of 5 to 7 days. The longer therapy is wise in an effort to prevent the Herxheimer reaction. Terramycin or similar antibiotics may be used in the patient sensitive to penicillin.

(3) Tertiary Syphilis—Gumma and Syphilitic Ulcer. Although the characteristic tertiary syphilitic lesion is the gumma, and although this may occur on the vulva, its tendency to necrosis and ulceration is so great that the most common tertiary lesion is the syphilitic ulcer. Such lesions are rarely seen today.

Granuloma Inguinale

This "venereal disease" presents primarily as single or multiple small ulcerations affecting the vulva and adjacent perineum. It is found especially in the tropics and the southern section of the U.S. It is of interest that granuloma may at times affect various extragenital sites, particularly the skin and bone.

The incubation period of this disease varies widely from a few days to several months. It usually begins as a small papular lesion on the labia minora or in the inguinal region, followed, in a few weeks, by ulceration which tends to assume a characteristic serpiginous form. The surface is reddish and granular and there is a considerable seropurulent exudate. By contrast with some of the other chronic ulerative vulvar lesions, the lesions of granuloma tend to remain superficial. Inguinal lymphadenopathy with suppuration rarely occurs.

The microscopic picture of the disease is characterized by an initial stage of subcutaneous infiltration with plasma cells, leukocytes, and large mononuclear cells, after which typical granulation tissue is formed. There is now general agreement that the disease can be transmitted by the Donovan inclusion, variously believed to be viral, bacterial (the Donovan virus or bacillus), or protozoal (Fig. 9.3). This can be stained in tissues in 100% of the cases (von Haam) during the

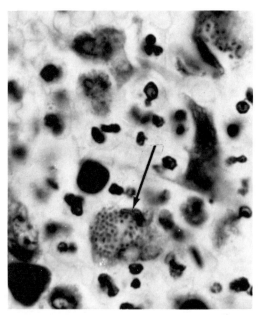

Figure 9.3. Donovan inclusions on smear or tissue specimen from acute or subacute lesion of granuloma inguinale.

acute stages of the disease. The Donovan inclusions are described as small encapsulated bodies resembling a "closed safety pin" as the result of the bipolar staining of the inclusions. In various southern clinics, a proportion of cases of vulvar carcinoma have been found to have been produced by granulomatous disease (Fig. 9.4).

Diagnosis. The diagnosis is made from the characteristic picture of the superficial granular inguinal lesion, together with the microscopic demonstration of the Donovan bodies. The lesion is generally more superficial and less painful than chancroid. Carcinoma and tuberculosis can be excluded by microscopic examination of excised tissue specimens.

Syphilis does not often produce lesions which resemble those of granuloma; however, as noted previously, all such ulcers must be studied by dark-field examination and serological test. Lymphogranuloma inguinale may present the greatest difficulty in its differentiation from granuloma. The former, however, is characterized by the frequent occurrence of subcutaneous suppurative foci, commonly diagnosed as acute, ulcerative, inguinale lymphadenitis, and which, in the later stages, are characterized by cicatricial stricture of the rectum or urethra.

Treatment. Antibiotics have superseded the heavy metals as effective therapeutic agents and usually 10 g of chloromycetin, either 1 g per day for 10 days or 2 g per day for 5 days, will result in complete regression of the local lesion. Other "mycins" have also proven to be effective therapeutic agents in the acute stage. In the chronic stages such therapy is less effective, and surgery may be necessary if the lesion is localized enough to permit removal. Extragenital dermatological, osseous, and ophthalmological manifestation of granuloma inguinale have been reported and may prove fatal.

Lymphopathia Venereum (Lymphogranuloma)

This chlamydial infection begins as an initial ulcerative lesion in the vagina, on the cervix, or on the external genitalia. The initial papule or pustule quickly disappears and is almost always overlooked. It is followed, however, by the appearance of inguinal suppuration or bubo formation. The condition seems to be essentially a disease of the lym-

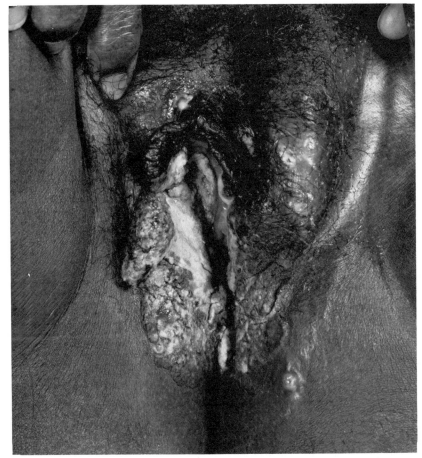

Figure 9.4. Carcinoma of vulva which has developed in granuloma inguinale (right labium). Donovan bodies were readily demonstrable.

phatics and/or associated with hypertrophic changes, lymphedema, and draining sinuses (Fig. 9.5).

If the ulcerative process dominates the picture, a large, ragged ulcer may be produced, surrounded by fibrous induration and edema. On the other hand, when the hypertrophic process predominates, marked lymphedema with leathery thickening of the skin produce a characteristic elephantiasis similar to the condition resulting from filariasis (Fig. 9.6). As with granuloma, extragenital lesions, particularly in the bowel and meninges, have been reported. During the stage of bubo formation, constitutional symptoms such as fever and malaise are commonly seen.

Mention has already been made in the preceding section that carcinoma has occasionally developed on the basis of either

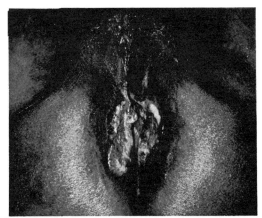

Figure 9.5. Carcinoma which has developed in lymphogranuloma venereum of vulva and vagina, extending up rectovaginal septum. In this case a 10-year salvage was achieved by vulvectomy plus posterior exenteration.

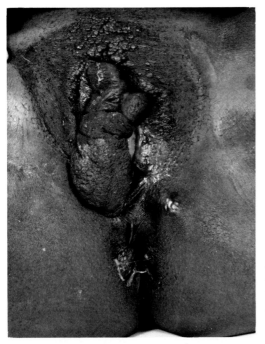

Figure 9.6. Elephantiasis of right labia and over mons with draining sinuses in left perineal and perirectal areas.

preexisting lymphopathia or granuloma (Fig. 9.5).

Diagnosis. Microscopically, the chief features are an extensive inflammatory reaction with focal microabscess formation. The latter produce the common "draining sinuses" (Fig. 9.6). Endothelial proliferation with pseudotubercle formation is characterized by central collections of polymorphonuclear cells rather than a "giant cell." The most striking feature is the proliferation and distortion of the epithelial rete pegs (pseudoepitheliomatous hyperplasia) (Fig. 9.7). Spread of the infecting agent through the lymphatics, with extensive inflammation and cicatrization of the endopelvic tissues, results in rectal and urethral strictures as well as fenestration of the vulvar structures.

The cause of lymphogranuloma is currently believed to be an organism of the Chlamydia family. The diagnosis is made by culture of the organism, *Chlamydia trachomatis.* Since the latter is an obligatory parasite, it must be grown in tissue culture. Skin reactions such as the Frei test or complement fixation may be used in the subacute or chronic phase.

Treatment. Tetracycline is the most effective during the early phases of the disease. Nevertheless, the local infection is generally self-limiting.

Surgical treatment is still occasionally necessary to excise the residual elephantitic masses. In the treatment of rectal strictures, colostomy may be required. With all granulomatous disease, multiple biopsy should be performed to exclude concomitant malignancy.

Virus Diseases

Among the many viruses that may attack the vulvar integument, the condyloma or wart virus and the herpes simplex (HSV) Type II are, at present, by far the most prevalent. The agents of molluscum contagiosum and undoubtedly other varieties of virus are probably extremely common but infrequently diagnosed.

Herpes Simplex (HSV)

Herpetic infections are probably one of the most common afflictions of the external genitalia. Nevertheless, the diagnosis is often not made since the initial vesicle is generally asymptomatic and the small, serpinginous superficial ulcerations are not recognized as the residuae of the ruptured and secondarily infected lesions (Figs. 9.8.) The latter ulcerations are often dramatic with extensive involvement of both labia, marked edema, and tender, enlarged inguinal lymph nodes. In view of the foregoing picture, care must be taken to rule out syphilis and granulomatous diseases.

The vagina and cervix may be simultaneously affected. Vaginal smears may demonstrate the presence of the typical intranuclear inclusions and multinucleate cell. Titers for herpes antibodies may be of value in differential diagnosis; however, the infections are so common that as high as 30 to 40% of any sexually active population may demonstrate positive reactions.

Pain is the most common complaint of the patient with vulvar herpes. On occasion, discomfort, fever, and malaise may be severe enough to demand hospitalization. Treatment of the secondarily infected vesicles with bed rest, local heat, and Burrow's solution (aluminum acetate) to reduce the edema produce much relief. Occasionally, hospitaliza-

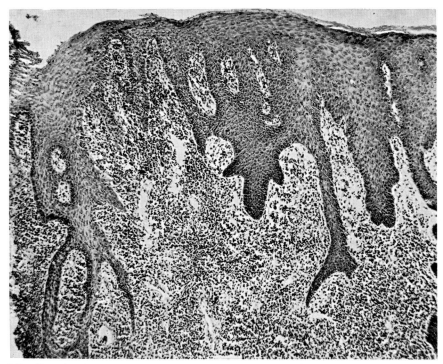

Figure 9.7. Pseudoepitheliomatous hyperplasia in granuloma inguinale showing marked elongation and irregularity of rete pegs suggesting anaplasia.

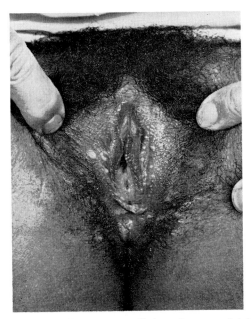

Figure 9.8. Numerous small, irregular, superficial ulcerations scattered over the inner surfaces of labia majora and adjacent perineum. Small vesicles could also be found in the immediate area.

tion for 24 to 48 hours is necessary to allow for concentrated therapy and rest. Unfortunately, antiviral agents such as Herplex, Stoxil, and the thiosemicarbazones are of little value after the vesicular stage. The use of tricyclic dyes such as 1% neutral red or 0.1% proflavin had been proposed as the treatment of choice. Double-blind studies have demonstrated that such agents afford no more relief than various topical medications, such as thymol (Listerine) and Betadine.

Latent herpes is common, although the recurrent lesions are usually less painful than the primary. The relationship between the viral diseases and cancer is circumstantial; nevertheless, the finding of specific antigens strengthens the case.

It must be recalled that although the acute disease probably produces only transient discomfort to the host, there is an additional problem during pregnancy more specifically at the time of delivery. Although the danger of infecting the newborn when an acute disease in the vulvovaginal area exists at the time of delivery may be minimal, nevertheless, that possibility should be kept in mind and cesarean section should be considered. (See Chapter 10.)

Molluscum Contagiosum

This viral infection is probably more common than generally appreciated since it rarely if ever produces symptoms except for a mild local irritation. The lesions are usually less than 1 cm in diameter and have a slightly umbilicated center. Treatment is accomplished by mere evacuation of the "waxy" core. Biopsy reveals the classic "molluscum bodies," which are intranuclear inclusions (Fig. 9.9).

For discussion of condylomata accuminata see "Benign Tumors of the Vulva."

WHITE LESIONS OF THE VULVA

Gross white appearance of the vulvar skin may be due to two general types of change,

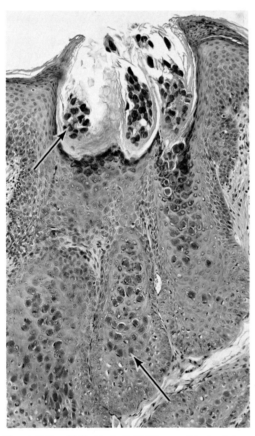

Figure 9.9. Molluscum contagiosum showing intranuclear inclusions (molluscum bodies) both at base and at surface (*arrows*) of the umbilication.

namely: (1) absence or loss of pigment and (2) increased keratinization (hyperkeratosis).

Classification of White Lesions

I. Depigmentation—leukoderma or vitiligo
II. Hyperkeratosis
  A. Chronic infections
  B. Benign tumors
  C. Dystrophies
    1. Lichen sclerosus
    2. Hyperplasia
      a. Typical
      b. Atypical
    3. Mixed (combination of 1 and 2)
  D. Carcinoma in situ
  E. Invasive cancer

Absence of Pigment or Depigmentation

Leukoderma or vitiligo may be due to a congenital or aquired absence of pigment. The congenital variety often appears at the menarche, suggesting a relationship between the pituitary gonadotrophes and the melanin-stimulating hormone. Frequently many areas of the body are involved, however the alterations seem to be more common in the anogenital area. Trauma, chronic infection, and radiation scarring are among the many causes of depigmentation.

Increased Keratinization (Hyperkeratosis)

Chronic Infection

The end result of chronic infection may be scarring, especially in those cases of the granulomatous diseases; however, the common dermatitides (eczamatoid, neuro, seborrheic, etc.) frequently demonstrate thickening of the skin with whitish change. Obviously, the latter description fits that of gross "leukoplakia"; unfortunately, the microscopic appearance also demonstrates the histologic characteristics suggested in most texts as typical of leukoplakia. Nevertheless, such changes are also typical of those seen with any chronic infection and have essentially no malignant potential.

Benign Tumors

Any of the papillomatous or verrucous lesions, in the chronic stages, may demonstrate areas of hyperkeratosis and whitish change.

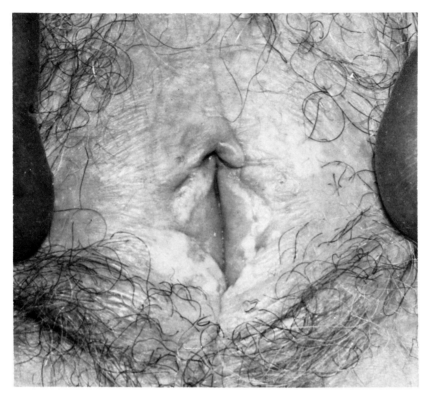

Figure 9.10. Markedly contracted introitus, with "leukoplakic" changes.

Dystrophies

Controversy as to the pathogenesis, clinical course, and particularly the malignant potential of these so-called primary hyperkeratotic lesions, frequently described as the leukoplakias, has been a continuing issue in the study of vulvar disease.

The many terms that have been applied to these primary hyperkeratoses need some interpretation (Figs. 9.10–9.12).

Leukoplakia has been used to describe a variety of whitish lesions since the term could be applied to any "white patch." Thus, because it has been so widely and poorly used, such a descriptive term cannot be applied to any specific lesion and thereby relay to the clinician information as to the degree of anaplastic potential. Consequently the general term of *dystrophy* has been substituted in an effort to develop a more clinicopathologically significant terminology. As noted in the "Classification of White Lesions," these alterations are divided into these with a thin parchment-like appearance (lichen sclerosus) and those covered with a thick layer of keratin and associated with varying degrees of

epithelial proliferations. Not infrequently the two varieties are appreciated in the same section.

Lichen Sclerosus. Lichen sclerosus applies to a skin lesion which begins as a small bluish white papule. Frequently coalescence of these papules produces a picture of diffuse whitish change over the entire vulva and perianal region (Fig. 9.13). In its terminal stage there

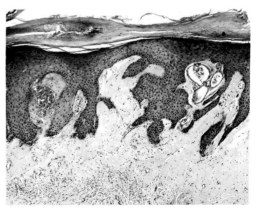

Figure 9.11. Hyperplastic alterations. Irregular rete pegs with collagenization of dermis, hyperkeratosis.

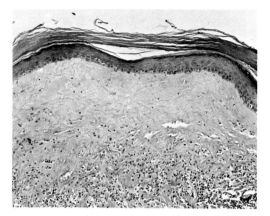

Figure 9.12. Lichen sclerosis with hyperkeratosis, thin epithelial layer, dermal collagenization, and inflammatory infiltrate.

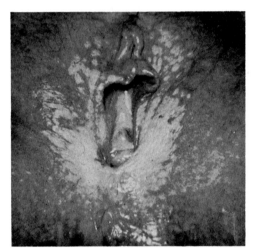

Figure 9.13. Lichen sclerosus in 56-year-old woman showing isolated lesions with confluence at fourchette.

is loss of the subcutaneous tissue with flattening of the labial folds and constriction of the outlet. The term "kraurosis" has been used to describe these terminal changes as if this was a specific disease. Actually kraurosis is simply a descriptive term meaning "shrinkage." The microscopic pictures of atrophic leukoplakia, lichen sclerosus et atrophicus, and kraurosis are similar.

Lichen sclerosus commonly appears in the early postmenopausal years. Nevertheless, similar patterns may be seen prepuberal and at any time during the menstruating years. Interestingly, these lesions initially are essentially asymptomatic and may remain so unless the collagenization becomes extensive. Similar lesions are frequently seen in other

areas, such as beneath the breasts and the lower abdomen.

Although the term atrophy has been applied to these lesions, certain studies have indicated that the thinned epithelium is not metabolically inactive. Although metabolic activity cannot be correlated directly with anaplasia, the changes do not justify the designation of atrophy. Furthermore, these lesions must be followed carefully, because carcinoma can develop in this context (Fig. 9.14). It is important to remember that any irritative lesion may become malignant, although the thickened, elevated, hyperkeratotic type seems to be more prone to anaplastic alteration. Of major importance in the study and therapy of the lesions are the regular biopsy of suspicious, focal areas of hyperkeratosis or superficial ulceration; and the elimination of scratching with the use of antipruritics, particularly hydrocortisones, intravaginal estrogens postmenopausal, the treatment of specific vaginitis, the removal of local irritating agents, and if necessary some variety of nerve

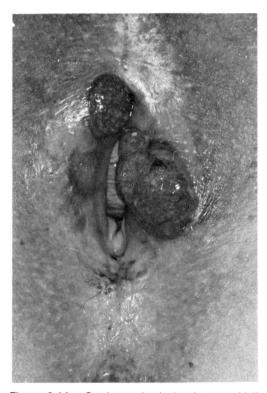

Figure 9.14. Carcinoma beginning in "atrophic" area. Patient had had partial excision of a lesion showing atypical hyperplasia and lichen sclerosus (mixed dystrophy) 4 years prior to the appearance of gross cancer.

block. Plastic procedures to increase the caliber of outlet are often necessary to eliminate
dyspareunia and allow for satisfactory coitus.
Vulvectomy is indicated only if anaplastic
changes are noted in the tissue study.

Hyperplasia. The term "hyperplasia" denotes an increase in the number of normal
cellular elements in a specific situation. More
specifically, to the term hyperplasia is added
the designations typical or atypical to connote
the degree of proliferation and its malignant
potential. Consequently, these terms have
been applied to the general designation of
"dystrophy" in order to assist the clinician in
his evaluation and treatment of the specific
case.

Obviously, in order to make such interpretation, *biopsy must be taken.* The importance
of this procedure cannot be overemphasized.
The instrument which seems most effective is
the Keyes punch, and the biopsy can be
performed under local anesthesia.

The malignant potential of hyperplastic
lesions obviously depends on the degree of
cellular aberration. Particularly significant is
the abnormal maturation of the epithelial
cells in the basal layer. It should go without
saying that the more active the therapy in
elimination of pruritus, the less the possibility
of the development of neoplasia.

Finally, it must be recognized that carcinoma in situ (Fig. 9.15) and invasive cancer
can and frequently do appear as whitish lesions. As a consequence, any hyperkeratotic
area must be biopsied and followed carefully.

Pruritus Vulvae

This term, in the past, has been used as if
it designated a specific disease entity. Obviously, however, pruritis describes only the
symptom of "itching." As noted previously,
almost all of the common dermatitides and
local irritants produce itching, inasmuch as it
is primarily due to an inflammatory reaction
about the underlying nerves. Various vaginal
infections produce a "reactive dermatitis"
with its concomitant pruritus. Systemic diseases associated with itching as well as gross
alterations such as lymphedema have been
described earlier. Thus the term "pruritus
vulvae" becomes a description of a symptom
and should *not* be used to identify a disease
entity.

Both estrogen and androgens have been
proposed as therapy for certain specific con-

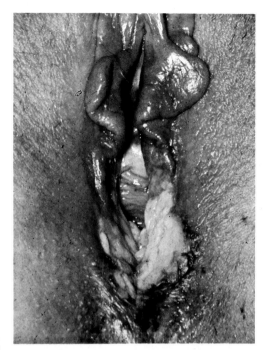

Figure 9.15. White, hyperkeratotic lesion occupying the area of the fourchette. Biopsy showed cancer
in situ.

ditions. It must be stated that, although local
estrogenic creams thicken the vaginal epithelium (see Chapter 10), they soften the integument and are not helpful in the treatment of
pruritus. Nevertheless, if the patient is postmenopausal, the elimination of the "weepy"
thin discharge from the thin vaginal epithelium by the use of intravaginal estrogen is an
important adjunctive therapy.

Conversely, local testosterone preparations
are most effective in the treatment of the
pruritus associated with the thin vulvar skin
of the patient with lichen sclerosus. Testosterone thickens the skin, improves the nutrition of the tissues, and eliminates or modifies
the pruritus in a majority of such cases. A 1
or 2% preparation used twice a day for a
month and then every day indefinitely is the
generally prescribed routine of therapy. Following this regime, if successful, the agent
should be used at intervals, possibly one to
two times a week to maintain the local reaction. It should also be noted that the troublesome symptom of "vulvar burning" may be
treated in this manner.

Alcohol Injection. The injection of 95% alcohol subcutaneously by the technique recommended by Stone for pruritus ani has been

employed also for pruritus vulvae. This procedure should only be used in chronic conditions when medications have failed. Unfortunately, it may be followed by sloughing in the vulvar or anal region if used inappropriately. Only 0.2 ml of 95% or absolute alcohol is injected beneath the dermis, needle punctures situated about 1 cm apart. Various plans of incising the labial skin at the outer border of majora with undercutting and disruption of the sensory nerves have been suggested by Mering, but it is important to evaluate each case very critically as the author suggests. Such procedures have the value of preserving normal anatomy. Vulvectomy should be performed only if biopsies demonstrate definite premalignant changes.

Whatever the type of therapy, abolition of the scratch reflex seems desirable, for it is possible that repeated mechanical trauma may be the stimulus that leads to carcinoma.

BENIGN TUMORS OF THE VULVA

Cystic
1. Bartholin duct cysts
2. Sebaceous or inclusion cysts
3. Mucinous cysts
4. Wolffian duct cysts
5. Cyst of the canal of Nuck
6. Endometriosis

Solid
1. Fibroma
2. Lipoma
3. Verrucous lesions (condyloma acuminatum)
4. Angioma
5. Hidradenoma
6. Granular cell myoblastoma
7. Nevus

Cystic

Bartholin Duct Cysts

These have been discussed under "Disease of the Vestibular Glands" in this chapter.

Sebaceous or Inclusion Cysts

These result from inflammatory blockage of the ducts of sebaceous glands and are usually small (Fig. 9.16). They contain a cheesy, sebaceous material and are prone to suppuration, with the formation of small furuncle-like abscesses. If very small and

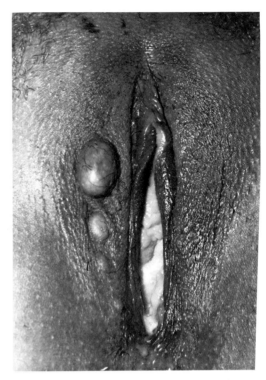

Figure 9.16. Inclusion cysts on right labium majus (usually the result of sebaceous gland infection).

asymptomatic, no treatment is necessary, but if they are sufficiently large to be annoying, or if they are recurrently infected, simple excision under local anesthesia is indicated.

In the infectious stage, the cavity has no specific lining but instead is filled with polymorphonuclear and foreign body giant cells. In the chronic stage, the cavity is lined by stratified epithelium and, thus, is classifed as an "inclusion" cyst.

Mucinous Cysts

Occasionally noted near the urethra or inner surfaces of the labia minora, mucinous cysts are probably of embryonic origin. The time of separation of the cloaca by the urorectal fold into urogenital sinus and rectum, elements, originally destined to be rectal endoderm, may be displaced toward the urogenital side and subsequently develop into cystic structures of various sizes, often pedunculated. Nevertheless, as noted by Friedrich and Wilkerson, most of the small cysts which appear at the outlet are mucinous, and probably represent dilation of the minor vestibular glands.

Wolffian Duct Cysts

These mesonephric remnants rarely appear on the vulva, but if they attain any size, they may project at the outlet.

Cyst of the Canal of Nuck (Hydrocele)

The round ligament inserts into the labium major and carries with it an investment of the peritoneum. The latter is usually firmly attached to its ligament, but it may at any point be divorced from its attachment and fluid may accumulate, forming a cystic dilation (Fig. 9.17). Such may present in the labium at the point of insertion and corresponds to the hydrocele in the male.

Endometriosis

Endometriosis in the vulva is rare and most commonly seen in the region of the Bartholin gland, suggesting possible implantation at the time of surgery or drainage of a cyst or abscess. Such lesions may develop in the inguinal canal and along the round ligament into the upper labium majus. Cyclic recurrence of a painful nodule should suggest this possible diagnosis.

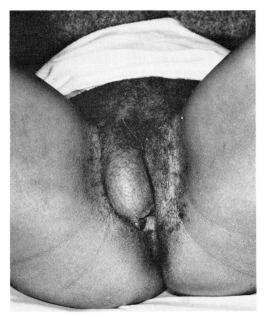

Figure 9.17.   Hydrocele of the canal of Nuck. Aspirated unsuccessfully and later excised.

Solid

Fibroma

Fibromas arise from the fibrous tissue of the vulva and are usually of small or moderate size (Fig. 9.18). They tend to become pedunculated, especially if large and lymphadenomatous, and tumors of this sort have sometimes reached almost unbelievable size, the classical case reported by Buckner (1851) attaining a weight of 268 pounds. The microscopic structure is that of fibrous tissue, usually light textured and edematous. Treatment is, of course, surgical.

Lipoma

In spite of the considerable amount of adipose tissue in the vulva, especially in the labia majora, lipoma is rare. It has the same clinical characteristics as those described for fibroma and the distinction is not always possible until microscopic examination. Both lipoma and the soft, nonpedunculated fibroma must be differentiated from the spongy varicocele.

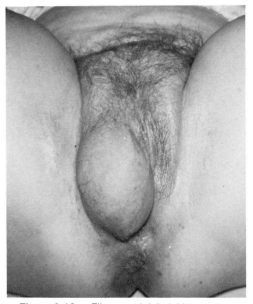

Figure 9.18.   Fibroma of right labium majus.

Verrucous Lesions

The most common form of vulvar verruca is that designated as condyloma acuminatum, to be distinguished from condyloma latum, the secondary syphilitic lesion. Pathologically the condyloma acuminatum has a treelike structure, with a central core of connective tissue covered with a hyperplastic epithelium characterized by elongated rete pegs (acanthosis) and superficial parakeratosis. The stroma is edematous and infiltrated with chronic inflammatory cells. Since they are of viral origin, transmission by coitus is the common mode of infection.

Clinically, condylomata acuminata appear in the form of warty growths of various sizes which are usually multiple and which are discretely scattered over the vulva, adjacent perineum, buttocks, and inner thighs (Fig. 9.19). They are also found in the vagina, and on the cervix.

When numerous, they tend to become confluent, forming large clusters. They undergo pronounced hypertrophy during pregnancy, sometimes forming huge cauliflower masses which may even offer obstacles to vaginal delivery. Actually, many regress spontaneously postpartum if removal is not necessary during pregnancy. Malignancy may develop in such lesions.

Topical applications of 20% podophyllin in tincture of benzoin are quite effective in the treatment of the smaller lesions. Treatment of associated infections, such as trichomoniasis and moniliasis, is of major significance to prevent recurrences. pH changes related to the use of oral contraceptives seem to promote the growth and recurrence of warts.

Surgical excision or fulguration may be necessary for larger lesions. More recently topical 5-FU (fluorouracil) has been used with effectiveness in some cases.

Angioma

Although angiomata are rare, the congenital type occasionally cause problems due to irritations of diapers, urine, and feces. It is important to remember that most of these congenital types regress as the child grows (Fig. 9.20), and therapy should not be instituted unless absolutely necessary.

Other angiomas, including the hyperkeratotic angiokeratoma, have been reported. Small hemorrhagic foci in the postmenopausal patient are usually tiny varicosities and may be the cause of postmenopausal bleeding. In the latter situation, however, other causes of the symptom must be ruled out.

Hidradenoma

Although this is a rare lesion, it is of importance because it is occasionally mistaken for adenocarcinoma microscopically (Fig. 9.21). The lesion arises from the vulvar sweat glands, and with rare exceptions it is benign.

Granular Cell Myoblastoma

This rather uncommon tumor, composed of irregular clumps of large pale-staining cells

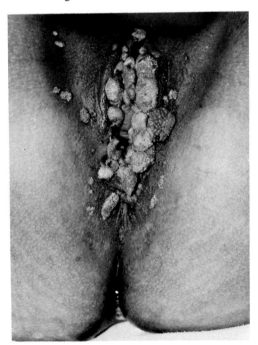

Figure 9.19.   Condylomata acuminata.

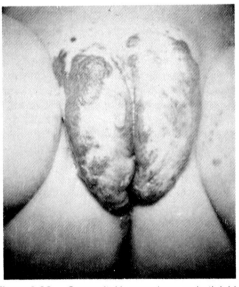

Figure 9.20.   Congenital hemangioma on both labia, appearing at 2 months of age. At 1 year it was much reduced without treatment.

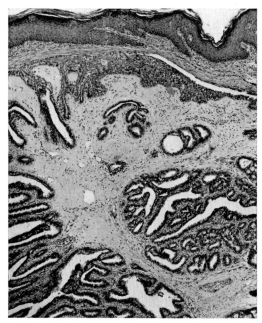

Figure 9.21. Hidradenoma of vulva. A rare lesion which may be mistaken for adenocarcinoma.

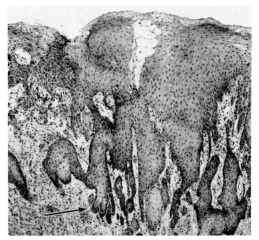

Figure 9.22. Granular cell myoblastoma showing extensive pseudoepitheliomatous hyperplasia simulating cancer. *Arrow* points to the underlying "granular" cells which lead to the correct diagnosis.

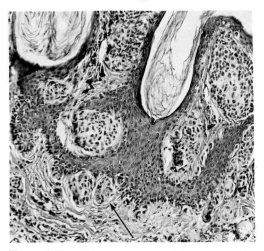

Figure 9.23. Nevus with marked junction activity (*arrow*).

with eosinophilic cytoplasmic granules, is most commonly noted in the tongue but has been recorded at many sites. Although called myoblastoma, the tumor is believed to arise from the myelin sheath of the nerve. Of interest is the pseudoepitheliomatous change in the overlying epithelium, suggesting and occasionally mistaken for cancer (Fig. 9.22).

Nevus

The nevus is an important lesion on the vulva. The vulvar skin makes up only 1–2% of the entire body surface, and 3 to 4% of malignant melanomata in the female occur on the external genitalia. Junction activity is common in the vulvar nevus and is of significance in the development of malignancy. Of particular significance is the flat, expanding pigmented lesion (Fig. 9.23). Biopsy of all pigmented lesions is of importance since only by this technique can malignancy be confirmed or eliminated.

CIRCULATORY DISEASES

Among circulatory disturbances involving the vulva, varices are perhaps the most common. They affect especially the labia majora and are more prominent unilaterally. Because the pampiniform plexus of veins is primarily involved, a varicocele, such as that so commonly seen in the male, may develop. A common cause of such venous distention is intrapelvic pressure from pregnancy or large tumors. The varices may become extremely large and may even rupture, with resultant bleeding. Most commonly however, the dilated veins appear as multiple small purplish elevations which simulate and are often mistaken for hemangiomata.

Edema of the vulva may be the result of intrapelvic pressure from large tumors, marked ascites, or metastatic tumor in the regional lymph nodes. Even furunculosis or the secondarily infected herpetic lesions may lead to significant degrees of vulvar edema or parasitic blockage of the vulvar lymphatics may cause "elephantiasis" most dramatically recognized in lymphogranuloma venereum. The edema of pregnancy is undoubtedly related to temporary lymphostasis resulting from pressure phenomena; nevertheless, local or diffuse swelling may be due to abnormal activity of the apocrine glands. It must be noted that, because the vulva is in the "milk line," normal breast tissue may be found in this area. Finally, lymphoedema may result from chronic debilitating disease such as anemia, multiple sclerosis, etc.

CARCINOMA OF THE VULVA

The most important of vulvar tumors is carcinoma, the third most common of all primary pelvic cancers, being exceeded in frequency only by uterine (cervix and corpus) and ovarian cancer. Vulvar cancer accounts for 3 to 4% of all primary malignancies of the genital canal.

Carcinoma *in situ* of the vulva is a definite entity, although far less common than its counterpart on the cervix. By definition, intraepithelial cervical cancer connotes full-thickness replacement of the lining epithelium by undifferentiated abnormal cells, often of basal type; similarly, intraepithelial cancer of the vulva shows abnormality of the lining epithelium with increased mitotic activity (Fig. 9.24). However, vulvar cancer is characteristically spinal in type, and some degree of differentiation of the component cells is often found despite undeniable intraepithelial anaplasia. A variety of terms such as Bowen's disease, erythroplasia of Quyrat, etc., have been used to describe types of in situ cancer, but basically the microscopic pictures are not sufficiently distinctive to be specific. Grossly, the anaplasias may appear as reddened, pigmented, whitish, or slightly elevated lesions and are commonly multicentric in origin.

With the apparent increase in the incidence of carcinoma in situ of the vulva has come the realization that certain lesions, histologically neoplastic, may in fact be reversible if, as noted by Friedrich, the alterations develop during pregnancy. Thus, it is obvious that, inasmuch as many are now noted in young women under 30 years of age, conservative therapy is in order.

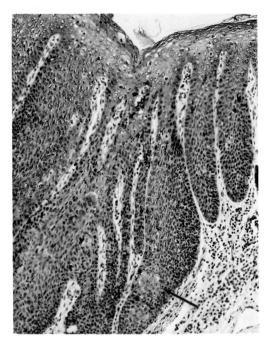

Figure 9.24. Microscopic appearance of carcinoma in situ with intraepithelial pearl formation and abnormal nuclear figures.

Treatment, in general, demands wide local excision if only a solitary lesion is present. Simple vulvectomy in the young patient rarely is necessary. It is imperative that the vulva and adjacent perineum, vagina, and cervix be thoroughly inspected, not only prior to any therapy, but also in the *follow-up* periods. Chemotherapy has been effective in certain instances. Most recently immunotherapy, in form of local DNCB(dinitrochlorobenzene) after sensitization of the patient has been employed.

Paget's disease is an uncommon multifocal disease which develops in the vulva and perineal area during the peri- and postmenopausal years (Fig. 9.25). The lesion is reddish with grayish white foci. Although 70 to 75% of such lesions are in situ, the involvement of the apocrine system is diffuse, and simple vulvectomy is the treatment of choice. Rarely in our estimation, is an underlying cancer found. Breasts should be thoroughly studied for the presence of occult cancer.

Invasive carcinoma is preeminently a disease of elderly women, the incidence being highest in the seventh decade. The exception occurs in those cases preceded by granulomatous disease where the average age is about 40 years as noted by Saltzstein et al., and

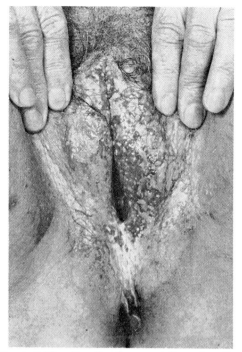

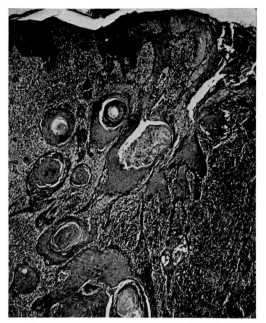

Figure 9.26.   Squamous cell carcinoma of the vulva showing classic "pearl formation."

Figure 9.25.   Paget's disease of the vulva. Dark areas are red in color, and white "leukoplakoid" areas are as seen.

Collins et al. The disease begins on any part of the vulva. The most common histological type is squamous cell carcinoma (Fig. 9.26), except in primary carcinoma of Bartholin's gland which may be either adenocarcinoma (cribriform), transitional, or epidermoid in character. In such instances a hard stony mass can be felt in the region of the gland.

The gross appearance may be whitish, ulcerated, or granulomatous depending on the primary lesion. As noted previously, several authors have reported the premalignant nature of the granulomatous and hyperplastic lesions.

Basal cell carcinoma is rare and appears as on the skin elsewhere as a superficial ulcer with "rolled" edges. Microscopically the cells "drop" from the basal layer of the epithelium and seem to invade the underlying tissue, however local excision results in a cure (Fig. 9.27).

In the usual forms of vulvar cancer, the initial lesion becomes steadily larger, with increasing induration, ulceration, and surrounding edema. Metastatic involvement of the superficial and deep inguinal and femoral glands soon develops.

The symptoms in the early stage are apt to

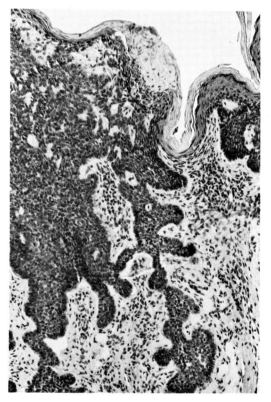

Figure 9.27.   Basal cell carcinoma showing the uniform basal cells "dropping" into the underlying tissue.

be very slight, consisting only of slight soreness and itching. In many instances, however, there is a history of long-standing pruritus antedating the appearance of carcinoma. As the ulceration and infiltration extend, the pain increases, and in advanced cases it may be persistent and intolerable.

Not uncommonly, there is an unfortunate delay of 1½ to 2 years between the appearance of symptoms and diagnosis of the disease. Much of this delay is due to reluctance of the older patient to seek medical consultation; however, in about one-third of the cases the physician is at fault. In the early stage the patient suffers very little discomfort, and the lesion may seem, even to the physician, a rather unimpressive one unless he is familiar with its potentialities. Biopsy and microscopic examination are of decisive importance. Upon this diagnostic procedure one must depend for the differentiation from other ulcerative lesions, such as tertiary syphilis or lymphogranuloma venereum.

Prophylaxis is of considerable importance, for it has been noted that both hyperplastic and various granulomatous or other irritative lesions are frequently percursors of cancer.

Treatment of Vulvar Cancer

The primary treatment for carcinoma of the vulva is surgery. Radical vulvectomy with inguinal and femoral lymphadenectomy is mandatory for invasive cancer. There is considerable difference of opinion as to how extensive the surgery should be. The presence of palpable nodes should not be the criterion, because in one-third of the cases nodal enlargement is due not to cancer but to infection. Likewise in one-third of the cases in which there is metastatic disease to the nodes, the nodes are not clinically enlarged.

The value of lymphadenectomy is argued, but does result in an increased 5-year salvage.

A one-stage vulvectomy and bilateral lymphadenectomy is accepted by most students as the procedure of choice (Fig. 9.28). Removal of, rather than undermining, the skin has resulted in better primary healing. The New Orleans approach (Collins et al.) is more radical, with an extended lymphadenectomy and freely performed exenteration if adjacent organs (vagina, urethra, or rectum) are involved without extrapelvic metastases. Many observers, believing that complete excision of the local disease is paramount to salvage, feel that vulvectomy with superficial node dissection (one-stage under local anesthesia) is adequate.

The lesion is slow to metastasize and usually does so in a superficial fashion. Consequently, for the well defined lesion, bilateral node dissection may not be necessary.

Other Vulvar Malignancies

Sarcoma of the vulva is exceedingly rare, only about 30 cases having been reported. Malignant melanoma is also rare; however, it is the second most common malignancy in the vulvar area. As in other parts of the body, its origin is usually in pigmented moles. Its tendency to widespread dissemination is well known, and a fatal termination is common. Symmonds et al. have reported improved results with early and radical surgery.

URETHRA

Although the urethra is technically not part of the genital canal, the diseases that affect the area commonly involve the genitalia. Urethral infection is often gonococcal. Actually the urethra may be the primary organ invaded by the gonococcus, but the symptoms are usually very transient. Residua may remain in the urethral glands or Skene's ducts.

Many other organisms also involve the posterior portion of the urethra, as well as of the trigone. The clinician must be mindful of the possibility that the suburethral gland infection may result in the formation of a diverticulum. Palpation of the urethra may reveal a saclike outpouching from which pus can be "milked out" through the urethral meatus. Occasionally, endoscopic examinations with urethrographic studies, are necessary.

Surgical excision of a diverticulum is the preferred treatment. Helpful, particularly in the low-grade, chronic infections, is the topical application of 2 to 5% silver nitrate. If the immediately adjacent Skene's glands are involved, as indicated by expression of pus on palpation, they may be easily fulgurated.

A real but frequently overlooked entity is the postmenopausal senile or atrophic urethritis (Fig. 9.29). This frequently occurs in conjunction with a similar type of vaginitis as a sequel to estrogen deprivation. There is a reddening of the meatus as edema and prolapse of the urethral mucosal lining occur, and the resultant appearance is much like a

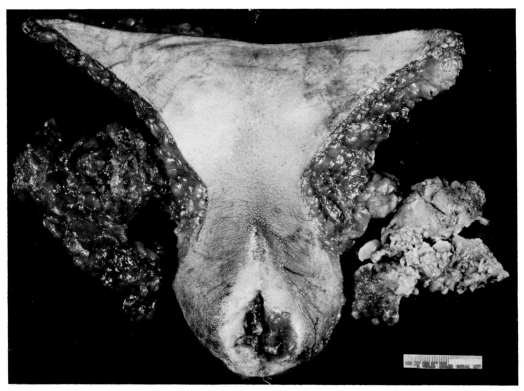

Figure 9.28.   Specimen from radical vulvectomy and node dissection. Lesion is seen on right lower vulva.

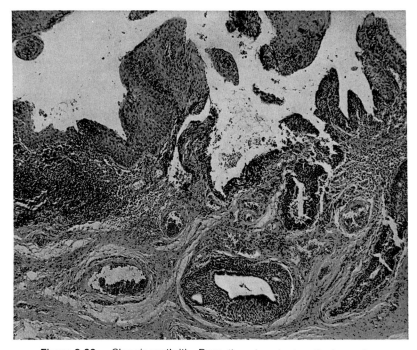

Figure 9.29.   Chronic urethriti⌣. Resection of marked urethral eversion.

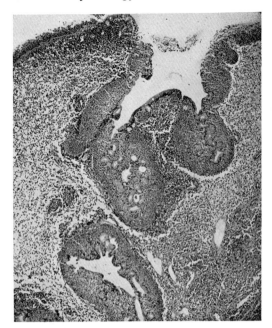

Figure 9.30. Microscopic appearance of uretnral caruncle of papillomatous type.

urethral caruncle. Local pain, terminal burning on urination, strangury, and even hematuria may occur, but prompt remission and relief are achieved by estrogen therapy. Fulguration, the preferred treatment for a caruncle, is not necessary in this form of urethral disease.

Benign tumors are uncommon, the most frequent being the caruncle (Fig. 9.30). This small, reddish, pedunculated lesion is occasionally tender and may bleed. Fulguration after biopsy is the treatment of choice.

The urethra may be the site of other pathological entities, such as stricture or fistula (frequently postirradiation or postoperative), granulomatous infection by lymphopathia or granuloma inguinale, prolapsed mucosa, and even carcinoma. Carcinoma is rare and carries a poor prognosis (less than 50%). Treatment is generally radiation, but occasionally radical surgical procedures are performed, particularly in the radiation-resistant lesion.

References and Additional Readings

Alexander, L. J., and Shields, T. L.: Squamous cell carcinoma of vulva secondary to granuloma inguinale. Arch. Dermatol., *67:* 395, 1953.

Birch, H. W., and Sondag, D. R.: Granular cell myoblastoma of the vulva. Obstet. Gynecol., *18:* 443, 1961.

Boschback, F. W.: Adenoid-cystic carcinoma of Bartholin gland. Geburtshilfe Frauenheilkd., *29:* 473, 1969.

Brack, C. B., and Dickson, R. J.: Carcinoma of the female urethra. Am. J. Roentgenol., *79:* 472, 1958.

Chung, J. T., and Greene, R. R.: Hidradenoma of vulva. Am. J. Obstet. Gynecol., *75:* 310, 1958.

Collins, C. G., Hansen, L. H., and Theriot, E.: Clinical stain for use in selecting biopsy sites in patients with vulvar disease. Obstet. Gynecol., *28:* 158, 1966.

Collins, C. G., Kushner, J., Lewis, G. N., and LaPointe, R.: Noninvasive malignancy of the vulva. Obstet. Gynecol., *6:* 339, 1955.

DiPaola, G. R., Balina, L. M., Gomez'Reuda, N. M., et al.: Treatment of lichen sclerosus et atrophicus of the vulva with topical testosterone. Rev. Argent. Ginecol. Obstet., *2:* 224, 1971.

DiSaia, P. J., Rutledge, F., and Smith, J. P.: Sarcoma of the vulva. Obstet. Gynecol., *38:* 180, 1971.

Friedrich, E. G.: Reversible vulvar atypia. Obstet. Gynecol., *39:* 173, 1972.

Friedrich, E. G.: *Vulvar Disease.* W. B. Saunders, Philadelphia, 1976.

Friedrich, E. G., Julian, C. G., and Woodruff, J. D.: Acridine orange fluorescence in vulvar dysplasia. Am. J. Obstet. Gynecol., *90:* 1281, 1964.

Freidrich, E. G., and Wilkerson, E. J.: Mucous cysts of the vulvar vestibule. Obstet. Gynecol. *42:* 407, 1973.

Hart, W. R.: Paramesonephric mucinous cysts of the vulva. Am. J. Obstet. Gynecol., *107:* 1079, 1970.

Hart, W. R., Norris, H. J., and Helwig, E. B.: Relation of lichen sclerosus et atrophicus of the vulva to development of carcinoma. Obstet. Gynecol., *45:* 369, 1975.

Hassim, A. M.: Bilateral fibroadenoma in supernumerary breasts of the vulva. J. Obstet. Gynaec. Br. Commonw., *76:* 275, 1969.

Hay, D. M., and Cole, F. M.: Post-granulomatous carcinoma of the vulva. Am. J. Obstet. Gynecol., *107:* 479, 1970.

Hester, L. J.: Granuloma venereum of cervix and vulva. Am. J. Obstet. Gynecol., *62:* 312, 1951.

Huffman, J. W.: Detailed anatomy of paraurethral ducts in adult human female. Am. J. Obstet. Gynecol., *55:* 86, 1948.

Hyman, A. B., and Falk, H. C.: White lesions of the vulva. Obstet. Gynecol., *12:* 407, 1958.

Japaze, H., Garcia-Bunuel, R., and Woodruff, J. D.: Primary vulvar neoplasia: A review of in-situ and invasive carcinoma, 1935–1972. Obstet. Gynecol., *49:* 404, 1977.

Jeffcoate, T. N. A.: Chronic vulval dystrophies. J. Obstet. Gynecol., *95:* 61, 1966.

Josey, W. E., Nahmias, A. J., Naib, Z. M., et al.: Genital herpes simplex infection in the female. Am. J. Obstet. Gynecol., *96:* 493, 1966.

Katayama, K. P., Woodruff, J. D., Jones, H. W., Jr., and Preston, E.: Chromosomes of condyloma acuminatum, Paget's disease, in-situ carcinoma, invasive squamous cell carcinoma and malignant melanoma of the human vulva. Obstet. Gynecol., *39:* 346, 1972.

Kaufman, R. H., Gardner, H. L., Brown, D., et al.: Vulvar dystrophies: an evaluation. Am. J. Obstet. Gynecol., *120:* 363, 1974.

Lang, W. R.: Genital infections in female children. Clin. Obstet. Gynecol., *2:* 428, 1959.

Langley, I. I., Hertig, A. T., and Smith, G. van S.: Relation of leucoplakic vulvitis to squamous carcinoma of vulva. Am. J. Obstet. Gynecol., *62:* 167, 1951.

Lipschutz, B.: Ulcus vulvae actum. In *Jadassohn's Handbuch der Haut-und Geschlechtskrankheiten.* Julius Springer, Berlin, 1927.

Marcus, S. L.: Basal cell and basal-squamous cell carcinomas of the vulva. Am. J. Obstet. Gynecol., *79:* 461, 1960.

Matthews, D.: Marsupialization of Bartholin's cysts. J. Obstet. Gynaecol., Br. Commonw., *73:* 1010, 1966.

McAdams, A. J., Jr., and Kistner, R.: The relationship of chronic vulvar disease, leukoplakia, and carcinoma in-situ to carcinoma of the vulva. Cancer. *11:* 740, 1958.

McBurney, R. P., and Bale, G. F.: Primary malignant melanoma of the female urethra. Surgery, *37:* 973, 1955.

McDonald, J. R.: Apocrine sweat gland carcinoma of vulva. Am. J. Clin. Pathol., *11:* 890, 1941.

Mering, J. H.: A surgical approach to intractable pruritus vulvae. Am. J. Obstet. Gynecol., *64:* 619, 1952.

Miller, N. F., Riley, G. M., and Stanley, M.: Leukoplakia vulvae. Am. J. Obstet. Gynecol., *64:* 768, 1952.

Neilson, D. R., Jr., and Woodruff, J. D.: Electron microscopy in "in-situ and invasive" vulvar Paget's disease. Am. J. Obstet. Gynecol., *113:* 719, 1972.

Newman, B., and Cromen, J. K.: Multicentric origin of carcinomas of the female anogenital tract. Surg. Gynecol. Obstet., 108: 273, 1959.

Newman, B., and Gray, D. B.: Primary carcinoma of Bartholin's gland. Am. J. Surg., *92:* 490, 1956.

Novak, E., and Stevenson, R. F.: Sweat gland tumors of vulva, benign (hidradenoma) and malignant (adenocarcinoma). Am. J. Obstet. Gynecol., *50:* 641, 1945.

Nowak, R. J.: Basal cell carcinoma of the vulva. Obstet. Gynecol., *4:* 392, 1954.

Palladino, V. S., Duffy, J. L., and Bures, G. J.: Basal cell carcinoma of the vulva. Cancer, *24:* 460, 1969.

Plachta, A., and Speer, F. D.: Apocrine gland adenocarcinoma and extra-mammary Paget's disease of the vulva. Cancer, *7:* 910, 1954.

Purola, E., and Widholm, O.: Primary carcinoma of Bartholin's gland. Acta. Obstet. Gynecol. Scand., *45:* 205, 1966.

Rainey, R.: Association of lymphogranuloma inguinale and cancer. Surgery, *34:* 221, 1954.

Richart, R. M.: A clinical staining test for the in vivo delineation of dysplasia and carcinoma in situ. Am. J. Obstet. Gynecol., *86:* 703, 1963.

Rubin, A.: Granular cell myoblastoma of the vulva. Am. J. Obstet. Gynecol., *77:* 292, 1959.

Rutledge, R., Smith, J. P., and Franklin, E. W.: Epidemiology of carcinoma of the vulva. Am. J. Obstet. Gynecol., *106:* 1117, 1970.

Sadler, W. P., and Dockerty, M. D.: Malignant myoblastoma vulvae. Am. J. Obstet. Gynecol., *61:* 1047, 1951.

Saltzstein, S. L., Woodruff, J. D., and Novak, E. R.: Postgranulomatous carcinoma of the vulva. Obstet. Gynecol., *7:* 80, 1956.

Siegler, A. M., and Greene, H. J.: Basal-cell carcinoma of vulva. Am. J. Obstet. Gynecol., *62:* 1219, 1951.

Stone, H. B.: A treatment for pruritus ani. Bull. Johns Hopkins Hosp., *27:* 242, 1916.

Symmonds, R. E., Pratt, J. H., and Dockerty, M. B.: Melanoma of the vulva. Obstet. Gynecol., *15:* 543, 1960.

Taussig, F.: *Diseases of Vulva.* Appleton-Century-Crofts, New York, 1921.

Thomas, W. A.: Clinical study of granuloma inguinale with a routine for the diagnosis of lesions of the vulva. Am. J. Obstet. Gynecol., *61:* 790, 1951.

Ulfelder, H.: Radical vulvectomy with bilateral inguinal, femoral and iliac node resection. Am. J. Obstet. Gynecol., *78:* 1074, 1959.

Wallace, H. J.: Vulva leukoplakia. J. Obstet. Gynecol. Br. Commonw., *69:* 865, 1962.

Way, S., and Hennigan, M.: Late results of extended radical vulvectomy for carcinoma of vulva. J. Obstet. Gynecol. Br. Commonw., *73:* 594, 1966.

Wharton, L. R., and Everett, H. S.: Primary malignant Bartholin gland tumors. Obstet. Gynecol. Surv., *6:* 1, 1951.

Woodruff, J. D.: Paget's disease of the vulva. Obstet. Gynecol., *5:* 175, 1955.

Woodruff, J. D., Borkowf, H. I., Holzman, G. B., Arnold, E. A., and Knaack, J.: Metabolic activity in normal and abnormal vulvar epithelia. Am. J. Obstet. Gynecol., *91:* 809, 1965.

Woodruff, J. D., and Hildebrandt, E. E.: Carcinoma in-situ of the vulva. Obstet. Gynecol., *12:* 414, 1958.

Woodruff, J. D., Julian, C. G., Puray, T., Mermut, S., and Katayama, P.: The contemporary challenge of carcinoma in-situ of the vulva. Am. J. Obstet. Gynecol., *115:* 677, 1973.

Woodruff, J. D., and Williams, T. J.: Multiple sites of anaplastic change in the lower genital system. Am. J. Obstet. Gynecol., *85:* 724, 1963.

Woodworth, H., Jr., Dockerty, M. B., Wilson, R. B., and Pratt, J. H.: Papillary hidradenoma of the vulva. Am. J. Obstet. Gynecol., *190:* 501, 1971.

Yackel, D. B., Symmonds, R. E., and Kempers, R. D.: Melanoma of the vulva. Obstet. Gynecol., *35:* 625, 1970.

Zelle, K.: Treatment of vulvar dystrophies with topical testosterone propionate. Am. J. Obstet. Gynecol., *109:* 570, 1971.

CHAPTER 10

Diseases of the Vagina

VAGINITIS

Vaginal infections are among the more common problems which challenge the gynecologist and the generalist. It is difficult for the clinician to be enthusiastic about such a patient, for, although she has a most valid and disturbing complaint, the infection is rarely of serious import, is often difficult to eradicate, and is frequently recurrent. During reproductive life, the vaginal epithelium is many cell layers thick. This fact, together with the absence of glands, makes gonorrheal infection very rare as compared to its incidence in the young child. In the latter, the Gonococcus finds a fertile field in the thin prepuberal vaginal epithelium. Again, in the postmenopausal phase of life, there is atrophy of the vaginal wall, so that various organisms, including the Gonococcus, are common invaders.

The normal flora of the vagina includes many organisms: Streptococcus, Staphylococcus, Döderlein's bacillus, the diphtheroids, and, not infrequently, fungi. Nevertheless, the full scope of the vaginal flora remains an unsolved puzzle.

Causes

Various agents are involved in the production of vaginal infections. During the menstrual years, the most frequent offenders are *Trichomonas vaginalis*, the Monilia or Candida, *Haemophilus vaginalis*, and herpes virus. In the prepubertal and postmenopausal years, the thin vaginal epithelium is easily infected by a variety of agents, including the Gonococcus and many nonspecific organisms.

As with the vulva, certain systemic diseases may predispose to vulvovaginitis. In the dia-

betic, monilial infections affect the epithelia of the entire area. In debilitating states, particularly cardiovascular disease, the vagina may be the site of "bleb" formation characteristic of vaginitis emphysematosa. This interesting alteration in the subepithelial tissues is most commonly seen in pregnancy and often associated with trichomoniasis. In the infant, the acute exanthematous diseases may be found both in the vagina and on the vulva, the most frequent offender probably being chicken pox. Foreign bodies are a particular hazard during early childhood when various agents may be introduced into the vagina without knowledge of the parents. On other occasions, pessaries, inserted in the treatment of prolapse may produce a severe reactive vaginitis, and deep fissures may result with the embedding of the agent in the vaginal mucosa. Various douches present on the market may produce reactions in certain individuals who are sensitive to the ingredients. This is particularly true when the agent contains high quantities of chlorine or caustics.

Symptoms and Signs

The primary symptom of vaginitis is a discharge commonly called leukorrhea. It must be appreciated that during the normal cycle there are well known variations in this discharge, depending on the time in the cycle at which the woman is observed. During the pre- and postmenstrual days, the "flow" is often milky and may appear as small, white clumps of "material." Conversely, at midcycle, the prominent cervical mucus component becomes dominant and the discharge is thick and mucilaginous.

With most vaginal infections, in addition to the discharge, the patient commonly complains of vulvar irritation and itching; these symptoms are especially prominent on urination. The importance of a "clean catch" urine and thorough examination is obvious.

Investigation usually reveals that the vaginal mucosa is extremely erythematous and congested, as is the epithelium of the introitus, the urethral meatus, and often the vulvoperianal areas.

Nonspecific Vaginitis

In the past, this has been a common designation for the vaginal infection for which there seems to be no definable infecting agent. At present, it would seem only realistic that the diagnosis of "nonspecific vaginitis" should be relegated to those reactions occurring in the prepubertal and postmenopausal years during which the thin vaginal epithelium is quite susceptible to a variety of irritative phenomena and many nonspecific infective agents. Conversely, during the menstrual years, the mature vaginal epithelium resists the inroads of these nonspecific bacteria as well as the Gonococcus, and every effort should be made to arrive at a specific cause for the vaginitis. With present sophisticated techniques for study of any disease process, an epitaph should be written for the diagnosis of nonspecific vaginitis during the menstrual years. Obviously, the correct therapeutic agent for the specific infective agent will lead to better results.

Treatment

Obviously the treatment of "nonspecific" vaginitis entails first a thorough study to rule out a "specific." Cleansing, hot vinegar douches in an attempt to restore normal acidity are an adjunct to any local or systemic treatment, appreciating that they should not be employed immediately after the use of intravaginal medications.

The true nonspecific vaginitis of the prepubertal or postmenopausal patient is best treated with the use of local estrogen. These agents thicken the thin stratified epithelium of these periods of life and, in most instances, will spontaneously effect a "cure." Particularly in the postmenopausal years, it is important to instruct the patient to continue with the insertion of the local agent once a week, in order to prevent recurrence of the problem. Usually one-half of an applicator full of the cream is sufficient.

Trichomonas Vaginitis

Although the organism known as the *Trichomonas vaginalis* was described by Donne as far back as 1836, its importance as the etiological factor in a frequent and troublesome form of vaginitis was not appreciated until recent years.

Incidence

The infection is extremely common. In a report of 5,712 obstetrical and gynecological patients examined routinely for the Trichomonas, Peterson states that 24.6% of the smears were positive. Others have shown that the infection is exceedingly common in pregnant women, when it may be associated with vaginitis emphysematosa.

Symptoms

The chief manifestation of Trichomonas vaginitis is leukorrhea, commonly associated with vaginal soreness, burning, and itching.

Speculum examination commonly reveals a pool of thin, greenish-yellow, foamy or bubbly discharge in the dependent vaginal fornix. The mucous membrane is diffusely reddened and the posterior fornix often presents a granular or strawberry-like appearance which is almost pathognomonic. Small petechial erosions are seen on the epithelium of the vagina and portio of the cervix.

Diagnosis

The diagnosis is made by demonstration of the Trichomonas. The patient is cautioned to take no douche on the day of examination. A bivalve speculum is introduced without the use of a lubricant, as this destroys the activity of the parasite. A drop of pus is taken, and a smear is then made on a warm slide, using normal saline solution to dilute the pus and to avoid too rapid drying out of the smear.

The slide is examined under moderately high power, part of the illumination being cut off. The organisms, when present, are readily recognizable as motile, pear-shaped parasites, with long flagellae at the narrow end and with an undulating cell membrane. The active movements of the flagellae are readily seen but must be distinguished from sperm.

Methods of Infection

The source of vaginal infection with Trichomonas has been discussed ad infinitum. Nevertheless, at present, the evidence that the organisms are transmitted through coitus is convincing.

Treatment

In view of the frequency of the infection and of recurrences, a tremendous variety of therapies have been proposed. Basically, these have been designed to increase the acidity of the vagina, appreciating that, with the normal pH of 4.5 to 5, the Trichomonas does not survive.

In recent years, metronidazide or Flagyl has proven to be a most effective trichomonacide. The usual dosage is 500 mg twice a day for 5 days. More recently a single dose of 2,000 mg has proven to be successful, although such a concentrated dose often produces gastrointestinal complaints. It should go without saying that, because this disease is transmitted by sexual contact, the partner or partners must be treated with the patient, particularly if recurrences develop. Certainly, there is no possibility of eliminating any venereal disease without treatment of the source.

Treatment in Pregnancy

As already mentioned, Trichomonas infection is extremely common in pregnant women. At the present moment, there is no evidence that Flagyl will produce any abnormality in the fetus. Nevertheless, it has generally been proposed that this agent not be used during the first 3 months of pregnancy. As a result, it is more common to use a variety of local agents during this period of time along with cleanliness and protection of the patient during coitus. Concentrated salt solution washes usually kill the organism. The methods of treatment are essentially the same as in the nonpregnant condition, and they can be carried out with safety until the last month of pregnancy, when they should be discontinued.

Mycotic Vaginitis (Fungous or Monilial Vaginitis)

As with Trichomonas infection, the frequency and importance of mycotic vaginitis has been recognized only in recent years. Various names are applied to the causative organism, such as *Monilia albicans*, *Saccharomyces albicans*, *Oidium albicans*, but it is usually believed that the *Candida albicans* is the one most commonly involved.

Symptoms

The disease is characterized by a discharge which varies from a thin watery to a thick purulent character, pruritus which may be intense, local irritation, and marked reddening of the entire vaginal or vulvovaginal mucous membrane. In addition, there are often thrushlike patches on the vagina or vulva or both. When the vulva is extensively involved, its surface may show large whitish or graying areas of the aphthous deposit, and itching may be exceedingly distressing, so that scratch marks are often present.

Diagnosis

Although the above described clinical picture should at once suggest the probability of the mycotic etiology, the diagnosis is made positive by microscopic demonstration of the fungi. A smear is made from the exudate, and potassium hydroxide (KOH) is added to the preparation. The fungi appear in the form of long threadlike fibers or mycelia, to which are attached the tiny buds or conidia. For confirmation, the organism may be cultured on Sabouraud's or Nickerson's medium (Fig. 10.1).

Methods of Infection

As with Trichomonas, the mode of contamination is rarely clearly explainable, although it seems certain that dissemination is by means of the hands, towels, coitus, clothing, bath water, bowel contents, or instruments. The organism grows readily in moist atmospheres and at a pH of more than 5. Thus the Lactobacillus is almost routinely absent in smear with Monilia. Furthermore, the use of systemic or local antibiotics promotes the growth of this agent, because the normal flora of the vagina is often destroyed by these medications.

Treatment

Gentian violet has been the most commonly used agent over the years and had become almost "specific" for such infections.

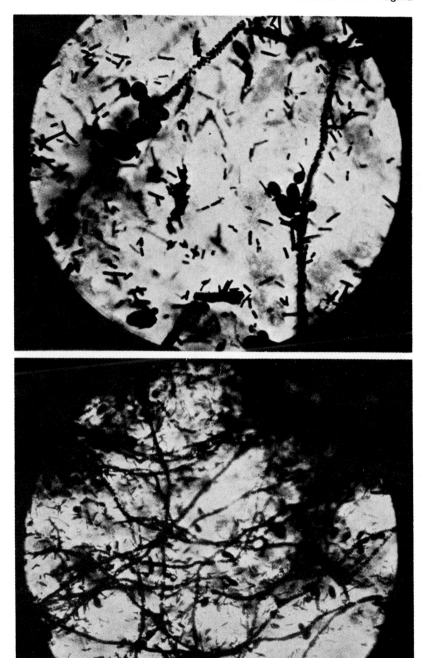

Figure 10.1.   Monilia in a vaginal smear. *Above*, high-dry power; *below*, mycelial forms with budding elements as well as other organisms (oil immersion). (From E. D. Plass: In *Gynecology and Obstetrics*, edited by C. H. Davis. W. F. Prior Company, Inc., Hagerstown, Maryland, 1933.)

To avoid complications, it is wise for the physician to apply the 1% aqueous preparation in the office and allow the medication to dry before the patient is allowed to ambulate.

More recently, various fungicides have been introduced into the market, and Myco-statin has proven to be one of the more effective agents. Excellent results have also been obtained with the use of such agents as Monistat and Lotrimin. It is recommended that the agent be used through at least three cycles and on a most rigid program during the intermenstrual period, possibly once to twice a week. Mycolog cream is effective to reduce the local reactive vulvar irritation and itching.

Haemophilus vaginalis Vaginitis

This agent as a sole or contributory cause of vaginitis has been noted by Gardner and Dukes (1955). Culture is taken with the use of Casman's blood agar medium, as well as thioglycolate broth. Possibly the most important diagnostic test is the simple vaginal smear. Conversely, in the preparation from the patient with Haemophilus infection, the lactobacilli are almost routinely absent and a number of other organisms are reduced greatly, as are the numbers of "pus cells." The Haemophilus, being a nonmotile, short gram-negative bacillus, agglutinates to the epithelial cells to form the so-called "clue cells." In the preparation, these groups of cells are noted along the epithelial border in large or small nests, almost appearing as "whiskers." Careful survey of the slide will make the diagnosis in a majority of cases (Fig. 10.2).

In cases of Haemophilus infection, the patient usually complains of an offensive discharge with little or no discomfort or itching. Inspection of the vagina frequently reveals local evidence of infection in the epithelium and a very slight creamy discharge.

Treatment

Haemophilus vaginalis vaginitis may respond to local therapy with sulfonamides. Triple sulfa cream used over a protracted period of time, at least 3 to 4 weeks, will frequently give relief of the symptoms. Conversely, at least one-half of the cases resist this therapy. Most recently, Flagyl has proven to be an effective agent. Since *Haemophilus vaginalis* vaginitis is classified as a venereal disease, all contacts of the patient must be treated in order to prevent recurrences.

Herpetic Vaginitis

Herpetic infections of the vulva are well documented, and recent years have seen a tremendous increase both in the frequency of the disease and the diagnosed cases. The part that such infections may play in the development of cervical neoplasia has furthered interest in the disease process. A final concern

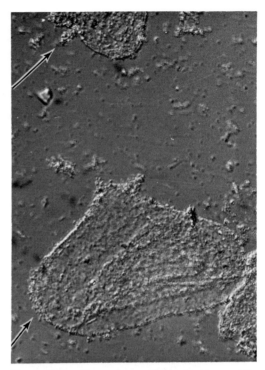

Figure 10.2.   Smear from patient with *Haemophilus vaginalis* vaginitis. Note the absence of lactobacilli and the paucity of pus cells. *Arrows* denote the accumulation of organisms at the edge of the epithelial cell—"clue" cells.

has been the possibility that delivery of the fetus through an infected "birth canal" may lead to viremia in the newborn with a variety of complications developing therefrom, including neonatal death.

Classically, the herpetic vaginitis is asymptomatic, although a nonspecific discharge may be present. Nevertheless, close inspection, particularly in those patients with vulvar herpes, will reveal numerous tiny, serpiginous ulcerations classic of those present on the vulva. On rare occasions deeper, phagadenic ulcers may develop.

The diagnosis is usually made by thorough inspection of the vagina. The vaginal smear may demonstrate the presence of acidophilic nuclear inclusions since herpes is a DNA virus.

Basically the disease is transmitted by sexual contact, so the patient's partner may also have evidence of such lesions on the foreskin or glans penis.

Treatment for the vaginal lesions is difficult and usually unnecessary inasmuch as the patient is asymptomatic.

Gonorrheal Vulvovaginitis in Children

Although the histological structure of the adult vagina, with its many layers of squamous epithelium and its lack of glands, protects it from attacks of the Gonococcus, this is not true of the immature vagina of the young child, with its thin mucous membrane covered with only a few layers of epithelial cells.

Mode of Infection

The disease is spread through contact with infected persons, often other children.

Symptoms

The chief and often the only symptom is persistent vaginal discharge, producing a soiling of the child's clothing. The course of the disease if untreated is extremely chronic, with alternation of periods of remission and exacerbation, but the tendency is to disappearance of the vaginal inflammation and discharge with the onset of puberty.

Diagnosis

There is no question that many errors of diagnosis occur. The criteria for diagnosis are the microscopic demonstration of the Gonococcus and a positive culture.

Treatment

Results are uniformly good with either intramuscular or even oral penicillin for 3 to 4 days.

Postmenopausal Vaginitis

The atrophy of the vaginal mucosa which takes place normally at the time of the menopause makes it very prone to infection. In seeking the cause of slight postmenopausal bleeding, senile vaginitis must be borne in mind as a not infrequent one. The most characteristic symptoms, however, are discharge, itching, burning, and soreness in the vaginal region. The discharge is usually rather thin, and it may, as already mentioned, be blood tinged.

Treatment

Here again estrogenic therapy is often invoked with benefit, and this should be local unless there is some other reason for oral administration. Vaginal suppositories of stilbestrol (0.5 mg) or some form of estrogenic vaginal cream, used two to three times per week, will usually relieve the symptoms promptly. It should be appreciated that treatment must be continued, possibly at weekly intervals, if recurrences are to be avoided.

Ulcerations

There are undoubtedly many causes for vaginal ulcerations. However, one of the "nonspecific" alterations occurs in the patient with a total prolapse. In this situation the vaginal epithelium (Fig. 10.3) is frequently keratinized and skinlike with superficial and deep ulcerations resulting from the decubitus situation. Furthermore, atypical cytologic findings are often associated with this condition.

Emphysematous Vaginitis

Vaginitis emphysematosa is a rare condition. It has been recognized during pregnancy and with heart failure. It is characterized by the appearance of bleblike, gas-filled cysts in the submucous layers of the upper vagina.

Inasmuch as the alterations seen with vaginitis emphysematosa are usually associated with other infections, primarily Trichomonas,

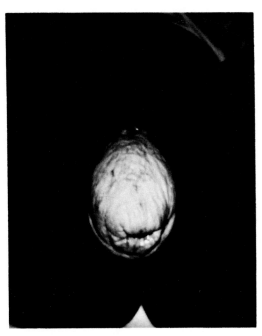

Figure 10.3. Total prolapse of the vagina with keratinization of the vaginal epithelium.

treatment should be directed at the specific disease.

NEOPLASMS OF THE VAGINA

These fall into two categories, namely, cystic or solid. Aside from a few rare cases produced by distention of an anomalous blind ureter or of a rudimentary unfused Müllerian duct, cysts of the vagina arise in one of two ways.

Inclusion Cysts

These cysts, occurring at the lower end of the vagina and usually on the posterior surface, arise from inclusion beneath the surface of tags of mucosa resulting from perineal lacerations or from imperfect denudation in the course of surgical repair of the perineum. Occasionally, such cysts are found at the apex of the vagina posthysterectomy in the region of the scar (Fig. 10.4). They are lined by a stratified squamous epithelium, and the content is usually cheesy.

Gartner Duct Cysts

These arise from the vestigial remains of the Wolffian or mesonephric system, which, as the so-called Gartner ducts, course along the outer anterior aspect of the vaginal canal. The resulting cysts may be small, or they may become so large as to bulge from the vaginal outlet (Fig. 10.5). Microscopically they are lined with a varying type of epithelium, cuboidal or columnar, ciliated or nonciliated, and sometimes stratified.

Solid Tumors

The most common of the solid tumors is the *acuminate wart*. These have been described extensively in Chapter 9, and most cases of vaginal condylomata are associated with similar vulvar lesions. The vaginal tumors may become exuberant during pregnancy and cause problems with bleeding during delivery. Thus, cesarean section must be considered in cases of extensive involvement. Generally it is wiser to treat the commonly associated infections and remove the larger lesions surgically.

Endometriosis may on rare occasions occur as a diffuse process and simulate adenosis. More commonly it penetrates through the cul-de-sac of Douglas and may appear as an area of subepithelial nodularity or as an irregular hemorrhagic mass (Figs. 10.6). Treatment follows the general pattern of that described for endometriosis elsewhere in the pelvis. Positive biopsy diagnosis is obviously of importance prior to the institution of any therapy.

The benign solid tumors include the *fibromyoma* and *leiomyoma*. The latter may represent a subserous uterine tumor which has developed extraperitoneally, divorced itself from the fundus, and is finding its way outside.

Adenosis vaginae is demonstrated by roughened areas in which mucus-secreting glands are found microscopically (Fig. 10.7). Congenital hydrocolpos or hematocolpos may occur in the newborn.

Aside from the occasional large growth, there are usually no symptoms produced by the benign vaginal tumors. These neoplasms are properly treated by surgical excision.

Adenosis Vaginae

Adenosis has taken on new clinicopathologic significance with the discovery of an unique malignancy developing in young women whose mothers receive estrogens, usually synthetic, during pregnancy. Admittedly this "mesonephroid" tumor has been de-

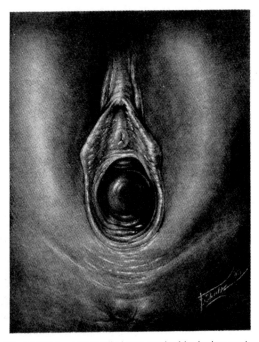

Figure 10.4. Unusually large vaginal inclusion cyst.

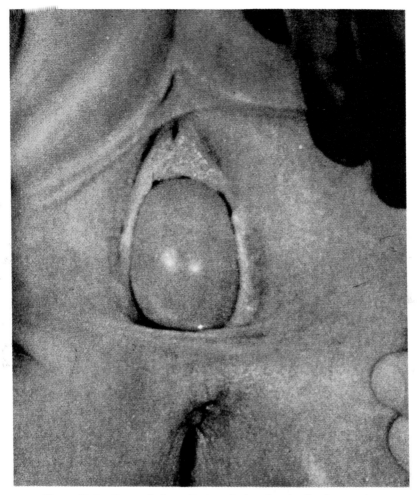

Figure 10.5.   Unusually large Gartner duct cyst protruding from vagina.

scribed previously in both the ovary and the lower genital canal; however, the recent increase in incidence suggests a developmental pathophysiologic alteration that is unique. The possibility that the administration of estrogens to the mother during the earliest stages of development of the urogenital canal might alter the point of junction between the urogenital and paramesonephric systems and eventually place the zone of transformation lower in the vaginal canal now seems a logical explanation for the development of adenosis. Studies by Herbst and others suggest that the unique mesonephroid or clear cell carcinoma is of paramesonephroid origin (Fig. 10.8). At present, it would seem wise to carefully observe such patients at risk but to perform no ablative surgery because of the difficulty in delineating the extent of the condition and the hazards of complications to the nearby bladder and rectum.

The 400 cases of "clear cell" or mesonephroid carcinoma of the vagina have been described in young women, generally between the ages of 13 and 25 years, and they have been largely asymptomatic.

MALIGNANT TUMORS

Primary vaginal neoplasia is rare, accounting for about 0.5 per cent of all primary malignancy arising in the genital canal.

Clinical Features

Primary carcinoma is usually found in the patient in the early sixth decade of life. Obviously this figure excludes the adenocarcinoma noted above which is found in the young woman.

The primary symptom is, as with cervical cancer, a bloody discharge. Late symptoms are the presence of a protruding mass and pain, the latter usually due to extension of the tumor.

The lesion occurs most commonly on anterior or posterior vaults. It is grossly either exfoliative and friable or ulcerative. Obviously there is early invasion of the bladder, rectum, or adjacent cervix. Lesions involving the cervix are generally classified as primary cervical lesions, regardless of the apparent differential in size.

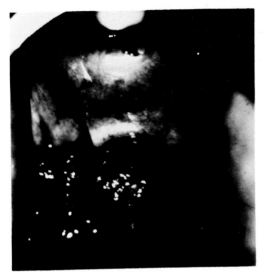

Figure 10.6. Endometriosis penetrating through the cul de sac. (From E. R. Novak and J. D. Woodruff: *Gynecologic and Obstetric Pathology*, W. B. Saunders Company, Philadelphia, 1974.)

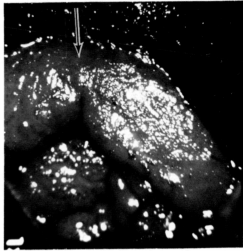

Figure 10.8. "Cockscomb" appearance of adenosis. The *arrow* is not at the squamocolumnar junction of the ovary, but well out on the vagina. Vagina is stained with iodine to demonstrate the transition.

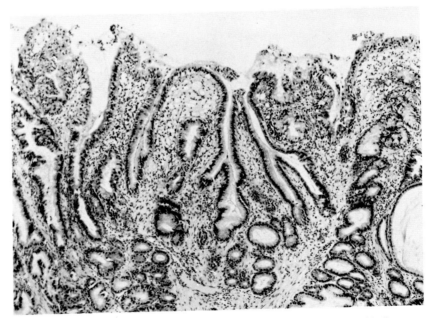

Figure 10.7. Adenosis of vagina. Glands lined by mucus-secreting epithelium.

Pathology

Squamous cell carcinoma comprises approximately 92–95% of all primary vaginal neoplasia. The remainder of the lesions are adenocarcinoma, sarcoma, or melanoma, but all are extremely rare. The lesions may be well differentiated or more epidermoid in nature.

Treatment

Radiation therapy is the treatment of choice in most clinics. If surgery is employed, the procedure is usually extensive, involving removal of the uterus, vagina, and either adjacent bladder or rectum or both, with the formation of urinary or bowel diversions. Prognosis obviously depends on the extent of the disease, thus salvage rates vary with the International Federation of Gynecology and Obstetrics (FIGO) staging of the disease (Table 10.1).

Carcinoma in situ

As with invasive, carcinoma in situ of the vagina is rare. Of interest has been the appearance of such lesions in conjunction with

an apparent "regional response to a carcinogen." Thus the in situ disease of the vagina is often found with or subsequent to the discovery of cervical or vulvar neoplasia and is not uncommonly multicentric. Thus, in the follow-up of any malignancy in the adjacent area, the vagina should be inspected thoroughly for evidences of malignant alterations.

Therapy has consisted largely of either surgery or irradiation. Most recently local chemotherapeutic agents have been used successfully in a majority of reported cases.

Secondary Carcinoma

This is common, chiefly because of the frequency with which carcinoma of the cervix extends to the surrounding vaginal wall. Adenocarcinoma of the corpus in its later stages may metastasize to the vagina, as may chorionephithelioma and carcinoma of distant organs.

Sarcoma

Sarcoma is infrequent but may occur at any age.

Melanoma

Rarely melanoma may arise primarily in the vagina. As one might expect, the prognosis is poor and preinvasive disease is rarely diagnosed.

Germ Cell Tumors

Rare cases of endodermal sinus tumor have been reported in the vagina. These lesions occur in the first decade of life and present grossly as sarcoma botryoides. Biopsy is necessary to confirm the diagnosis, and it is of major importance in order to institute the appropriate treatment, namely triple chemotherapy.

Table 10.1
FIGO Classification of Vaginal Cancer

Preinvasive Carcinoma of the Vagina	
Stage 0	Carcinoma in situ, intraepithelial carcinoma.
Invasive Carcinoma of the Vagina	
Stage I	The carcinoma is limited to the vaginal wall.
Stage II	The carcinoma has involved the subvaginal tissue but has not extended on to the pelvic wall.
Stage III	The carcinoma has extended on to the pelvic wall.
Stage IV	The carcinoma has extended beyond the true pelvis or has involved the mucosa of the bladder or rectum; however, bullous edema as such does not permit one to classify a case as Stage IV.

Cases should be classified as carcinoma of the vagina when the primary site of the growth is in the vagina. A growth that involves the cervix should be classified as carcinoma of the cervix.

A growth that has extended to the vulva should be classified as carcinoma of the vulva. A growth that is limited to the urethra should be classified as carcinoma of the urethra.

References and Additional Readings

Ariel, I. M.: Malignant melanoma of the vagina. Report of a successfully treated case. Obstet. Gynecol., *17:* 222, 1961.
Ariel, I. M.: Five-year cure of a primary malignant melanoma of the vagina by local radioactive isotope therapy. Am. J. Obstet. Gynecol., *82:* 405, 1961.
Arronet, G. H., Latour, M. P. A., and Tremblay, P. C.: Primary carcinoma of the vagina. Am. J. Obstet. Gynecol., *79:* 445, 1960.
Ayre, J. E.: Cyclic ovarian changes in artificial vagina. Am. J. Obstet. Gynecol., *48:* 690, 1944.
Batsakis, J. G., and Dito, W. R.: Primary malignant melanoma of vagina. Obstet. Gynecol., *20:* 109, 1962.
Bivens, M. D.: Primary carcinoma of vagina—a report of 46 cases. Am. J. Obstet. Gynecol., *65:* 390, 1963.

Boatwright, D. C., and Moore, V.: Suburethral diverticula in the female. J. Urol., *89:* 581, 1963.

Boutselis, J. G., Ullery, J. C., and Bair, J.: Vaginal metastases following treatment of endometrial carcinoma. Obstet. Gynecol., *21:* 622, 1963.

Brack, C. B., Merritt, R. I., and Dickson, R. J.: Primary carcinoma of the vagina. Obstet. Gynecol., *12:* 104, 1958.

Brenner, P., Sedlis, A., and Cooperman, H.: Complete imperforate transverse vaginal septum. Obstet. Gynecol., *25:* 135, 1965.

Burt, E. P., Roark, S. P., and Couri, P. J.: Vaginitis emphysematosa. Obstet. Gynecol., *4:* 335, 1954.

Burt, R. L., Prichard, R. W., and Kim, B. S.: Fibroepithelial polyp of the vagina. Obstet. Gynecol., *47:* 525, 1976.

Copenhaven, E. H., Salzman, F. A., and Wright, K. A.: Carcinoma in situ of the vagina. Am. J. Obstet. Gynecol., *89:* 962, 1964.

Daniel, W. W., Koss, L. G., and Brunschwig, A.: Sarcoma botryoides of the vagina. Cancer, *12:* 74, 1959.

Diercks, K.: Der normale mensuelle Zyklus der menschlichen Vaginalschleimhaut. Arch. Gynaekol., *130:* 46, 1927.

Duckett, H. C., Davis, C. D., and McCall, J. B.: Sarcoma botryoides. Obstet. Gynecol., *10:* 517, 1957.

Forsberg, J. G.: Estrogen, vaginal cancer and vaginal development. Am. J. Obstet. Gynecol., *113:* 83, 1972.

Forsberg, J. G.: Cervicovaginal epithelium: its origin and development. Am. J. Obstet. Gynecol., *115:* 1025, 1973.

Gardner, H. L.: Trichomoniasis. Obstet. Gynecol., *19:* 279, 1962.

Gardner, H. L., and Dukes, C. D.: Hemophilus vaginalis vaginitis. Am. J. Obstet. Gynecol., *69:* 962, 1955.

Gardner, H. L., and Fernet, P.: Etiology of vaginitis emphysematosa. Am. J. Obstet. Gynecol., *88:* 680, 1964.

Gardner, H. L., and Kaufman, R. H.: *Benign Diseases of the Vulva and Vagina.* C. V. Mosby, St. Louis, 1969.

Geist, S. H.: Cyclical changes in vaginal mucous membrane. Surg. Gynecol. Obstet., *51:* 848, 1930.

Graham, J. B., and Meigs, J. V.: Residual carcinoma in vaginal cuff after radical hysterectomy with bilateral pelvic lymph node dissection. Am. J. Obstet. Gynecol., *64:* 402, 1952.

Gray, L. A., and Barnes, M. L.: Vaginitis in women—diagnosis and treatment. Am. J. Obstet. Gynecol., *92:* 125, 1965.

Greenwalt, P., Barlow, J. J., Nasea, P. C., and Burnett, W. S.: Vaginal cancer after maternal treatment with synthetic estrogens. N. Engl. J. Med., *285:* 392, 1971.

Herbst, A. L., Green, T. H., Jr., and Ulfelder, H.: Primary carcinoma of the vagina—an analysis of 68 cases. Am. J. Obstet. Gynecol., *106:* 210, 1970.

Herbst, A. L., Robboy, S. J., MacDonald, G. J., and Scully, R. E.: The effects of local progesterone or stilbestrol-associated vaginal adenosis. Am. J. Obstet. Gynecol., *118:* 607, 1974.

Herbst, A. L., and Scully, R. E.: Adenocarcinoma of the vagina in adolescence. Cancer, *25:* 745, 1970.

Hummer, W. K., Mussey, E., Decker, D. G., and Dockerty, M. B.: Carcinoma in situ of the vagina. Am. J. Obstet. Gynecol., *108:* 1109, 1970.

Koss, L. G., Melamed, M. R., and Daniel, W. W.: In situ epidermoid carcinoma of the cervix and vagina following radiotherapy for cervical cancer. Cancer, *14:* 353, 1961.

Lang, W. R.: Premenarchal vaginitis. Obstet. Gynecol., *13:* 723, 1959.

Lash, S. R., and Rubenstone, A. I.: Adenocarcinoma of the rectovaginal septum probably arising from endometriosis. Am. J. Obstet. Gynecol., *78:* 299, 1959.

Laufe, L. E., and Bernstein, E. D.: Primary malignant melanoma of the vagina. Obstet. Gynecol., *37:* 148, 1971.

Marcus, S. L.: Müllerian mixed sarcoma (sarcoma botryoides) of the cervix. Obstet. Gynecol., *15:* 47, 1960.

Merrill, J. A., and Bencer, W. T.: Primary carcinoma of the vagina. Obstet. Gynecol., *11:* 3, 1958.

Norris, H. J., and Taylor, H. B.: Melanomas of the vagina. Am.

J. Clin. Pathol., *46:* 420, 1966.

Norris, H. J., and Taylor, H. B.: Polyps of the vagina—a benign lesion resembling sarcoma botryoides. Cancer, *19:* 227, 1966.

Novak, E., Woodruff, J. D., and Novak, E. R.: Probable mesonephric origin of certain genital tumors. Am. J. Obstet. Gynecol., *68:* 1222, 1954.

Ober, W. B., and Edgcomb, J. H.: Sarcoma botryoides in the female urogenital tract. Cancer, *7:* 75, 1954.

Ober, W. B., Smith, J. A., and Rovilland, F.: Congenital sarcoma botryoides: report of 2 cases. Cancer, *11:* 620, 1958.

Plaut, A., and Dreyfuss, M. L.: Adenosis and its relation to primary adenocarcinoma. Surg. Gynecol. Obstet., *71:* 756, 1940.

Randall, C. L., Birtsch, P. K., and Harkins, J. L.: Ovarian function after the menopause. Am. J. Obstet. Gynecol., *74:* 719, 1957.

Ruffolo, E. H., Foxworthy, D., and Fletchner, J. C.: Vaginal adenocarcinoma arising in vaginal adenosis. Am. J. Obstet. Gynecol., *110:* 167, 1971.

Rutledge, F.: Cancer of the vagina. Am. J. Obstet. Gynecol., *97:* 635, 1967.

Sandberg, E. C., Danielson, R. W., Cauwet, R. W., and Bonar, B. E.: Adenosis vaginae. Am. J. Obstet. Gynecol., *93:* 209, 1965.

Sandberg, E. C.: The incidence and distribution of occult vaginal adenosis. Am. J. Obstet. Gynecol., *101:* 322, 1968.

Schiller, W.: Mesonephroma ovarii. Am. J. Cancer, *35:* 1, 1939.

Searle, G. C.: Symposium on Flagyl. Research, *56:* 26, 1964.

Sheets, J. L, Dockerty, M. B., Decker, D. G., and Welch, J. S.: Primary epithelial malignancy in the vagina. Am. J. Obstet. Gynecol., *89:* 121, 1964.

Silverberg, S. G., and Digiorgi, L. S.: Clear cell carcinoma of the vagina (a clinical, pathologic and electron microscopic study). Cancer, *29:* 1680, 1972.

Stafl, A., and Mattingly, R.: Vaginal adenosis: A precancerous lesion. Am. J. Obstet. Gynecol., *120:* 666, 1974.

Stafl, A., Mattingly, R. F., Foley, D. V., and Fetherston, W. C.: Clinical diagnosis of vaginal adenosis. Obstet. Gynecol., *43:* 118, 1974.

Stieve, H.: Das Schwangerschaftswachstum und die Gerburtserweiterung der menschlichen Scheide. Z. Mikros. Anat. Forsch., *3:* 307, 1925.

Stieve, H.: Uber angebliche zyklische Veranderungen des Scheidenepithels. Zentralbl. Gynaekol., *55:* 194, 1931.

Studdiford, W. E.: Vaginal lesions of adenomatous origin. Am. J. Obstet. Gynecol., *73:* 641, 1957.

Taussig, F. J.: Metastatic tumors of vagina and vulva. Surg. Clin. North Am., *18:* 1309, 1938.

Tobon, H., and Murphy, A. I.: Benign blue nevus of the vagina. Cancer, *40:* 3174, 1977.

Traut, H. F., Block, P. W., and Kuder, A.: Cyclical changes in the human vaginal mucosa. Surg. Gynecol. Obstet., *63:* 7, 1936.

Veridiano, N. P., Weiner, F. A., and Tancer, M. L.: Squamous cell carcinoma of the vagina associated with vaginal adenosis. Obstet. Gynecol., *47:* 639, 1976.

Westerhout, F. C., Hodgman, J. E., Anderson, G. V., and Sack, R. A.: Congenital hydrocolpos. Am. J. Obstet. Gynecol., *89:* 957, 1964.

Whelton, J., and Kottmeier, H. L.: Primary carcinoma of the vagina: a study of a Radiumhemmet series of 145 cases. Acta Obstet. Gynecol. Scand., *41:* 22, 1962.

Whitacre, F. F., and Wang, Y. Y.: Biological changes in squamous epithelium transplanted to pelvic connective tissue. Surg. Gynecol. Obstet., *79:* 192, 1944.

Woodruff, J. D., and William, T. J.: Multiple sites of change in the lower genital system. Am J. Obstet. Gynecol., *85:* 724, 1963.

Zondek, B., and Friedmann, M.: Are there cyclical changes in the human vaginal mucosa? J. A. M. A., *106:* 1051, 1939.

CHAPTER 11

Benign Conditions of the Cervix

ACUTE CERVICITIS

Pathology

In the acute stage, which clinically is seen in most typical form in acute gonorrheal infection, the cervix is reddened, congested, and somewhat swollen, while from the canal there escapes a profuse, purulent exudate, sometimes white and sometimes yellowish. *Microscopically*, this phase is characterized by intense polymorphonuclear infiltration of the mucosa and immediately underlying tissue, hyperemia, and more or less edema. The gland lumina may be distended with an exudate consisting of large numbers of dead leukocytes, desquamated epithelial cells, and mucus.

Clinical Symptoms

By far the most constant and usually the only symptom of cervicitis is *leukorrhea*. In the acute stage this is purulent, and in the gonorrheal type, especially where there is associated urethritis, there may be much vaginal and urinary irritability, suggesting cystitis. During this stage the infection is very active, and, in the gonorrheal cases, if no antibiotic has been given, the causative organisms can be readily found in large numbers in the purulent discharge.

There may be a slight elevation of body temperature, with a sensation of congestion in the vaginal region, combined with urinary irritability and burning if there is an associated urethritis.

Acute cervicitis is seldom seen as an isolated condition. Most often it is seen in patients who also have an acute infection of other segments of the generative tract, especially of the fallopian tubes.

Diagnosis

The diagnosis of acute cervicitis must be made by inspection of the cervix by means of a speculum. The cervix, on exposure, will be seen to be reddened and irritated and frequently friable. Gram-stained smears of the cervical discharge often reveal the classic gram-negative intracellular diplococci, and cultures on Thayer-Martin agar may be positive for gonococcus. Acute gonorrheal cervicitis is rarely diagnosed until there is adnexal involvement.

Identification of the specific organism in patients with nongonococcal cervicitis is difficult, because gram-stained smears and cultures usually show a wide variety of bacteria that are common inhabitants of the cervix in asymptomatic women.

Treatment

Antibiotics have become the most important part of the therapy of acute cervicitis of the gonorrheal variety. Penicillin is the drug of choice, although certain drug-resistant strains seem to be on the increase. The general principles and the dosages are discussed in Chapter 19 "Pelvic Inflammatory Disease."

CHRONIC CERVICITIS

This is perhaps the most common of all gynecological lesions and is, along with vaginitis, the most frequent cause of leukorrhea. Although it may represent a residual phase of gonorrheal infection, it is even more frequently due to infection by any of the other organisms found in the vagina, especially streptococci and staphylococci, which ascend to involve an injured cervix.

Pathology

The chronic stage is characterized grossly by any one of a number of pathological pictures, such as:

(1) The cervix is quite normal in appearance on its vaginal surface, but the endocervix is thickened and produces a whitish pus.

(2) The anatomical cervical os is surrounded by a reddish area which may vary in diameter from a centimeter or so to several centimeters. Within this, or without it also, the vaginal surface may show a number of small or large *retention cysts* of the cervical glands (Nabothian cysts). These may be translucent when they contain a clear mucus, or they may appear as opaque whitish blebs when the content is a viscid pus.

(3) When the cervix has been deeply lacerated, as is often the case, it is likely to be large and hypertrophic, sometimes enormously so. Eversion of the endocervical mucosa may occur.

Microscopic

The microscopic picture of chronic cervicitis is that of chronic inflammation, with round cell infiltration, often intense, not only in the mucous membrane, but usually invading the deeper structure of the cervix as well (Fig. 11.1). Especially interesting are the changes that occur in the so-called *transformation zone* between the original squamous epithelium of the exocervix and the columnar epithelium of the endocervix. This is an area of active change where columnar epithelium covering the surface and lining the glands is replaced by squamous epithelium (Fig. 11.2). This process is called *metaplasia* or *epidermidization* and is a normal change seen in the cervix. It may also be involved in the development of cervical cancer; this aspect is discussed more fully in the following chapter.

Symptoms

In the chronic stages of the disease the prominent and sometimes only symptom in most cases is persistent *leukorrhea*. The discharge may be thick, viscid, and like white of an egg, but it is often mucopurulent in character. Where the cervix is quite vascular, slight *staining* may occur after coitus.

Lower abdominal discomfort and dyspareunia caused by motion of the cervix may be eliminated by the successful treatment of chronic cervicitis. Such symptoms seem to be due to a focus of infection in the cervix with low-grade pelvic lymphangitis.

Diagnosis

Speculum examination of the cervix usually reveals evidence of changes in the pars vaginalis, as has already been discussed. Occasionally the chronic infection may involve the endocervical mucosa alone, so that the diagnosis is based upon the presence of a thick, glairy exudate in conjunction with a normal-appearing portio. One must be aware that the early degrees of cervical malignancy show no gross abnormality; occasionally an infected hypertrophic cervix appears more ominous than an early malignancy.

Cytologic smears or colposcopic examination can be helpful, but only a biopsy can make the definitive diagnosis.

Cultures are rarely helpful, because the pathogenic organisms are almost always those that normally inhabit the vagina and cervix.

Treatment

In former years the treatment of chronic cervicitis consisted of the *application of antiseptic or caustic chemicals.*

Systemic therapy with antibiotics is sometimes useful and worth trying, especially in cases of infertility when the infected cervix seems to produce mucus hostile to sperm. In general, however, physical destruction of the infected abnormal epithelium is in vogue.

Cryotherapy. Destruction of cervical epithelium by freezing is a common technique for the management of chronic cervicitis. Refrigerants such as nitrous oxide, Freon, or liquid nitrogen are passed through a probe that is placed in contact with the cervix. Prior to any destructive therapy, careful evaluation to rule out neoplasia must be done. A thorough visual inspection and a negative Pap smear constitute a minimum work-up.

Cauterization. Electrocautery or hot cautery has long been an effective method of therapy for chronic cervicitis, although it has

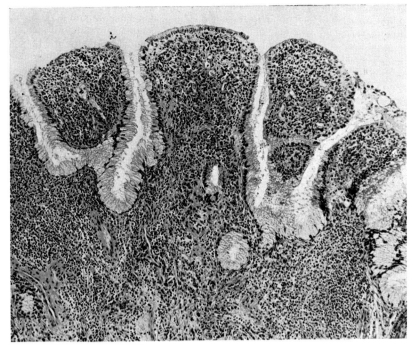

Figure 11.1.   Microscopic appearance of chronic cervicitis.

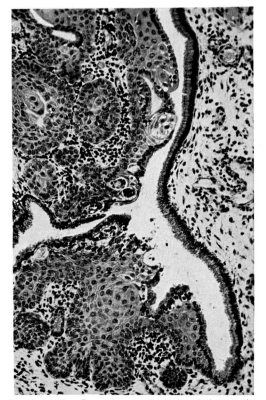

Figure 11.2.   Squamous metaplasia of the cervix. Note how squamous cells undermine columnar epithelium.

almost completely been replaced by cryotherapy today.

Conization. Although destruction by heat or cold is the simplest, most effective, and most generally applicable method of treatment of chronic cervicitis, extensive endocervicitis with profuse discharge but a normal-appearing portio may be treated by means of conization. This is especially indicated if the Pap smear is abnormal, because the cone biopsy is both diagnostic and therapeutic.

NONBACTERIAL INFECTIONS OF THE CERVIX

Infection of the generative tract by viruses and allied organisms has become more frequently recognized. The infection of the cervix is to be considered only a part of a more general infection of the generative tract.

Herpes progenitalis has long been used to designate herpetic lesions of the external genitalia. Josey et al. have described the variegated manifestations, which may consist of edema, vesicles, ulcers and, in extreme cases, granulomatous lesions. These lesions may involve the cervix as part of the more general involvement. Herpetic infection of the upper generative tract does not seem to have been observed.

The clinical manifestation of the lesion in the cervix is self-limited and endures no more than 2 to 3 weeks. No specific therapy is known.

The diagnosis is based on the history, cultures, the gross appearance of the lesion, and specific changes in exfoliated vaginal and cervical cells. Genital herpetic infection is venereally transmitted.

The diagnosis of lower genital tract herpes is important during pregnancy because of the possibility of transmission of the infection to the child if vaginal delivery is allowed.

Chlamydia trachomatis is a microorganism intermediate between a bacteria and a virus that has been isolated from the cervix in 12 to 31% of women studied. It is often associated with a vaginal discharge, and clinically the patient may have a reddened cervix. *C. trachomatis* can also produce salpingitis; thus, the patient and her partner should be treated when the diagnosis is made by culture. The organism is sensitive to tetracycline and trimethoprim sulfamethoxazole according to studies by Ripa et al. They found excellent clinical and microbiological results in symptomatic patients treated for 10 days.

T-mycoplasma and *Mycoplasma hominis* have also been implicated in genital infections in women, including acute infections of the fallopian tubes. There seems to be no specific gross clinical manifestation of mycoplasmic infection of the cervix.

Although syphilis must often involve the cervix, it is rare today to see a primary lesion. *Tuberculous cervicitis* is an uncommon lesion and is, with a few exceptions, secondary to tuberculous infection in the tubes and uterus, although it may be contracted through coitus. It may bring about a hyperplastic or ulcerative lesion which grossly *can be mistaken for the far more common carcinoma* of the cervix. The microscopic appearance is that of tuberculosis elsewhere, with characteristic tubercles, giant cells, and epithelioid cells.

CONDYLOMA ACUMINATUM

Condylomata generally involve the external genitalia, are much less common in the vagina, and are a relatively uncommon finding in the cervix. Condyloma may appear as a pale white, raised irregular plaque on the cervix.

Meisels et al. described the cytologic, colposcopic, and histologic appearance of cervical condyloma (Fig. 11.3). With increasing use of the colposcope to examine the cervix, smaller condyloma, perhaps earlier in their natural history, are being seen more frequently. Biopsy of these lesions with careful histologic examination may be necessary to differentiate them from dysplasia.

CERVICAL STENOSIS

Stenosis of the cervical canal with obstruction of uterine drainage may occur with atrophy of age or scarring from trauma or surgery. Blood may be trapped within the uterine cavity, producing an *hematometra*; or, if the intrauterine contents become infected, a *pyometra* is formed. Cervical stenosis due to atrophy is usually not symptomatic, because this condition is almost always associated with an inactive endometrium. However, if malignancy of the uterine fundus occurs, blood or mucus may fill the cavity and cause pain and cramping. The distended uterus may be felt on examination. The uterus may become greatly enlarged, and misdiagnosis is frequent, because the soft cystic consistency is suggestive of an ovarian cyst. The diagnosis of hematometra or pyometra in an older patient should always suggest the possibility of an associated malignancy. Occasionally, exogenous estrogen therapy may stimulate the endometrium above a stenotic cervix, producing an hematometra.

Cervical stenosis may also occur after lacerations, cone biopsy, cryotherapy, or cervical cauterization. In menstruating women the chief symptom is dysmenorrhea. On examination, the cervical os is noted to be pinpoint, and a sound or probe cannot be passed. Dilatation under paracervical block or regional or general anesthesia is usually adequate therapy. Radiation therapy for cervical cancer almost always results in cervical stenosis.

CERVICAL POLYP

Cervical polyps are generally pedunculated tumors that usually arise from the intracervical mucosa but that may at times spring from the external or vaginal surface of the cervix.

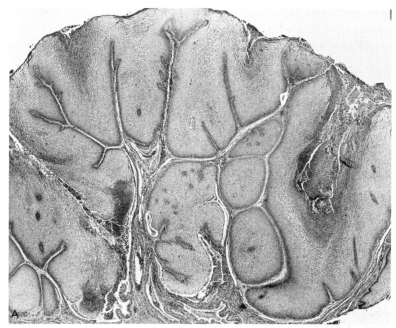

Figure 11.3. Condyloma acuminatum on cervix in pregnancy. (Courtesy of Dr. M. E. Marsh.)

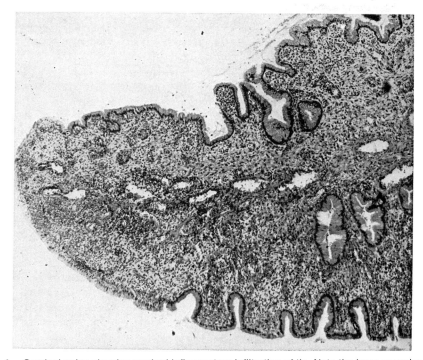

Figure 11.4. Cervical polyp showing marked inflammatory infiltration of tip. Note the large vascular channels in the central core.

They are single or multiple, usually of bright red color, and of rather fragile, spongy structure. Clinically they present as small, bright red growths which peep or protrude from the cervical canal.

The *histological structure* of the cervical polyp is in general that of the mucosa from which it springs. In the most common variety, therefore, the microscope reveals a covering epithelium made up of a single layer of the very tall columnar cells which characterize the normal endocervix, the typical cervical glands, and a stroma of light connective tissue which often shows much edema and round cell infiltration. Not infrequently there is ulceration of the tip of the polyp which, with the vascular congestion, explains the bleeding which such tumors may cause (Fig. 11.4).

Many cervical polyps originating in the endocervix show extensive squamous metaplasia, which, with superimposed infection, may mimic early cancer.

Symptoms

Cervical polyps are frequently revealed in the course of routine examinations for other indications, and they often cause no symptoms when very small. As a rule, however, the larger polyps produce intermenstrual staining and the contact type of bleeding, which occurs especially after coitus.

Diagnosis

Inspection of the cervix through a bivalve speculum usually will reveal even small polyps. It is important to stress that the finding of cervical polyps should not close one's eyes to the possibility of other more serious causes of the bleeding in any particular case, especially if the bleeding is rather free, because such free bleeding is relatively rare with the smaller polyps. A Pap smear should always be done, and biopsy of the cervix and endometrium should be considered if bleeding persists.

Treatment

Removal of the polyps is indicated, and this is a simple procedure. Where the polyp is fairly large and the pedicle easily demonstrable, it can be twisted off and the base touched up with a cautery point. If they are multiple and the canal appears to be crowded with them, it is best to dilate and curette the canal very thoroughly. Pathological study of the polyp and adjacent cervix should be routine.

References and Additional Readings

Bolognese, R. J., et al.: Herpesvirus hominis type II infections in asymptomatic pregnant women. Obstet. Gynecol., 48: 507, 1976.

Farrar, H. K., Jr., and Nedoss, B. R.: Benign tumors of uterine cervix. Am. J. Obstet. Gynecol., 81: 124, 1961.

Hofmeister, F. J., and Gorthey, R. L.: Benign lesions of cervix. Obstet. Gynecol., 5: 504, 1955.

Josey, W. E., Nahmias, A. J., Naib, Z. M., Ucley, E. M., McKenzie, W. M., and Coleman, M. D.: Genital herpes simplex infections in females. Am. J. Obstet. Gynecol., 96: 493, 1966.

Matthews, D.: T-Mycoplasma genital infection: effect of doxycycline therapy on human unexplained infertility. Fertil. Steril., 30: 98, 1978.

McCormack, W. M., Rankin, J. S., and Lee, Y. H.: Localization of genital mycoplasma in women. Am. J. Obstet. Gynecol., 126: 920, 1972.

Meisels, A., Fortin, R., and Roy, M.: Condylomatous lesions of the cervix. II. Cytologic colposcopic and histopathologic study. Acta Cytol., 21: 379, 1977.

Miller, J. F., and Elstein, M.: A comparison of electrocautery and cryocautery for the treatment of cervical erosions and chronic cervicitis. J. Obstet. Gynaecol. Br. Commonw., 80: 658, 1973.

Ostergard, D. R., Townsend, D. E., and Hirase, F. M.: Comparison of electrocauterization and cryosurgery for the treatment of benign disease of the uterine cervix. Obstet. Gynecol., 33: 58, 1969.

Ripa, K. T., Svensson, L., Mardh, P. A., and Westrom, L.: Chlamydia trachomatis cervicitis in gynecologic outpatients. Obstet. Gynecol., 52: 698, 1978.

Schachter, J., Hanna, L., Hill E. C., Massad, S., Sheppard, C. W., Conte, J. Jr., Cohen, S., and Meyer, K. F.: Are chlamydial infections the most prevalent venereal disease? J. A. M. A., 231: 1252, 1975.

Stevenson, C. S.: Tuberculosis of cervix, with report of so-called primary case. Am. J. Obstet. Gynecol., 36: 1017, 1938.

CHAPTER 12

Carcinoma of the Cervix

Carcinoma of the cervix uteri is one of the most important diseases with which the gynecologist must contend. This is true, not only because of the frequency with which the preinvasive and invasive forms of the disease are encountered, but also because much is known about the natural history of this cancer which may serve as a model for the early diagnosis and treatment of other cancers.

INCIDENCE

The recognition of the potential malignancy of intraepithelial lesions of the cervix together with the ability to diagnose them by a relatively inexpensive and painless test, the *Papanicolaou (Pap) smear*, has resulted in a significant reduction in the incidence of invasive cancer of the cervix.

The incidence rate, as well as the mortality from cervical cancer is related to age, race, and ethnic background. The data presented in Figure 12.1 from the Third National Cancer Survey demonstrate an increasing incidence of invasive cervical cancer with age, with a small peak at age 48 and a broad hump above the age of 70. Carcinoma-in-situ, on the other hand, is a disease of young women, being more common in ages 25–40. In the United States, blacks are more frequently affected than whites. Their age-adjusted incidence rate is 33.6/100,000, whereas whites experience only 15.0 cases/100,000. The association of cervical cancer with low socioeconomic status has been demonstrated by many studies and it is difficult to separate such factors as race, customs, and socioeconomic status.

ETIOLOGICAL FACTORS

In a biological sense the cause of carcinoma of the cervix, like the cause of all cancer, is unknown. However, certain circumstances are so closely associated with it that they may be regarded as etiological factors.

Within the past decade some half-dozen major studies have examined the relationship between coitus or marriage and cervical cancer. All studies agree that cervical cancer risk is increased by early marriage or by first coitus at an early age.

The impression has been held for many years that the childbearing woman is far more prone to cervical cancer than the unmarried one.

Thus, it is very likely that childbearing per se is not the important etiological event, but rather it is sexual exposure. In this sense, epidermoid carcinoma of the cervix may be regarded as a venereal disease.

Epidemiologic evidence has implicated early sexual exposure, especially with multiple partners, as an important etiological factor in the development of cervical cancer. This has naturally led to the suspicion that an infective agent may be involved. At one time or another, sperm, smegma, trichomonas, chlamydia, and condyloma have all been under suspicion. Coppleson et al. have presented evidence which suggests that the etiologic agent is spermatozoon DNA.

Recently, Schacter et al. have reported a frequent association of chlamydial infection of the lower genital tract and cervical dysplasia. Josey et al. have reviewed the association of viruses in general and lower genital tract

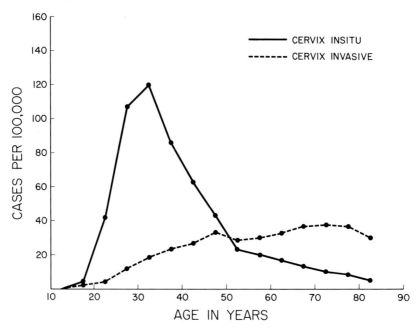

Figure 12.1. Age-specific incidence rates for carcinoma-in-situ and invasive cervical cancer for white women 1969–1970. (Reproduced with permission from the Third National Cancer Survey, Cramer and Cutler, *American Journal of Obstetrics and Gynecology, 118:* 448, 1974.)

cancer, and Tobin, et al. have summarized the evidence linking herpes simplex virus and cervical cancer.

It appears as if many different DNA-containing agents are associated with cervical cancer, but if the relation is one of cause and effect rather than the incidental association of a common infective agent in sexually active women, it has yet to be proved.

PATHOLOGICAL TYPES

There are two principle pathological types of cervical cancer, corresponding to one or another of the two types of epithelium found in the cervix. It will be recalled that the epithelium covering the external or vaginal surface of the *pars vaginalis* of the cervix is of stratified squamous variety, continuous with the stratified squamous epithelium of the vagina. Corresponding to this type of cervical epithelium is the *squamous cell* or *epidermoid carcinoma*. On the other hand, the columnar epithelium of the cervical canal gives rise to *adenocarcinoma* of the cervix. Squamous cell lesions account for approximately 90% of all cervical cancers.

Some tumors have been found to have both adenomatous and squamous cell components and are referred to as *adenosquamous* or *ad-*

enoepidermoid carcinoma of the cervix. Such tumors seem to carry a more serious prognosis than either pure squamous cell tumors or adenocarcinoma.

GROSS PATHOLOGY

Preclinical Stage

There are no distinctive pathological changes which help to identify an intraepithelial carcinoma of the cervix on gross inspection. In fact, some examples of chronic cervicitis present a more abnormal appearance than a cervix with intraepithelial carcinoma.

Early Stage

In its early clinical stage, cervical cancer presents most often as a small lesion at or near the external os, i.e. at the squamocolumnar junction. It appears as a small, hardened, granular area, which to the palpating finger is often slightly raised above the surrounding surface. On speculum examination, the surface of the area is granular or slightly elevated and bleeds on touch. Sometimes the surface may, even in this stage, be covered with a fine papillary outgrowth. The surrounding cervix may be normal, but more frequently it is a seat of chronic inflammatory disease.

Indeed, as with intraepithelial carcinoma, it should be emphasized that it is frequently impossible to make a visual distinction between early invasive cancer and such benign lesions as so-called erosions and eversions.

Moderately Advanced Stage

From its original site, the cancer spreads until it involves the whole or the greater portion of one lip of the cervix, or portions of both lips. As it grows, it exhibits one of two chief characteristics. The papillary tendency may predominate, the growth being chiefly above the surface, so that the lesion takes the form of the so-called cauliflower growth. This constitutes the everting or *exophytic* variety. On the other hand, there may be little or no surface growth, with the lesion extending into the cervical tissues, producing a very hard, sometimes almost stoney induration, although practically always there is some ulceration. To this type of lesion, the designation of inverting or *endophytic* is applied. The infiltrating growth may already involve the adjoining vaginal fornix, and the broad ligaments may show infiltration.

Advanced Stage

In its late stages, the progress of the cancerous process brings about increasing destruction of the cervix, which may be replaced by an excavated ulcerating cavity with ragged, friable walls, so that free bleeding is caused by any but the gentlest examination.

Where the growth is chiefly exophytic, a huge cauliflower mass is formed which may almost fill the vagina. In this variety there may be surprisingly little gross infiltration of the adjoining tissues even when the cervical growth is very large. The further progress of the disease is one of advancing involvement and destruction, producing more and more broad ligament infiltration, with blockage of one or both ureters and not infrequently involving the bladder or rectum, and with the production of fistulous openings between either of these organs and the vagina.

Metastatic Disease

As the disease advances, metastases to the pelvic lymph nodes occur and eventually aortic and distant nodal involvement develops.

The lungs, liver, bone, and brain are also sites for metastases in advanced disease. Ureteral obstruction from enlarging pelvic cancer with resultant renal failure is the most common cause of death in patients with cervical cancer. Sepsis, respiratory failure, hemorrhage, and hepatic failure are also common.

MICROSCOPIC PATHOLOGY OF EPIDERMOID CARCINOMA

Pathogenesis

More is known about the natural history of squamous cell carcinoma of the cervix than about the course of any other cancer. In spite of this, the exact sequence of neoplastic transformation in the cervix remains a subject of controversy. One of the significant findings in very early microscopic carcinoma is the constancy of its origin at the squamocolumnar junction.

In the prepubertal female, the *portio vaginalis* or *exocervix* is composed of cervical stroma without glands, covered by mature or *native squamous epithelium*. The *endocervix*, which is anatomically the canal lying above the external cervical os and below the internal os, is covered by *columnar epithelium* which lines not only the surface of the canal, but the endocervical glands which lie within the stroma (Fig. 12.2).

Prior to menarche, the junction between the squamous epithelium of the exocervix and the columnar epithelium of the endocervix is usually sharp and distinct. However, with the growth of the cervix during menarche, and especially with the physiologic eversion of the endocervix during pregnancy, the columnar epithelium and the glands of the endocervix are everted onto the anatomic exocervix.

This columnar epithelium which is now found on the exocervix is exposed to the vaginal environment. Because of the environmental influence, probably due in part to the pH, the exocervical columnar epithelium is gradually replaced by squamous epithelium. The anatomic zone on the cervix where this occurs is referred to as the *transformation zone*. It is in this dynamic transformation zone that the earliest squamous epithelial abnormalities which are thought to be forerunners of invasive carcinoma are first seen.

Exactly how this process occurs is still a subject of debate despite years of intense study by many investigators.

Whatever the cell or origin however, there

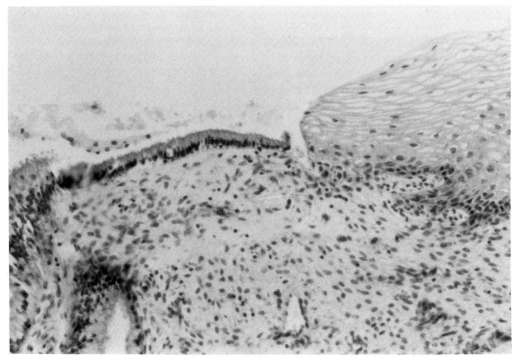

Figure 12.2.   The squamocolumnar junction. The stratified squamous epithelium of the exocervix (*on the right*) gives way to the columnar epithelium which lines the endocervical canal. The anatomic location of the squamocolumnar junction changes with menarche, pregnancy, and other hormonal and mechanical events. (Courtesy of Dr. Eileen B. King, San Francisco.)

is good evidence to suggest that neoplasia of the cervix originates from a single cell rather than multiple sites. Park and Jones, using women who were heterozygous for the A and B form of glucose-6-phosphate dehydrogenase, found that cancer tissue had only the A or B form. Since the locus of the gene for this enzyme is on the X chromosome, the result can be explained by the development of the tumor mass from a single cell which was active for one or the other form of this enzyme.

Intraepithelial Neoplasia

Carcinoma-in-situ has been classically defined as a microscopic pattern in which the full thickness of the lining squamous epithelium *must be completely replaced* by undifferentiated abnormal cells morphologically indistinguishable from cancer (Fig. 12.3). One must not infer, however, that the diagnosis of intraepithelial cancer is simple and clear-cut; on the contrary, it may be one of the most complex and difficult which the pathologist must make. Squamous metaplasia, tangential cuts, condylomata, and other patterns may

be misleading, but unquestionably the most confusing pictures are those due to varying degrees of epithelial hyperactivity and dysplasia.

The incomplete degrees of aberration which involve less than the full thickness of the squamous epithelium have been previously referred to as "atypical cervical epithelium," "atypia," "anaplasia," "basal cell hyperplasia," and many other terms. Most gynecologists and pathologists today refer to these intraepithelial changes as *dysplasia*. Various classifications have been proposed and diagnoses are somewhat subjective, but *mild dysplasia* is said to exist when only the lower one-third of epithelium is replaced by immature undifferentiated cells with frequent mitoses. When the middle third is involved, a diagnosis of *moderate dysplasia* is made and if the upper third of the epithelium is involved, but there is still some maturation on the surface, then a diagnosis of *severe dysplasia* is appropriate. Richart has referred to these changes as *cervical intraepithelial neoplasia*, (C.I.N.) which he has subdivided into clinical-pathologic groups (Fig. 12.4). The natural history of these intraepithelial changes has been the subject of much investigation.

Early Stromal Invasion

Diagnosis of early degrees of stromal invasion is difficult, for buds of tumor may completely replace glands in the absence of true invasion. If the framework of the gland is well preserved and smooth, there is no invasion. If the outline is grayed and hazy, possibly there is beginning stromal invasion (Fig. 12.5). Almost always, the invading squamous cells appear more mature with in-

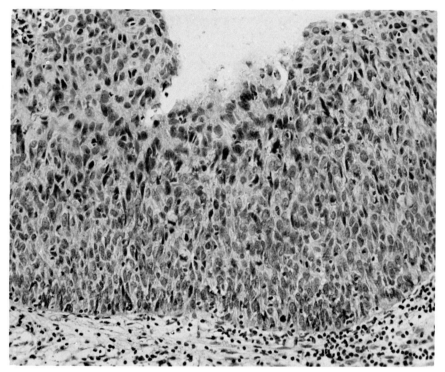

Figure 12.3.   Carcinoma in situ (intraepithelial carcinoma).

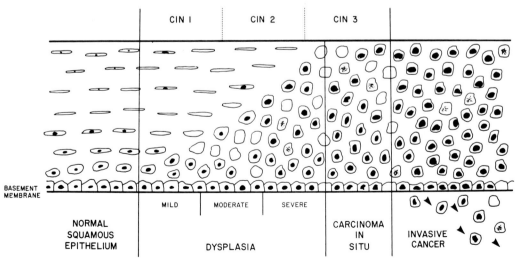

Figure 12.4.   Diagram of cervical epithelium showing the various terminology used to characterize progressive degrees of cervical neoplasia. (Modified from Richart; Can. J. Med. Tech. *38:* 117, 1976).

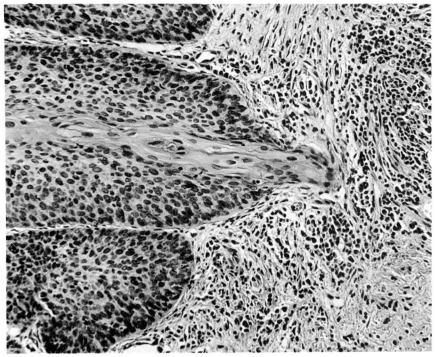

Figure 12.5. Microinvasive carcinoma. Note the eosinophilic cytoplasm of the more mature invading cells. (H & E × 200). (From H. W. Jones, Jr. et al.: *Obstetrics and Gynecology, 30:* 790, 1967.)

creased eosinophilic cytoplasm when compared with the undifferentiated basal-like cells of carcinoma-in-situ. Tangential sections, gland involvement, and poor tissue preparation frequently make this diagnosis extremely difficult.

Invasive Carcinoma

As with carcinoma elsewhere, the microscopic diagnosis of invasive carcinoma of the cervix is based on two chief characteristics: (1) an abnormal pattern or architecture, and (2) abnormalities in the constituent cells.

In the normal epithelial surface, the epithelial cells are sharply demarcated from the stroma by the basement membrane; in cancer, the latter is broken through, so that the epithelium pushes into the stroma, at first in small buds, but later in the form of long columns which grow deep into the stroma much as the roots of a tree grow down into the soil. In all but the earliest phases, therefore, a reasonably certain diagnosis can usually be made with a low power alone, as this suffices to reveal the disorderly and illegitimate invasion of the stroma by the epithelium. It is this invasiveness with the dissemi-

nation of cells by the lymphatics which is responsible for the characteristics traditionally associated with malignancy, such as local infiltration, metastases, and recurrence after incomplete removal.

ADENOCARCINOMA AND ADENOSQUAMOUS CARCINOMA OF THE CERVIX

Cervical adenocarcinoma is less common than the squamous cell variety. It accounts for approximately 10% of all cervical cancers according to recent studies. While it usually begins within the cervical canal, the initial lesion may appear at or near the external os, and in the later stages it may form a large vegetative growth presenting on the vaginal surface of the cervix. More characteristically, the growth produces increasing involvement of the cervix and adjoining tissues without extensive external lesions on the vaginal surface.

Microscopically, it is characterized by the atypical gland patterns so distinctive of adenocarcinoma, in striking contrast with the orderly distribution and appearance of the normal cervical glands. In some cases the departure from normal is moderate, in others the abnormal gland pattern is intricate and highly atypical (Fig. 12.6).

At times, tumors arising from the cervix will contain malignant elements of both squamous and glandular epithelium.

CLINICAL CHARACTERISTICS OF CERVICAL CARCINOMA

The mean age of patients with symptomatic carcinoma of the cervix is about 45 years. In contrast, patients with intraepithelial carcinoma average 32 years of age and it is not uncommon to see patients in their teens or early twenties with this diagnosis. Intraepithelial carcinoma is almost always asymptomatic, the diagnosis being made at the time of routine cervical smear.

Pain is not a symptom of cervical carcinoma until the late stages of the disease. Ignorance of this fact is one of the most important obstacles in the campaign for the early recognition of cancer. In the majority of cases the first symptom is bleeding, although this is usually slight. Characteristically, it is of intermenstrual type if the patient is still within the reproductive years. It is apt to be noted after coitus, severe exertion or the straining of defecation. The contact bleeding following coitus or simple pelvic examination is especially characteristic. Unfortunately, in some cases bleeding does not occur until the disease has obtained a fairly good foothold and extended into the lymphatics, so that even an alert and intelligent patient may have advanced disease before the appearance of symptoms. If the tumor is located in the endocervix, moreover, bleeding is apt to be later in appearance because of the more protected position of the lesion.

Abnormal discharge, frequently pinkish or blood tinged, may at times be noted even before the appearance of the bleeding, especially with adenocarcinoma. As the disease advances, both bleeding and discharge become more persistent and perfuse and the increasing ulceration and secondary infection make the discharge increasingly offensive. Other symptoms such as *bladder irritability,* may arise from involvement of the vesicovaginal septum with corresponding *rectal discomfort* from posterior extension. Heavy, aching *pain* is an ominous symptom and may become severe as the disease advances. Persistent lumbosacral pain, especially when accompanied by lymphedema of the leg, is a very serious prognostic sign. The "terrible triad" of sacral pain, unilateral lymphedema, and unilateral ureteral obstruction indicates far advanced, usually incurable disease. Fistulas into the bladder or rectum may develop, adding tremendously to the patient's misery. Increasing lateral infiltration obstructs the ureters and *uremia is the cause of death* in perhaps the largest proportion of cases.

DIAGNOSIS OF CERVICAL CANCER

Pap Smear

The development of an accurate cytological method for assessing an asymptomatic woman with a completely normal appearing cervix has lead to the diagnosis of many cases of early cancer long before symptomatology or overt pathological abnormalities are apparent. Every sexually active woman should have a cancer smear. Nevertheless, a thorough history regarding intermenstrual or contact bleeding should be taken and careful palpation of the cervix and speculum examination should be performed. *Where there is a visible lesion present on the cervix, it should be*

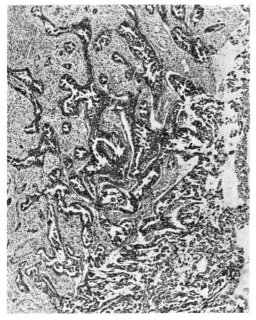

Figure 12.6.   Adenocarcinoma of cervix.

biopsied in addition to obtaining a smear whether or not the lesion looks like cancer.

Papanicolaou and Traut initially introduced the technique of cytology into clinical medicine in 1943. Many different techniques have been described for obtaining cytologic specimens, the so-called *Papanicolaou or "Pap" smear* (Fig. 12.7). Regardless of the procedure used, several principles should be borne in mind: (1) the sampling technique should be optimal for obtaining cells which will provide the most accurate information about the condition under investigation; (2) the specimen should be *immediately* and properly fixed to allow for the best interpretation; and (3) the cytopathologist must be informed of any unusual clinical findings or history, and any specific questions or concerns should be noted. Thus, if screening for cervical cancer is the object, a good sample from the area of the squamocolumnar junction of the cervix is in order, but if evaluation of the hormonal status of a patient is desired, a scraping from the lateral vaginal wall is preferable. In order to provide the most ac-

curate and helpful interpretation of the specimen, it is important to list such facts as the patient's age, last menstrual period, type of contraception (if any), and previous diagnoses or treatment such as biopsy or radiation therapy.

The technique we have used for cervical cancer screening is illustrated in Figure 12.8. Either the pipette shown or a cotton-tipped applicator twirled within the endocervical canal can be used to collect the endocervical sample.

Studies by Silbar and Woodruff, among others, have indicated that cervical cytology has a false negative rate of 10–20%. The gynecologist must always be aware of this problem in counseling patients and in making recommendations about the frequency of examinations.

Schiller Test

This simple test is based on the fact that cancer epithelium contains no glycogen and hence does not take up iodine as does the

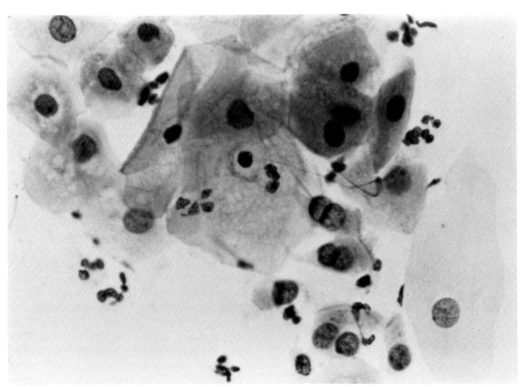

Figure 12.7. Microphotograph of a cervical cytology smear. In this sample, there are large flake-like superficial cells with a small central, dark, nucleus. An intermediate cell is seen on the *lower right*. There is still a large amount of cytoplasm, but the nucleus is larger and the chromatin is finely granular. A few parabasal cells are seen in the *upper left*. There are also some polys and columnar cells in this smear. (Courtesy of Dr. Eileen B. King, San Francisco.)

VAGINAL POOL, CERVICAL AND ENDOCERVICAL SPECIMENS REQUIRED

Complete cytology request forms
Label fixative bottle and frosted end of each slide with patient's name
Gloves must be free of powder
Insert dry or saline rinsed speculum -no lubricant

VAGINAL POOL SPECIMEN OBTAINED FIRST

1. Label slide "V" with lead pencil on frosted end
2. Scrape the posterior fornix pool
3. Spread uniformly on slide with spatula
4. Fix immediately in 95% ethyl alcohol

CERVICAL SPECIMENS OBTAINED SECOND

1. Label slide "C" and attach paper clip
2. Scrape squamocolumnar junction area
   in entirety (360°) using cervical scraper
3. Spread uniformly on slide with cervical scraper
4. Fix immediately in 95% ethyl alcohol

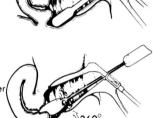

ENDOCERVICAL SPECIMENS OBTAINED THIRD

1. Label slide "E" and attach paper clip
2. Aspirate from the external os
   with disposable glass pipette
3. Expel contents of pipette onto slide
   and spread uniformly with edge of pipette
4. Fix immediately in 95% ethyl alcohol

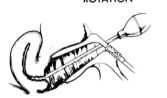

360°
ROTATION

Note: Both ectocervical and endocervical specimens
may be placed on a single slide as shown:

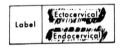

Label | Ectocervical | Endocervical

Figure 12.8.   Technique of obtaining routine gynecological cytology.

normally glycogen-rich epithelium of the cervix or vagina. Thus, application of an iodine solution (Schiller's 0.3% or Lugol's 5%) may show normal epithelium in a deep mahagony color, whereas areas of dysplasia and cancer are unstained and present a sharp distinction.

Unfortunately, columnar epithelium and various benign inflammatory processes may also fail to stain leading to a "positive Schiller test," and more liberal use of smears, colposcopy, and biopsy have, to a certain extent, limited its employment. However, it has a definite value, especially where smears are positive and biopsies inclusive or, when colposcopy is not available, it points out logical targets for biopsy.

Colposcopy

The colposcope is an instrument by which the cervix may be visualized in bright light under a 10–40× magnification. The examination technique is rapid, requiring almost the same time as inspection of the cervix with the naked eye. Special attention is directed to visualizing the *squamo-columnar junction* and the entire *transformation zone* where cervical neoplasia begins and is found in its' early stages.

In recent years, cytological techniques have become so refined that more and more problems are presented in finding small suspect areas on the cervix for clinical investigation. With the discovery of earlier and earlier lesions during routine examination and population screening, the colposcope is assuming an increasingly important place in the sophisticated management of patients with abnormal cytology.

Biopsy

Our own preference is to obtain a colposcopically directed biopsy when the Pap smear is abnormal or if a cervical lesion is visible grossly or with the colposcope. It should be apparent that the pathologist can assess only the material presented to him, and it is paramount to obtain adequate bits of tissue, although biopsy may sometimes be technically difficult.

In the event a trained colposcopist is not available, the technique of *multiple punch biopsy,* with bites of the forceps at 12 and 6 o'clock—the most frequent sites of beginning neoplasia—or a so-called "four quadrant biopsy" with bites at 12, 3, 6, and 9 o'clock of the cervical circumference at the squamocolumnar junction, has been widely adopted. However, this is not a very satisfactory method of evaluating the cervix. Therefore, unless these more or less random punch biopsies show invasive cancer, it is usually necessary to do a large circumferential biopsy called a *cone biopsy* to be sure that a focus of invasive cancer has not been missed.

What has been said above does not apply to the more advanced cases, in which a biopsy from any part of the gross lesion will show cancer, and usually nothing but cancer. Even in the most advanced cases, a biopsy is advisable in order to determine the exact pathological type of the lesion and also to eliminate the rare case in which such lesions as cervical tuberculosis may simulate the gross picture of cancer.

Conization of the Cervix

When the squamocolumnar junction cannot be visualized with the colposcope, the lesion extends into the canal and the upper limits cannot be seen, or if the smear, the colposcopic evaluation, and the directed biopsy do not agree, then a cone biopsy is indicated. If colposcopy is not available and there is no gross lesion on the cervix or no nonstaining areas with the Schiller test, a diagnostic conization is also indicated.

The diagnostic conization is useful not only in establishing the diagnosis of carcinoma-in-situ, but it is vitally important in excluding the possibility of invasive cancer, for it must constantly be borne in mind that carcinoma-in-situ frequently exists at the periphery of a true invasive cancer. A cervical cone biopsy merely involves removing a conical shaped piece of tissue from the cervix which will include the entire area of abnormality (Fig. 12.9). From the pathologic standpoint, the main points to be remembered are: (1) to be sure that the tissue is excised in such a way as to reveal the endocervical mucous membrane as well as the squamous epithelium of the

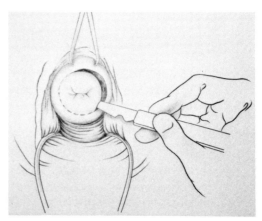

Figure 12.9.   Cone biopsy. The size and shape of the cone is variable and depends on the size and shape of the dysplastic epithelium.

portio vaginalis and the necessary underlying stroma and glands, and (2) to cut a sufficient number of blocks and sections at various levels to be sure that a small area of early invasive carcinoma is not overlooked.

In pregnant patients, morbidity from hemorrhage (9.4%) and premature labor (7.4%) complicated cone biopsy among 180 patients reported by Averette et al. Colposcopic evaluation of pregnant patients with abnormal Pap smears has almost completely eliminated the need for cone biopsy in this group.

CLINICAL CLASSIFICATION OF CERVICAL CANCER

It is obvious that for comparative study of the statistical reports and treatment results of cervical cancer there must be a uniform staging system to provide grouping of similar patients. Since many patients with cervical cancer are treated by radiation therapy and never undergo exploratory laparotomy or lymph node biopsy, the staging system must be clinical rather than surgical to allow for inclusion of patients treated with all modalities. Several different classifications have been proposed through the years, but the international classification which has been adopted by the International Federation of Gynecology and Obstetrics (FIGO) is now widely used (Table 12.1). Patients are staged prior to any therapy utilizing only commonly available diagnostic techniques such as biopsy, examination under anesthesia, cystoscopy, proctoscopy, chest x-ray, intravenous pyelogram, and barium enema. Exploratory laparotomy with lymph node biopsy and lymphangiography, two commonly used techniques in some areas, are not permitted to be considered in staging a patient within the international classification. That does not mean, of course, that such diagnostic tests should not be done or that one cannot take the results into account in planning therapy, but merely that they cannot be considered in the official staging of patients with cervical cancer.

Every patient with cervical cancer should undergo the appropriate diagnostic evaluation and be formally staged prior to the start of therapy. Once so staged, the stage may not be changed as new developments occur in the course of treatment or follow-up.

TREATMENT OF INTRAEPITHELIAL CARCINOMA

The treatment of carcinoma-in-situ of the cervix is far from standardized and many factors enter into the therapeutic decision. Although radiation therapy is rarely used, it is effective therapy and might be considered for a patient who could not tolerate surgery as a result of medical condition or age.

For the average patient who has completed her family and has no objection to hysterectomy, acceptable surgery for carcinoma-in-situ should be total hysterectomy with care 'taken to remove the entire cervix and with preservation of one or both ovaries in the young woman. The hysterectomy may be done abdominally or vaginally. Careful preoperative evaluation by colposcopy and the Schiller test will delineate the extent of the lesion and dictate some variation in the amount of vaginal cuff, if any, which must be removed.

If the patient desires preservation of her reproductive potential or objects to a hysterectomy on whatever grounds, conization, cauterization, or cryotherapy can be used as an alternative to hysterectomy. It is important to involve the patient in this decision, which should be explained to her as clearly as possible.

Table 12.1
Staging Classification for Carcinoma of the Cervix as Adopted by the International Federation of Gynecology and Obstetrics (FIGO)

Preinvasive carcinoma	
Stage 0	Carcinoma in situ, intraepithelial carcinoma
	Cases of Stage 0 should not be included in any therapeutic statistics for invasive carcinoma
Invasive carcinoma	
Stage I	Carcinoma strictly confined to the cervix (extension to the corpus should be disregarded)
Stage Ia	Microinvasive carcinoma (early stromal invasion)
Stage Ib	All other cases of Stage I. Occult cancer should be marked "occ"
Stage II	The carcinoma extends beyond the cervix, but has not extended on to the pelvic wall. The carcinoma involves the vagina, but not the lower third
Stage IIa	No obvious parametrial involvement
Stage IIb	Obvious parametrial involvement
Stage III	The carcinoma has extended on to the pelvic wall. On rectal examination there is no cancer-free space between the tumor and the pelvic wall. The tumor involves the lower third of the vagina. All cases with a hydronephrosis or non-functioning kidney should be included, unless they are known to be due to other cause.
Stage IIIa	No extension on to the pelvic wall.
Stage IIIb	Extension on to the pelvic wall and/or hydronephrosis or nonfunctioning kidney.
Stage IV	The carcinoma has extended beyond the true pelvis or has clinically involved the mucosa of the bladder or rectum. A bullous edema as such does not permit a case to be allotted to Stage IV.
Stage IVa	Spread of the growth to adjacent organs
Stage IVb	Spread to distant organs

Conization

Therapeutic conization has been used much longer than the other two simple methods and was first used as an alternative to hysterectomy with a view to preserving fertility. Although one of the advantages of conization is the preservation of fertility, the conization itself may adversely affect reproductive function.

Bleeding is the main complication of cone biopsy. Pelvic infection and cervical stenosis are occasionally seen. Induction of labor is a risk in the pregnant patient.

Cauterization and Cryosurgery

The treatment of cervical atypia and intraepithelial neoplasia by cauterization or freezing is a more recent development and has the great advantage of being possible on an outpatient basis.

Long-term results are not available from either of these methods but, as judged by persistent positive smears after treatment, Wilbanks et al. found that with cauterization atypia was cured in 84% of patients.

It is important to realize that the potential for persistent or recurrent epithelial neoplasia exists following this or any other therapy, including hysterectomy, for carcinoma-in-situ.

MICROINVASIVE CARCINOMA

Stage Ia, i.e. microinvasive carcinoma, represents a special situation. The definition of this lesion is just as controversial as is the treatment. In the FIGO classification, Stage Ia is defined as "early stromal invasion," but exactly what constitutes "early" is not specified. Historically, stromal invasion up to 5 mm has been accepted as "microinvasive carcinoma" or Stage Ia. The Society of Gynecologic Oncologists has recommended that Stage Ia cervical cancer be defined as cases in which the neoplastic epithelium invades the stroma in one or more places to a depth of 3 mm or less below the base of the epithelium and in which lymphatic or vascular involvement is not demonstrated. Depth of invasion, the importance of a confluent pattern, and lymphatic or vascular space involvement are all controversial points. All agree that *a cone biopsy with adequate margins is essential to making an accurate diagnosis of microinvasive carcinoma.*

Because of the difficulties of making the correct diagnosis, recommendations for therapy must be flexible to allow for such variables as the amount and depth of invasion, the suitability of the patient for surgery, and the attitude of the gynecologist. For patients with penetration less than 3 mm below the basement membrane with no lymphatic space involvement and no confluent pattern, a simple hysterectomy, either abdominal or vaginal, is adequate. The studies of Boyes et al., Christopherson et al. and Ng and Reagan indicate that recurrences are rare and survival rates approach 100% when simple hysterectomy is used to treat patients with a small isolated focus of cancer with up to 5 mm invasion and no lymphatic space involvement.

However, with a large area of tumor invasion, with lymphatic space involvement, or when the depth of invasion is in the 3–5 mm range or greater, we have generally recommended radical hysterectomy or radiation.

INVASIVE CERVICAL CANCER— RADIATION THERAPY

General Principles

In the treatment of cervical cancer, both external and intracavitary radiation are generally used but other techniques such as radioactive needles and implantable seeds may be used in special circumstances. Although this treatment is usually managed by trained radiotherapists today, it is important for the gynecologist to understand the principles and techniques involved so that he may work with the radiotherapist and the patient to provide the optimum treatment possible. As a general principle, external radiation which delivers a uniform dose to the whole pelvis is emphasized in the treatment of large tumors with spread to the paracervical tissues and a high probability of pelvic lymph node metastases. Intracavitary radiation, which consists of radioactive sources placed within the uterus and lateral vaginal fornices, produces high intensity radiation. However, the extent of the radiation is very limited so that it is utilized as the main treatment component in patients with small tumors or after a large primary lesion has been reduced in size by external irradiation.

Therapy Techniques

Radiation therapy for cervical cancer usually involves *external radiation* which is administered to the whole pelvis with the purpose of destroying tumor in the parametrial tissues, pelvic wall, and lymph nodes of the pelvis (Fig. 12.10).

Patients are usually treated via anterior and posterior "portals," or treatment fields, each day although in some instances lateral fields or a rotational technique may be used. Each treatment, or "fraction," is usually from 170 to 200 rads/day and thus the average total duration of external therapy for a patient who is to receive a standard dose of 4000 rads is 4–5 weeks.

During the therapy, patients have few side effects and usually are able to continue their regular routine. Many patients experience some diarrhea due to the irritation of the rectal mucosa and occasionally some urinary frequency and urgency.

Intracavitary radiation is also an important part of the therapy for cervical cancer and was one of the first successful therapeutic applications of radium. The hollow, thin tube, or *tandem,* with the correct pelvic curvature is inserted into the uterus in the operating room under general or regional anesthesia. Two vaginal cylinders called *colpostats*

or *ovoids* are next selected depending on the vaginal size and placed in the lateral vaginal fornices. With great care to be sure that the applicators are correctly positioned, they are then packed in place with gauze packing. Anterior-posterior, and lateral placement x-rays are then taken in the operating room and checked to be sure that the applicators are in satisfactory position (Fig. 12.11). They are readjusted if necessary, and the patient is returned to her room after recovery from anesthesia. Finally, with appropriate radiation safety precautions, the radioactive sources are loaded into the applicators. This *afterloading technique* greatly reduces the radiation exposure to hospital personnel and allows unhurried placement of the applicators which greatly improves the precision of the application, allowing a maximum dose to the cervix with a tolerable dose to the bladder and rectum.

The patient is kept at bedrest with catheter drainage and low residue diet until the radioactive sources and applicators have been removed—usually 48–72 hours. The length of the application and the radiation dose to the points of interest such as the cervix, bladder, rectum, and pelvic lymph nodes are calculated by computer dosimetry. Most clinics use low-dose heparin, 5000 units subcutaneously every 8–12 hours, preoperatively and throughout the period of bedrest, until the patient is fully ambulatory again.

Depending on the size and anatomy, external irradiation may be given initially or may follow intracavitary radiation, or a split course of external irradiation interrupted by one or two intracavitary applications may be utilized. Occasionally, the anatomy will dictate that the patient be treated entirely by external therapy or, in some early lesions, only intracavitary radiation may be used. In still other cases, it may be preferable, as discussed below, to add hysterectomy to the radiation, and so a good working relationship with regular communication between the radiotherapist and the gynecologist is essential.

Results and Complications

There can be no doubt that radiation therapy is effective treatment for carcinoma of the cervix. The 5-year survival rates presented in Table 12.2 show results reported from different clinics throughout the world.

Despite all precautions, it is inevitable that

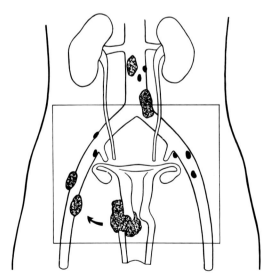

Figure 12.10. Typical external radiation field for cervical cancer. The treated area includes the primary tumor and the regional lymphatics of the pelvis.

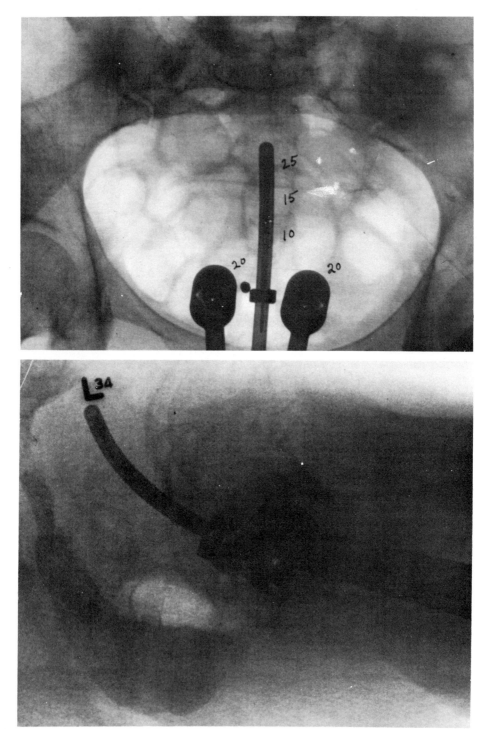

Figure 12.11. (*Top*) An anterior posterior roentgenogram showing a satisfactory application of the tandem and ovoids in a patient with carcinoma of the cervix. The numbers are the milligrams of radium equivalents of cesium in the tandem and ovoids. (*Bottom*) A lateral view of a satisfactory cesium application. A small amount of barium has been introduced in the rectum to show its location.

Table 12.2
Results of Radiation Therapy for Carcinoma of the Cervix[a]

City	Patients	Treated by Radiation	Absolute 5 Year Survival			
			Stage I	Stage II	Stage III	Stage IV
		%	%	%	%	%
Innsbruck, Austria	439	90.6	88	76	49	9
Toronto, Canada	671	82	77	70	36	6
Munich, Germany	415	98	91	76	38	12
Rotterdam, Netherlands	508	99	80	67	39	5
Warsaw, Poland	1251	97	76	60	31	17
Stockholm, Sweden	924	91	85	58	27	11
Cape Town, South Africa	711	93	57	43	25	4
Manchester, England	1501	99	72	55	35	8
Danville, United States	106	82	75	67	20	0
Totals for all patients treated with radiation alone	6526		75	57	31	9

[a] Adapted from *Annual Report on the Results of Treatment in Gynecological Cancer*, vol. 17, International Federation of Gynecology and Obstetrics, Stockholm, 1969–1972.

radiation should have some complications. Every clinic must experience a certain percentage of complication or the salvage rate will be poor. It has often been said that "the worst complication of therapy is recurrent cancer." Almost the only mortality associated with radiation therapy is the occasional patient who dies from a pulmonary embolus during a radium application. However, many women experience varying degrees of bladder irritability, diarrhea, skin changes, and occasional rectal bleeding during and after therapy, but most of these cases are transitory and short-lived. Far more distressing and troublesome are the bowel or bladder fistulas that may occur at any stage after treatment, even in the complete absence of cancer.

The incidence of radiation complications is directly related to the dose which, for the most part, is related to the stage of disease or tumor volume. In addition, it seems probable that radiation tolerance is variable from one individual to another, and when a patient seems unduly sensitive based on her early response, it seems prudent to consider a reduction in the total dose.

INVASIVE CERVICAL CANCER— SURGICAL THERAPY

The resurgence of surgery as a primary treatment for cancer of the cervix is directly attributable to such medical advances as improved anesthesia, well equipped blood banks, antibiotic drugs, etc., which have made it possible to perform extensive radical surgery with minimal operative mortality.

Meigs, and others, suggested the routine use of an extended radical Wertheim-type hysterectomy and pelvic lymphadenectomy in medically fit women with Stage I and Stage II lesions (Fig. 12.12). There is no question that a skilled operator can perform this procedure with negligible mortality but, even in expert hands, there is some irreducible morbidity.

There are few clinics in which all patients with Stage I and early Stage II disease are treated by surgery. Thus, surgical series are selected and end results must be interpreted with this in mind. The 5-year figures shown in Table 12.3 for abdominal radical hysterectomy and pelvic lymphadenectomy may be considered representative.

The curability of lymph node metastases by surgery has received special attention just as it has with radiation. There is no doubt that lymph node involvement is of ominous prognostic significance. About 15% of all patients with Stage I cervical cancer will have spread to the pelvic nodes, and it is not clear if radiation therapy following radical hysterectomy and pelvic lymphadenectomy can increase the survival rate in this group of patients. Survival rates of 50–60% have been reported for these patients with and without adjunctive postoperative radiation.

Surgical therapy, like radiation, is associated with complications—principally to the urinary tract. Ureteral or vesicle fistulas have been reported in up to 10% of patients in some older series, but with more case selection and improvement in technique most recent series report fistula rates of 5% or less (Table 12.3).

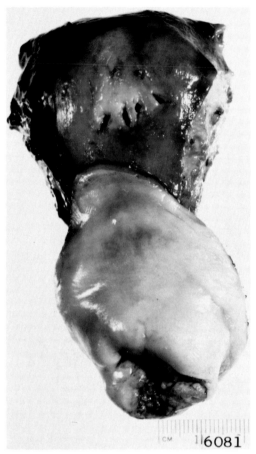

Figure 12.12. Specimen from epidermoid carcinoma of the cervix clinical Stage Ib. Note the very large vaginal cuff and the fact that the tubes and ovaries were not removed. In operations for Stage Ia and Ib about one-half of the patients, depending on the age, have the tubes and ovaries left in situ.

COMBINED RADIATION AND SURGERY

It is our feeling that this should not be a routine form of treatment, and for two different reasons. First, there is no doubt that irradiation, by virtue of its tendency to cause increased vascularity, edema, and scarring, makes subsequent surgery more difficult with a resultant increase in complicating fistula. Of even more importance, however, is the tendency of surgery to undo one of the most important and vital irradiation effects. In addition to an immediately destructive and lethal affect on cancer, both radium and x-ray lead to later fibrosis and scarring that may entrap and hold in check microscopically viable appearing tumor cells. Surgery tends to cut across and break down these fibrotic barriers with dissemination of malignant cells into lymphatic and vascular channels. We have observed this apparent sequence in more than one instance.

We cannot recommend this form of therapy for the routine case.

In some cases of large, endocervical tumors and perhaps in cases with involvement of the uterine fundus or unusual histology such as adenosquamous carcinoma, adjunctive *simple* hysterectomy may improve survival by removing bulky central disease—the so called barrel lesion—which cannot be sterilized by radiation therapy.

CARCINOMA OF THE CERVICAL STUMP

With the contemporary use of total hysterectomy carcinoma of the cervical stump is becoming an increasingly less common problem, although it is by no means rare to see

Table 12.3
Results of Radical Hysterectomy for Stage Ib Cervical Cancer

Author	Patients	Pelvic Nodes	Operative Mortality	Fistula Rate	5-Year Survival
		%	%	%	%
Liu and Meigs	116	17.7	1.7	9.0	78.4
Christensen et al.	168	17.2	0.5	8.8	82.7
Brunschwig	202	13.4	1.1	10.0	81.5
Masterson	120	10.0	1.1	4.4	87.5
Hoskins et al.	224	9.8	0.9	2.2	87.0
Morley and Seski	156	12.6	1.4	4.8	87.2
Webb and Symmonds	304	14.5	0.3	2.5	90.0
Total	1290	13.4	0.9	5.4	85.5

such cases today. In previous reports, close to 50% of patients with malignancy of the cervical stump have been diagnosed less than a year following subtotal hysterectomy, making it appear probable that the cancer was present at the time of the incomplete and inadequately studied hysterectomy. Routine prehysterectomy Pap smears should certainly be the rule and an especially careful evaluation, possibly including colposcopy and/or biopsy should be undertaken if a subtotal operation is contemplated (as is rarely necessary today).

The recent series of Nass et al. and Wimbush and Fletcher suggest minimal morbidity with survival rates comparable to those reported for patients with an intact uterus when modern radiation therapy techniques are utilized.

In early cases, just as with cancer of the intact cervix, radical surgery can be used. Radical cervicectomy and pelvic lymphadenectomy is somewhat more difficult since the landmarks may be altered and the convenient "handle" of the uterine fundus is absent.

CANCER OF THE CERVIX IN PREGNANCY

Fortunately, cancer of the cervix in the pregnant woman is relatively rare.

If careful study of the cervix by cytology, colposcopy, and directed biopsy and occasionally by cone biopsy, as outlined in the section on diagnosis, indicates that the disease is intraepithelial, the pregnancy may be allowed to go to term with normal vaginal delivery, and treatment deferred until the postpartum period. For more advanced cancer, the disease should be treated without regard to the pregnancy unless the pregnancy is 26 weeks or more. After 28 and 30 weeks, the baby can be delivered by classical cesarean section and then treatment instituted.

In general, if the cancer is recognized in the early stages of pregnancy the disease is treated promptly and the pregnancy disregarded. For Stage Ib and early Stage II cases, radical surgery may be used (Fig. 12.13). For other stages, irradiation therapy is the best plan starting with external irradiation. Spontaneous abortion usually follows. Others prefer to do a therapeutic abortion or hysterotomy, followed by either irradiation or radical operation depending on the stage of disease and the personal predilection of the physician. In the later stages of pregnancy, one can wait a short time for viability or, if this has been reached, deliver the baby by a classical cesarean section followed by radical hysterectomy or irradiation. The prime motive is to treat the cancer as promptly and as normally as possible and to avoid vaginal delivery.

TREATMENT OF RECURRENT OR METASTATIC CANCER

Clearly, not all patients with cervical cancer are cured by their initial therapy. By definition, cancer which is diagnosed within 6 months of primary therapy is called *persistent* disease whereas tumor diagnosed after that time is referred to as *recurrent* disease, despite the fact that in most cases the tumor cells which grew into a tumor mass eventually diagnosed as recurrent cancer have been present since the original tumor was diagnosed and treated.

Halpern et al. reviewed a series of 134 patients with recurrent cervical cancer seen at the Sloane Hospital for Women in New York. He found that 60% of patients destined to develop recurrent disease were diagnosed in the first 2 years following therapy and by 5 years more than 90% of those who would fail had been diagnosed (Fig. 12.14). It is interesting to note that the most common presenting symptom in this group of patients with recurrent cancer of the cervix was *no symptoms*—that is, they are asymptomatic when diagnosed at the time of a routine follow-up visit. The importance of careful follow-up is even more clearly seen when we realize that of the 14 patients in this group who were apparently cured by secondary therapy for this recurrence, 4 (28.5%) were in this asymptomatic group. Other common symptoms included bleeding (13%), back or leg pain (19%), weight loss (9.7%), and obstructive uropathy (8.2%). From an analysis of the common sites of recurrence and the treatability of these recurrences, it seems that a good interval history, careful pelvic examination, and cytologic smear are the only tests that should be "routine" at follow-up visits. The patient's weight and blood pressure are recorded and the lymph nodes of the supraclavicular areas and groins are palpated, and a breast exam is done, but these procedures usually pick up other medical diseases or occasional distant metastases rather than early, treatable recurrence.

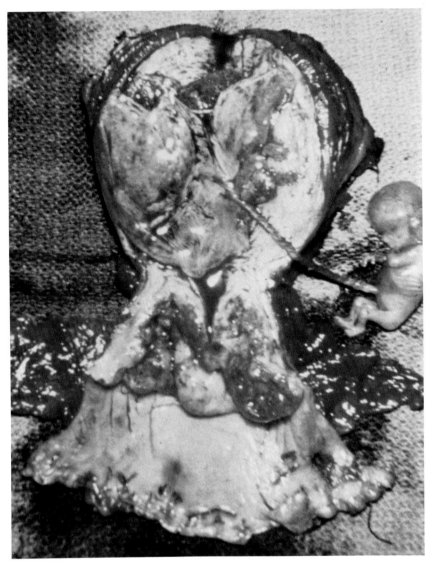

Figure 12.13.   Radical hysterectomy in a patient with Stage Ib carcinoma of the cervix at 12 weeks pregnancy.

Diagnosis

Although recurrent cervical carcinoma may be easily diagnosed when the smear is positive or a granular lesion is seen at the vaginal apex, at times the diagnosis may be extremely difficult and equivocal. It should be emphasized that a distinction must be made between potentially curable recurrences such as those at the vaginal vault or central pelvis and probably incurable metastases such as pelvic sidewall masses, which call for a less urgent definite diagnosis.

In addition to the Pap smear and biopsy, there are several other techniques helpful in confirming a diagnosis of recurrent cancer. The *thin needle biopsy* or more accurately, aspiration for cytology, is a useful technique to sample the nodular, indurated perimetria or the pelvic or abdominal mass. Chest x-ray and IVP are frequently helpful, but barium enema is rarely worthwhile unless some specific symptom suggests obstruction. Cystoscopy and proctoscopy may be useful in selected cases. New techniques such as ultrasound and CT scanning of the pelvis or abdomen may be helpful. Radionucleotide bone, liver, and occasionally brain scans are

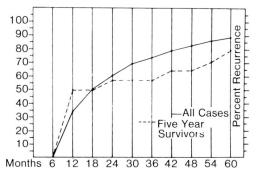

Figure 12.14. Recurrent carcinoma of the cervix. Months from initial treatment until the diagnosis of recurrence. The dashed line represents those patients who were retreated and survived at least 5 more years. (From T. F. Halpern et al.: *American Journal of Obstetrics and Gynecology, 114:* 755, 1972.)

indicated in some patients. It must be remembered, however, that a good history and careful physical examination will help select those tests which will be most helpful and diagnostic.

Treatment of Recurrence

Once the diagnosis of recurrent cancer has been confirmed, what are the options?

Radiation

After full-course modern radiation therapy for treatment of the original primary cancer, *reirradiation of the pelvis* is frought with hazard. T. K. Jones, et al. reported only a 3.8% 5-year survival in 53 patients with a curative attempt at reirradiation for recurrent cervical cancer. The urinary tract and rectovaginal fistula rate was 34%. Almost identical figures have been reported by Keettel et al. The survival rates are essentially the same as for patients who were not treated at all and the high fistula rate is certainly not palliative.

On the other hand, patients who have been treated primarily by radical surgery and have not previously received pelvic irradiation are good candidates for radiation therapy for recurrent disease. In addition, radiation therapy to focal lesions outside the previous radiation fields may well be palliative and rarely curative. Bone metastases or supraclavicular nodes are a good example of metastatic lesions which can be very effectively managed with small field radiation therapy.

Surgery

Radical surgery, however, provides the most likely hope of cure for a few patients with recurrent cervical carcinoma following primary radiation therapy. The surgical approach depends on the extent and location of the recurrence and to some extent the amount of previous radiation. If early, a *radical hysterectomy with pelvic lymphadenectomy* may be utilized, but this is insufficient for all but the smallest central recurrences. It should be remembered that the radiation-induced endarteritis has produced poor vascularity in the pelvis with resultant poor healing and high fistula rate.

Ultraradical surgery, as proposed by Brunschwig, is sometimes a lifesaving procedure in these circumstances. The procedure of *total pelvic exenteration* involves removal of all pelvic organs including the uterus, tubes, ovaries, bladder, and rectum with transplantation of the ureters into an exteriorized colon or illial segment as well as removal of the pelvic lymph nodes (Fig. 12.15). This operation involves considerable morbidity and a definite mortality even if done by trained gynecologic oncologists. With recurrent or resistant irradiated cancer, one must admit that there is no chance for cure other than by surgery.

Since the pioneering work of Brunschwig, the indications for pelvic exenteration have been refined, surgical and postoperative care greatly improved, and the limits of practicality have been generally accepted. Great improvements have been made in reducing morbidity and mortality and the survival rates in most recent series are in the 30–40% range with a mortality rate related to the surgery of less than 5%. Since this is essentially a "last hope" attempt in most patients, there is a temptation to bend a little so that there are no absolute contraindications to pelvic exenteration, but Rutledge lists several relative contraindications: (1) tumor spread beyond the pelvis, fixed to the pelvic bones, or with multiple nodes involved; (2) poor surgical candidate due to medical condition, obesity, or age greater than 70; (3) more than 7000 rads external radiation; (4) psychological instability. This type of ultraradical surgery should be done by trained gynecologic oncologists at a center where such operations are done with reasonable frequency since the

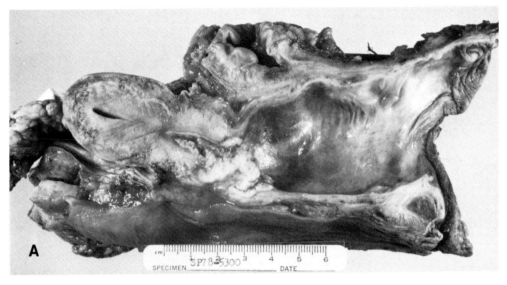

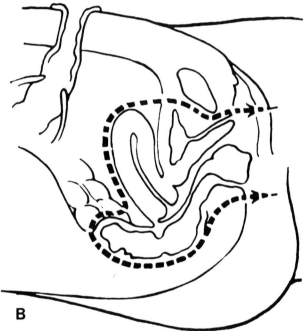

Figure 12.15. Total pelvic exenteration. The uterus, cervix, vagina, bladder, and rectum are removed *en block* and a urinary conduit and colostomy are constructed. *A.* Lateral view of the gross specimen. *B.* Diagram of excised organs.

perioperative care and rehabilitation of these patients requires considerable experience.

PALLIATIVE THERAPY

Based on the collected statistics of the FIGO Annual Report, slightly more than one-half of all patients with Stages I–IV cer-

vical cancer are cured. This means that about one-half are not cured and it becomes the responsibility of the physician to see that these patients have sympathetic and responsible attention.

Death from cancer of the cervix is most often due to uremia secondary to ureteral obstruction. Infection, hemorrhage, and malnutrition are also common. In some patients, pain is the most troublesome symptom to combat.

Systemic or regional chemotherapy has been disappointing for most patients with epidermoid carcinoma of the cervix. However, modest improvement is sometime noted and Smith et al. reported a 19% objective response in 107 patients treated with cyclophosphamide, which they found to be the safest and most easily administered chemotherapeutic agent among many which they investigated. Although no cures were noted and doubtful prolongation of life was obtained, the patients reported an improved sense of well being and required less narcotic. Newer agents such as *cis*-platinum and Adriamycin and various drug combinations are presently under investigation.

As noted above, relief of pain is often the most serious problem. Characteristically, the pain may begin in the sacroiliac region from infiltration of the pelvic lymph nodes with resultant pressure on the nerves to the legs. Such pain radiating down the leg, and especially when accompanied by lymphedema and ureteral obstruction, is an exceedingly serious prognostic finding. For any patient with localized pain and a predicted life span of more than 3 or 4 months, some consideration should be given to a chordotomy, if liberal use of narcotics is ineffective. Oral or rectal pain medication such as narcotics, Schlessenger's Solution and Brompton's Mixture may be helpful. Emotional support by the physician, family members and friends, and such organizations such as the Hospice movement are often invaluable.

References and Additional Readings

Annual Report on the Results of Treatment in Gynecological Cancer, FIGO Stockholm, Vol. 17, 1969–1972.

Andras, E. T., Fletcher, G. H. and Rutledge, F. N.: Radiotherapy of carcinoma of the cervix following simple hysterectomy. Am. J. Obstet. Gynecol., *115:* 647, 1973.

Aurelian, L.: Varions and antigens of herpes type 2 in cervical carcinoma. Cancer Res., *33:* 1548, 1973.

Averette, H. E., Nasser, N., Yankow, S. L., and Little, W. A.: Cervical conization in pregnancy. Am. J. Obstet. Gynecol. *106:* 543, 1970.

Averette, H. E., Nelson, J. H., Jr., Ng, A. B. P., Hoskins, W. J., Boyce, J. G., and Ford, J. H., Jr.: Diagnosis and management of microinvasive (Stage Ia) carcinoma of the uterine cervix. Cancer *38:* 414, 1976.

Bjerre, B., Eliasson, G., Linell, F., Soderberg, H., and Sjoberg, N. O.: Conization as the only treatment for carcinoma-in-situ of the uterine cervix. Am. J. Obstet. Gynecol. *125:* 143, 1976.

Boyes, D. A., Worth, A. J., and Fidler, H. K.: The results of treatment of 4389 cases of pre-clinical cervical squamous carcinoma. J. Obstet. Gynaecol. Br. Commonw. *77:* 769, 1970.

Brunschwig, A.: Complete excision of pelvic viscera for advanced carcinoma; a one-stage abdominoperineal operation with end colostomy and bilateral ureteral implantation into the colon above the colostomy. Cancer, *1:* 177, 1948.

Brunschwig, A.: Surgical treatment of stage I cancer of the cervix. Cancer, *13:* 34, 1960.

Brunschwig, A.: Surgical treatment of carcinoma of the cervix, recurrent after irradiation of the combination of irradiation and surgery. AJR, *99:* 365, 1967.

Brunschwig, A.: Some reflections on pelvic exenterations after twenty years' experience. In *Progress in Gynecology,* edited by S. H. Sturgis, and M. L. Taymor, Vol. 5, p. 416. Grune & Stratton, Inc., New York, 1970.

Christensen, A., Lange, p., and Neilsen, E.: Surgery and radiotherapy for carcinoma of the cervix: surgical treatment. Acta Obstet. Gynecol. Scand (Suppl) *43:* 59, 1964.

Christopherson, W. M., Gray, L. A., and Parker, J. E.: Microinvasive carcinoma of the uterine cervix: a long-term followup study of eighty cases. Cancer *38:* 629, 1976.

Coppleson, M., Pixley, E., and Reid, B.: *Colposcopy: A Scientific and Practical Approach to the Cervix in Health and Disease.* Charles C Thomas, Springfield, Ill., 1971.

Coppleson, M., and Reid. B.: The pathogenesis of cervical intraepithelial neoplasia in *The Colposcopist.* American Society for Colposcopy and Cervical Pathology, March, 1979.

Cramer, D. W. and Cutler, S. J.: Incidence of histopathology of malignancies of the female genital organs in the United States. Am. J. Obstet. Gynecol. *118:* 443, 1974.

Creasman, W. T., Weed, Jr., J. C., Curry, S. L., Johnston, W. W., and Parker, R. T.: Efficacy of cryosurgical treatment of severe cervical intraepithelial neoplasia. Obstet. Gynec., *41:* 501, 1973.

De Petrillo, A. D., Townsend, D. E., Morrow, C. P., et al.: Colposcopy evaluation of the abnormal Papanicolaou test in pregnancy. Am. J. Obstet. Gynecol. *121:* 441, 1975.

Doll, R., Payne, P., and Waterhouse, J. (eds): Cancer incidence in five continents. *International Union Against Cancer,* Vol. 2. p. 1966. Springer-Verlag, Berlin, 1972.

Dudan, R. C., Yon, J. L., Ford, J. H., and Averette, H. E.: Carcinoma of the cervix and pregnancy. Gynecol. Oncol. *1:* 283, 1973.

Durrance, F. Y.: Computer dosimetry of radium dosage to pelvic lymph nodes, In *Cancer of the Uterus and Ovary,* edited by F. N. Rutledge, p. 204. Year Book Medical Publishers, Chicago, 1969.

Durrance, F. Y., Fletcher, G. H., and Rutledge, F.: Analysis of central recurrent disease in stages I and II squamous cell carcinomas of the cervix on intact uterus. AJR, *106:* 831, 1969.

Fletcher, G. E.: *Textbook of Radiotherapy.* Lea & Febiger, Philadelphia, 1973.

Fox, C. H.: Biologic behavior of dysplasia and carcinoma-in-situ. Am. J. Obstet. Gynecol. *99:* 960, 1967.

Frick, H. C.: Cancer of the cervix: treatment. In *Corscaden's Gynecologic Cancer,* edited by S. B. Gusberg and H. C. Frick, Ed. 5, p. 241, Williams & Wilkins Co., Baltimore, 1978.

Gagnon, F.: Contribution to study of etiology and prevention of cancer of cervix of uterus. Am. J. Obstet. Gynecol., *60:* 516, 1950.

Haenszel, W., and Hillhouse, M.: Uterine cancer morbidity in New York City and its relation to the pattern of regional variation within the United States. J. Natl. Cancer Inst., *22:* 1157, 1959.

Hall, J. E., and Walton, L.: Dysplasia of the cervix: a prospective tudy of 206 cases. Am. J. Obstet. Gynecol. *100:* 662, 1968.

Halpern, T. F., Frick, H. C., et al.: Critical points of failure in the therapy of cancer of the cervix. Am. J. Obstet. Gynecol. *114:* 755, 1972.

Hoskins, W. J., Ford, J. H., Jr., Lutz, M. H., and Averette, H. E.: Radical hysterectomy and pelvic lymphadenectomy for the management of early invasive cancer of the cervix. Gynecol. Oncol. *4:* 278, 1976.

Ingersoll, F. M., Ulfelder, H.: Pelvic exenteration for carcinoma of the cervix. New Engl. J. Med. *274:* 648, 1966.

Joelsson, I.: Experience at Radiumhemmet in treatment of carcinoma of the uterine cervix. Gynecol. Oncol., *1:* 17, 1972.

Johnson, L. D., Easterday, C. L., Gore, H., and Hertig, A. T.: The histogenesis of carcinoma in situ of the uterine cervix. Cancer, *17:* 213, 1964.

Jones, H. W., Jr., Katayama, K. P., Stafl, A., and Davis, H. J.: The chromosomes of cervical atypia, carcinoma in situ and invasive carcinoma of the cervix. Obstet. Gynecol., *30:* 790, 1967.

Jones, T. K. McDonald, I., and Brestlow, L.: Epidemiologic factors in carcinoma of the cervix. Am. J. Obstet. Gynecol., *76:* 1, 1958.

Jones, T. K., Jr., Levitt, S. H. and Krug, E. R.: Restraint of persistent and recurrent carcinoma of the cervix with irradiation. Radiology 95: 167, 1970.

Josey, W. E., Nahmias, A. J., and Naib, Z. M.: The epidemiology of type 2 (genital) herpes simplex virus infection. Obstet. Gynecol. Surv., 27: 295, 1972.

Julian, C. G., Daikoku, N. H., and Gillespie, A.: Adenoepidermoid and adenosquamous carcinoma of the uterus. Am. J. Obstet. Gynecol, *128:* 106, 1977.

Kaufman, R. H., and Irwin, J. F.: The cryosurgical therapy of cervical intraepithelial neoplasia. III. Continuing follow-up. Am. J. Obstet. Gynecol. *131:* 381, 1978.

Keettel, W. C., Van Voorhis, L. W., and Latourette, H. B.: Management of recurrent carcinoma of the cervix. Am. J. Obst. Gynecol. *102:* 671, 1968.

Kessler, I. I.: Human cervical cancer as a venereal disease. Cancer Res. *36:* 783, 1976.

Ketcham, A. S., Deckers, P. J., Sugerbaker, E. V., Hoye, R. C., Thomas, L. B., and Smith, A. R.: Pelvic exenteration for carcinoma of the uterine cervix. Cancer *26:* 513, 1970.

Kim, K., Rigal, R. D., Patrick, J. R., Walters, J. K., Bennett, A., Nordin, W., Claybrook, J. R., and Parekh, R. R.: The changing trends of uterine cancer and cytology: a study of morbidity and mortality trends over a twenty year period. Cancer *42:* 2439, 1978.

Kiselow, M., Butcher, H. R. Jr., and Bricker, E. M.: Results of the radical surgical treatment of advanced pelvic cancer: a fifteen-year study. Ann. Surg. *166:* 428, 1967.

Kolstad, P., and Klem, V.: Long-term follow-up of 1121 cases of cervical carcinoma-*in-situ*. Obstet. Gynecol. *48:* 125, 1976.

Kullander, S., and Sjööberg, Nils-Otto: Treatment of carcinoma in situ of the cervix uteri by conization. Acta Obstet. Gynecol. Scand., *50:* 153, 1971.

Liu, W., and Meigs, J. V.: Radical hysterectomy and pelvic lymphadenectomy. Am. J. Obstet. Gynecol., *69:* 1, 1955.

Lohe, K. J., Burghardt, E., Hillemanns, H. G., Kaufmann, C., Ober, K. G., and Zander, J.: Early squamous cell carcinoma of the uterine cervix. Gynecol. Oncol. *6:* 31, 1978.

Lurain, J. R., and Gallup, D. G.: Management of abnormal Papanicolaou smears in pregnancy. Obstet. Gynecol. *53:* 484, 1979.

MacVicar, J., and Willocks, J.: The effect of diathermy conization of the cervix on subsequent fertility, pregnancy and delivery. J. Obstet. Gynaecol. Br. Commonw., *75:* 355, 1968.

Martimbeau, P. W., Kjorstad, K. E., and Kolstad, P.: Stage Ib carcinoma of the cervix, The Norwegian Radium Hospital, 1968–1970: results of treatment and major complications I. Lymphedema. Am. J. Obstet. Gynecol. *131:* 389, 1978.

Masterson, J. G.: The role of surgery in the treatment of early carcinoma of the cervix. Clin. Obstet. Gynaecol. *10:* 922, 1967.

Meigs, J. V.: *Surgical Treatment of Cancer of the Cervix.* Grune & Stratton Inc., New York, 1954.

Mikuta, J. J., Giuntoli, R. L., Rubin, E. L., and Mangan, C. E. The "problem" radical hysterectomy. Am. J. Obstet. Gynecol., *128:* 119, 1977.

Morley, G. W., and Seski, J. C.: Radical pelvic surgery versus radiation therapy for stage I carcinoma of the cervix (exclusive of microinvasion). Am. J. Obstet. Gynecol. *126:* 785, 1976.

Nass, J. M., Brady, L. W., Glassburn, J. R., and Prasasvinichai, S.: The radiotherapeutic management of carcinoma of the cervical stump. Int. J. Radiat. Oncol. Biol. Phys. *4:* 279, 1978.

Nelson, A. J., Fletcher, G. H., and Wharton, J. T.: Indications for adjunctive conservative extrafascial hysterectomy in selected cases of carcinoma of the uterine cervix. AJR *128:* 91, 1975.

Ng, A. B. P., and Reagan, J. W.: Microinvasive carcinoma of the uterine cervix. Am. J. Clin. Path., *52:* 511, 1969.

Papanicolaou, G. N., and Traut, H. F.: *Diagnosis of Uterine*

Cancer by the Vaginal Smear, The Commonwealth Fund, New York, 1943.

Park, I. J., and Jones, H. W., Jr.: Glucose 6-phosphate dehydrogenase and the histogenesis of epidermoid carcinoma of the cervix. Am. J. Obstet. Gynecol., *102:* 106, 1968.

Photopulos, G. J., Shirley, R. E. L., Jr., and Ansbacher, R.: Evaluation of conventional diagnostic tests for detection of recurrent carcinoma of the cervix. Am. J. Obstet. Gynecol. *129:* 533, 1977.

Plentyl, A., and Friedman, E.: *Lymphatic System of the Female Genitalia,* W. B. Saunders, Philadelphia, 1971.

Rawles, W. E., Thompkins, W. A. F., Figueroam, E., and Melnick, J. L.: Herpes virus type 2 association with carcinoma of the cervix. Science, *151:* 1255, 1968.

Richart, R.: Cervical intraepithelial neoplasia. Pathology Annual, *8:* 301, 1973.

Rotkin, I. D.: A comparison review of key epidemiological studies in cervical cancer related to current searches for transmissible agents. Cancer Res., *33:* 1353, 1973.

Rutledge, F. N., Smith, J. P., Wharton, J. T., and O'Quinn, A. G.: Pelvic exenteration: An analysis of 296 patients. Am. J. Obstet. Gynecol. *129:* 881, 1977.

Schachter, J., Hill, E. C., King, E. B., Coleman, V. R., Jones, P., and Meyer, K. F.: Chlamydial infection in women with cervical dysplasia. Am. J. Obstet. Gynecol. *123:* 753, 1975.

Sedlis, A., Sall, S., Tsukada, Y., Park, R. Mangan, C., Shingleton, H., and Blessing, J.: Microinvasive carcinoma of the uterine cervix: a clinical-pathologic study. Am. J. Obstet. Gynecol. *133:* 64, 1979.

Sevin, B., Ford, J. H., Girtanner, R. D., Hoskins, W. J., Ng, A. B. P., Nordqvist, S. R. B., and Averette, H. E.: Invasive cancer of the cervix after cryosurgery. Obstet. Gynecol. *53:* 465, 1979.

Silbar, E. L., and Woodruff, J. D.: Evaluation of biopsy, cone, and hysterectomy sequence in intraepithelial carcinoma of the cervix. Obstet. Gynecol. *17:* 89, 1966.

Smith, J. P., Rutledge, F., Burns, B. C., Jr., and Soffar, S.: Systemic chemotherapy for carcinoma of the cervix. Am. J. Obstet. Gynecol., *97:* 800, 1967.

Stafl, A., and Mattingly, R. F.: Colposcopic diagnosis of cervical neoplasia. Obstet. Gynecol. *41:* 168, 1973.

Stafl, A., and Mattingly, R. A.: Vaginal adenosis—a precancerous lesion. Am. J. Obstet. Gynecol., *120:* 666, 1974.

Strockbine, M. F., Hancock, J. E., and Fletcher, G. H.: Complications in 831 patients with squamous cell carcinoma of the intact cervix treated with 3000 rads or more whole pelvis irradiation. AJR, *108:* 293, 1970.

Surwit, E., Fowler, W. C., Jr., Palumbo, L., Koch, G., and Gjertsen, W.: Radical hysterectomy with or without preoperative radium for stage Ib squamous cell carcinoma of the cervix. Obstet. Gynecol., *48:* 130, 1976.

Symmonds, R. E., Pratt, J. H., and Webb, M. J.: Exenterative operations: experience with 198 patients. Am. J. Obstet. Gynecol., *121:* 907, 1975.

Talebian, F., Krumholz, B. A., Shayan, A., and Mann, L. I.: Colposcopic evaluation of patients with abnormal cytologic smears during pregnancy. Obstet. Gynecol., *47:* 693, 1976.

Talebian, F., Shayan, A., Krumholz, B. A., Palladino, V. S., and Mann, L. I.: Colposcopic evaluation of patients with abnormal cervical cytology. Obstet. Gynecol., *49:* 670, 1977.

Tobin, S. M., Fish, F. E. N., Cooter, N. B. and Papsin, F. R.: Relation of HVH-II to cervical carcinoma, Obstet. Gynecol., *53:* 553, 1979.

Townsend, D. E.: Colposcopy and cryotherapy for cervical intraepithelial neoplasia. Presented at the Annual Meeting, Society of Gynecologic Oncologists, Key Biscayne, Fla. 1978.

Villasanta, U., and Durkan, J. P.: Indications and complications of cold conization of the cervix: Observations on 200 consecutive cases. Obstet. Gynecol. *27:* 717, 1966.

Walton, R. J., et al.: Cervical cancer screening programs—Report of the Canadian Task Force. Can. Med. Assoc. J. *114:* 1003, 1976.

Wasserman, T. H., and Carter, S. K.: The integration of chemotherapy into combined modality treatment of solid tumors: cervical cancer. Cancer Treat. Rev. *4:* 25, 1977.

Webb, M. J., and Symmonds, R. E.: Wertheim hysterectomy: a

reappraisal. Obstet. Gynecol., *54:* 140, 1979.

Wentz, W. B., and Lewis, G. C., Jr.: Correlation of histologic morphology and survival in cervical cancer following radiation therapy. Obstet. Gynecol., *26:* 228, 1965.

Wertheim, E.: The radical abdominal operation in carcinoma of the cervix uteri. Surg. Gynecol. Obstet., *4:* 1, 1907.

Wharton, J. T., Jones, H. W. III, Day, T. G., Jr., Rutledge, F. N.: Preirradiation celiotomy and extended field irradiation for invasive carcinoma of the cervix. Obstet. Gynecol. *49:* 333, 1967.

Wilbanks, G. D., Creasman, W. T., Kaufmann, L. A., and Parker, R. T.: Treatment of cervical dysplasia with electrocautery and tetracycline suppositories. Am. J. Obstet. Gynecol., *117:* 460, 1973.

Wimbush, P. R., and Fletcher, G. H.: Radiation therapy of carcinoma of the cervical stump. Radiol. *93:* 655, 1969.

CHAPTER 13

Relaxations, Incontinence, Fistulas, and Malpositions

STRUCTURE OF THE VAGINAL OUTLET

The pelvic floor, closing the outlet of the pelvis, is made up of a number of muscular and fascial structures which are pierced by the rectum, vagina, and urethra as these canals pass to the exterior of the body. The most important of the muscles is the levator ani, which forms a broad muscular sheet, concave above and convex below, and which extends like a diaphragm from one side of the pelvis to the other. It consists of a pubic portion that arises from the pubic bone anteriorly and passes backward to encircle the rectum, whereas the iliac portion arises from the so-called white line of the pelvis and passes downward to meet its fellow of the opposite side in the midline, extending to the tip of the coccyx behind. Most of its fibers pass behind the rectum and, according to the majority of anatomists, few or no fibers pass between the vagina and the rectum.

Even more important in the support of the pelvic organs is the fascia. The superior or pelvic fascia covers the upper surface of the muscular diaphragm, extending from the white line of the pelvis on one side to that of the other and giving off fascial coverings to the vaginal and rectal canals as they pass through the pelvic floor.

The inferior or external pelvic fascia, found beneath the levator diaphragm, is divisible into two parts, one *anterior* and one *posterior* to a line between the tuberosities of the ischia. The posterior covers the under surface of the levator muscles, whereas the anterior constitutes the so-called urogenital diaphragm or inferior triangular ligament. This is a dense fascial sheet which fills in the triangle formed by the pubic arch, the rami, and a line drawn between the two tuberosities. It is composed of a superficial and a deep layer. The superficial perineal muscles are placed superficial to the urogenital diaphragm, but the deeper group, with other important structures, is situated in the space between the two layers (Figs. 13.1–13.3).

LACERATIONS OF THE PERINEUM

These are best subdivided into those of the *incomplete* and *complete* varieties. In the former, the laceration does not involve the sphincter ani, whereas in the latter this muscle is partly or completely torn. Incomplete tears are sometimes subdivided into those of *first* and *second degree*, according to their extent, the complete variety being considered as of the *third degree*. In the overwhelming majority of cases, *lacerations of the genital canal* are due to childbirth, often complicated, but other forms of trauma, such as coitus, attempted rape, or external violence may at times be responsible.

CERVICAL LACERATIONS

Cervical lacerations are findings in the woman who has had complicated labors. Lacerations may be slight or deep with extension into the vaginal fornices or even into the base of the broad ligament. They may be unilateral, bilateral, or stellate. Unless such lacerations cause cervical incompetence they are of little clinical significance.

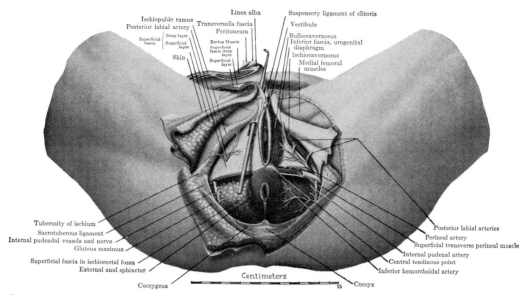

Figure 13.1. The female perineum. On the right half of the urogenital triangle the superficial fatty layer has been turned aside to display the deep layer of the superficial fascia; the latter, on the left half, has been reflected to show the contents of the superficial perineal compartment.

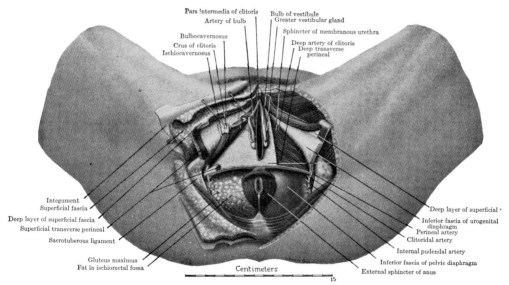

Figure 13.2. On the right half of the urogenital triangle the cavernous bodies in the superficial compartment have been exposed by partial removal of the superficial perineal muscles; on the left, the inferior fascia of the urogenital diaphragm has been reflected to show the musculature in the deep perineal compartment. In the anal triangle, on the left side, the superficial (fatty) tissue has been removed from the ischiorectal fossa.

RELAXATION OF THE VAGINAL OUTLET (RVO)

A relaxed vaginal outlet is usually a sequel to mere overstretching of the perineal supporting tissues, generally as a result of previous parturition. Varying degrees of perineal laceration may be apparent, but even without visible evidence there may be extensive submucosal laceration and division of the muscular and fascial supports.

Cystocele and *rectocele* (Fig. 13.4) are frequent concomitants as may be *prolapse of the uterus*, and actually these three generally oc-

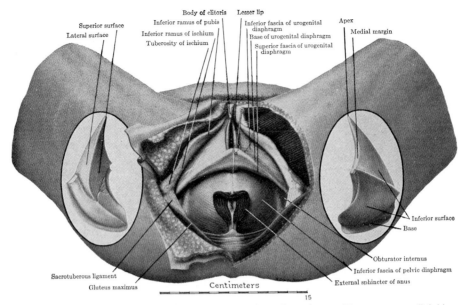

Figure 13.3. The urogenital and pelvic diaphragms in the female perineum. The more superficial layers have been removed to show the urogenital diaphragm; the latter has been drawn forward, revealing the anterior continuation of the ischiorectal fossa, the superior boundary of which is the pelvic diaphragm. *Inserts:* upper and lower aspects of plaster cast of the left ischiorectal fossa showing the extent and shape of the space.

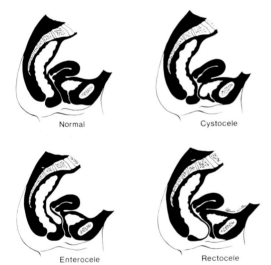

Figure 13.4. Sagittal diagram of relation of bladder and urethra to uterus and vagina and to rectum. *Upper left*, normal relation; *upper right*, a cystocele of moderate degree; *lower left*, an enterocele; *lower right*, a rectocele of moderate degree.

cur in association with one or the other being predominant.

SYMPTOMS OF GENITAL RELAXATION

Even extensive relaxation of the outlet may be entirely symptomless, whereas in other cases there is a complaint of *pressure and heaviness in the vaginal region*, especially after prolonged standing. The patient not infrequently describes her symptoms as a sensation of "everything dropping out." There may be some *bearing-down discomfort in the lower abdomen* and *backache*. However, troublesome backache should always lead to a search for such more frequent causes as abnormalities of the back itself.

Where relaxation is associated with *complete perineal laceration*, at least partial *fecal incontinence* is produced. In the latter, the patient may have fairly good control, but, if the stools are rather loose, distressing incontinence develops.

Although moderate *cystocele* often causes no symptoms, the more marked degrees bring about increasing *difficulty in emptying the bladder*. In extreme cases the patient may be unable to void unless the bladder is first pushed back in the vagina with the finger. In the more marked cases, the bladder may contain much residual urine, and *cystitis* is almost always the result, with the possibility of ascending infection. There is, therefore, a complaint of *increased frequency of urination*, with perhaps *tenesmus*, the symptoms being most troublesome during the day and improved by night or when the patient is in the recumbent position. *Incontinence of urine* is frequent and this *incontinence* is usually of the *stress* variety, with escape of urine on coughing, laughing, sneezing, or other muscular effort. Although stress incontinence may occur with cystocele or urethrocele, it may occur with no obvious relaxation and from many causes.

Rectocele, like cystocele, may produce few symptoms. However, when the protruding rectal pouch is large, there may be a deflection of feces into the pouch, with increasing *difficulty of defecation* and *constipation,* because of the impaired overstretched rectal wall. *Hemorrhoids* frequently develop, adding to the patient's discomfort. Finally, in cases associated with *prolapse of the uterus,* there is added the strain of symptoms characterizing the latter, especially the discomfort produced by the *protrusion* of the uterus, bladder, and rectum.

Diagnosis

The simpler *relaxations of the vagina* are usually evident, even on simple inspection, from the gaping appearance of the orifice and the separation of the anterior and posterior vaginal walls, normally in juxtaposition. Where there has been extensive laceration, scar tissue may be plainly visible, either in the midline or in one or both sulci. When the examining fingers are introduced and the patient is asked to strain down, one can at once note the *absence of the resistance of the muscles* surrounding the lower vagina.

Cystocele and rectocele, when large, may be at once visible on inspection, but often they recede when the patient is lying flat. It is always important to ask the patient to strain, this bringing out the cystocele and rectocele so that their extent can be seen. The presence of *urethrocele* is indicated by marked bulging just below the urethral orifice. This must be distinguished from a suburethral diverticulum.

The demonstration of a *rectocele* can be made more striking by introducing a finger into the rectum and pushing it upward and forward into the rectal pouch. By thrusting the finger forward, the anterior rectal wall can be hooked outward from the vagina, the rectovaginal septum being exceedingly thin and atrophic in such cases. On occasion it may be difficult to distinguish between a high rectocele and enterocele; a light of some kind placed up the rectum will suggest an *enterocele,* if there is no observed vaginal transillumination (Altchek).

When *complete laceration* exists, there is often a deep midline cleft from the posterior vaginal margin through the perineum into the rectum, and sometimes extending upward into the anterior rectal wall. Under such circumstances, the rectal mucosa is commonly everted, presenting as a bright red spongy area. Even when the anus seems intact, the sphincter may have been injured. Here, as in the case of the vagina, a demonstration of the adequacy or inadequacy of the sphincter control may be made by asking the patient to "draw in" on a finger inserted into the anus.

Treatment

Correction of any of these forms of genital relaxation is possible only by surgical procedures, but in a large proportion of cases operations may be deferred for long periods of time, and in the less pronounced cases they may be avoided altogether. Jeffcoate points out the frequency of dyspareunia, if injudicious, too snug, posterior repair is utilized. Our own tendency is to avoid posterior repair in the younger woman unless there are major degrees of relaxation.

Reparative Surgery

When any type of vaginal plastic procedure is contemplated, the rational gynecologist will at once consider the possibility of *vaginal hysterectomy* with appropriate repair. As to the age-old question, "Isn't she too young?" the informed gynecologist will reply that only a rare woman is "too young" for hysterectomy if she has completed her family. Admittedly, one stroke of lightning could wipe out that family with the woman unable to have more children, but this is certainly a pessimistic approach to life in general. Nevertheless, the conscientious gynecologist will discuss this possibility with the patient and her husband.

Above all, it should be emphasized that pelvic repair is an elective procedure that should generally be deferred until after the desire for children has been satisfied. On occasion, judicious use of pessaries may obviate the necessity for any operative intervention until the family has been completed, at which time, irrespective of age, definitive surgery can be accomplished. There is nothing urgent about cystocele, rectocele, or prolapse, and only if these are symptomatic should surgery be contemplated.

STRESS INCONTINENCE

Orientation

Stress incontinence is the leakage of urine through the urethra after a sudden increase in intraabdominal pressure, and thereby intravesical pressure, without a compensating increase in intraurethral pressure. It is due to abnormal function of the sphincter mechanism.

Symptoms and Signs

For the most part stress incontinence is a problem of the vaginally delivered parous woman. However, there is an interesting racial variation in susceptibility to this problem. Thus, the northern European Caucasian is much more likely to be troubled by stress incontinence after several pregnancies than the black African, probably because of the superior muscular development of the latter. Obesity certainly complicates the problem.

The typical history is of involuntary loss of urine in spurts associated with stress, i.e., coughing, running, jumping, or other forms of athletic or other activity.

The pelvic examination, except in nulliparous patients, will show various degrees of cystocele or urethrocele or both. However, these relaxations may occur in patients who have no stress incontinence so that they are not, per se, the cause of the incontinence, but rather are associated with the damage to the pelvic-supporting structures including the sphincter mechanism.

With about 250 cc of urine or water in the bladder in the prone examining (lithotomy) position, a spurt of urine will emerge from the urethral meatus if the patient coughs or strains on request.

That this is due to loss of support of the bladder neck may be confirmed by either the Bonney test or the Marchetti test. In the Bonney test, two fingers in the vagina with the tips on either side of the urethra at approximately the urethrovesical junction make upward pressure. When this is done, if coughing is not followed by a spurt of urine in a patient who had such a spurt without the upward pressure, it may be assumed that the stress incontinence is due to damage to the supporting structures of the urethra. The Marchetti test is essentially the same except that local anesthesia is used in the vagina and Allis clamps are used instead of the fingers.

Pathology

In the process of the normal emptying of the female bladder, the patient voluntarily increases her intraabdominal pressure and relaxes her levator muscles, with the result that there is descent of the bladder base. This causes a small amount of urine to descend into the proximal urethra. At this point, a reflex contraction seems to be initiated in the detrusor bladder muscle and further relaxation of the voluntary muscles of the urogenital diaphragm takes place. This causes an emptying of the bladder.

In the patient with stress incontinence, cinefluoroscopy and other radiological methods of examination of the bladder have shown that the bladder base is usually much lower than in the normal situation and that the caliber of the urethra may be more patulous. It is likely that these changes may predispose to the loss of urine. Unfortunately, there is considerable variation in the findings of patients who seem on history and physical examination to fit into the category of stress incontinence.

Diagnosis

The history of involuntary leakage of urine with stress is a key point in arriving at the diagnosis of stress incontinence. As will be further emphasized in the section on differential diagnosis, particularly important is the history of absence of an urge to void and the history of absence of involuntary emptying of the bladder. It is to be noted that stress incontinence is not related to the amount of urine in the bladder.

The finding of some pelvic relaxation and a positive Bonney or Marchetti test as described above are very helpful in arriving at an accurate diagnosis.

There is some difference of opinion as to whether roentgenography and/or urodynamic studies are an essential part of the work-up of the patients suspected of having stress incontinence.

Essentially all studies have confirmed the fact that in stress incontinence there is no abnormality in intravesical pressure and that the basic defect is a decreased intraurethral pressure.

It goes without saying that in order to make a diagnosis of urinary stress incontinence the urine must be free of infection. In addition, there should be no intrinsic disease of the bladder or disease of the pelvic structures influencing the bladder.

Differential Diagnosis

Urge Incontinence

By definition, urge incontinence is characterized by a sudden overwhelming desire to empty the bladder because of a feeling of pressure or pain. The patient generally voids in an uncontrolled fashion, often before she can get to a commode, and the voiding usually continues until the bladder is empty.

This is the type of disorder which women experience with acute cystitis, with foreign bodies or calculi in the bladder, or with other abnormalities such as trigonitis and urethral disturbances. However, by definition, patients are characterized as having urge incontinence when they are free of disorders of this type.

In urge incontinence, there seems to be some neurological difficulty with the bladder, and a good many authors have believed that a psychosomatic component was important in this disorder.

Anticholinergic drugs theoretically and practically seem to be most useful for this condition (Bentyl, Probanthine, Orinade, etc.). In this disorder, urodynamic studies are helpful in arriving at the diagnosis, as almost invariably there is some increase in intravesical pressure with increasing amounts of urine in the bladder.

Dyssynergic Bladder

The existence of the dyssynergic bladder has been the source of some controversy. There are those who distinguish this from the problem of urge incontinence by pointing out that in the dyssynergic bladder there is no prior urge to void. Thus, the patient experiences true episodes of voiding with no prior warning thereof rather than short spurts as produced by stress. In most cases, however, the triggering mechanism is a critical bladder volume. It is often triggered by such things as running water and there is often a long-standing history of difficulty of urinary control, for example, bedwetting for a prolonged period of time in childhood. The patient profile is one of an emotionally labile female with a progressively deteriorating bladder picture.

The diagnosis of dyssynergia is made by the history plus a urodynamic study.

The treatment of dyssynergia is basically the same as that of stress incontinence.

As with stress and urge incontinence, patients labeled with a diagnosis of bladder dyssynergia must be free of urinary tract infection.

Treatment

A great variety of surgical operations have been devised for the treatment of urinary stress incontinence. It has been stated that there are more than 50 different techniques to attack this problem. This alone would indicate that the treatment is less than perfect.

For patients with pure stress incontinence, the two most frequently used procedures are either (1) vaginal repair or (2) periurethral suspension by an abdominal approach. The vaginal approach consists of a repair of any accompanying cystocele and urethrocele and a plication of the vesical sphincter. The abdominal approach with suspension of the urethra can be done by a variety of techniques including variations of the procedure originally described by Marshall, Marchetti, and Krantz.

Primary treatment of urinary stress incontinence is, as indicated, by no means limited to these approaches. For example, Stamey et al. have devised a cystoscopically controlled suspension of the vesical neck. In this technique, a periurethral suspension is done while the vesical neck is visualized through the cystoscope. Many other types of procedures could be cited.

For patients who have had failure of the first operative attempt to cure urinary stress incontinence, various procedures have been advocated. The Marshall-Marchetti-Krantz procedure is frequently used after failure of a vaginal approach. On the other hand, some type of strap operation has been a stand-by for recurrent disease for a number of years. In addition, there are special types of operations, such as the one designed by Ingelman-Sunberg of a transplant of the pubococcygeal muscle, the Zacharin abdominoperineal urethral suspension, and others too numerous to mention.

The results from the secondary operations are, as might be expected, not quite as good as from the first operation for urinary stress incontinence. However, the results that have been reported by a number of authors vary from 80 up to 90%.

FISTULAS

Genital Fistulas

A genital fistula is an abnormal communication between some part of the genital canal, on the one hand, and either the urinary or intestinal tract or both.

Etiology

By far the most common cause of genital fistulas in past years was *obstetrical trauma*, especially in cases of prolonged and difficult labor. In such cases the fistula was due to necrosis and sloughing of the genital canal, usually the vagina, and also of the wall of the subjacent viscus, generally the bladder. The great improvement in obstetrical management which has occurred in recent years has essentially eliminated fistulas due to this group of causes.

On the other hand, *radical surgery* and *radiation* have led to a not inconsiderable incidence of genital fistulas. The majority of fistulas seen nowadays are the result of injury to the bladder, ureter, or rectum in the course of radical hysterectomy, or they result from necrosis and sloughing produced by radiation. Other causes are the *destruction of tissue by malignant tumors, ulceration due to foreign bodies*, especially vaginal pessaries, and occasionally, *hysterectomy for benign disease* or *cystocele repair.*

Urinary Fistulas

Even the most accomplished gynecological surgeon will at one time or another inadvertently damage the urinary tract. The abnormal communication may involve various portions of the urinary and genital canals. The following are the chief varieties: (1) vesicovaginal, (2) urethrovaginal, (3) ureterovaginal, and (4) combinations thereof.

Of these the most frequent variety is the *vesicovaginal.* The fistulous communication between the bladder and the vagina may be of such tiny size that it is difficult to demonstrate, or it may involve destruction of the whole base of the bladder, not infrequently extending to the urethra below or the ureter above.

The locations of the other types of fistula are indicated by their designations, and they are depicted in the accompanying diagrams (Figs. 13.5) so that they need not be described

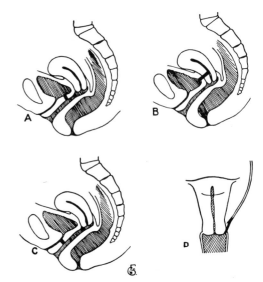

Figure 13.5. Diagram of chief varieties of urinary fistula. *A*, vesicovaginal; *B*, vesicouterine; *C*, urethrovaginal; *D*, ureterovaginal.

in detail. The *ureterovaginal* merits special mention, because it is the type most often resulting from accidental injury to the ureter during the operation of hysterectomy, especially where radical surgery for malignant disease is being performed. *Urethrovaginal* fistulas are more likely to be sequelae of anterior repair and plication or excision of a suburethral diverticulum than an obstetrical injury (Gray).

Symptoms

The characteristic symptom is *leakage of urine from the vagina.* This, with small fistulas, may be only in the form of a slight dribble, more noticeable in some postures than others. In other cases, the flow of urine is constant and profuse, and none may be voided through the meatus in such cases. The distress of the patient is increased by the *irritation of the vagina, vulva, and perineum* produced by such constant leakage, to say nothing of the unpleasant *ammoniacal odor.* Unless meticulous cleansing is observed, phosphatic incrustations may develop about the fistula, thus further adding to the local irritation.

Diagnosis

The diagnosis of urinary fistula is usually comparatively simple, although varying amounts of the usual postoperative vaginal discharge may confuse the issue. In any case, it is not always so easy to determine the exact location and nature of the fistula. Leakage of urine may be the result of extreme relaxation of the vesical sphincter, without a fistula. When this occurs after difficult delivery or after operation, it may make one apprehensive that a fistula exists. With simple *sphincter atony* the leakage is apt to be intermittent and it often occurs only after such straining efforts as coughing, sneezing, or laughing.

Vesicovaginal fistula presents no difficulty in diagnosis unless it is very small or unless it is in an inaccessible location high up in the vagina, where it may be concealed by extensive cicatricial deposits following operation. In the ordinary case, the fistula can be readily seen when the patient is examined in the knee-chest position, which gives an excellent view of the whole anterior vaginal wall and fornix. For that matter, the larger fistulas are readily palpated by the finger in the vagina. The smaller, more inaccessible fistulas can be demonstrated by filling the bladder with *methylene-blue colored sterile water* and observing the escape of the bluish fluid from the abnormal opening. Cystoscopic examination, often gives valuable information as to the location of the fistula and its relation to the ureters.

In the not infrequent *ureterovaginal* fistula the demonstration of urinary leakage from within the vagina and the elimination of a vesical source by such simple methods as have been described leave little doubt as to the existence of leakage from the ureter. This should be verified by more intensive urological study, often including intravenous or retrograde pyelograms or both.

Treatment

Small fistulas, unless produced by malignant disease, occasionally close spontaneously, and this may often be facilitated by postural treatment, limitation of fluids, urinary antiseptics, and the employment of a retention catheter with suction. Such a happy outcome, however, is *not* the rule, and surgical treatment must almost always be resorted to. The operation must be adapted to the indications of the particular case, but the well versed gynecologist will probably prefer a vaginal to a transvesical approach. Without detailing the operative methods which may

be called for, suffice it to say that by the utilization of such principles as partial closure of the vagina (Latzko) or free mobilization of the bladder, there are few cases in which the trained operator cannot effect cure (Blaikley).

A cardinal rule, frequently overlooked, is the *desirability* of waiting 4 to 6 months after injury before attempting any kind of reparative procedure. This delay is not easy to justify to the patient, but sufficient time must be allowed for subsidence of edema and induration if there is to be any chance of a successful surgical outcome. Where there is evidence of severe upper tract damage, nephrostomy is preferable to premature attempts to restore lower urinary tract integrity. Collins and Jones have suggested cortisone to minimize fibrosis and speed up the time needed before repair. Local palliative measures and antibiotics are also used preoperatively.

Vaginal Fecal Fistula

Rectovaginal fistula is by far the most common form of vaginal fecal fistula. The possible *causes* are in the main the same as those concerned in the etiology of urinary fistula, namely, irradiation, obstetrical trauma, and surgery (especially vaginal). The operations which are most apt to be followed by the development of such a fistula are vaginal puncture for pelvic abscess, perineorrhaphy, and hemorrhoidectomy. Lymphogranuloma inguinale is another possible cause. Much less frequently the fecal fistula may involve the sigmoid colon, or small intestine, the usual cause being malignancy, diverticulitis, or operations upon either the pelvic organs or the intestine, although *posterior colpotomy* for a postoperative infected pelvic hematoma seems a frequent agent in the causation of vaginal fecal fistulas.

A rectovaginal fistula may be very tiny, producing only occasional escape of gas or fecal matter from the vagina, and even this may be noted only when the stools are soft or liquid, as after purgatives. Such small fistulas may close spontaneously. In the larger fistulas, the lot of the patient may be made distressing by continuous leakage of fecal material, with resulting irritation and a constantly offensive odor. The *treatment* is surgical, the operation being done by the vaginal route in the rectovaginal type. Occasionally, temporary colostomy is advisable to permit the badly infected tissues to undergo some preliminary improvement as regards healing properties.

Abdominal procedures are required for the closure of vaginal fistulas involving other parts of the intestinal tract; rarely suction ("sump") drainage will close a high fistula but will often minimize autodigestion of the adjacent tissues. The site of the intestinal component of the fistula should be ascertained by barium and other studies; obviously, a colostomy would be valueless for an ileovaginal fistula, and this type of defect warrants prompt surgery without a prolonged waiting period. Bowel "prep" should be routine.

MALPOSITIONS

Normal Supports of the Uterus

The normal position of the uterus is maintained by three factors.

(1) The Pelvic Floor. The fascial planes of the pelvic floor are inserted at about the level of the internal os, the strongest band being the fasciomuscular condensation in the base of the broad ligament, constituting the so-called ligament of Mackenrodt or cardinal ligament.

(2) The Uterine Ligaments. Of these the most important in the support of the uterus are the *broad* and the *uterosacral* ligaments. This is true particularly because in the base of the former is the fascial condensation above alluded to as the cardinal ligament, whereas the uterosacral ligament likewise includes a strong fascial band stretching backward to the junction of the second and third sacral vertebrae. The round ligaments, formerly spoken of picturesquely as exerting a guyrope function on the fundus, are now looked upon as having little supporting function except perhaps during pregnancy, when they become thick and hypertrophic and may even, as some believe, help to direct the presenting part of the child downward toward the pelvic canal during labor. In the nonpregnant uterus, their laxity and their circuitous course make it difficult to believe that they can have a supporting function, although they may become extremely hypertrophic when there is an enlarged myomatous uterus.

(3) Intraabdominal Pressure. Normally this considerable force is directed upon the posterior surface of the uterus, driving it downward and forward, and thus tending to accentuate the normal position of the organ. Intestinal loops are, so to speak, deflected into the posterior cul-de-sac and are not normally found between the uterus and bladder. The same intraabdominal force can become a power for evil if the uterus is displaced backward, as it is then exerted on the anterior uterine surface, tending to crowd the uterus farther backward and downward.

Displacements of the Uterus

Of great importance to the gynecologist are the *retrodisplacements*. These may be either *congenital or acquired*, the latter being the more important, especially when complicated by other pelvic lesions, such as pelvic inflammatory disease or endometriosis.

Types and Degrees

Retroversion refers to the retrodisplacement in which the uterus is tilted backward on its transverse axis to a greater or lesser degree. When comparatively slight, so that the fundus is about vertical or pointing no farther back than the sacral promontory, the retroversion is spoken of as of *first degree.* When the fundus is within the hollow of the sacrum but not below the level of the cervix, the designation of *second degree* is commonly used. Finally, when the uterus is so far back that the fundus is below the level of the cervix, the retroversion is *third degree.*

Retroflexion, simply defined, is a bending backward of the uterus, *i.e.*, of the body upon the cervix. The latter may still be directed normally downward and backward, but more frequently has tilted downward and forward (erect position of the woman) toward the symphysis as the fundus falls backward (Fig. 13.6).

Causes

The causes of retrodisplacements of the uterus may be grouped as follows.

(1) Congenital. This condition often persists into adult life, probably as a result of developmental deficiencies.

(2) Acquired. Retrodisplacement of a previously normally placed uterus may occur from a number of causes, the most important of which may be grouped as follows.

(a) Puerperal. This group embraces a considerable number of possible factors which may develop following full term and especially

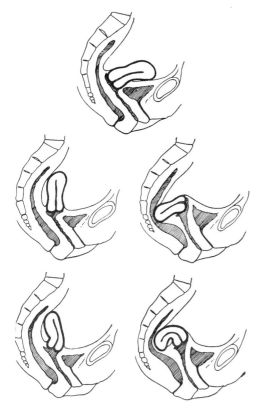

Figure 13.6. Degrees of retroposition. *Top,* normal position of uterus; *center left,* slight retroversion (1st degree); *center right,* marked retroversion (3rd degree); *bottom left,* slight retroflexion; *bottom right,* marked retroflexion.

Symptoms

Simple uncomplicated retrodisplacements of the uterus are often entirely symptomless, although dysmenorrhea and *backache* may be noted. Certainly every gynecologist, in the course of routine examinations, encounters innumerable cases of even marked retrodisplacement in which not the slightest menstrual cramps, backache, or any other symptom has been complained of which might be linked up with the displacement. Even when backache is a symptom, it is often due to causes other than the position of the uterus.

Diagnosis

The symptoms of retroposition are of little value in diagnosis. Certainly the mere existence of backache is anything but characteristic, contrary to the lay view. Careful elimination of postural, spinal, and other causes is essential before one is justified in attributing backache to a retrodisplacement.

Pelvic examination is necessary for diagnosis, and this is usually easy (Fig. 13.7). The cardinal points are as follows.

(1) The cervix points toward the symphysis, instead of downward and toward the sacrum.

(2) The fundus cannot be felt anteriorly, where it should be placed, but it can be palpated posteriorly. Occasionally, anesthesia may be required for satisfactory evaluation.

Differential Diagnosis

Although the diagnosis is usually easy enough, there are certain cases in which it may be exceedingly difficult, even if the conditions for palpation are satisfactory. A *myoma of the posterior wall* may be difficult to distinguish from a retroflexed fundus, whereas, on the other hand, a sharply retroflexed fundus may feel like a myoma. A firm *inflammatory mass densely adherent to the posterior wall* may likewise simulate a retroflexed uterus. A *pregnant retroflexed fundus* may even be mistaken for an ovarian cyst, and various other possibilities for error may be encountered. In the occasional case where differentiation is important, it may be necessary, under strict aseptic preparations, to insert a uterine sound in order to determine the position of the uterus. It need scarcely be said that this is not to be done when there is any suspicion of pregnancy.

complicated delivery, or, much less frequently, miscarriage.

(b) Adnexal Disease. The complicated form of retroflexion is as a rule associated with adnexal disease, either inflammatory or endometriosis.

(c) Neoplasms. The effect of pelvic neoplasms of one sort or another in producing retrodisplacements is a mechanical one. For example, a large myoma developing in the anterior wall of the uterus will tend to push the uterus backward

(d) Trauma. The question of whether acute displacement can occur as a result of trauma is not infrequently of medicolegal importance. The protected position of the uterus and the nature of its support make it difficult to believe that any but the most severe trauma could bring about displacement. However, the burden of medicolegal proof rests on the certainty that trauma has led to retrodisplacement, bleeding, and abortion.

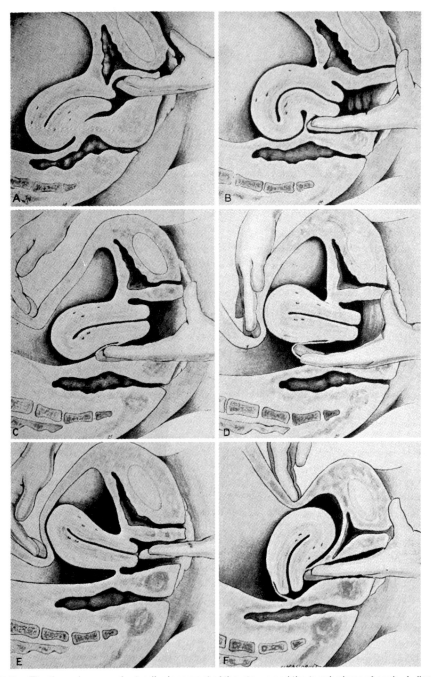

Figure 13.7.   The three degrees of retrodisplacement of the uterus and the touch signs of each. *A,* first degree, corpus out of reach of examining fingers, both above and below; *B,* second degree, vaginal fingers feel posterior surface of corpus uteri extending directly back; *C,* third degree, vaginal fingers impinge on corpus uteri turned down into the posterior cul-de-sac; *D,* grasping the fundus through the abdominal wall and pushing it upward with internal finger; *E,* further replacement by pushing backward and upward on cervix; *F,* continuing this maneuver to full replacement.

Suspension Operations

In the past many suspension operations were carried out for a variety of complaints, including backache. Many of these failed to alleviate the complaints, and the operation has fallen into disrepute.

Although there is some difference of opinion, most gynecologists feel that an occasional suspension operation is indicated in the correction of *infertility*. This is justifiable only when all the usual sterility tests have been performed and found normal, and when there has been a 2-year span of infertility after all minor defects have been corrected.

Prolapse of the Uterus (Descensus Uteri)

This is an extremely common condition, being far more frequent in elderly than in young patients. This is explained by the increasing laxity and atony of the muscular and fascial structures in later life. The effects of childbirth injuries may thus make themselves evident, in the form of uterine prolapse, many years after the last pregnancy. Pregnancy in a prolapsed uterus may lead to numerous complications, as noted by Piver and Spezia.

The important factor in the mechanism of prolapse is undoubtedly injury or overstretching of the pelvic floor, and especially of the cardinal ligaments (Mackenrodt) in the bases of the broad ligaments. Combined with this there is usually extensive injury to the perineal structures, producing marked vaginal relaxation and also frequent injury to the fascia of the anterior or posterior vaginal walls, with the production of cystocele or rectocele. Usually, various combinations of these conditions are seen, although at times little or no cystocele or rectocele is associated with the prolapse. Occasional cases are seen, for that matter, in women who have never borne children, and in these the prolapse apparently represents a hernia of the uterus through a defect in the pelvic fascial floor. When the cervix of the prolapsed uterus, usually pointing in the axis of the vagina because of the associated retrodisplacement, is well within the vaginal orifice, the prolapse is spoken of as of *first degree*. In prolapse of *second degree*, the cervix is at or near the introitus. Finally, when the cervix protrudes well beyond the vaginal orifice, the prolapse is of *third degree* (*procidentia uteri*). Complete prolapse of the posthysterectomy (abdominal or vaginal) vagina may occur and is often difficult to repair if a functioning vagina is desired, as noted by Lee and Symmonds.

Pathology

Aside from the prolapse of the uterus and the frequently associated cystocele or rectocele, there are other possible pathological sequelae of this condition. Ulceration (*decubitus ulcer*) of the cervix not infrequently occurs as a result of friction against the patient's thighs, her clothing, or the protective napkins which many of these patients wear. *Hypertrophy* of the cervix is another frequent concomitant, this portion of the uterus often being enormously elongated; however, this condition may occur without prolapse, even in the nulliparous woman, apparently as a congenital malformation.

When the relaxation is marked, there may be complete inversion of the vagina, the canal being literally turned inside out. The drying effect of the air produces a skinlike thickening of the vaginal mucosa, with ulceration and bleeding. In addition, marked degrees of prolapse and cystocele may lead to angulation of the ureter at the urethrovesical junction, with significant degrees of upper tract dilatation. Pyelograms should be routine with complete procidentia.

Symptoms of Prolapse

As with other forms of uterine displacement, there are marked individual differences in the symptomatology. Even the most complete prolapse may be associated with no symptoms except for the discomfort produced by the mechanical protrusion of the uterus. In most cases, however, there is likely to be some degree of bearing down and heaviness in the lower abdomen and some backache, both of these being probably due to traction on the uterine ligaments and the venous congestion produced by the prolapse. Cystocele and rectocele are often associated and productive of their respective symptoms (Fig. 13.8).

Diagnosis

The diagnosis is usually simple, and, as a matter of fact, the usual complaint of the

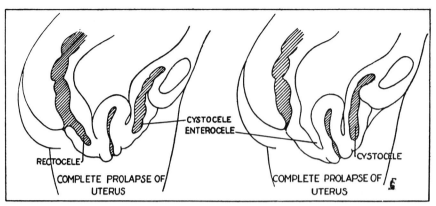

Figure 13.8.   Sagittal section to show anatomical relations with prolapse of uterus. *On the left*, the prolapse is associated with cystocele and rectocele. *On the right*, the prolapse is associated with cystocele and enterocele.

patient when she presents herself is that she has "falling of the womb." Although the history of difficult or instrumental labors is suggestive, it is of no great value in diagnosis, which must be made from pelvic examination.

Inspection will, in many cases, reveal the prolapse at once, if this is of the complete type. In such cases the cervix, even with the patient lying down, protrudes beyond the outlet, often occupying a position between a soft boggy cystocele anteriorly and a pouch-like protrusion of the rectocele posteriorly, should these coexist. When massive degrees of prolapse, cystocele, rectocele, and enterocele are present, there may be such a mass of bulging, billowy mucosa presenting at the introitus that it is sometimes difficult to be certain of "how much of what type of relaxation is present." Marked edema and sometimes partial strangulation may occur.

Even in cases of complete prolapse, however, the protrusion usually recedes when the patient lies down, whereas in first or second degree prolapse no external protrusion exists. In such cases the patient is asked to strain, this bringing the cervix far down into the vagina and perhaps beyond the introitus. The same straining effort will ordinarily reveal the cystocele and rectocele, should they be present. In the complete variety, if straining does not restore the protrusion, gentle traction on the cervix with a light tenaculum will usually do so.

Differential Diagnosis

The chief source of error is to mistake for prolapse the *simple hypertrophy of the cervix* which is seen at times, even with little or no vaginal relaxation. The cervix may become so elongated as to present at or beyond the introitus. Careful examination, however, will show that the cervical elongation is all below the cervicovaginal junction, and that the latter is still high up in the vaginal canal. Cystocele and rectocele are usually not present. Remarkable degrees of *vaginal prolapse* or *inversion* may exist with only minor degrees of cystocele, rectocele, or uterine prolapse.

Treatment

Among the factors which influence the management of this condition are the patient's age, marital status, and general health, on the one hand; and on the other, the degree of the prolapse and the presence or absence of any associated pathological conditions.

Surgical. This is best deferred until the family has been completed, for further pregnancy, even over an adequately repaired pelvic floor, will often undo the best surgical results. Although many operations have been devised for the correction of prolapse, 99% of such cases are satisfactorily handled by any one of the following procedures (along with appropriate repairs).

(1) Vaginal Hysterectomy (see Chapter 5). This is suitable for all but the most massive degrees of prolapse and, if combined with adequate anterior or posterior repair, gives excellent results. Furthermore, it removes the usual site of later cancers, tumors, or bleeding and is obviously sterilizing. It should be stressed that abdominal hysterectomy and suspension of the vaginal vault from above is *not* the proper operation for prolapse; re-

moval from below with adequate building up of the weakened and attenuated structures is the only feasible surgical approach. The *composite operation*, which preserves the uterine isthmus while removing fundus and cervix, has won no wide support.

(2) Operations Which Preserve the Uterus. The *Manchester* procedure, named for the English city where it was first used, consists of amputation of the cervix and shortening of the cervical ligaments. It is used only infrequently today even in Manchester. However, it may be useful in a poor-risk patient because it can be quickly accomplished.

Curettage to exclude malignancy should precede the operation, and it should rarely be done in the childbearing era, because cervical amputation (although not included in the original Manchester procedure) seems an integral part of the operation.

(3) Colpocleisis (Le Fort Operation). Occasional cases of massive procidentia, often failures by other procedures, require closing the vagina. Colpocleisis is generally easily and quickly performed and may, of course, be preceded by vaginal hysterectomy. This type of surgery should be a last resort, but is almost infallible if properly performed. Stress incontinence may be incurred if approximation of the vaginal walls includes the region of the bladder neck.

Nonsurgical. There are a few elderly women who are poor operative risks and have a limited life-span, and these represent the main indication for pessary treatment. With modern anesthesia (local, block, and low spinal), such easily performed procedures as the Le Fort operation are usually preferred; but there is a small number of cases in which operation is not feasible or desirable.

References and Additional Readings

Altchek, A.: Diagnosis of enterocele by negative intrarectal transillumination. Obstet. Gynecol., *26:* 636, 1965.

Beck, R. P., Arnusch, D., and King, C.: Results in treating 210 patients with detrusor overactivity in continence of urine. Am. J. Obstet. Gynecol., *125:* 593, 1976.

Blaikley, J. B.: Colpocleises for difficult vesicovaginal and rectovaginal fistulas. Am. J. Obstet. Gynecol., *91:* 589, 1964.

Collins, C. G., and Jones, F. B.: Preoperative cortisone for vaginal fistulae. Obstet. Gynec., *9:* 533, 1957.

Diaz-Bazan, N.: Cervical carcinoma with procidentia in El Salvador. Obstet. Gynecol., *23:* 281, 1964.

Enhörning, G.: Simultaneous recording of intravesical and intraurethral pressure. Acta Chir. Scand., Suppl. 276, 1961.

Fantl, J. A., Hurt, W. G., and Dunn, L. J.: Dysfunctional detrusor control. Obstet. Gynecol. Surv., *33:* 294, 1978.

Graber, E. A.: Stress incontinence in women. A review 1977. Obstet. Gynecol. Surv., *32:* 565, 1977.

Gray, L. A.: Urethrovaginal fistulas. Am. J. Obstet. Gynecol., *101:* 28, 1968.

Green, T. H.: Development of a plan for the diagnosis and treatment of urinary stress incontinence. Am. J. Obstet. Gynecol., *83:* 632, 1962.

Hodgkinson, C. P., Doub, H. P., and Kelly, W. T.: Urethrocystograms: metallic bead chain technique. Clin. Obstet. Gynecol., *1:* 668, 1958.

Jeffcoate, T. N. A.: Posterior colpoperineorrhaphy. Am. J. Obstet. Gynecol., *77:* 490, 1959.

Kelly, H. A.: *Operative Gynecology.* Appleton-Century-Crofts, Inc., New York, 1928.

Kittzmiller, J. L., Manzer, G. A., Nebel, W. A., and Lucas, W. E.: Chain cystourethrogram and stress incontinence. Obstet. Gynecol., *39:* 333, 1972.

Latzko, W.: Postoperative vesicovaginal fistulas. Am. J. Surg., *58:* 211, 1942.

Lee, R. A., and Symmonds, R. E.: Repair of posthysterectomy vault prolapse. Am. J. Obstet. Gynecol., *112:* 953, 1972.

Lund, C. J. (Editor): Symposium on urinary incontinence in the female. Clin. Obstet. Gynecol., *6:* 125, 1963.

Marchetti, A. A., Marshall, V. F., and Shultis, L. D.: Simple vesicourethral suspension. Am. J. Obstet. Gynecol., *74:* 57, 1957.

McCall, M. L.: Posterior culdoplasty. Obstet. Gynecol., *10:* 595, 1957.

Ostergard, D. R.: The neurological control of micturition and voiding reflexes. Obstet. Gynecol. Surv., *34:* 147, 1979.

Ostergard, D. R.: Effects of drugs on the lower urinary tract. Obstet. Gynecol. Surv., *34:* 424, 1979.

Piver, M. S., and Spezia, J.: Uterine prolapse during pregnancy. Obstet. Gynecol., *32:* 765, 1968.

Rud, T., Ulmsten, U., Andersson, K.-E.: Initiation of voiding in healthy women and both with stress incontinence. Acta Obstet. Gynecol. Scand., *57:* 457, 1978.

Stamey, T. A., Schaeffer, A. J., and Condy, M.: Clinical and roentgenographic evaluation of endoscopic suspension of the vesical neck for urinary incontinence. Surg. Gynecol. Obstet., *140:* 355, 1975.

Tompkins, P.: In defense of suspension of the uterus in treatment of infertility. Fertil. Steril., *7:* 317, 1956.

Zacharin, R. F.: Abdomino-perineal urethral suspension. A 10-year experience in the management of recurrent stress incontinence of urine. Obstet. Gynecol., *50:* 1, 1977.

CHAPTER 14

Hyperplasia of the Endometrium and Endometrial Polyps

HYPERPLASIA

The condition designated as *hyperplasia* of the endometrium was, at one time, rather distinctively correlated with *functional* (or, *dysfunctional*) *uterine bleeding*, and this association is frequent but far from invariable. Actually, *functional* bleeding is purely a clinical term, and endometrial hyperplasia is a pathological classification.

In the postmenopausal woman, hyperplasia is usually a result of hormone therapy. Where there is no history of this, an ovarian or adrenal source of estrogen is often the cause.

Etiology

The histological pattern of hyperplasia in the menstrual years is produced by *persistent estrogen stimulation in the absence of progesterone.* This implies that it is associated with an *anovulatory* type of cycle. A single follicle may fail to rupture and instead continue to grow and to function beyond the usual ovulation period, so that an abnormal growth effect is produced upon the endometrium. In other cases of anovulatory menstruation, a group of follicles continues to mature to various levels and to produce estrogen, with pronounced stimulation of the endometrium.

The *characteristic changes in the ovary*, therefore, are an absence of functioning corpora lutea and the presence of either a single, persistent, functioning follicle or a considerable group of smaller, functionally active follicles. In the latter case, the ovaries may be grossly cystic, but the small cysts are lined with an intact granulosa. There is a thick cortex with no or rare evidence of a recent corpus luteum and, indeed, there may be a close resemblance to the so-called Stein-Leventhal ovary. Where a single large follicle seems to dominate the picture, it may present clinically as a follicle cyst of considerable size, although there is a well preserved granulosa-theca zone and an active estrogenic function.

Endometrial hyperplasia is also a common cause of *postmenopausal bleeding*. It seems that estrogenic stimulation of the endometrium is the culprit here too, although the ovary is probably not the main source. In an elegant series of experiments Siiteri and MacDonald have demonstrated that peripheral conversion of androstenedione to estrone is the principal source of postmenopausal estrogen.

Still another cause of endometrial hyperplasia is *exogenous estrogen therapy*. This will be discussed in the following chapter in relation to endometrial carcinoma, but it is clear that all forms of hyperplasia of the endometrium may result from estrogenic medication (Fig. 14.1).

Microscopic Appearance of Hyperplasia

A common histologic pattern of endometrial hyperplasia is referred to as *cystic hyperplasia* or the *Swiss-cheese type* (Fig. 14.2), because of the disparity in size of the gland lumina. Some are large and cystic, whereas

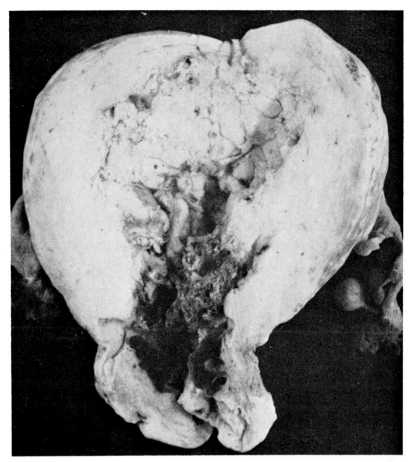

Figure 14.1. Marked polypoid hyperplasia (histologically benign) following prolonged estrogen therapy. (Courtesy of Dr. Derek Tacchio, New Castle, England.)

others, perhaps in the same microscopic field, are small in caliber. The epithelium is cuboidal or columnar, with heavily stained nuclei, and in the small glands there may even be some stratification. The stroma is abundant and hyperplastic, so that an endometrial sarcoma may be simulated. Mitoses are numerous in the epithelium and not infrequent in the stroma. The epithelium shows an *absence of the secretory activity* produced by progesterone. The finding of ciliated tubal-like epithelium is not at all uncommon in endometrial hyperplasia.

This type of cystic hyperplasia must be differentiated from *cystic atrophy*, which is characterized by the same type of dilated glands but has a hypocellular, atrophic, and often fibrotic stroma.

Focal Hyperplasia

Occasionally, patches of hyperplastic endometrium may be found in conjunction with a general secretory reaction. It must be borne in mind that the basalis endometrium is not responsive to the biphasic hormonal stimulus. Where an intact endometrium is available for study, as in a hysterectomy specimen, one often finds that there are occasionally patches of superficial immature basal tissue that have not acquired the capacity of response to progesterone and hence exhibit a proliferative or hyperplastic pattern, despite a biphasic cycle (Fig. 14.3).

Proliferative Hyperplasia

In a majority of cases the microscopic pattern of hyperplasia is a frankly benign one. In a small proportion, however, markedly proliferative and adenomatous pictures are produced, sometimes diffusely involving the whole endometrium but more often only certain focal areas. *Adenomatous hyperplasia*, as defined by Gore and Hertig, is characterized by glandular proliferation with projection

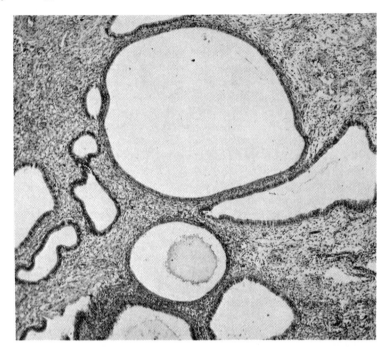

Figure 14.2.   An example of hyperplasia with characteristic Swiss-cheese pattern.

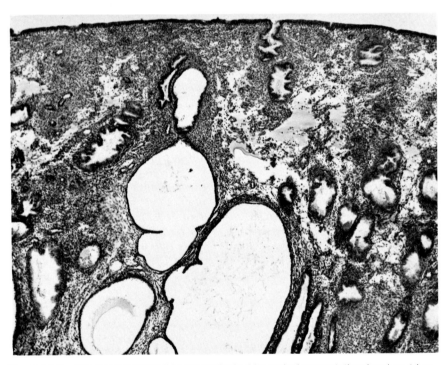

Figure 14.3.   ''Focal hyperplasia'' in *center* flanked by typical progestational endometrium.

into the surrounding stroma. The finger-like projections extend into the supporting endometrial stroma, forming complex and convoluted glands. These outpouchings may be-

come pinched off, forming many small glands with very little intervening stroma (Fig. 14.4). The epithelial cells lining the glands are often pale staining and become piled up or "pseudostratified" instead of the single layer usually seen in endometrial glands. As this process continues, the glandular proliferation tends to crowd out the stroma so that the glands become "back to back." There is more epithelial proliferation with intraluminal budding, papillary formation, and bridging across glands by the epithelium.

When cellular abnormalities are added to those marked proliferative changes, the term *atypical adenomatous hyperplasia* is often used (Fig. 14.5). The individual cells are usually enlarged, and there is an increase in nuclear size with clumping of the chromatin. Large nucleoli are often seen. Gusberg and Kaplan described these changes many years ago and has reported his observations on the transition of endometrial hyperplasia to cancer in many publications. Although we have preferred not to use the term because diagnostic criteria are so imprecise, Hertig and his colleagues have referred to the more severe forms of atypical adenomatous hyperplasia as *carcinoma in situ of the endometrium.*

It is often very difficult to separate these advanced hyperplasias from well differentiated endometrial carcinoma. When there is serious doubt, the safe plan is that expressed in the dictum of Halban, "Nich Karzinom, aber besser heraus!" (Not carcinoma, but better out!) In the milder degrees of proliferative overactivity, however, there is rarely any difficulty in excluding malignancy, and conservative treatment is indicated.

Differentiation of Progestational and Hyperplastic Endometrium

It may on occasion be extremely difficult to distinguish between certain progestational endometria and various forms of proliferative hyperplasia. Both exhibit abundant evidence of secretory activity, considerable infolding and intraluminal tufting by tall pale-staining cells, and extensive proliferation of the glands. If a well developed decidual-like stroma is present, there is considerable support for recent ovulation and progesterone influence. If not, one must consider an atypical hyperplasia, especially if there are associated areas of the benign cystic ("Swiss cheese") variety. This matter of distinction is of more than academic importance, because these proliferative endometrial patterns seem to be a *precursor to adenocarcinoma* or to coexist in conjunction with a true malignancy.

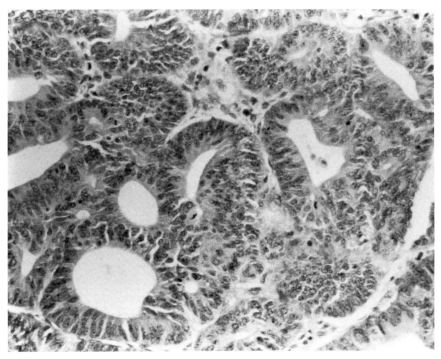

Figure 14.4.   High power of severe adenomatous hyperplasia with atypia. The glands are "back to back" with epithelial bridging and cellular atypia.

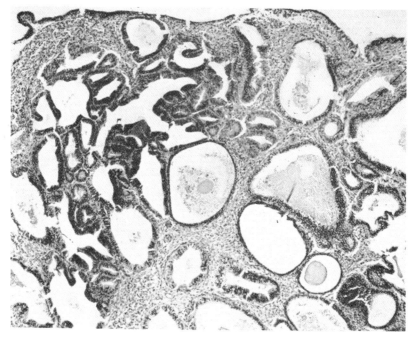

Figure 14.5.   An example of an atypical hyperplasia (*left*) with associated cystic hyperplasia.

Squamous Metaplasia (Acanthosis)

It is by no means rare to find *squamous metaplasia or acanthosis* in conjunction with endometrial hyperplasia and various other benign conditions of the endometrium. In such cases, however, it is the glandular element that determines the malignant potential, because the squamous cells are well differentiated and quite benign.

Squamous metaplasia of the endometrium may be a sequel of chronic infection, radium, any long-standing irritant such as intrauterine contraceptive devices (IUD) or foreign bodies, various hormonal stimuli, vitamin A deficiency, or other causes. It seems that a mature epithelial cell can be converted into a squamous cell, for we have seen all types of seeming transition between the lining epithelium and a mature squamous cell with frank pearl formation (Fig. 14.6).

On occasion, the whole endometrial surface may be converted into a stratified squamous surface, the so-called "icthyosis uteri." Malignant degeneration may occur with the production of the rare primary epidermoid cancer of the endometrium, or combined adenosquamous lesions may occur.

Squamous cells in the endometrium are not indicative of any malignant trend as long as the epithelioid cells are mature and well developed.

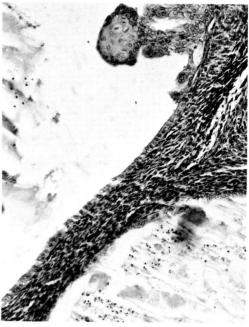

Figure 14.6.   Syncytial bud of squamous cells seemingly arising by metaplasia of the lining epithelium.

Diagnosis and Management of Hyperplasia

It has already been pointed out that endometrial hyperplasia is a pathologic diagnosis that cannot be made on clinical evaluation but only by histologic examination of the tissue. Therefore, it should be obvious that tissue must be obtained in order to make the diagnosis or eliminate it. *Abnormal uterine bleeding* is the only real symptom of this condition, and *this symptom must be investigated by fractional dilatation and curettage or endometrial biopsy.* It should be remembered that endometrial hyperplasia frequently coexists with carcinoma. Therefore, only by a thorough and careful dilatation and curettage can one rule out the possibility of carcinoma when hyperplasia is found on biopsy.

Endometrial hyperplasia in the menstrual era is usually an innocuous and self-limited process that frequently reverts to normal after curettage. When anovulation is the cause, intermittent therapy with progestational agents or induction of ovulation will usually result in elimination of the hyperplasia and the troublesome bleeding which often accompanies it. Unless the more severe forms of adenomatous hyperplasia are diagnosed, medroxyprogesterone acetate tablets, 10 mg per day for 5 to 10 days each month, should establish a normal bleeding pattern with elimination of the hyperplasia. Other progestogens or ovulation induction can be used as indicated in Chapter 31 on "Abnormal Uterine Bleeding."

When the diagnosis of adenomatous hyperplasia is made, especially in the postmenopausal patient, more vigorous therapy is in order, i.e., high-dose progestational therapy, Such as depomedroxyprogesterone acetate, 1000 mg per week for 4 weeks followed by 5 months of monthly therapy of 400 mg per month. Other drugs and dosage schedules include 17-α-hydroxyprogesterone caproate, 500 mg per day for 2 weeks and then 2 g weekly for an additional 5 months, and megesterol acetate, 80 mg daily for 6 to 12 weeks. Excellent results, at least for the short term, have been reported by Kistner, Wentz, and Eichner and Abellera. Follow-up biopsy or dilatation and curettage is necessary to evaluate the effectiveness of therapy, which is usually given over a 6-month period. For patients with persistent hyperplasia, especially if it is increasingly severe, or for patients whose symptoms of bleeding are not controlled, or for those women who cannot or will not take the hormonal therapy, hysterectomy is advised. Indeed, in many cases of atypical adenomatous hyperplasia, both the gynecologist and the patient will prefer to treat the condition by hysterectomy, thereby removing any possibility of malignant transformation.

ENDOMETRIAL POLYPS

The term polyp is a clinical one, referring to tumors attached by a stem or pedicle. Thus a polypoid tumor within the uterus may be a myoma, carcinoma, or sarcoma, or it might be made up of retained placental tissue (placental polyp). The common *endometrial polyp* is made up of endometrial tissue. Such polyps may be single or multiple, small, or large enough to fill the uterine cavity. The pedicle may become so long that the growth projects beyond the cervix, and, in rare cases, beyond the vaginal introitus.

Microscopic Structure

The microscopic structure of these polyps is like that of the endometrium from which they spring, with some qualification on the basis of the *functional* or *nonfunctional* type of the constituent epithelium. In some polyps the endometrial tissue shows a *functional* cyclical response paralleling that of the general uterine mucosa (Fig. 14.7). When the latter exhibits a progestational picture, for example, so does the endometrium of the polyp.

In a far larger proportion of cases, however, the polyp is made up of an *immature or unripe* type of endometrium, like that seen in the basalis, that is not responsive to progesterone. Such polyps, therefore, show a proliferative picture, often with a typical Swiss-cheese hyperplasia pattern, at all phases of the menstrual cycle, even when the surrounding endometrium is in a progestational phase.

Clinical Characteristics

Unless they become large enough to protrude from the cervix, or unless secondary degenerative or ulcerative changes develop, endometrial polyps are apt to be entirely asymptomatic, although the constituent immature endometrium may lead to various types of abnormal bleeding. As a matter of fact, a proportion are not discovered until uteri removed for other indications are opened.

In the larger polyps or those that obtrude into the cervical or vaginal canals, *bleeding* is almost always a symptom, because of the secondary ulcerative changes that develop.

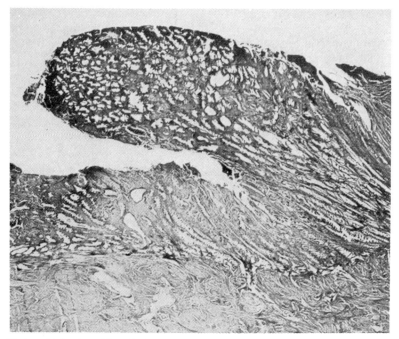

Figure 14.7. Endometrial polyp of functioning type showing premenstrual secretory activity of glands similar to that in surrounding endometrium.

As a rule, it is of metrorrhagic type and moderate degree, but, in some cases, it may be quite profuse. In a series of 401 patients with postmenopausal bleeding, Pacheco and Kempers found that 23% had endometrial polyps as the cause.

Premalignant Potentialities of Endometrial Polyps

It has generally been assumed that endometrial polyps have little tendency to be associated with or to evolve into fundal adenocarcinoma, and there seems little doubt that this view is correct in regard to women *during menstrual life*. In the *menopausal* and *postmenopausal eras*, however, there would seem to be considerable question as to whether such lesions can be regarded with complete equanimity.

Indeed, analysis of some 1,100 polyps in our clinic revealed that 10 to 15% were *associated* with malignancy in postmenopausal women.

Treatment

The polyps which manifest themselves by protrusion through the cervical canal are readily diagnosed, although it is not always

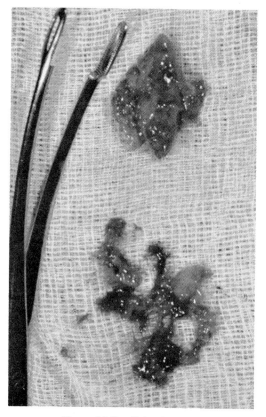

Figure 14.8. Polyp forceps.

easy to be sure whether they spring from the cervix or from the endometrium. The distinction is not usually of practical importance, because the method of treatment is the same for both types. For the endometrial growths, especially those of larger size, the cervix should be dilated and the growth removed, followed by curettage, to make sure that other small polyps are not present. It is wise to follow any curettage with the introduction of a long narrow forceps (Fig. 14.8) to "fish around" for a possibly overlooked polyp. This may easily happen, despite the most thorough uterine scraping.

References and Additional Readings

Chamlian, D. L., and Taylor, H. B.: Endometrial hyperplasia in young women. Obstet. Gynecol., *36:* 659, 1970.

Cope, E.: Management of abnormal bleeding. Br. Med. J., *2:* 700, 1971.

Eichner, E., and Abellera, M.: Endometrial hyperplasia treated by progestins. Obstet. Gynecol., *38:* 739, 1971.

Gore, H., and Hertig, A. T.: Premalignant lesions of the endometrium. Clin. Obstet. Gynecol., *5:* 1148, 1962.

Gusberg, S. B., and Kaplan, H. G.: Precursors of corpus cancer. Am. J. Obstet. Gynecol., *87:* 662, 1963.

Hertig, A. T., Sommers, S. C., and Bengloff, H.: Genesis of endometrial carcinoma. III. Carcinoma in situ. Cancer, *2:* 964, 1949.

Israel, R., Mishell, D. R., and Labudovich, M.: Mechanism of uterine bleeding. Clin. Obstet. Gynecol., *13:* 386, 1972.

Kistner, R. W.: Treatment of carcinoma in situ of the endometrium. Clin. Obstet. Gynecol., *5:* 1166, 1962.

Ober, W. B., Sobrero, A. J., Korman, R., and Gold, S.: Endometrial morphology and polyethylene intrauterine devices; a study of 200 endometrial biopsies. Obstet. Gynecol., *32:* 782, 1968.

Overstreet, E. W.: Clinical aspects of endometrial polyps. Surg. Clin. North. Am., *42:* 1013, 1962.

Pacheco, J. C., and Kempers, R. D.: Etiology of postmenopausal bleeding. Obstet. Gynecol., *32:* 40, 1968.

Schenker, J. G., Weinstein, D., and Okon, E.: Estradiol and testosterone levels in the peripheral and ovarian circulations in patients with endometrial cancer. Cancer, *44:* 1809, 1979.

Scommegna, A., and Dmowski, W. P.: Dysfunctional uterine bleeding. Clin. Obstet. Gynecol., *16:* 221, 1973.

Siiteri, P. K., and MacDonald, P. C.: Role of extraglandular estrogen in human endocrinology. In *Handbook of Physiology,* Sect. 7, *Endocrinology,* edited by R. O. Greep and E. A. Astwood, Vol. II, Part I, Ch. 28, p. 615. American Physiological Society, Washington, D. C., 1973.

Sippe, G.: Endometrial hyperplasia and uterine bleeding. J. Obstet. Gynaecol. Br. Commonw., *69:* 1015, 1962.

Sobrina, L. G., and Kase, N.: Endocrinologic aspects of dysfunctional uterine bleeding. Clin. Obstet. Gynecol., *13:* 400, 1970.

Vellios, F.: Endometrial hyperplasias, precursors of endometrial carcinoma. In *Pathology Annual,* edited by S. C. Sommers. Appleton-Century-Crofts, New York, 1972.

Wallach, E. E. (Editor): Dysfunctional uterine bleeding. Clin. Obstet. Gynecol., *13:* 363, 1972.

Welsh, W. R., and Scully, R. E.: Pre-cancerous lesions of the endometrium. Hum. Pathol., *8:* 503, 1977.

Wentz, W. B.: Treatment of persistent endometrial hyperplasia by progestins. Am. J. Obstet. Gynecol., *95:* 999, 1966.

CHAPTER 15

Endometrial Carcinoma

Endometrial carcinoma is the most common invasive gynecologic malignancy in the United States today. This is due not only to an increase in the number of cases of endometrial cancer but also to a significant decline in the incidence of invasive cervical cancer. Invasive carcinoma of the cervix, which has for years been the most common primary site of gynecologic cancer, has now been replaced by carcinoma of the corpus or uterine fundus, more than 90% of which is adenocarcinoma of the endometrium. Weiss et al. surveyed the incidence of endometrial cancer in eight areas of the United States and found an increase in all sections of the country.

This increased incidence has been due to several factors. First, the greater longevity of the population in general is a consideration. With better nutrition, health care, and living conditions more women are living long enough to develop endometrial carcinoma. This cancer is most common in the postmenopausal patient. The average age at diagnosis is 59 years, which is more than 10 years older than the average age for cervical cancer. Second, increased awareness on the part of both physicians and patients has led to increased surveillance, with earlier and more accurate diagnosis; therefore, patients with adenocarcinoma of the endometrium are being diagnosed earlier and correctly. Third, and perhaps most important, increased use of estrogen replacement therapy for the menopause has probably led to an increase in endometrial adenocarcinoma.

Relationship of Estrogen to Endometrial Carcinoma

The concept that estrogen might produce hyperplastic and even malignant changes in hormone-sensitive tissues is not a new one. Estrogens have been known to produce tumors in a variety of experimental animals in such tissues as the uterus, vagina, and breast.

Feminizing Ovarian Tumors

Patients with granulosa-theca cell tumors of the ovary have a high incidence of endometrial carcinoma (Table 15.1). These uncommon ovarian tumors are capable of estrogen production, and the greatly increased incidence of adenocarcinoma associated with these tumors is quite suggestive. The risk is even more striking when only postmenopausal patients are considered.

Polycystic Ovarian Disease

Endometrial cancer is predominantly a disease of postmenopausal women, with only about 5% of all cases occurring in women under the age of 40. Among these young women there is a very high incidence of *anovulation*. According to several reviews noted in Table 15.2, the typical polycystic ovary of the Stein-Leventhal syndrome is found in 19–25% of young women with endometrial carcinoma (Fig. 15.1). Anovulation, with the resultant lack of a corpus luteum and thus a lack of progesterone synthesis, leads to prolonged unopposed estrogen stimulation of the endometrium.

Estrogen Therapy

As suggested earlier, exogenous estrogen therapy has been shown to be associated with an increased risk of developing endometrial carcinoma. With the availability of oral estrogen preparations, the use of estrogen "replacement" therapy as a routine matter for the postmenopausal patient became widespread. Some authors advocated the use of estrogens in all postmenopausal women, be-

Table 15.1
Incidence of Endometrial Carcinoma in Patients with Granulosa Cell Tumors

All Patients		Postmenopausal Patients	
Author	Endometrial Cancer	Author	Endometrial Cancer
	%		%
Greene	3.5	Ingram & Novak	12
Kottmeier	5.6	Larson	15
Diddle	6.1	Greene	23
Mansell and Hertig	15	Hertig and Sommers	24
Smith et al. (1975)	16	Dockerty et al.	27
Speert	18		

Table 15.2
Incidence of Polycystic Ovarian Disease in Women Under Age 40 with Endometrial Cancer

Author	Incidence of Polycystic Ovarian Disease
	%
Speert	21
Sommers et al.	25
Dockerty et al.	19
Silverberg et al.	20

cause increasing life expectancy now allows women to "outlive their ovaries," with a resulting decline in endogenous estrogen production during the postmenopausal years. It has been argued that this hypoestrogenic state is abnormal and should be treated, just as one would treat hypothyroidism or diabetes.

Although several early studies failed to demonstrate any association between endometrial cancer and exogenous estrogen therapy, since 1975 many studies have clearly found an increased use of estrogen among patients with endometrial cancer (Table 15.3). These recent studies used more appropriate control groups than the earlier studies. Estrogen therapy is well known to cause endometrial hyperplasia, and the older studies had used women with uterine bleeding, some of whom had estrogen-induced hyperplasia, as control patients. For long-term estrogen users the risk of developing cancer of the endometrium seems to be increased about 3- to 12-fold (Fig. 15.2). The dose of estrogen and the duration of exposure seem to be related to the degree of increased risk.

The studies noted above have all been concerned with estrogen therapy, largely with conjugated estrogens, in postmenopausal women. However, McCarroll et al. and Roberts and Wells among others, have reported endometrial cancer in young women treated with the nonsteroidal estrogen, diethylstilbesterol, for gonadal dysgenesis. Rosenwaks et al. have also reported endometrial hyperplasia in a series of 46 hypogonadal patients treated with long-term estrogen therapy.

Silverberg and associates reported on 30 women under the age of 40 who developed endometrial carcinoma while taking oral contraceptives, mostly sequential agents. These sequential oral contraceptive agents utilize synthetic estrogens, usually ethinyl estradiol, for 21 days followed by 5 days of a progestogen. It seems that the estrogenic stimulation of the endometrium produced by these pills in some women was not modified sufficiently by the short course of progestogen. Sequential oral contraceptives have been removed from the market; there is no evidence that such a problem exists with the combination type of oral contraceptives, which have a predominantly progestational effect.

It seems clear that estrogens—steroidal and nonsteroidal, estrogens from a bottle or estrogens from the patient's own ovary—can all lead to hyperplasia and endometrial cancer in some women. Underwood et al. suggest that most, but not all, estrogen-associated cancers are early, and the survival rates after treatment are excellent. The current indications and risks of exogenous estrogen therapy are still extremely controversial, and it behooves the prudent gynecologist to keep abreast of the latest developments. If estrogen therapy is to be used, the lowest dose possible to relieve symptoms for the shortest time is indicated in order to minimize risk.

Relationship of Endometrial Hyperplasia to Carcinoma

On the previous pages, we have alluded to the association between endometrial hyper-

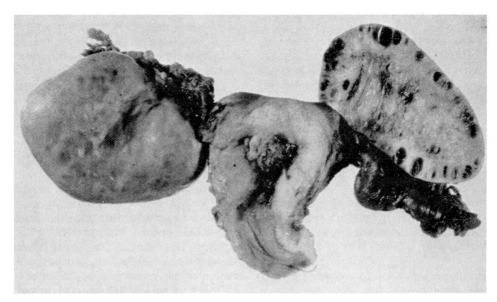

Figure 15.1. Polycystic ovaries associated with endometrial carcinoma in a 15-year-old girl. (Courtesy of Dr. R. Greenblatt, Augusta, Georgia.)

Table 15.3
Association of Exogenous Estrogens with Endometrial Carcinoma

Authors	Cancer Patients	On Estrogens	Control Patients on Estrogens	Relative Risk
		%	%	
Smith et al.	317	48	17	7.5
Ziel and Finkle	94	57	15	7.6
Mack et al.	63	89	50	8.0
McDonald et al.	145	17	8	2.3
Gray et al.	205	16	6	3.1
Horowitz et al.	119	30	3	12.0
Antunes et al.	339	19	5	4.3

plasia and endometrial carcinoma. Although endometrial hyperplasia in the menstruating woman, and especially cystic hyperplasia, is almost always benign, several lines of evidence suggest that "atypical" hyperplasia is a precursor of endometrial cancer. Studies concerning the relationship between hyperplasia and cancer have been fraught with difficulty due to the lack of clearly defined terminology for the various forms of endometrial hyperplasia. The terminology and controversy have been well reviewed by Welch and Scully and by Vellios. It is important to consider both the over-all architecture of the glands and stroma as well as the individual cellular characteristics.

The study of McBride suggests that the malignant potential of cystic hyperplasia is very low. He followed 544 postmenopausal women up to 24 years after a diagnosis of cystic hyperplasia and found that only two patients in the group went on to develop endometrial cancer. However, with more proliferative forms of hyperplasia, which have both architectural and cellular atypia, the prognosis is more worrisome (Fig. 15.3). Sherman and Brown reported a prospective study of 216 women over age 50 who underwent dilatation and curettage for bleeding and were found to have "adenomatous hyperplasia" (113), "atypical adenomatous hyperplasia" (91), or "carcinoma in situ" (12). Subsequent curettage or hysterectomy 2–18 years later showed progression to adenocarcinoma in 22.1% of the women with "adenomatous hyperplasia," 57.1% of the women

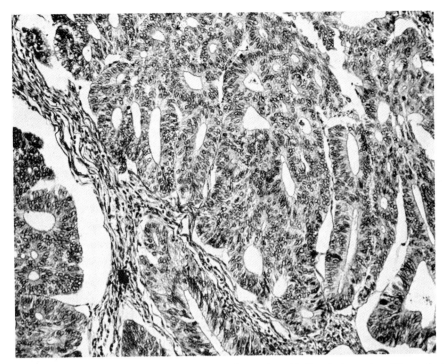

Figure 15.2   High power of well differentiated adenocarcinoma found in the uterine polyp of the patient treated with long-term estrogens.

with "atypical adenomatous hyperplasia," and 58.5% of the women with an original diagnosis of "carcinoma in situ." In a series of 97 premenopausal woman with endometrial hyperplasia, many of whom were anovulatory, Chamlian and Taylor found 14% progressed to endometrial carcinoma in 1–14 years.

Retrospective studies of women with endometrial carcinoma who have had endometrial sampling years prior to the diagnosis of cancer have also shown a high incidence of hyperplasia. Sherman and Brown reported adenomatous hyperplasia in 72.3% of 235 women over age 60 who had a curettage specimen from 1 to 10 years before the diagnosis of carcinoma of the endometrium.

A third line of evidence linking endometrial hyperplasia to cancer is the frequent presence of the two lesions in the same uterus. In patients with a diagnosis of invasive endometrial carcinoma, Gray et al. found associated proliferative hyperplasias in the uterus of 42.6% of 192 hysterectomy specimens.

Although none of this evidence is "proof" of the malignant potential of endometrial hyperplasia, it seems clear that patients with

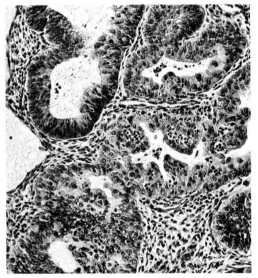

Figure 15.3.   Marked adenomatous ("back-to-back") crowding with beginning stratification and proliferation of lining epithelium with small papillae. This lesion might be called "carcinoma in situ" by some.

hyperplasia—especially those with glandular proliferation, irregular architecture, and cytologic abnormalities—are at increased risk for the development of endometrial carcinoma and should be carefully followed or treated as outlined in Chapter 14.

PATHOLOGY

Gross Pathology

Adenocarcinoma may arise from any portion of the uterus and may appear grossly as a diffuse fungating overgrowth with surface ulceration and necrosis or occasionally as a very circumscribed lesion.

Microscopic Diagnosis

We have already alluded to the difficulty of making the diagnosis in some cases of well differentiated carcinoma. The microscopic appearance is quite critical and is of considerable prognostic significance in endometrial cancer. The diagnosis is made on the basis of two chief criteria:

(1) The Pattern or Architecture. The small crowded glands of adenomatous hyperplasia obliterate the intervening stroma ("back-to-back" crowding), and cellular proliferation within individual glands leads to stratification, papillary formation and eventually obliteraton of the gland pattern (Fig. 15.4).

(2) Individual Cell Changes. In adenocarcinoma, the cells show varying degrees of immaturity and dedifferentiation with abnormal pleomorphic nuclei; many of the latter show hyperchromatosis, abnormal mitotic activity, and other evidences of anaplasia.

Histologic Grading

The degree of histologic differentiation has long been known to be an important factor in the prognosis of endometrial cancer. Mahle was the first to document the relationship between survival and degree of differentiation of the tumor. He grouped 136 patients in four grades and found that all the patients with Grade 1 (well differentiated) cancers were living, 71% of Grade 2, 38% of Grade 3, and 0% of the few patients with Grade 4 (undifferentiated) tumors. These findings have been confirmed by many investigators, and Ng and Reagan among others have demonstrated that survival is related to degree of differentiation when extent of disease is held constant.

The majority of patients with endometrial adenocarcinoma have Grade 1 or Grade 2 tumors, and only about 15–20% have poorly differentiated lesions. With increasing cell dedifferentiation, there is progressive loss of the rather delicate adenomatous pattern due to proliferation of the epithelial lining cell. As this stratification continues there may be obliteration of the glandular pattern with little resemblance to an adenocarcinoma, so that

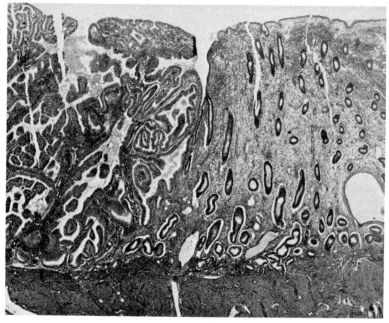

Figure 15.4. Microscopic picture of adenocarcinoma (*left*) as contrasted with normal endometrium (*right*).

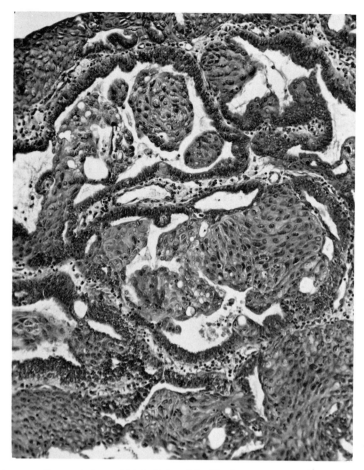

Figure 15.5. Adenoacanthoma of uterus. This is distinguished by the presence of plaques of well differentiated, obviously benign, squamous cells in association with adenocarcinoma.

the lesion mimics an epidermoid or an undifferentiated carcinoma. However, examination of other areas may suggest glandular acini, indicating a high grade adenocarcinoma.

Adenoacanthoma of the Uterus

This specific variant of endometrial adenocarcinoma is characterized by the presence of many squamous cells, filling the gland lumina and/or lining and replacing the surface endometrium. The squamous cells are well differentiated, generally uniform, and obviously benign. In 1961 Marcus suggested the term *adenoacanthoma of the endometrium* for lesions with extensive benign squamous metaplasia together with malignant adenomatous elements (Fig. 15.5). The lesion is malignant, although not because of the squamous cells. It is the *glandular component* that

is decisive, and indeed this same squamous metaplasia may occur with benign endometrial hyperplasia, in which event the lesion is benign.

Most recent reports suggest that the *prognosis of patients with adenoacanthoma is dependent on the degree of differentiation of the adenocarcinomatous element of the tumor.* Charles and Javert and Renning reported a worse prognosis, while Liggins and Way and Silverberg et al. have described a better prognosis than pure adenocarcinoma. Recent studies which have matched patients for the degree of differentiation of the adenocarcinoma have found similar survival statistics for both lesions, as pointed out by Salazar et al. They found that there was a tendency for adenoacanthomas to have a well differentiated adenocarcinoma component. Seventy-six percent of the lesions with squamous metaplasia were accompanied by a well differentiated adenocarcinoma, while only 49% of the pure adenocarcinomas were Grade 1.

Adenosquamous or Mixed Carcinoma of the Endometrium

When both the adenomatous and squamous components are malignant, the lesion is known as *adenosquamous carcinoma*, or adenoepidermoid or mixed carcinoma (Fig. 15.6). Ng and Reagan have noted this variety of endometrial cancer has been encountered with increasing frequency in the past two decades. In their experience, adenosquamous carcinoma accounted for less than 5% of all endometrial cancer prior to 1956. Since then there has been a steady increase, through the period 1967–1971, when it accounted for 32.8% of all endometrial neoplasms seen in their laboratory. Other observers, including Salazar et al., have found that there has been no change in the incidence of adenosquamous carcinoma of the endometrium and have suggested that the apparent increase was due to the overdiagnosis of poorly differentiated adenocarcinoma. This would also explain the poor prognosis associated with these lesions. Ng et al. reported a

19% 5-year survival for patients with adenosquamous carcinoma, while the more recent series by Silverberg et al. found a 5-year salvage of 35%. In contrast to these figures are those of the Rochester group in which Salazar reports a 5-year survival of 80%— exactly the same as for pure adenocarcinoma. We suspect that all these variations are merely a result of different diagnostic criteria for the different lesions and, again, the degree of differentiation of the adenocarcinomatous elements is the most important histologic prognostic factor. Mixed adenosquamous lesions, in distinct contrast to adenoacanthoma, tend to have a poorly differentiated adenocarcinoma component.

CLINICAL CHARACTERISTICS

Endometrial carcinoma is typically a disease of the postmenopausal woman, with roughly 75% of all patients being beyond the menopause, 15% perimenopausal, and only 10% still menstruating. There are certain clinical characteristics associated with endometrial carcinoma which have been used to identify a high risk group. An excellent review of

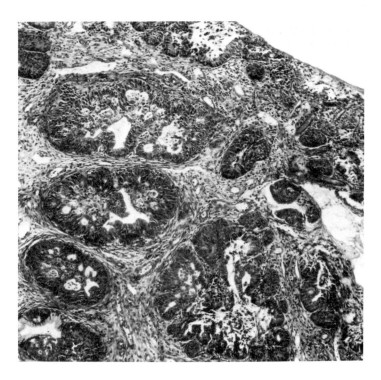

Figure 15.6. Adenosquamous carcinoma of the endometrium. Glandular areas with malignant squamous epithelium in the lower right.

these characteristics, which include obesity, impaired fertility, and glucose intolerance, has been published by Lucas.

Wynder found 21% of patients with endometrial cancer were 21–50 pounds overweight, a highly significant rate of obesity when compared with a control group. McDonald et al. were able to calculate that the relative risk of developing endometrial cancer was 3.5 times greater in women who were 30% above the upper limit of ideal weight than in matched controls.

Many authors have noted that women with endometrial cancer seem to be of low parity or are nulliparous. Dunn and Bradbury found a 25% incidence of nulliparity among married women with cancer while only 4.8% of married control patients were childless. In the study of women with endometrial cancer in Olmsted County, Minnesota, McDonald and his colleagues calculated a 1.9 fold increased risk among nulliparous woman.

Although many clinicians have had the impression that diabetes and hypertension are more common among women with endometrial cancer, recent studies have not supported these opinions. In a prospective study, Benjamin and Romney reported a 32% incidence of endometrial cancer among patients with diabetes and an additional 32% among those who had abnormal glucose tolerance tests. This was significantly greater than the 22% of the control population who had abnormal glucose tolerance. However, neither Dunn and Bradbury or McDonald et al. found an increased incidence of abnormal glucose metabolism in endometrial cancer patients.

The association of exogenous estrogen therapy with endometrial cancer has already been discussed.

The only important symptom is *abnormal bleeding*, commonly postmenopausal. Among all women with postmenopausal bleeding, uterine malignancy is the cause in 15–25%, according to most studies. In the case of women still in the menstruating age, *menorrhagia* is frequently observed. Next to bleeding, the most significant symptom is an *abnormal discharge*, at first watery, but soon admixed with blood.

On occasion there may be no abnormal bleeding but pressure symptoms due to a uterus massively distended by blood which cannot escape due to some obstruction in the lower genital tract. Arrata and Zarou find that about one-third of their cases of postmenopausal hematometra are due to an endometrial carcinoma.

DIAGNOSIS

The first thought of every physician when confronted with a case of *postmenopausal bleeding* should concern cancer of the uterus, either of the cervix or of the body. Cervical cancer can usually be eliminated by careful inspection and office smears and biopsy.

Assuming, however, that a cervical or vaginal source for the bleeding can be eliminated, an intrauterine source should be assumed. As a matter of fact, it is often possible to observe a blood-stained discharge or a trickle of blood escaping from the cervical canal. Even then, it is by no means certain that adenocarcinoma exists, this being found in only 15–25% of all cases of postmenopausal bleeding. Other possible causes are benign polyps or hyperplasia (often estrogen induced), submucous myoma, or senile vaginitis.

Evaluation of the different methods of endometrial sampling has been reported by Creasman and Weed. One thing is certain. *The standard cervical-vaginal Pap smear is not an adequate method of evaluating uterine bleeding.* Various estimates indicate that a smear will be positive in only 35–80% of all patients with endometrial cancer, with most authors finding about a 65% correlation.

Over 50 years ago Dr. Howard Kelly proposed a "curettage without anesthesia on the office table" as a solution to the problem of obtaining an adequate tissue sample from the endometrium. This type of *outpatient endometrial biopsy* has been championed by Hofmeister, who has performed over 20,000 office biopsies using only a small amount of intrauterine lidocaine anesthetic (Fig. 15.7). Most of these cases were asymptomatic women, and he diagnosed 197 endometrial cancers by this biopsy procedure. More recently, this technique has been adapted for use with a small office suction machine which connects to a very thin hollow curette. Both the endometrial biopsy and the Vabra aspirator have a diagnostic accuracy of greater than 90% and provide a tissue sample which can be processed and examined by the pathologist in the usual way.

Despite these office procedures for endometrial sampling, many patients with abnormal uterine bleeding will require a *fractional*

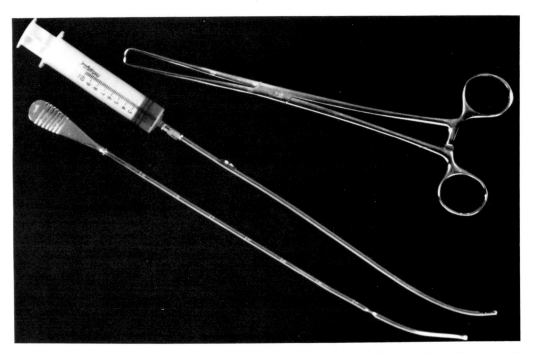

Figure 15.7. Endometrial biopsy instruments. The uterus is sounded and then the thin hollow curette is inserted and suction applied with the syringe during curettage.

dilitation and curettage under anesthesia. The importance of a *fractional* curettage should be stressed, since correct staging of endometrial cancer requires knowing if the cervix is involved or not. Cervical biopsies and endocervical curettage are done individually and sent as separate specimens before the uterine cavity is sounded and curettage of the uterine corpus is done. Such a procedure need not be done on an inpatient basis if the patient is in otherwise good health, since most gynecologists today have access to outpatient surgical facilities where patients "come and go" on the same day for minor procedures under anesthesia. In addition to allowing a thorough curettage of the endometrial cavity, anesthesia provides the opportunity for a good pelvic examination, for even the most experienced clinician may be unable to perform an adequate examination on an obese, anxious patient in the office.

STAGING

Once the diagnosis of endometrial carcinoma has been made, the patient must be "staged" or classified as to the extent of disease for therapeutic, prognostic, and statistical purposes. The classification system generally accepted throughout the world today is the one proposed by the International Federation of Gynecology and Obstetrics, which is shown in Table 15.4. As with all other gynecological malignancies except those involving the ovary, the classification is a *clinical staging system* which does not permit consideration of findings obtained by laparotomy or hysterectomy. This is to allow for comparable staging of patients treated by radiation alone where the surgical findings are never known. Routine evaluation with examination, dilitation and curettage, cystoscopy, proctoscopy, as well as standard radiological examinations, are performed.

In a thorough review, H. W. Jones has noted that stage, uterine size, degree of tumor differentiation, depth of myometrial penetration, lymph node metastases, and age are all correlated with prognosis. Endometrial carcinoma is one of the most favorable types of cancer to have by virtue of its tendency to remain confined to the surface. Myometrial extension may occur, and increased degrees impair the prognosis. *Ovarian involvement* by tubal or lymphatic extension is evident in 10% of most large series. Vaginal, especially suburethral, tumor was frequent in the preirradiation days. But a review by Boutselis, et al. confirms the relative infrequency of vaginal metastasis in irradiated patients, and Ingersoll has carried out a more recent study. The prognosis where the vagina is involved is poor, perhaps because this type of lesion is generally quite undifferentiated.

In occasional cases, the peritoneum may be the seat of implantation and peritoneal lavage for cytology appears to have prognostic importance. *Distant metastases* to such locations as the liver or lungs are not uncommon in advanced disease.

In attempting evaluation of metastatic disease, one must be cognizant of Bailar's observations that almost 5% of women with endometrial cancer had another extrauterine malignancy. Breast cancer is much more fre-

quent, and lower bowel lesions are disproportionately common.

Lymph node metastases: Studies have shown that pelvic lymph node metastases occur in about 11% of all patients with Stage I endometrial cancer (Table 15.5). In a series of 107 women who were treated by radical hysterectomy and pelvic lymphadenectomy for Stage I disease, Lewis et al. found the incidence of lymph node metastases varied with the degree of tumor differentiation and depth of myometrial penetration of the tumor.

Recently, a cooperative effort by Creasman et al. has examined the incidence of aortic as well as pelvic lymph node metastases in patients with Stage I endometrial carcinoma. A

Table 15.4
Staging Classification for Carcinoma of the Uterine Corpus Adopted by the International Federation of Gynecology and Obstetrics (FIGO)

Stage 0	Carcinoma in situ. Histological findings suspicious of malignancy.
	Cases of Stage 0 should not be included in any therapeutic statistics.
Stage I	The carcinoma is confined to the corpus including the isthmus.
Stage Ia	The length of the uterine cavity is 8 cm or less.
Stage Ib	The length of the uterine cavity is more than 8 cm.
	The Stage I cases should be sub-grouped with regard to the histological type of the adenocarcinoma as follows:
	G1—highly differentiated adenomatous carcinoma
	G2—moderately differentiated adenomatous carcinoma with partly solid areas
	G3—predominantly solid or entirely undifferentiated carcinoma.
Stage II	The carcinoma has involved the corpus and the cervix, but has not extended outside the uterus.
Stage III	The carcinoma has extended outside the uterus, but not outside the true pelvis.
Stage IV	The carcinoma has extended outside the true pelvis or has obviously involved the mucosa of the bladder or rectum. A bullous edema as such does not permit a case to be allotted to Stage IV.
Stage IVa	Spread of the growth to adjacent organs as urinary bladder, rectum, sigmoid, or small bowel.
Stage IVb	Spread to distant organs.

Table 15.5
Incidence of Pelvic Lymph Node Metastases in Patients with Endometrial Carcinoma[a]

Author	Stage I		Stage II	
	Patients (No.)	Positive Nodes	Patients (No.)	Positive Nodes
Liu and Meigs	33	4	14	7
Lefebre	37	3	1	1
Schwartz and Brunschwig	14	2	12	4
Roberts	22	5	8	2
Hawksworth	64	8	11	6
Rickford	36	2	9	2
Lees	56	3	8	4
Lewis et al.	107	12	22	5
TOTAL	369	39 (10.6%)	85	31 (36.5%)

[a] From Morrow et al., *Obstetrics and Gynecology, 42:* 399, 1973.

total of 161 patients underwent aortic lymph node sampling and 17, or 10.5% had metastatic tumor in the aortic nodes. Only three patients had aortic node involvement with negative pelvic nodes, suggesting that spread along the ovarian lymphatics is a possible, although uncommon, pathway of metastasis for endometrial cancer. More significantly, 14 of 23 patients (60.8%) who had pelvic lymph node metastases also had positive aortic nodes. This indicates that involvement of pelvic lymph nodes with metastatic cancer is often indicative of widespread disease, an important point to bear in mind when treatment approaches are considered.

TREATMENT AND RESULTS

Despite an enormous volume of literature on the subject, the treatment of adenocarcinoma of the endometrium still remains controversial. The results of treatment which have been reported in the last 20 years have generally been very good regardless of the treatment method employed. In addition to a seemingly endless variety of treatment plans, different investigators have used different staging systems and different methods of analyzing their results. These factors have combined to make it extremely difficult to compare the results of treatment methods and have made many gynecologists reluctant to abandon the type of therapy they have been using in search of a few percentage points in the 5-year survival statistics.

Surgery Alone

Surgical therapy alone was the original treatment method for endometrial carcinoma and is still widely used today. Several types of operations have been used including vaginal hysterectomy and radical hysterectomy with pelvic lymphadenectomy, but the most common procedure employed has been total abdominal hysterectomy and bilateral salpingooophorectomy. Many studies have shown a 5–12% incidence of ovarian metastases and for this reason removal of the adnexa should be carried out at the time of hysterectomy whenever possible. Because of the high incidence of vaginal recurrences following surgery for endometrial carcinoma, most investigators have recommended taking a wide vaginal cuff when no radiation is included in the treatment plan.

Radical hysterectomy and pelvic lymphadenectomy for endometrial carcinoma was introduced by Meigs and Brunschwig, who popularized its use for cervical cancer. Radical surgery for endometrial carcinoma has also been popular in England following the tradition of Victor Bonney. The rationale for pelvic lymphadenectomy comes from the figures on the incidence of pelvic lymph node metastases noted previously in Table 15.5. The results of treatment in several radical surgical series are shown in Table 15.6. The overall 5-year survival rate in 376 patients is a very respectable 76.7% for all stages. However, in the 45 patients with positive nodes, the 5-year survival rate falls to only 24.3%, despite the fact that most of the patients with positive nodes were also treated with postoperative pelvic irradiation. Thus, the survival rates for patients with or without positive nodes, treated by radical surgery are no better than with simple hysterectomy and the morbidity is considerably greater.

Total abdominal hysterectomy and bilateral salpingooophorectomy alone was the original method of treatment for adenocarcinoma of the endometrium. Today, hysterectomy is frequently combined with radiation in some form. However, controversy exists concerning the value of adjunctive radiation in early lesions.

Current trends favor the use of primary hysterectomy in patients with Stage I endometrial carcinoma with subsequent postoperative radiation reserved for those patients with high risk factors, such as deeply invasive cancers, cervical involvement, or poorly differentiated tumors. There is general agreement that hysterectomy to remove the pri-

Table 15.6
Results of Radical Hysterectomy and Pelvic Lymphadenectomy in the Treatment of Endometrial Carcinoma[a]

Author	Over-all		Positive nodes	
	Patients	5-Year Survival	Inci-dence	5-Year Survival
		%	%	%
Brunschwig	57	87	17	37
Parsons	52	79	8	50
Lees	76	68	17	15
Lewis	129	71	13	33
Park	62	90	1.6	0
	376	77	12	24

[a] From Jones, H.W.

mary tumor is an important aspect of the treatment of most patients with endometrial cancer.

Radiation Therapy

Radiation therapy alone for endometrial carcinoma is not commonly used in the United States, but in other countries many women are quite successfully treated with this modality.

In cases where the entire treatment is to be delivered by radiation therapy, both external and intracavitary radiation is used. Because carcinoma of the endometrium usually involves the fundus, it is necessary to concentrate the radioactive sources in the uterine cavity, against the tumor. When the uterus is not enlarged, this can be done quite adequately with a single intrauterine "tandem." However, with an enlarged uterus, an adequate dose cannot be delivered by this technique. In the 1920s Professor Heyman at the Radiumhemmet in Stockholm developed a technique of packing the uterine cavity with multiple radium capsules. This technique, called the "Stockholm Method," or "Heyman

packing," is extremely helpful in the treatment of a patient with a grossly enlarged uterus (Fig. 15.8). Although there is not much occasion for using this packing technique today, it should be available and utilized in patients who are to be treated solely by radiation therapy or when the uterus is quite enlarged.

Patients treated with radiation alone for endometrial cancer should receive at least 4000 rads external radiation to the whole pelvis and one or two intracavitary applications, preferably Heyman packings if the uterus is enlarged. The dose to the vaginal vault should be about 8000 rads.

The effacacy of radiation therapy for carcinoma of the endometrium has long been debated. It has proven almost impossible to find comparable groups for comparison of results since patients referred for radiation are often older and have more medical problems, making them poor operative candidates, and frequently have more advanced disease.

We have reserved radiation therapy alone for the treatment of those patients where

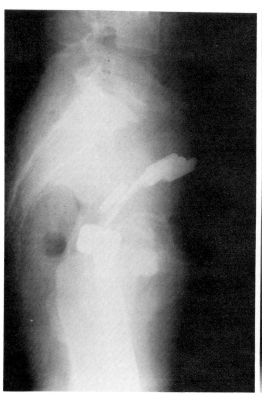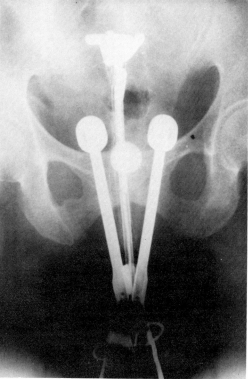

Figure 15.8. X-ray placement films of Heyman packing. Note that in addition to the multiple intrauterine capsules, a rigid intrauterine tandem and vaginal colpostats (or ovoids) are utilized.

advanced disease or poor medical condition makes hysterectomy impossible.

Radiation Plus Surgery

The proven effectiveness of both surgery and radiation in the treatment of endometrial carcinoma has led many gynecologists to employ a combination of the two approaches. A wide variety of treatment schemes using both external or intracavitary radiation or both has been used either preoperatively or following hysterectomy. Despite this extensive experience there is a surprising lack of hard data to support the general feeling that combined therapy produces better results than does surgery alone. Although the difference in survival is not significant, there are two reasons why adjunctive radiation has been favored in patients with endometrial carcinoma. First, it reduces the incidence of vaginal cuff recurrences and second, it may cure metastatic tumor in pelvic lymph nodes.

Both external and vaginal radiation are effective in reducing this type of recurrence, which is probably due to paravaginal lymphatic involvement in most cases. Both vaginal recurrences and lymph node metastases are related to the degree of differentiation, depth of myometrial invasion, and presence or absence of lower uterine segment involvement.

In recent years the value of intrauterine and vaginal radiation has also been questioned.

Current treatment for Stage I endometrial carcinoma is in a state of flux and most treatment methods seem to produce excellent results. In our clinic we favor primary hysterectomy but utilize both preoperative intrauterine and vaginal radiation for patients with poorly differentiated tumors and external radiation postoperatively for those with deep myometrial invasion.

In patients with more advanced disease a combination of preoperative radiation and hysterectomy is generally used if the patient is a surgical candidate. Gagnon et al. have reported an actuarial 5-year survival of 81% for patients with Stage II endometrial cancer treated in this way. The results shown in Table 15.7 are reported from the Seventeenth Annual Report, which collates treatment results from throughout the world.

RECURRENT AND METASTATIC CANCER

Patients who develop recurrent or metastatic adenocarcinoma of the endometrium are candidates for chemotherapy. Since Kelley first reported regression of endometrial carcinoma in two of three patients treated with progesterone in 1951, progestational agents have been widely used in the treatment of metastatic carcinoma of the endometrium. Many different compounds have been used, but the greatest experience has been with Depo-Provera (medroxy-progesterone acetate), Delalutin (17-alphahydroxyprogesterone caproate) and Megase (megesterol acetate). An excellent review by Kohorn found an over-all objective response rate of 32% with a significant relationship between tumor differentiation and response. Well differentiated tumors seem to respond best. Although some authors have suggested that pulmonary metastases respond more favorably, Reifenstein was not able to find any correlation between tumor site and response (Fig. 15.9). Many different dosage schedules have been used, but Depo-Provera, 400 mg per week for at least 12 weeks is frequently recommended. If the patient responds to therapy the drug should be continued, at reduced dosage, for life. Some authors recommend a "loading dose" of at least a gram a week for 4 weeks.

Estrogen and Progesterone Receptors

Since Jensen et al. reported that the absence of estrogen receptor proteins in the cytosol of breast cancers was indicative of a lack of responsiveness of that tumor to hormonal therapy, much work on both estrogen and progesterone receptors in hormonally sensitive tumors has been done. The characteristics of these receptors and their relationship in both benign and malignant endometrium has been reviewed by Pollow et al. As with breast cancer, Young et al. have reported

Table 15.7
Five-year Absolute Survival Results for Endometrial Carcinoma Collected by the 17th Annual Report from Stockholm.

	Patients Treated	5-year Survival
		%
Stage I	8009	73.6
Stage II	1426	55.7
Stage III	895	31.3
Stage IV	359	9.2
TOTAL	10689	65.5

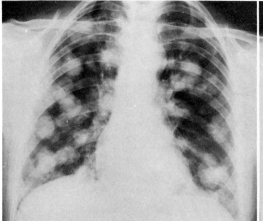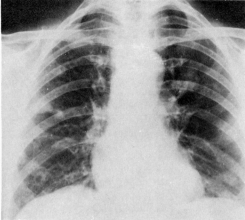

Figure 15.9. *Left,* Recurrent Stage II adenocarcinoma 1-year postirradiation and surgery with biopsy-proven metastasis. *Right,* X-ray 8 months later after large dose progesterone. Patient now has complete 6-year remission. (Courtesy of Dr. P. A. Nilsen, Oslo, Norway.)

that endometrial cancer patients with low levels or a lack of progesterone receptors do not respond to progestational chemotherapy. While this work is still preliminary, it may be significant and may tell us more about the control mechanisms of malignant tumors, as well as being predictive of the response to hormonal therapy.

Cytoxic chemotherapy for endometrial cancer has not been widely used, but Donovan reported response rates of about 25% to both cyclophosphamide and 5-Fluorouracil as single agents. A recent Gynecologic Oncology Group study reported by Thigpen et al. found a 38% response rate to Adriamycin. Trials with combination chemotherapy are now underway.

References and Additional Readings

Annual Report on the Results of Treatment in Carcinoma of the Uterus, Vol. 17, Stockholm, 1979.

Antunes, C. M. F., Stolley, P. D., Rosenshein, N. B., Davies, J. L., Tonascia, J. A., Brown, C., Burnett, L., Rutledge, A., Pokempner, M., and Garcia, R.: Endometrial cancer and estrogen use. N. Engl. J. Med., *300:* 9, 1979.

Arrata, W. S., and Zarou, G. S.: Postmenopausal hematometra. Am. J. Obstet. Gynecol., *85:* 959, 1963.

Badib, A. C., et al.: Biologic behavior of adenoacanthoma of the endometrium. Am. J. Obstet. Gynecol., *106:* 205, 1970.

Bailar, J. C.: Multiple tumors with uterine cancer. Cancer, *16:* 842, 1963.

Bean, H. A., et al.: Carcinoma of the endometrium in Saskatchewan: 1966 to 1971. Gynecol. Oncol., *6:* 503, 1978.

Benjamin, F., and Romney, S. L.: Disturbed carbohydrate metabolism in endometrial carcinoma. Cancer, *17:* 386, 1964.

Bickenbach, W., Lochmuller, H., Dirlich, G., Ruland, G., and Thurmayr, R.: Factor analysis of endometrial carcinoma in relation to treatment. Obstet. Gynecol, *29:* 632, 1967.

Boronow, R. C.: A fresh look at corpus cancer. Obstet. Gynecol., *42:* 448, 1973.

Bouteselis, J. G., Ullery, J. C., and Bain, J.: Vaginal metastases

following treatment of endometrial carcinoma. Obstet. Gynecol., *21:* 622, 1963.

Bruckman, J. E., et al.: Combined irradiation and surgery in the treatment of stage II carcinoma of the endometrium. Cancer, *42:* 1146, 1978.

Chamlian, D. L., and Taylor, H. B.: Endometrial hyperplasia in young women. J. Obstet. Gynecol., *36:* 659, 1970.

Charles, D.: Endometrial adenoacanthoma. Cancer, *18:* 737, 1965.

Creasman, W. T., Boronow, R. C., and Morrow, C. P.: Adenocarcinoma of the endometrium; its metastatic lymph node potential. Gynecol. Oncol., *4:* 239, 1976.

Creasman, W. T., and Weed, J. C.: Screening techniques in endometrial cancer. Cancer, *38:* 436, 1976.

Cutler, B. S., et al.: Endometrial carcinoma after stilbestrol therapy in gonadal dysgenesis. N. Engl. J. Med., *287:* 628, 1972.

Diddle, A. W.: Granulosa and theca cell ovarian tumors: Prognosis. Cancer, *5:* 215, 1952.

Donovan, J. F.: Nonhormonal chemotherapy of endometrial adenocarcinoma: A review. Cancer, *34:* 1587, 1974.

Dunn, L. J., and Bradbury, J. T.: Endocrine factors in endometrial carcinoma. Am. J. Obstet. Gynecol., *97:* 465, 1967.

Frick, H. C., et al.: Carcinoma of the endometrium. Am. J. Obstet. Gynecol., *115:* 663, 1973.

Gagnon, J. D., et al.: External irradiation in the management of stage II endometrial carcinoma. A logical approach. Cancer, *44:* 1247, 1979.

Gore, H., and Hertig, A. T.: Carcinoma in situ of the endometrium. Am. J. Obstet. Gynecol., *94:* 134, 1966.

Gray, L. A., et al.: Estrogens and endometrial carcinoma. Obstet. Gynecol., *49:* 385, 1977.

Greenwood, S. M., and Wright, D. J.: Evaluation of the office endometrial biopsy in the detection of endometrial carcinoma and atypical hyperplasia. Cancer, *43:* 1474, 1979.

Gusberg, H. B.: Hormone dependence of endometrial cancer. Obstet. Gynecol., *30:* 287, 1967.

Hofmeister, F. J.: Endometrial biopsy: another look. Am. J. Obstet. Gynecol., *118:* 773, 1974.

Heyman, J.: The so-called Stockholm method and the results of treatment of uterine cancer at the Radiumhemmet. Acta Radiol., *16:* 129, 1935.

Homesley, H. D., Boronow, R. C., and Lewis, J. L., Jr.: Stage II endometrial adenocarcinoma. Memorial hospital for cancer, 1949–1965. Obstet. Gynecol., *49:* 604, 1977.

Horwitz, R. I., and Feinstein, A. R.: Alternative analytic methods for case-control studies of estrogens and endometrial cancer. N. Engl. J. Med., *299:* 1089, 1978.

Ingersoll, F. M.: Vaginal recurrence of corpus cancer. Am. J. Surg., *121:* 473, 1971.

Javert, C., and Renning, E.: Endometrial cancer; survey of 610 cases treated at Women's Hospital (1919–1960). Cancer, *16:* 1057, 1963.

Jensen, E. V. T., et al.: *Steroid Dynamics.* Academic Press, New York, 1966.

Jones, H. W., III: Treatment of adenocarcinoma of the endometrium. Obstet. Gynecol. Surv., *30:* 147, 1975.

Keller, D., Kempson, R., Levine, G., and McLennan, C.: Management of the patient with early endometrial carcinoma. Cancer, *33:* 1108, 1974.

Kelley, R. M.: Proceedings of the second conference on steroids and cancer, p 116. American Medical Association, Chicago, 1951.

Kohorn, E. I.: Gestagens and endometrial carcinoma. Gynecol. Oncol., *4:* 398, 1976.

Larson, J. A.: Estrogens and endometrial cancer. Obstet. Gynecol. *3:* 551, 1954.

Lewis, G. C., Jr., Mortel, R., and Slack, N. H.: Endometrial cancer. Cancer, *39:* 959, 1977.

Lewis, B., Stallworthy, J. A., and Cowdell, R.: Adenocarcinoma of the body of the uterus. J. Obstet. Gynaecol. Br. Commonw., *77:* 343, 1970.

Liggins, G. C., and Way, S.: A comparison of adenoacanthoma and adenocarcinoma of the corpus uteri. J. Obstet. Gynaecol. Br. Commonw., *67:* 294, 1960.

Lucas, W. E.: Causal relationships between endocrine-metabolic variables in patients with endometrial carcinoma. Obstet. Gynecol. Surv., *29:* 507, 1974.

Mack, T. M., et al.: Estrogens and endometrial cancer in a retirement community. N. Engl. J. Med., *294:* 1262, 1976.

Mahle, A.: The morphological histology of adenocarcimona of the body of the uterus in relation to longevity. Surg. Gynecol. Obstet. *36:* 385, 1923.

Marcus, S. C.: Adenoacanthoma of the endometrium: a report of 24 cases and a review of squamous metaplasia. Am. J. Obstet. Gynecol., *81:* 259, 1961.

McBride, J. M.: Premenopausal cystic hyperplasia and endometrial hyperplasia. J. Obstet. Gynaecol. Br. Comm., *66:* 288, 1959.

McCarroll, A. M., et al.: Endometrial carcinoma after cyclical oestrogen-progestogen therapy for Turner's syndrome. Br. J. Obstet. Gynaecol., *82:* 421, 1975.

McDonald, T. W., et al.: Exogenous estrogen and endometrial carcinoma: Case-control and incidence study. Am. J. Obstet. Gynecol., *127:* 572, 1977.

McLennan, C.: Results of various types of treatment in adenocarcinoma of the endometrium. Am. J. Obstet. Gynecol., *50:* 254, 1945.

Morrow, C. P., DiSaia, P. J., and Townsend, D. E.: Current management of endometrial carcinoma. Obstet. Gynecol., *42:* 399, 1973.

Ng, A. B. P., and Reagan, J. W.: Incidence and prognosis of endometrial carcinoma by histological grade and extent. Obstet. Gynecol., *35:* 437, 1970.

Ng, A. B. P., Reagan, J. W., Storaasli, J. P., Wentz, W. B.: Mixed adenosquamous carcinoma of the endometrium. Am. J. Clin. Pathol., *59:* 765, 1973.

Piver, M. S., et al.: A prospective trial comparing hysterectomy, hysterectomy plus vaginal radium, and uterine radium plus hysterectomy in stage I endometrial carcinoma. Obstet. Gynecol., *54:* 85, 1979.

Pollow, K., Schmidt-Gollwitzer, M., and Nevinny-Stickel, J.: *Progesterone Receptors in Normal Human Endometrium Car-* *cinoma,* edited by W. L. McGuire, et al., p. 313, Raven Press, New York, 1977.

Reifenstein, E. C., Jr.: The treatment of advanced endometrial cancer with hydroxyprogesterone caproate. Gynecol. Oncol., *2:* 377, 1974.

Roberts, G., and Wells, A. L.: Oestrogen-induced endometrial carcinoma in a patient with gonadal dysgenesis. Br. J. Obstet. Gynaecol., *82:* 417, 1975.

Rosenwaks, Z., et al.: Endometrial pathology and estrogens. Obstet. Gynecol., *53:* 403, 1979.

Salazar, O. M., et al.: Adenosquamous carcinoma of the endometrium. Cancer, *40:* 119, 1977.

Schwartz, A. E., and Brunschwig, A.: Radical panhysterectomy and pelvic node excision for carcinoma of corpus uteri. Surg. Gynecol. Obstet., *105:* 675, 1957.

Sherman, A. I., and Brown, S.: The precursors of endometrial carcinoma. Am. J. Obstet. Gynecol., *134:* 947, 1979.

Siiteri, P. K., and MacDonald, P. C.: Role of extraglandular estrogen in human endocrinology. In *Handbook of Physiology—Endocrinology II,* Part 1. Ch. 28, p. 615.

Silverberg, S. G., Bolin, M. G., and De Giorgi, L. S.: Adenoacanthoma and mixed adenosquamous carcinoma of the endometrium. Cancer, *30:* 1307, 1972.

Silverberg, S. G., Makowski, E. L., and Roche, W. D.: Endometrial carcinoma in women under 40 years of age. Cancer, *39:* 592, 1977.

Smith, G. V. W., Johnson, L. C., and Hertig, A. T.: Relation of ovarian stromal hyperplasia and thecoma of the ovary to endometrial hyperplasia and carcinoma. N. Engl. J. Med., *226:* 365, 1942.

Smith, D. C., et al.: Association of exogenous estrogen and endometrial carcinoma. N. Engl. J. Med., *293:* 1164, 1975.

Spanos, W. J., Jr., Fletcher, G. H., Wharton, J. T., and Gallages, H. S.: Patterns of pelvic recurrence in endometrial carcinoma. Gynecol. Oncol., *6:* 495, 1978.

Stallworthy, J. A.: Surgery of endometrial cancer in the Bonney tradition. Ann. R. Coll. Surg. Engl., *48:* 293, 1971.

Surwit, E. A., Fowler, W. C., Jr., and Rogoff, E. E.: Stage II carcinoma of the endometrium. Obstet. Gynecol., *52:* 97, 1978.

Thigpen, J. T., Buchsbaum, H. J., and Blessing, J. A.: Phase II trial of adriamycin in the treatment of advanced or recurrent endometrial carcinoma: A gynecologic oncology group study. Cancer Treat. Rep., *63:* 21, 1979.

Underwood, P. B. Jr., Finn, J. O., Keene, W., and Travis, E.: Adenocarcinoma of the endometrium. Gynecol. Oncol., *2:* 71, 1974.

Underwood, P. B., Miller, M. C., Kreutner, A., Joyner, C. A., and Lutz, M. H.: Endometrial carcinoma: the effect of estrogens. Gynecol. Oncol., *8:* 60, 1979.

Vellios, F.: Endometrial hyperplasias, precursors of endometrial carcinoma. In Pathology Annual, edited by S. C. Sommers, Appleton-Century, Crofts, New York, 1972.

Weiss, N. S., Szekely, D. R., and Austin, D. F.: Increasing incidence of endometrial cancer in the United States. N. Engl. J. Med., *294:* 1259, 1976.

Welch, W. R., and Scully, R. E.: Precancerous lesions of the endometrium. Hum. Pathol., *8:* 503, 1977.

Young, P. C., Ehrlich, C. E., and Cleary, R. E.: Progesterone binding in human endometrial carcinomas. Am. J. Obstet. Gynecol., *125:* 353, 1976.

Ziel, H. K., and Finkle, W. D.: Increased risk of endometrial carcinoma among users of conjugated estrogen. N. Engl. J. Med., *293:* 1167, 1975.

CHAPTER 16

Myoma of the Uterus

GENERAL CHARACTERISTICS

By far the most common tumor of the uterus is the myoma. It is estimated that fully 20% of all women over 35 years of age harbor uterine *myomas*, although frequently without symptoms. For unknown reasons the incidence of myoma is much higher in the black than in the white race, epecially between the ages of 30 and 45, although Barber and Graber note a case in an 11-year-old female. New tumors rarely develop after the menopause, and already existing growths diminish in size, although they do not always disappear. Postmenopausal increase in sze is almost always indicative of secondary degeneration and should lead to the suspicion of sarcomatous change.

Myomas are frequently spoken of as *fibroids* but are of smooth muscle cell origin and not derived from fibrous tissue elements.

Myomas of the uterus may be single or, more frequently, multiple. They may be microscopic or of mammoth proportions, weighing over 100 pounds. They are of dense structure, well encapsulated and form small or large nodules which can be peeled out from the surrounding muscular wall of the uterus. On cutting into such a tumor its surface is seen to be of a glistening white color, with a characteristic whorl-like trabeculation so that it stands out in sharp contrast to the surrounding muscularis.

LOCATION

The location of the tumors may be *cervical* or *corporeal*, the former being much less common. When they reach very large size they impinge on the bladder and may bring about urinary retention through blockage of the urethra. Such large cervical tumors not infrequently become impacted in the pelvic cavity, and the technical difficulty in their removal is apt to be much greater than with the more movable tumors of the corpus uteri.

TYPES

From the standpoint of their position as regards the various layers of the uterine wall, myomas are divisible into three groups (Fig. 16.1).

Submucous tumors, developing just beneath the endometrium, push the latter before them as they grow. They constitute about 5% of all myomas, but are much more likely than either of the other varieties to cause profuse bleeding and to require hysterectomy, even though small. Their presence can usually be detected by feeling the curette "bump" over the protruding surface, although they are generally too firmly embedded to be removed by the curette. The hazard of sarcomatous degeneration is likewise greater with this group. The covering mucous membrane becomes thin, atrophic, and ulcerated.

Although some submucous tumors, even of large size, are sessile, others become pedunculated as a result of the expulsive action of the uterine muscle and may protrude from the cervix (Fig. 16.2) or even from the vagina. The surface of these *pedunculated submucous* tumors frequently becomes ulcerated, infected, and even infarcted.

Interstitial or *intramural* myomas are situated in the muscular wall, with no close propinquity to either the mucosa or serosa. When large or multiple, they cause marked uterine enlargement and a nodular contour and consistency.

Subserous or *subperitoneal* tumors, like the submucous, may be sessile or pedunculated. On occasion, large veins overlying the surface

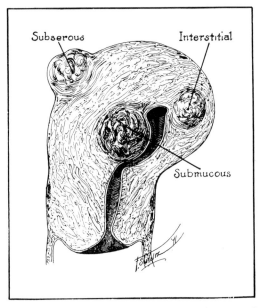

Figure 16.1. Sketch showing the various types of myomata.

of the fibroid may rupture with massive intraperitoneal bleeding; Saidi and associates have tabulated 26 cases, a few of which have occurred during pregnancy. Often subserous tumors grow out between the folds of the broad ligament (*intraligamentary*), even impinging on the ureter and iliac vessels and sometimes giving rise to difficult problems in diagnosis and operative treatment.

In some such cases the tumor receives more and more blood supply from the omental vessels and less and less from the uterine vessels. Gradually the tumor may be weaned away from the uterus entirely, the pedicle becoming thinner and thinner and finally disappearing. Such *parasitic* myomas are rare but may present interesting diagnostic problems.

MICROSCOPIC STRUCTURE

The characteristic histological picture of myoma is that of spindle muscle cells arranged in an interlacing or whorl-like pattern (Fig. 16.3). The cells are uniform in size, if one makes allowance for the different angles at which they are cut, and there is a variable

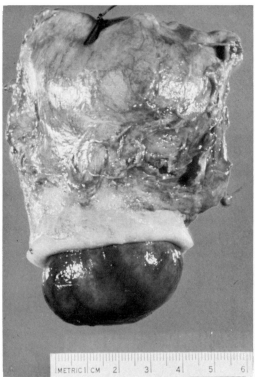
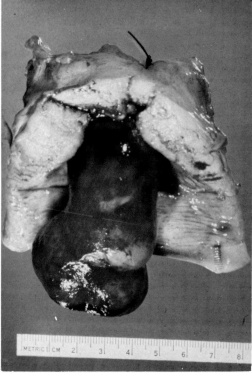

Figure 16.2. *Left,* large infarcted submucous myoma protruding through and distending cervix. *Right,* opened uterus. Thick sessile base would have made vaginal removal difficult.

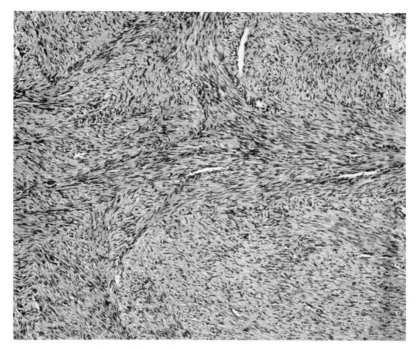

Figure 16.3.   Microscopic appearance of myoma.

amount of connective tissue. There is no definite capsule about the myomatous elements, but they are usually sharply marked off from the surrounding uterine musculature by a pseudocapsule of light areolar tissue."Mast cells," presumably containing heparin, are often present in the myometrium and should not be interpreted as neoplastic or giant cells (Fox and Abell).

UNUSUAL VARIANTS OF APPARENTLY BENIGN MYOMAS

Intravenous Leiomyomatosis

This represents a most unusual variant of benign myomas. It is manifest pathologically by polypoid extension of benign smooth muscle tumor into the pelvic veins. These are most commonly in close proximity to the uterus, with the frequency of venous involvement decreasing with increasing distance from this organ. It has been suggested that the tumors arise in situ from the smooth muscle wall of the uterine veins, but some believe that the tumors emanate from adjacent myomas. The fact that the lesions can be seen arising from the vein walls with no association with adjacent tumor support the former view. It is, however, most unusual to

see this situation in the absence of myomata uteri. Harper and Scully note the difficulty in distinguishing this from certain malignant processes such a (endometrial) sarcoma or stromatosis. It is, however, a benign abnormality that does not produce metastases. The only deaths are related to venous embolization.

Leiomyomatosis Peritonealis Disseminata

In 1965 Taubert et al. reported three cases of this very rare pathologic entity and referred to several other cases in the literature that met their diagnostic criteria. As the name implies, multiple histologically benign myomas are found to involve subperitoneal surfaces (Fig. 16.4). Goldberg et al., in 1976, reported a new case and added seven others from the world literature. Five of the eight women involved were either pregnant at the time of diagnosis or postpartum. The association with pregnancy has led some investigators to presume that this particular myoma represents fibrosis of a decidual reaction throughout the peritoneal cavity. Electron microscopic studies by Goldberg and his group strongly suggest that these are of smooth muscle origin. All cases have oc-

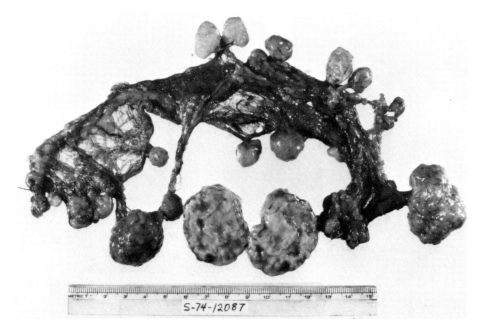

Figure 16.4. Leiomyomatosis peritonealis diseminata. Multiple omental lesions. (Courtesy of M. F. Goldberg.)

curred in females in the reproductive age group and estrogen dependency is intimated by the fact that regression has been noted following castration.

Benign Metastasizing Myomas

This nomenclature is used to describe a curious and rare situation characterized pathologically by metastatic lesions that appear microscopically to represent benign smooth muscle tumors. It is felt by many that this condition is related to intravenous leiomyomatosis. Although microscopically benign, it is generally felt that this myoma is a variant to low-grade leiomyosarcoma.

SECONDARY CHANGES IN MYOMA

Hyaline Degeneration

This, the most common of all secondary changes, is seen to some degree in almost all myomas, except those of very tiny size. The hyaline change may involve broad areas of the tumor, or it may occur in long intercommunicating strands and columns which appear to tease apart the muscle bundles (Fig. 16.5). Whether the so-called "plexiform tumorlet," as noted by Larbig et al., Buddinger and Greene, and most recently Patchevsky,

is a tumor of stromal origin or a form of hyaline degeneration seem uncertain.

Cystic Degeneration

The tendency of hyaline degeneration is toward liquefaction, and in extreme cases practically all of the original tumor is thus involved, being converted into a large cystic cavity. The clinical impression may thus simulate pregnancy or an ovarian cyst. Extreme edema and engorgement of the lymphatics may occur and simulate a lymphangiomatous pattern (Fig. 16.6).

Calcification

This is especially likely to occur where there is some circulatory disturbance, as in the myomas of old women. Where extreme, the myoma may be converted into a hard, stony mass, the "wombstone" of the older writers. Preoperative flat plate may reveal multiple foci of calcium deposits (Fig. 16.7).

Infection and Suppuration

This is most common in the submucous variety of myoma, which is so prone to thinning and ulceration of the overlying mucosa, thus giving access to organisms from the uterine canal.

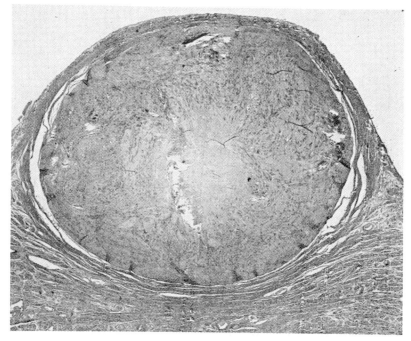

Figure 16.5. Hyaline change in small myoma.

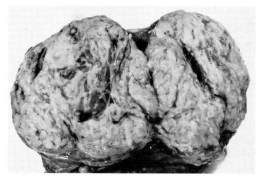

Figure 16.6. Extensive degeneration with early cystic changes.

Necrosis

This is commonly due to impairment of the blood supply or to severe infection. Pedunculated tumors may become necrotic through torsion of the pedicle. An interesting form of necrosis is the so-called *carneous* or *red degeneration*, seen most often but not always in association with pregnancy. Its cause is not definitely known, although many believe it to be explained by an aseptic degeneration associated with hemolysis or local tissue ischemia (Fig. 16.8).

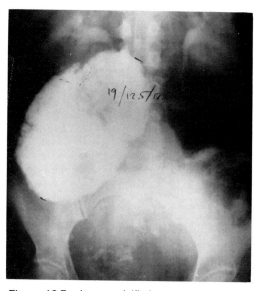

Figure 16.7. Large calcified myomatous tumor as visualized by intravenous pyelogram.

Fatty Degeneration

This is rare, but may occur with advanced hyaline degeneration. In other cases, large areas of genuine fat in the substance of a

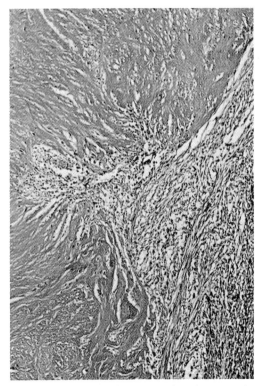

Figure 16.8. Margin of myoma undergoing necrosis.

more or less antiestrogenic and antitumorigenic. Their growth, however, is somewhat estrogen-dependent. They do not appear until menarche and usually diminish in size after menopause. With the use of estrogen-containing birth control pills in the last decade and a half, we have learned that myomas can suddenly increase in size while the patient is taking these medications. Therefore, replacement therapy by estrogen in the postmenopausal individual with known myomata should warrant due consideration. On occasion myomata will grow after the menopause. When this occurs, the possibility of sarcomatous change must be considered. We now know that, even in the absence of exogenous estrogen, peripheral conversion of androgen to estrogen by adipose tissue can provide significant stimulation to growth.

SYMPTOMS AND PHYSICAL SIGNS

The presence of myoma does not necessarily produce any symptoms, and every practitioner knows that even large growths may be entirely symptomless.

Palpable Mass

In a considerable proportion of cases the patient is impelled to seek advice because she or her physician has noticed a lump in the lower abdomen or, in the case of large tumors, a general enlargement of the abdomen.

Bleeding

The main symptom characteristic of fibroids, though not always present, is excessive or prolonged menstruation. One must always be on the alert for an associated lesion, such as adenocarcinoma or polyp or a functional factor, for endometrial hyperplasia is frequently associated with myomata.

The mechanism by which myomata produce menorrhagia is still open to some dispute. Clearly, even in the absence of submucous myomas, the uterine cavity is significantly expanded by the tumors. Such an effect produces a markedly enlarged endometrial surface from which to bleed. Some authors suggest that veinous congestion of the endometrium is caused by intramural myomata whatever the cause, menorrhagia is the characteristic bleeding abnormality, and this is most profound when submucous tumors are present. Submucous myomas can give rise

myoma are probably due to the fact that the tumor is of mixed variety.

Sarcomatous Change

This important type of change is discussed in Chapter 18, "Sarcoma of the Uterus," but is so rare, as not to influence the usual management of myomata. Even less common is metastasis to a myoma by a distant malignancy noted by Banooni and associates.

ETIOLOGY AND HISTOGENESIS

Nothing definite is known of the etiology of uterine myomas, although it is established that they are of muscle histogenesis. Most investigators accept Meyer's view that the source is not from mature muscle elements but from immature cells.

Evidence for a possible role of the ovarian hormones in the causation of uterine myoma is far from convincing. No explanation has been suggested as to why they occur in some women and not in others, since estrogen is produced in practically all women. Furthermore, a good many women with myomas ovulate, producing progesterone, supposedly to intermenstrual bleeding as well as menorrhagia but it is dangerous to assume that this variety of bleeding is due to the myomas unless other causes have been ruled out by adequate endometrial sampling. Subserous growths do not ordinarily produce abnormal bleeding.

Pain

Pain is not a characteristic symptom of myoma, although it is often present. Concomitant pelvic inflammatory disease or endometriosis, as well as various genitourinary or gastrointestinal causes of pain, must be considered. The most frequent form seen with the larger tumors is a *sensation of weight* and *bearing-down or dysmenorrhea.*

Pressure Effects

The larger myomas impinge on the bladder, producing *irritability, increased frequency of urination*, and possibly *dysuria.* When impacted in the pelvis they may bring about *retention of urine* through blockage of the urethra. *Hydroureteronephrosis* may ensue, along with a real possibility of damage to the urinary tract at operation. The pressure effects upon the rectum are less conspicuous, although *constipation* and occasionally *pain on defecation* may be produced. Very large growths into the upper abdomen may produce *digestive disturbances*, and in extreme cases pressure upon the vena cava or iliac veins may even cause *edema* of the lower extremities.

MYOMA AND PREGNANCY

There is a considerable difference of opinion as to the role of myoma in the production of infertility. No one would doubt that even very large myomata are perfectly compatible with uncomplicated pregnancy and normal delivery. On the other hand, most students, such as the late Isodore Rubin, feel strongly that fibroids may on occasion be a factor in impairing fertility and consequently mandate myomectomy, *after other causes for sterility are excluded.*

The incidence of pregnancy following myomectomy is 40–50% according to Babaknia, et al., far higher than nonoperated sterile women might achieve, even after prolonged exposure to pregnancy. The size, number, and location of fibroids in relation to the cornua and endometrial cavities are obvious variables so that no guarantee can be given to any woman in whom myomectomy is contemplated. Ingersoll summarizes the indications for and results with myomectomy.

A patient should never be promised myomectomy before operation; the surgeon may find it desirable or even necessary to remove the uterus, because of excessive bleeding. The careful clinician will assure the woman that he is cognizant of her wishes and will do his best to abide by them, but the ultimate decision must be his. He should likewise point out that myomectomy will not assure pregnancy, and there is a definite possibility, 25–35% (Brown, A. L., et al., and Brown, J. M., et al.) that subsequent hysterectomy may be required. If, however, within that interim a pregnancy or two should intervene, most women will gladly accept a second operation. In addition to producing infertility, myomas may be a factor in causing a disproportinately high incidence of abortion, generally in the first trimester.

In the *second trimester* pain and tenderness may occur in a previously asymptomatic myoma, with fever, leukocytosis, and development of a surgically acute abdomen. This is generally due to *carneous (red) degeneration*, a curious phenomenon of pregnancy which is probably related to impaired or inadequate circulation in the fibroid, although other degenerative changes or causes of an acute abdomen must be considered. Should expectant conservative treatment not avail, exploration with myomectomy is reluctantly carried out. Curiously enough, most of these surgically treated women do not go into labor or bleed, and such bland behavior may occur even when the uterine cavity is entered. Nevertheless, many obstetricians will give large doses of prophylactic progesterone. Similarly, many will later elect cesarean section, although it is our own opinion that myomectomy itself would not always contraindicate delivery from below.

In the *third trimester* and at delivery a fibroid may cause premature bleeding, uterine inertia, or mechanical blockage to normal passage through the birth canal. Postpartum hemorrhage due to an atonic uterus and infection of the endometrium and adjacent myoma is more common after vaginal delivery. Cesarean section with hysterectomy is performed frequently these days and is probably easier and preferable to multiple myomectomy when procreative desires are complete. Total hysterectomy immediately following cesarean section is generally simple for the well trained gynecologist. Although the tissues are quite vascular, planes of cleavage are extraordinarily good. At operation the cervix is so soft that it is difficult to feel within the vagina; if a subtotal hysterectomy is first accomplished, the operator's finger can then be placed down into the endocervical canal, allowing for easy identification and removal of the cervix.

The clinician should recall, however, that small myomas may increase remarkably in size during the course of pregnancy and yet regress when it is terminated. Whether this is due to an increased hormonal stimulus or simply to a better blood supply is uncertain, although the latter seems likely. Full consideration of the temporary but evanescent growth of fibroids should precede any final decision to perform hysterectomy at the time of cesarean section.

PHYSICAL SIGNS

Abdominal Palpation

In some cases a presumptive diagnosis of uterine myoma can be made by palpating the tumor through the abdominal wall, especially when the latter is not too obese. Such tumors are hard, generally of irregular nodular contour, movable unless so large that they fill most of the abdomen, and not tender.

Bimanual Pelvic Examination

In many cases the diagnosis of myoma is extremely easy, especially when bowel and bladder are empty. One or more nodular outgrowths on the uterine surface can be felt between the examining fingers within the vagina and the external hand. The problem, however, is not always so simple, and examination under anesthesia is occasionally necessary. In obese or highly nervous women, where the uterus is hard to outline, it may be difficult to determine whether a firm globular mass felt behind the cervix is a myoma of the posterior wall or merely a rather large retroflexed fundus. Again, when a firm, solid mass is felt laterally, it is not always easy to decide between a pedunculated subserous myoma and a solid tumor of the ovary. Adnexal masses, either inflammatory or neoplastic,

may be so firmly adherent to the uterus that they may simulate uterine myoma. When there is any question that the intrapelvic tumor is ovarian rather than uterine in origin, laparascopy or, if necessary, laparotomy should be performed because of the dismal nature of many ovarian lesions.

One of the most important diagnostic problems presented to the gynecologist is to differentiate between myoma and early pregnancy, or to decide whether or not pregnancy exists in an obviously myomatous uterus. Nowadays the problem has been much simplified because of the accuracy of even early "quick" pregnancy tests, and it is desirable to obtain such tests whenever there is any suspicion of pregnancy. However, even the most astute clinician may on rare occasion find that a presumed "pelvic tumor" will be a pregnant uterus. Sonograms may be of considerable assistance.

The submucous variety of myoma presents special difficulties in diagnosis; being concealed within the uterus, they may show no appreciable enlargement or irregularity. In such cases *diagnostic curettage* is indicated in an effort to determine the cause of the patient's bleeding, which may be due to any one of a number of causes, such as submucous myoma, incomplete abortion, polyp, adenocarcinoma, or a functional factor. The diagnosis is often made by noting the curette to "bump over" a protruding intracavitary nodule which is too firmly embedded to be removed, unlike the usual polyp. The use of hysteroscopy or hysterograms may be useful.

TREATMENT

Expectant Treatment with Periodic Examination

Not all myomas call for surgery, but since they all present some potentiality for subsequent problems, an expectant plan of treatment should always be combined with the advice that periodic examination be sought at regular 6-month intervals. When menstrual function ceases, a myoma rarely causes difficulty, often involuting. Thus, in the immediately premenopausal woman, simple observation is all the treatment that an only slightly symptomatic myoma warrants. In every case, age, procreative desires, the likelihood of an incipient menopause, etc. should be factors to consider, even when symptoms suggest surgery.

We feel it unwise, however, to allow even an asymptomatic myoma to grow larger than a 12- to 14-week pregnancy, particularly when the woman is young and the tumor has a long time to grow, or when there is evidence of rapid growth. Very large myomas can be difficult surgical problems, and when ultimate hysterectomy seems inevitable, it is best performed before the possibility of operative complications is increased.

In the postmenopausal era, a myomatous uterus is rarely symptomatic. However, any postclimacteric growth of a myoma suggests either sarcomatous change or the possibility that the supposed uterine tumor is really ovarian. In either case exploration is indicated.

Surgical Treatment

Myomectomy has its great field in the removal of tumors in cases where the preservation of reproductiveness is of importance. However, there are disadvantages to be considered, such as subsequent tumor formation. Lock has summarized the indications and techniques of myomectomy. Myomectomy should always be preceded by diagnostic curettage if there has been abnormal bleeding, as the latter may be due to an intrauterine lesion, like adenocarcinoma, and not to the myoma.

On the other hand, in the presence of large and numerous myomatous nodules, the chances for the patient to bear children are so slight, and the risks of subsequent trouble so real, that hysterectomy is unquestionably the wiser procedure. When hysterectomy is performed upon younger women, there is no question as to the advisability of leaving one or both ovaries. In discussing pathology found in postsurgical preserved ovaries, Randall et al. indicate that there is a certain risk of subsequent neoplasm, but conservation of ovarian tissue is worth the risk.

References and Additional Readings

Abithol, M. M.: Submucous fibroids complicating pregnancy labor, and delivery. Obstet. Gynecol., *10:* 529, 1957.
Ariel, I. M., and Trinidad, S.: Pulmonary metastases from a uterine "leiomyoma." Am. J. Obstet. Gynecol., *94:* 110, 1966.
Babaknia, A., Rock, J. A. and Jones, H. W. Jr.: Pregnancy success following abnormal myomectomy for infertility. Fertil. Steril. *30:* 644, 1978.
Banooni, F., Labes, J., and Goodman, P. A.: Uterine leiomyoma containing metastatic breast carcinoma. Am. J. Obs. Gynecol., *111:* 427, 1971.
Barber, J. R. K., and Graber, E. A.: Gynecological tumors in childhood and adolescence. Obstet. Gynecol. Surv. *28:* 357, 1973.
Boyce, C. R., and Buddhev, H. N.: Pregnancy complicated by metastasizing leiomyoma. Obstet. Gynecol., *42:* 252, 1973.
Brown, A. L., Chamberlain, R. W., and TeLinde, R. W.: Myomectomy, Amer. J. Obstet. Gynec., *71:* 759, 1956.
Brown, J. M., Malkasian, G. D., and Symmonds, R. E.: Abdominal myomectomy. Amer. J. Obstet. Gynec., *99:* 126, 1967.
Buddinger, J. M., and Greene, R. R.: A distinctive myometrial tumor of undetermined origin. Cancer, *17:* 1155, 1964.
Edwards, D. L., and Peacock, J. F.: Intravenous leiomyomatosis of the uterus. Obstet. Gynecol., *27:* 176, 1966.
Everett, H. S.: Effect of uterine myomas on the urinary tract. Clin. Obstet. Gynecol., *1:* 429, 1958.
Farrer-Brown, G., Beilby, J. O. W., and Tarbit, M. H.: Vascular patterns in myomatous uteri. J. Obstet. Gynaecol. Br. Comm., *77:* 917, 1970; Venous changes in the endometrium of myomatous uteri. Obstet. Gynecol. *38:* 743, 1971.
Fox, J. E., and Abell, M. R.: Mast cells in uterine myometrium and leiomyomatous neoplasms. Am. J. Obstet. Gynecol., *91:* 413, 1965.
Faulkner, R. L.: Red degeneration of myomas. Am. J. Obstet. Gynecol., *53:* 474, 1947.
Gerbie, A. B., Greene, R. R., and Reis, R. A.: Heteroplastic bone and cartilage in the female genital tract. Obstet. Gynecol., *11:* 573, 1958.
Goldberg, M. F., Hurt, W. G., and Feable, W. J.: Leiomyomatosis peritonealis disseminata. Obstet. Gynecol., *49:* (Suppl.) 46S, 1977.
Harper, R. S., and Scully, R. E.: Intravenous leiomyomatosis of the uterus. Obstet. Gynec. *18:* 519, 1961.
Ingersoll, F. M.: Myomectomy and fertility. Fer. Steril., *14:* 596, 1963.
Kelly, H. A., and Cullen, T. S.: *Myomata of the Uterus.* W. B. Saunders Co., Philadelphia, 1909.
Larbig, C. G., et al.: Plexiform tumorlets of endometrial stromal origin. Am. J. Clin. Pathol., *44:* 32, 1965.
Lardaro., H. H.: Extensive myomectomy. Am. J. Obstet. Gynecol., *79:* 43, 1960.
Lock, F. R.: Multiple myomectomy. Am. J. Obstet. Gynecol., *104:* 642, 1969.
Meyer, R.: Die pathologische Anatomie der Gerbarmutter. In Handbuch der spezielle pathologische Anatomie und Histologie, edited by F. Henke and O. Lubarsch, Vol. 7, Part 1, Julius Springer, Berlin, 1930.
Novak, E. R.: Benign and malignant changes in uterine myomas. Clin. Obstet. Gynecol., *1:* 421, 1958.
Patchevsky, A. S.: Plexiform tumorlet of the uterus. Obstet. Gynecol. *35:* 592, 1970.
Puukka, M. J., Kontula, K. K., Kauppila, A. J., Janne, O. A., and Vihko, R. K.: Mol. Cell. Endocrinol., *6:* 35, 1976.
Randall, C. L., Hall, D. W., and Armenia, C. S.: Pathology in the preserved ovary after unilateral oophorectomy. Am. J. Obstet. Gynecol., *84:* 1233, 1962.
Rubin, I. C.: Uterine fibromyomas and sterility. Clin. Obstet. Gynecol., *1:* 501, 1958.
Saidi, F., Constable, J. D., and Ulfelder, H.: Massive intraperitoneal hemorrhage due to uterine fibroids. Am. J. Obstet. Gynecol., *82:* 367, 1961.
Sampson, J. A.: Blood supply of uterine myomata. Surg. Gynecol., *14:* 215, 1912.
Schwartz, O.: Benign diffuse enlargement of the uterus. Am. J. Obstet. Gynecol., *61:* 902, 1951.
Stearns, H. C., and Sneeden, V. D.: Observations on the clinical and pathological aspects of the pelvic congestion syndrome. Am. J. Obstet. Gynecol., *94:* 718, 1966.
Steiner, P. R.: Metastasizing fibroleiomyoma of the uterus. Am. J. Pathol., *15:* 89, 1939.
Taubert, H. D., Wissner, S. E., and Haskins, A. L.: Leiomyomatosis peritonealis disseminata. Obstet. Gynecol., *25:* 561, 1965.
Wright, C. J. E.: Solitary malignant lymphoma of the uterus. Am. J. Obstet. Gynecol., *117:* 114, 1973.

CHAPTER 17

Adenomyosis of the Uterus

Adenomyosis of the uterus is characterized by histologically benign invasion of the uterine musculature by the endometrium, which normally is found lining only the uterine cavity. There are many points of similarity between adenomyosis and pelvic endometriosis, although adenomyosis characteristically affects the 40-year-old, parous woman, and endometriosis the younger infertile patient. In both, however, there is ectopic growth of endometrial tissue. For that matter, adenomyosis was at one time spoken of as *endometriosis interna*, to distinguish it from *endometriosis externa* or pelvic endometriosis.

With adenomyosis of the uterus we apparently deal with an exaggerated growth activity of the endometrium, which pushes down into the underlying muscle. With this endometrial invasion is combined a marked, generalized overgrowth of the muscle elements.

Incidence

Bird et al. record a 61.5% incidence of adenomyosis in 200 consecutive hysterectomies, an excessive figure compared to such studies as those of Molitor (8.8%). However, nearly one-half of Bird's cases occurred less than one low power field below the basal endometrium; even if these are deleted, the resultant figure of 38.5% seems much greater than the incidence usually quoted in the literature (10–20%).

Pathology

The enlargement of the uterus produced by adenomyosis is diffuse and not nodular, as in the case of myoma. There is often enormous thickening of the uterine wall, usually asymmetrical, the posterior wall usually being more extensively involved than the anterior

(Fig. 17.1). Never, however, does the uterus reach the large proportions seen in many cases of myoma, rarely being larger than a grapefruit. It should not be forgotten, however, that myoma and adenomyosis often coexist.

The distinctive *microscopic* characteristic is the presence of islands of typical endometrial tissue scattered throughout the muscle, often far beneath the endometrial surface, and sometimes extending to the peritoneal surface. The endometrial glands in the ectopic tissue are surrounded by typical endometrial stromal cells. Occasionally the endometrium is of *functioning type*, menstruating just as does the normal surface endometrium. In such cases collections of chocolate-colored menstrual blood are seen throughout the wall, constituting miniature uterine cavities (Fig. 17.2).

More frequently the endometrium is of the immature, *nonfunctioning type*, often presenting a typical Swiss-cheese hyperplasia pattern. When the endometrium penetrates to the peritoneum, it may continue to propagate itself, sometimes producing extensive pelvic endometriosis. In such cases, the uterus is often densely adherent to the rectum and other surrounding organs. The muscle tissue shows marked hyperplasia, with a whorl-like tendency not unlike that seen in myoma. Pregnancy may bring about decidual changes (Fig. 17.3) in the invading endometrium quite like those noted in the uterine mucosa proper.

Sandberg and Cohn have indicated that superficial adenomyosis rarely shows decidual changes, whereas this is relatively frequent in the more extreme degrees of myometrial invasion. The most logical explanation is that continued growth has allowed the aberrant endometrium to mature and achieve

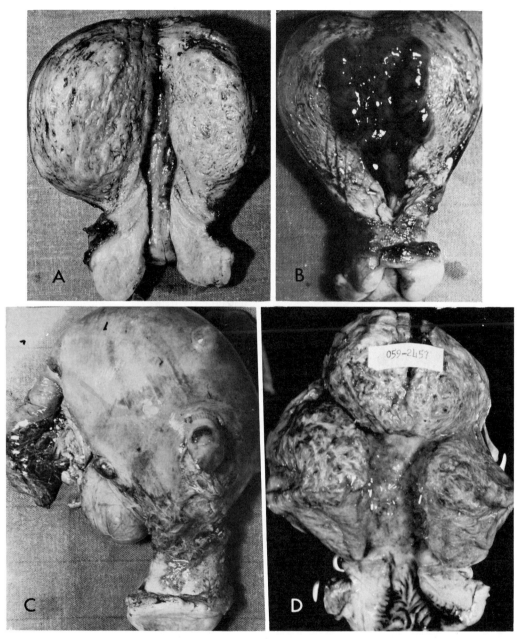

Figure 17.1.   *A*, extensive adenomyosis of posterior wall. *B*, marked endometrial hyperplasia with large uterus, although no significant adenomyosis. *C*, adenomyosis and myomas. *D*, extensive diffuse adenomyosis extending into cervix. (Courtesy of L. Emge: Elusive adenomyosis of the uterus. Am. J. Obstet. Gynecol., *83:* 1541, 1962, C. V. Mosby Co., Publishers.)

the faculty of progesterone response, and indeed this is one of several possibilities noted by the authors.

It would thus seem that adenomyosis may be compared to an inverting polyp, composed of a mature responsive form of endometrium or more often an immature juvenile tissue completely incapable of response to progesterone. Hyperplasia in conjunction with a biphasic cycle is common, but *adenocarcinoma* developing in these aberrant islands has been reported on only a few occasions (Novak and Woodruff).

In any case, a frequent and difficult prob-

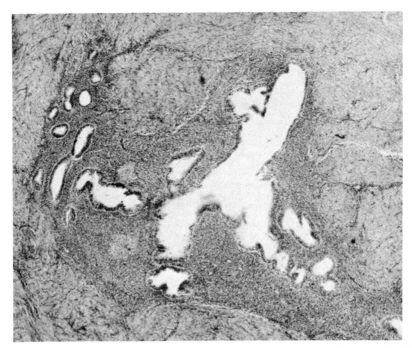

Figure 17.2. Microscopic appearance of adenomyosis in which the invading endometrium is of functioning (secretory) type.

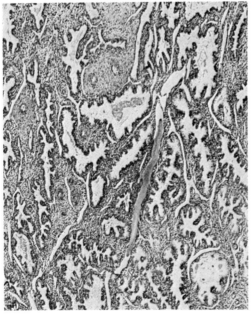

Figure 17.3. Decidual changes in adenomyosis associated with pregnancy.

lem to the pathologist is distinction between well differentiated endometrial adenocarcinoma with early invasion and superficial malignancy with associated adenomyosis. If, however, there is no observed evidence of direct invasion with reaction on the part of the invaded myometrium or if the ectopic endometrium is obviously better differentiated than the surface adenocarcinoma, it is probable that there is merely associated adenomyosis. The presence of benign stroma in conjunction with adenocarcinoma situated in the myometrium indicates the development of adenocarcinoma within adenomyosis. This does not have the same negative prognostic implications as does actual myometrial invasion.

The range of coassociations with other lesions is wide. In discussing the diagnostic approach to adenomyosis, Emge points out the suggestive importance of associated endometrial hyperplasia which is frequently but not inevitably found in conjunction with adenomyosis. Seemingly this is an estrogen-dependent disease process.

Histogenesis

The histogenesis of aberrant endometrium was formerly widely discussed, but it is now clearly established, as a result of the work of Cullen and others, that it has its source from downward growth of the surface endometrium. Histological studies often show direct continuity of the deep islands with the surface mucosa, although the overgrowth of muscle elements may nip off the connecting endometrial process. Endometrial islands should be noted at least one HPF (high-power field) below the level of the basal layer to warrant the diagnosis of *adenomyosis*.

Clinical Characteristics of Adenomyosis

The two most frequent symptoms are *menorrhagia* and *dysmenorrhea*, generally increasingly severe in the older (fifth decade) woman who has borne children. The former may be partly explained by the increased amount of endometrium, but is often due to the ovarian dysfunction so frequently associated. The dysmenorrhea is typically of colicky nature, due to the painful contractions of the uterine muscle induced by the menstrual swelling of the endometrial islands. When pelvic endometriosis is present, it often involves the uterosacral ligaments, and the menstrual swelling of the endometrium in the region produces *pain* referred to the rectum or the lower sacral region. Where endometriosis is present there may be some intermenstrual discomfort, but this is not nearly as characteristic as the menstrual symptoms.

Novak and De Lima indicated that pelvic endometriosis and adenomyosis coexist with relative frequency. Benson and Smeeden stated that pelvic endometriosis occurs in only 13% of cases of adenomyosis; he also added that surface endometrial hyperplasia is a rare accompaniment, which differs from Emge's findings and our own impressions.

Diagnosis

Although the diagnosis is not usually made until after pathological examination, there is a group of cases in which at least a strongly presumptive diagnosis can be made clinically. When one finds a moderately and diffusely enlarged uterus firmly fixed in the pelvis, with one or more small nodules palpable in the region of the uterosacral ligaments, and when these findings are combined with menorrhagia and a colicky dysmenorrhea referred to the rectum or lower sacral or coccygeal regions in a parous woman, there will be little doubt of the presence of adenomyosis, probably combined with endometriosis. In a proportion of cases, however, pelvic endometriosis does not coexist, and preoperative diagnosis is often not possible. A symmetrically enlarged uterus with the proved absence of pregnancy in a 40-year-old woman with increasing dysmenorrhea and menorrhagia should be highly suggestive of adenomyosis.

Treatment

Because, like myoma, this disease is usually dependent on continued ovarian function, minor symptoms in the premenopausal woman require only palliative treatment. Where symptoms are extreme, however, the proper treatment is surgical. Hysterectomy is indicated, the fate of the ovaries being decided on the basis of such factors as the age of the patient and the presence or absence of ovarian or general pelvic endometriosis.

Stromal Adenomyosis or Endometriosis (Stromatosis)

Hunter and Lattig have called attention to a form of adenomyosis in which the invading tissue is altogether stromal, with no gland elements, and which some clinicians designate as *stromatosis*, although a better designation would seem to be *stromal endometriosis* or *adenomyosis*. Although such stromal invasion occurs, it is relatively rare, and it should not be assumed unless the study of many sections demonstrates an actual absence of glands. Various authors speak of benign and malignant forms, but the latter is better looked upon as akin to a low-grade endometrial sarcoma (see Chapter 18, "Sarcoma of the Uterus").

Publications on the subject of this lesion, frequently referred to as *stromatosis*, have clarified many of its pathological and clinical characteristics, although its comparative rarity suggests the need for only a short discussion. It has been suggested that there are three categories of cases, with all intermediate gradations. (1) The simplest is identical with ordinary adenomyosis, except that the invading endometrium is made up entirely of stroma, with no glands. It is clinically entirely benign (Fig. 17.4). (2) In this group the endometrial stroma invades not only the musculature but may also exhibit endolymphatic and intravascular penetrativeness, growing in a rubbery, wormlike fashion into both lymphatics and veins (Figs. 17.4 and 17.5). It may thus become at least locally invasive, pushing into the broad ligaments, but it has no tendency to distant metastases. According to Henderson, cases of this kind can often be tem-

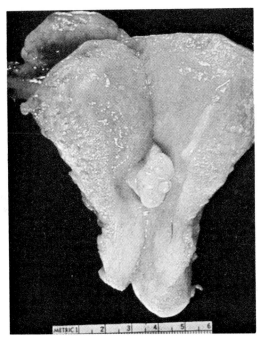
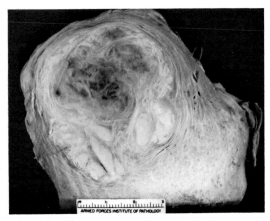

Figure 17.4. *Left,* benign stromatosis; compare lack of invasion with that shown in Figure 17.6. (Courtesy of Dr. D. Nichols, Buffalo, New York.) *Right,* cut surface of a uterus containing a stromal tumor with a pushing margin. Note the circumscription and lack of infiltration of myometrium at the periphery of the tumor. (Courtesy of H. J. Norris and H. B. Taylor: Mesenchymal tumors of the uterus. I. A clinical and pathological study of 53 endometrial stromal tumors. Cancer, *19:* 755, 1966.)

porarily cured even if the removal of tumor tissue is not altogether complete, although death may occur from local extension. (3) The definitely malignant group, speaking histologically, is also malignant clinically (Fig. 17.5). For this reason, we prefer to classify such cases as *endometrial sarcoma*, in spite of the fact that the morphological characteristics of the sarcoma cells are remindful of the stroma from which they arise. The histological differences between these three types are exceedingly tenuous, and there is considerable logic in accepting only benign stromatosis or a malignant type which is a low-grade variant of endometrial sarcoma.

Ideal initial therapy for patients with endolymphatic stromal myosis is total surgical excision of all grossly apparent tumor. Care should be taken to search for intravascular extension. Supracervical hysterectomy is inadequate surgical treatment for this disease because of frequent recurrence of the lesion in the cervical stump. The common finding of intravascular extension into the broad ligaments and adnexa and the occasional regression of widespread disease when the ovaries are removed indicate that bilateral adnexal extirpation is ideal. Exceptions to this can be

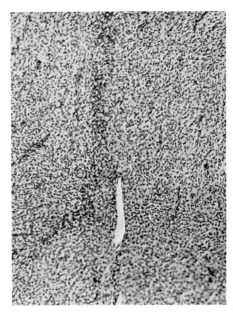

Figure 17.5. Stromal adenomyosis. The invading stroma in this case shows malignant characteristics.

made in young patients with disease confined to the uterus.

Among patients with extrauterine extension, there are occasional instances of retro-

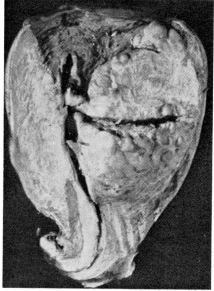
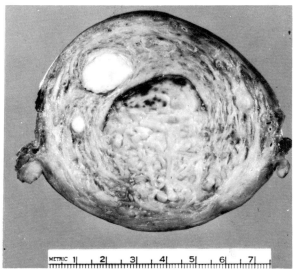

Figure 17.6. *Left,* gross appearance of uterus with malignant stromatosis; compare with benign stromatosis in Figure 17.4. (Courtesy of Harper Hospital, Detroit.) *Right,* cross section of a uterus containing a stromal tumor with infiltrating margins (endolymphatic stromal myosis). There is poor circumscription, and poorly defined extensions of the tumor bulge above the cut tumor, infiltrate the myometrium, and obliterate the endometrial cavity. (Courtesy of H. J. Norris, and H. B. Taylor: Mesenchymal tumors of the uterus. I. A clinical and pathological study of 53 endometrial stromal tumors. Cancer, *19:* 755, 1966.)

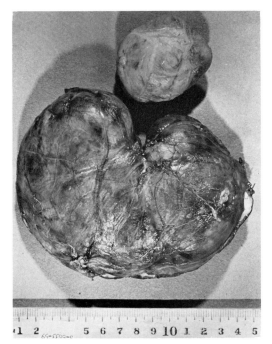

Figure 17.7. Intraligamentary hemangiopericytoma *(below)* with myoma. (Courtesy of Dr. Albert Brown, Wilmington, N. C.)

peritoneal ureteral compression. This may require ureteral diversion with ureteroneocystostomy. It is not uncommon for the surgeon to come upon this condition without prior knowledge of it, but, when this diagnosis is considered, intravenous pyelography is indicated.

Because of the low-grade nature of this neoplasm, reexploration with excision of recurrent disease is frequently fruitful in terms of prolonging survival and decreasing morbidity. At times the tumor clearly seems to be estrogen dependent, and anecdotal examples of response to progestational therapy have been reported.

Although these lesions arising from the endometrial stroma are not common, one would presume that some beneficial effects might be expected from progesterone therapy, as in the case of some endometrial cancers, and such cases have been described by Baggish and Woodruff.

Hemangiopericytoma

On occasion the pathologist may encounter difficulty in distinguishing between stromal endometriosis and *hemangiopericytoma,* a vascular lesion closely related to a glomus tumor (Fig. 17.7). Histologically, it is characterized by a concentric arrangement of pericytes around capillaries, but such special stains as Massons, silver, and reticulum are often necessary. Grossly one may find a tumor much like a vascular myoma, generally unlike the wormlike buds of stromatosis. Hemangiopericytoma is generally regarded as a low-grade (20 to 25%) malignant tumor.

References and Additional Readings

Baggish, M. S., and Woodruff, J. D.: Uterine stromatosis. Obstet. Gynecol., *40:* 487, 1972.

Bensen, R. C., and Smeeden, V. D.: Adenomyosis; a reappraisal of symptomatology. Am. J. Obstet. Gynecol. *76:* 1044, 1958.

Bird, C. C., McElin, T. W., and Menalo-Estrella, P.: The elusive adenomyosis of the uterus—revisited. Am. J. Obstet. Gynecol., *112:* 583, 1972.

Cope, E.: Adenocarcinoma of the endometrium with malignant stromatosis. J. Obstet. Gynaecol. Br. Commonw., *65:* 58, 1958.

Cullen, T. S.: *Adenomyoma of Uterus.* W. B. Saunders, Philadelphia, 1908.

Cullen, T. S.: Distribution of adenomyomata containing uterine mucosa. Arch. Surg., *1:* 215, 1920.

Emge, L. A.: Elusive adenomyosis of uterus; its historic past and its present state of recognition. Am. J. Obstet. Gynecol., *83:* 1541, 1962.

Goldfarb, S., Richart, R. M., and Ogaki, T.: Nuclear DNA content in endolymphatic stromal myosis. Am. J. Obstet. Gynecol., *106:* 524, 1970.

Green, R. R., Gerbie, A. B., and Eckman, T. R.: Hemangiopericytoma of the uterus. Am. J. Obstet. Gynecol., *106:* 1020, 1970.

Hart, R. H., and Yoomessi, M.: Endometrial stromatosis of the uterus. Obstet. Gynecol., *49:* 393, 1977.

Henderson, D. N.: Endolymphatic stromal myosis. Am. J. Obstet. Gynecol., *52:* 1000, 1946.

Hunter, W. C., and Lattig, G. J.: Stromal endometriosis and uterine adenomyosis. Am. J. Obstet. Gynecol., *75:* 258, 1958.

Kinshen, E. J., Nattolin, F., and Benirschke, K.: Uterine hemangiopericytoma in a 19-year-old girl. Obstet. Gynecol., *40:* 652, 1972.

Kistner, R. W.: Endometriosis and adenomyosis. In *Gynecology and Obstetrics,* edited by C. H. Davis, Vol. II, Ch. 43. Harper & Row, Hagerstown, Md., 1968.

Koss, L. G., Spiro, D. H., and Bronschwig, A.: Endometrial stromal sarcoma. Surg. Gynecol. Obstet., *121:* 531, 1965.

Kumar, D., and Anderson, W.: Malignancy in endometriosis interna. J. Obstet. Gynaecol. Br. Commonw., *65:* 435, 1958.

Molitor, J. J.: Adenomyosis. Am. J. Obstet. Gynecol., *110:* 275, 1971.

Norris, H. J., and Taylor, H. B., Jr.: Mesenchymal tumors of the uterus. I. A clinical and pathological study of 53 endometrial stromal tumors. Cancer, *19:* 755, 1966.

Norris, H. J., and Taylor, H. B., Jr.: Postirradiation sarcomas of the uterus. Obstet. Gynecol., *26:* 689, 1965.

Novak, E., and De Lima, O. A.: A correlative study of adenomyosis and pelvic endometriosis, with special reference to the hormonal reaction of ectopic endometrium. Am. J. Obstet. Gynecol., *56:* 634, 1958.

Novak, E. R., and Woodruff, J. D.: Postirradiation malignancy of the pelvic organs. Am. J. Obstet. Gynecol., *77:* 667, 1959.

Sandberg, E. C., and Cohn, F.: Adenomyosis in the gravid uterus at term. Am. J. Obstet. Gynecol., *84:* 1457, 1962.

Scott, R. B.: Adenomyosis and adenomyoma. Clin. Obstet. Gynecol., *1:* 413, 1958.

Stearns, H. C.: Study of stromal endometriosis. Am. J. Obstet. Gynecol., *75:* 603, 1958.

Stout, A. P.: Hemangiopericytoma. Cancer, *2:* 1027, 1949.

Winkelman, J., and Robinson, R.: Adenocarcinoma of endometrium involving adenomyosis. Cancer, *19:* 901, 1966.

CHAPTER 18

Sarcoma of the Uterus

Sarcoma of the uterus is far less common than carcinoma; however, any precise statistics are difficult to assemble, for many clinics designate as low-grade sarcomas what others might consider as merely cellular myomas. Obviously, this discrepancy affects not only salvage but also the incidence. Although uncommon, it is a rather serious lesion because of its tendency to spread via the blood stream, so that lung and liver metastases as well as local invasion are common.

CLASSIFICATION

It is now generally accepted that sarcoma of the uterus may arise from any of the connective tissue elements of the uterine structure and that it may be of myogenic origin as well. Thus, it may arise from the myometrium, endometrium, blood vessels, or a myoma. Whether any lesion should be categorized as a leiomyosarcoma (of smooth muscle origin) or fibromyosarcoma (of connective tissue variety) seems of purely academic interest as compared to whether it is malignant or benign.

Ober, among others, has attempted to classify sarcoma on a histogenetic basis, and he proposes the following scheme (which is presented here only in outline form):

(1) Leiomyosarcoma
(2) Mesenchymal sarcoma
    (a) Pure homologous as endometrial sarcoma
    (b) Pure heterologous as rhabdomyosarcoma
    (c) Mixed homologous as carcinosarcoma
    (d) Mixed heterologous as carcinosarcoma plus other heterologous elements
(3) Blood vessel sarcomas
(4) Lymphomas
(5) Unclassified
(6) Metastatic

There are numerous subclassifications which are not necessary for a simple workable means of dividing these lesions.

LEIOMYOSARCOMA

Although *leiomyosarcoma* is a very infrequent complication of myoma, in the nature of 0.2% or less (Montague et al.), the prevalence of myomata still makes this the most common form of uterine sarcoma. *Sudden accelerated growth* of a previously static tumor or *postmenopausal enlargement* will always suggest the possibility of sarcoma and will indicate surgery despite any symptoms.

If the tumor is cut open after its removal, one will find an absence of the symmetrically whorled white, firm, surface. Instead there is apt to be a softer, yellowish consistency or, when necrotic changes are marked, a more pultaceous appearance with cystic and hemorrhagic degeneration. Although this may represent merely degenerative phenomena, it should impel the surgeon to increase the scope of his operation, i.e., hysterectomy rather than myomectomy.

With reference to the much discussed question of the *incidence* of sarcomatous changes in myomas, the wide discrepancy of figures quoted suggests that there is incomplete uniformity in recognition of the histological criteria of malignancy. The most common error is to mistake very cellular but benign myomas for sarcomas.

Microscopic Pattern

At least two mitotic figures per high power field should be encountered before considering a diagnosis of sarcoma.

Mitotic activity (Fig. 18.1), giant cell formation, and increasing degrees of pleomorphism, are frequent in leiomyosarcoma and often offer a distinctive contrast to the orderly pattern of myoma from which the malignancy may have arisen. Nevertheless, it is not always easy to be sure whether or not sarcoma is secondary to benign myoma. The mere

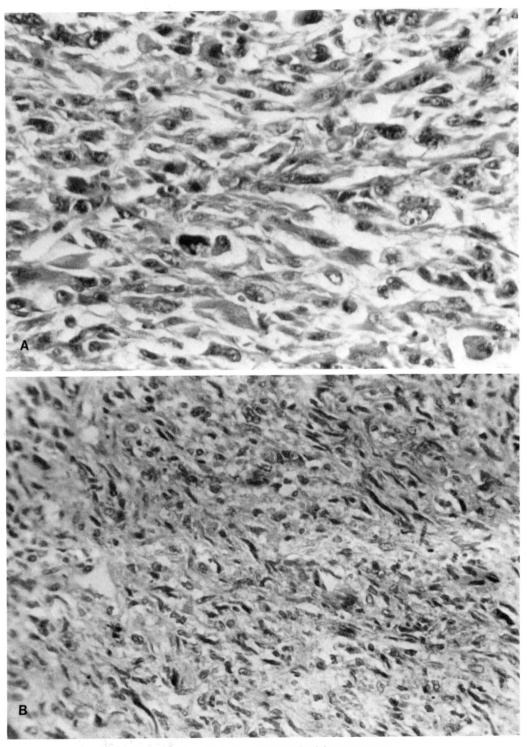

Figure 18.1.   *A* and *B*, representative leiomyosarcoma.

presence of myomas does not justify this assumption and, moreover, it must be remembered that sarcoma may arise as a rather nodular growth which might simulate a myoma. On the other hand, when a sarcoma is found developing in the interior of a myoma in which one can still find abundant evidence of the original benign tumor, the origin from such a tumor seems clear. In the late stages of the disease, however, such aids in determining the origin of the tumor are not available, and one can only speculate.

The incidence would seem less than 1% according to accrued statistics, but one must always be mindful of "what constitutes a sarcoma."

Such interpretation obviously dictates the salvage. The usual salvage lies in the 25-50% bracket.

Silverberg indicates that cellular atypia rather than a mitotic count is the most important prognostic factor. He likewise suggests that when the sarcoma is confined to the myoma, the results should be favorable; we are in complete agreement if there is no vascular invasion.

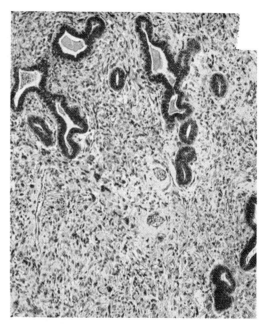

Figure 18.2. Endometrial sarcoma (occasional glands present).

MESENCHYMAL SARCOMA

This variety of uterine malignancy is usually diagnosed preoperatively since it arises from the endometrium and causes bleeding which necessitates curettage.

Endometrial sarcoma is less common but more malignant than leiomyosarcoma.

Microscopically endometrial sarcoma (Fig. 18.2) shows a marked proliferation of the stromal elements, with progressive loss of the endometrial glands. Marked nuclear hyperchromatosis, mitotic activity, and pleomorphism are present.

The tumor *grossly* presents a polypoid architecture (Fig. 18.3) like a cervical polyp. However, benign polyps are generally smoother and less friable than these endometrial lesions, which histologically show complete overgrowth of a proliferative stroma although an infrequent abnormal gland may be found. On occasion, both connective tissue and epithelium are stimulated to malignancy with the development of a *carcinosarcoma*. This should be regarded merely as a variant of endometrial sarcoma and is composed only of *homologous* elements (in contrast to the mixed mesodermal sarcoma).

There are all degrees of histological and clinical malignancy with endometrial sarcoma. As noted earlier, it may be very difficult to make a distinction between this and the locally invasive but nonmetastasizing *stromal endometriosis*, or *stromatosis* (see Chapter 17), which may be a rather completely benign process or locally malignant with venous and lymphatic extension but rarely distant metastasis. (The rare hemangiopericytoma may histologically represent a very difficult diagnostic problem.) More malignant degrees of stromal endometriosis or adenomyosis (*stromatosis*) merge imperceptibly into the patterns of an endometrial sarcoma, as noted by Symmonds et al. and Ober and Tovell. One should recall that there are certain benign epithelial-stromal tumors such as the rare papillary adenofibromas reported by Vellios.

Clement and Scully reported 10 cases of endometrial sarcoma that contained a number of essentially normal endometrial glands and regarded them as a specific entity. These *adenosarcomas* occur in older women and have a rather low degree of malignancy, with late local recurrence and only rare metastasis.

Mixed mesodermal tumors are stromal sarcomas that also contain such *heterologous* elements as bone, cartilage, and striated muscle. Williams and Woodruff point out the considerable confusion as to their nature and

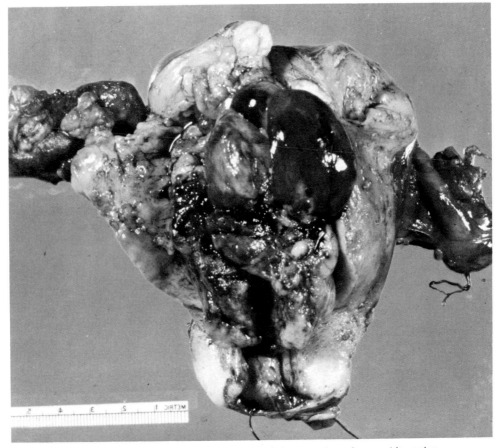

Figure 18.3.   Multipolypoid lesion may extend down cervix and present in vagina.

histogenesis, but today it is generally accepted that the foreign elements arise from a simple metaplasia of the common stem cell of the stroma.

The frequency of *preceding irradiation* has been noted in most reports of these tumors, and in reviewing 400 reported cases, Williams and Woodruff observed this in one-third. A case in association with bilateral thecoma has been reported by Laurain and Monroe. The prognosis is poor with frequent metastases to distant parts of the body as well as the regional nodes, and Taylor has noted only 6 survivors in 40 patients studied. Norris et al. record 19% salvage.

BLOOD VESSEL SARCOMAS

Hemangiopericytoma of the uterus is a vascular lesion not unlike a glomus tumor. It may be distinguished by a tendency toward concentric arrangements of pericytes around capillaries. Special stains (e.g., Masson's) are frequently helpful in distinguishing this tumor from other endothelial or mesothelial growths. Pedowitz et al. have noted a malignancy rate of around 25%, and Ziegerman, in a review, was able to document 10 fatal cases. The tumor must be regarded as a low-grade sarcoma.

Intravenous leiomyomatosis is characterized by multiple intravenous protrusions of a histologically benign, smooth muscle tumor of the uterus. These worm-like nodular lesions are generally grossly apparent, and obvious extrauterine extension into the pelvic veins was present in 10 of 14 patients reviewed by Norris and Parmley. Myometrial leiomyomas are frequently present in addition to the intravenous tumor, and the prognosis in most cases seems to be excellent, even when all gross tumor cannot be removed. There are two theories of origin of this tumor. One suggests that the condition results from vascular invasion by leiomyoma, while the other maintains that the neoplasm arises primarily from the wall of veins. It should be added that intravenous leiomyomatosis needs to be distinguished from other lesions which are characterized by worm-like involvement of the pelvic veins. The most common of these is so-called stromatosis, which more properly may be regarded as a low-grade stromal sarcoma. The prognosis for stromatosis was at one time considered to be excellent, but very late recurrences have been noted with disturbing regularity. The prognosis for intravenous leiomyomas with sarcomatous change is quite serious, although all of these intravenous tumors, even when malignant, seem to be relatively sluggish and characterized by recurrences which are relatively late.

LYMPHOMAS

The various lymphoid malignancies are rare in the uterus but still more commonly found than in the ovary. Ober and Tovell noted occasional cases of lymphosarcoma which present primarily in the uterus with no apparent evidence of this disease in other areas of the body, and, more recently, Wright recorded a "solitary malignant lymphoma." Leukemoid deposits may likewise involve the genital tract, but generally in connection with an extensive spread or infiltrates so that the prognosis is very poor. In any case the outcome with any pelvic lymphoma is guarded.

CLINICAL CHARACTERISTICS OF SARCOMA

The disease most frequently affects women during the middle period of life; our own series showed the highest incidence during the fifth decade. Most authors agree that the prognosis is better in the younger rather than in the postmenopausal patient. Any portion of the uterus may be the seat of the tumor, although the body is far more frequently involved than is the cervix.

The *symptomatology* is not distinctive and is usually that of myoma in which most sarcomas arise. The diagnosis is not made until operation, or even more frequently, not until the pathological examination. *Abnormal bleeding* may be entirely absent, especially when the endometrium is not involved. On the other hand, it may be of great significance, especially when it occurs after the

menopause and particularly when in these postmenopausal cases, the uterus is the seat of presumably myomatous enlargement. In younger women there may be either menstrual excess or intermenstrual bleeding, or both. Needless to say the hemorrhage is in any event only suggestive of possible malignancy, and carcinoma will be found more frequently to be its cause than sarcoma.

Abnormal discharge is common, but *pain* is usual only in advanced disease, along with *anemia, cachexia,* and *weakness. Rapid increase in the size of myomatous tumors,* especially when associated with bleeding, should suggest the possibility of sarcoma. Although recurrence and metastases with a fatal outcome are usually rapid, there are exceptions, such as that noted by Drake and Dobben. They reported a case with probable recurrence 18 years after complete operation and recovery, and their publication, with microscopic sections, would seem to suggest that it was a recurrent rather than a new malignancy.

Extension of the disease is by direct continuity, by the blood stream, and less commonly by the lymphatics. The hematogenous route is most important in metastasis, which therefore is more characteristically systematic than regional. Among the organs most frequently involved are the lungs and liver. Chest x-ray is routine when uterine sarcoma is diagnosed.

Prognosis, as with all malignant tumors, depends on the clinical extent of the disease. Because of their infrequency, a scheme with the clinical staging of sarcoma has not been popularly used. This has made the evaluation of treatment especially difficult. In order to improve this situation, the gynecologic oncology group has suggested the following clinical staging of sarcoma.

Clinical Staging of Sarcoma

Stage I:	Sarcoma confined to the corpus uteri.
Stage Ia:	The length of the uterine cavity is 8 cm or less.
Stage Ib:	The length of the uterine cavity is more than 8 cm.
Stage II:	The sarcoma has involved the corpus and cervix.
Stage III:	The sarcoma has extended outside the uterus but not outside the true pelvis.
Stage IV:	The sarcoma has extended

outside the true pelvis or has invaded the mucosa of the bladder or rectum.

TREATMENT

Because of the difficulties of diagnosis, the treatment of sarcoma is often a matter of expediency rather than of deliberate planning. Surgery has been, and still is, the backbone of treatment, especially since a large proportion of sarcomas are not discovered until operation for supposed myoma or until the laboratory examination of such supposedly benign tumors. The possibility of *sarcomatous change* in *myomas* must always be borne in mind by the surgeon, and it is a wise precaution to cut into the tumor masses as soon as the uterus is removed, for a presumptive diagnosis of sarcoma can sometimes be made from the gross appearance of the cut surface.

Occasionally sarcoma is found after myomectomy has been performed or, more frequently in earlier days, when subtotal hysterectomy was the operation of choice, yet many patients are cured with no further treatment. It would seem that the patient's salvation is due to the fact that many of the sarcomas developing in myomas are comparatively early and of a relatively low degree of malignancy, i.e., cellular myoma.

When endometrial sarcoma is diagnosed preoperatively by curettage, it is treated like adenocarcinoma, i.e., hysterectomy with possible subsequent irradiation. This type of lesion seems more radiosensitive than does leiomyosarcoma.

The recent case report by Pellillo in which a pulmonary metastasis from a recurrent "proliferative stromatosis" underwent a 2-year remission following *large dosage progesterone therapy* suggests that this hormone may be effective in certain cases where the malignancy involves not only the adenomatous but also the stromal portion of the endometrium.

The role of supplementary radiation therapy in uterine sarcoma has been the subject of conflicting reports. With available data so sketchy and the inability to categorize patients according to clinical stage, it is very difficult to be dogmatic about the role of radiation therapy in uterine leiomyosarcoma.

Our clinic has taken a middle course on practical grounds. If the uterus is free, no postoperative therapy is used. If there are adhesions or obvious tumor spread, postoperative therapy is used. It is very doubtful that it is really helpful, but it is often used on an empiric basis.

Endometrial sarcoma is another story. Gilbert's data show a nonrecurrence rate of this disease of a dismal 17%. However, enthusiasm for radiation, either preoperatively as for an endometrial cancer or postoperatively, stems from Gilbert's experience with 21 patients so treated, 17 of whom seemed to have been substantially helped and 8 of whom remained free of disease. Others have had the same experience. Therefore, with endometrial sarcoma in its various forms, adjunctive radiation therapy seemed helpful.

The role of adjunctive chemotherapy is even more uncertain than is the role of adjunctive radiotherapy. The gynecological oncology group is presently evaluating the role of chemotherapy by several alternate protocols; to date the data are not very meaningful. Barlow and his associates did suggest that adriamycin might be a possible value as an adjunctive therapeutic agent, and Buchsbaum and his associates thought that prophylactic chemotherapy in stages I and II uterine sarcoma might be helpful. Gottlieb et al. detected an increased response rate when adriamycin was used along with DTIC (Dimethyltriazenoimidazole carboxamide). Other experiences with chemotherapy were reviewed by Gallup and Cordray.

References and Additional Readings

Aaro, L. A., and Dockerty, M. B.: Leiomyosarcoma of the uterus. Am. J. Obstet. Gynecol., 77: 1187, 1959.

Badib, A. O., Vongtama, V., Kurohara, S. S., and Webster, J. H.: Radiotherapy in the treatment of sarcomas of the corpus uteri. Cancer, 24: 724, 1969.

Baggish, M. S.: Mesenchymal tumors of the uterus. Clin. Obstet. Gynecol., 17: 51, 1974.

Barlow, J. J., Piver, M. S., Chuang, J. T.: Adriamycin and Bleomycin alone and in combination in gynecologic cancers. Cancer, 32: 735, 1973.

Bartsich, E. G., O'Leary, J. A., and Moore, J. G.: Carcinosarcoma of the uterus. Obstet. Gynecol., 30: 518, 1967.

Bartsich, E. G., Bowe, E. T., and Moore, J. G.: Leiomyosarcoma of the uterus. Obstet. Gynecol., 32: 101, 1968.

Buchsbaum, H. J., Lifshitz, S., and Blythe, J.: Prophylactic chemotherapy in stages I and II uterine sarcoma. Gynecol. Oncol., 8: 346, 1979.

Clement, P. B., and Scully, R. E.: Müllerian adenosarcoma of the uterus: a clinicopathologic analysis of ten cases of a destructive type of Müllerian mixed tumor. Cancer, 34: 1138, 1974.

Drake, E. T., and Dobben, G. D.: Leiomyosarcoma of the uterus with unusual metastasis. JAMA 170: 1294, 1959.

Gallup, D. G., and Cordray, D. R.: Leiomyosarcoma of the uterus: Case reports and a review. Obstet. Gynecol. Surv., 34: 300, 1979.

Gilbert, H. A., Kagan, A. R., Lagasse, L., Jacobs, M. R., and Tawa, K.: The value of radiation therapy in uterine sarcoma. Obstet. Gynecol., 45: 84, 1975.

Gottlieb, J. A., Benjamin, R. S., and Baker, L. H.: Role of DTIC in the chemotherapy of sarcomas. Cancer Treat. Rep., *60:* 199, 1976.

Kelly, H. A., and Cullen, T. S.: *Myomata of the Uterus,* W. B. Saunders Co., Philadelphia, 1909.

Laurain, A. R., and Monroe, T. C.: Mixed mesodermal sarcoma of the corpus uteri with associated bilateral thecoma. Am. J. Obstet. Gynecol., *78:* 613, 1959.

Montague, A., Schwarz, D. P., and Woodruff, J. D.: Leiomyosarcoma originating in myoma. Am. J. Obstet. Gynecol., *92:* 421, 1965.

Norris, H. J., and Parmley, T.: Mesenchymal tumors of the uterus: Intravenous leio-yomatosis. A clinical and pathological study of 14 cases. Cancer, *36:* 2164, 1975.

Norris, H. J., Roth, E., and Taylor, H. B.: Mesenchymal tumors of the uterus. II. A clinical and pathological study of 31 mixed mesodermal tumors. Obstet. Gynecol., *28:* 57, 1966.

Ober, W. B.: Uterine sarcomas; histogenesis and taxonomy. Ann. N. Y. Acad. Sci., *75:* 568, 1959.

Ober, W. B.: Mesenchymal sarcomas of the uterus. Am. J. Obstet. Gynecol., *77:* 246, 1959.

Ober, W. B., and Tovell, H. M.: Malignant lymphomas of the uterus. Bull. Sloane Hosp., *5:* 65, 1959.

Pedowitz, P., Felmus, L. B., and Grayzeld, M.: Vascular tumors of the uterus: Benign vascular tumors. Am. J. Obstet. Gynecol., *69:* 1291, 1955.

Pedowitz, P., Felmus, L. B., and Grayzeld, M.: Vascular tumors of the uterus: Malignant vascular tumors. Am. J. Obstet. Gynecol., *69:* 1309, 1955.

Pellillo, D.: Proliferative stromatosis of the uterus with pulmonary metastases. Obstet. Gynecol., *31:* 33, 1968.

Pratt, J. H.: Some surgical considerations of retroperitoneal tumors. Am. J. Obstet. Gynecol., *87:* 956, 1963.

Silverberg, S. G.: Leiomyosarcoma of the uterus. Obstet. Gynecol., *38:* 613, 1971.

Symmonds, R. E., Dockerty, M. B., and Pratt, J. H.: Sarcoma and sarcoma-like proliferation of the endometrial stroma. Am. J. Obstet. Gynecol., *73:* 1054, 1957.

Taylor, C. W.: Mixed mesodermal tumors of the female genital tract. J. Obstet. Gynaecol., Br. Comm., *65:* 177, 1958.

Vellios, F., Ng, A. B. P., and Reagan, J. W.: Papillary adenofibroma of the uterus. Am. J. Clin. Pathol., *60:* 543, 1973.

Williams, T. J., and Woodruff, J. D.: Similarities in malignant mixed mesenchymal tumors of the endometrium. Obstet. Gynecol. Surv., *17:* 1, 1962.

Wright, C. J. E.: Solitary malignant lymphoma uterus. Am. J. Obstet. Gynecol., *117:* 114, 1973.

Zeigerman, J. H.: Vascular tumors of the uterus: Benign or malignant. JAMA, *176:* 108, 1961.

CHAPTER 19

Pelvic Inflammatory Disease

ACUTE PELVIC INFLAMMATORY DISEASE

In this chapter is considered sexually transmitted pelvic inflammatory disease (PID), which involves the uterus, fallopian tubes, ovaries, peritoneum or adjacent structures, or any extension from these organs.

Thus, the syndrome of genital infection is frequently a composite one, produced by various degrees of tubal involvement, with or without extension to the ovaries and pelvic peritoneum. As a rule, the uterus itself is more or less immune to the inflammatory impact, for although there may be a very definite pathological involvement of the endometrial surface, this contributes little to the general symptomatology. This composite clinical syndrome is usually designated as *pelvic inflammatory disease*, and although there are many exceptions, the usual tendency is to begin with a rather acute episode, followed by either complete resolution or else gradual subsidence into a more chronic process characterized by not infrequent acute or subacute resurgence.

Etiology

Pelvic inflammatory disease may be caused by a great variety of organisms. Not infrequently more than one is implicated. The four most important types of infection are:

(1) *Gonorrheal* due to infection by *Neisseria gonorrhoeae*. While gonorrhea may not be the most frequent venereal disease causing PID, it is potentially the most destructive to subsequent reproductive function, either by virtue of its damage to the fallopian tubes or by its association with other organisms of a pyogenic nature which cause widespread tubal damage.

(2) *Pyogenic* due to infection by a large variety of organisms such as the gram-negative aerobes including *Escherichia coli*, the gram-positive aerobes including *Streptococcus viridans* and the enterococci, and most importantly, the anaerobes including anaerobic cocci and *bacteroides fragilis*. Even now there is uncertainty as to whether these pyogenic organisms can cause pelvic inflammatory disease primarily or whether they are secondary invaders complicating a primary infection with a gonococcus. The traditional teaching has been that a primary infection by the gonococcus is necessary and, indeed, there is no evidence to contradict this view. Therefore, it is still currently thought that patients who have a pyosalpinx or a pelvic abscess due to these pyogenic organisms have so as a complication of an infection which is primarily gonorrhea.

In a review devoted primarily to anaerobic infections of the female generative tract, Chow et al. tabulated the various aerobic and anaerobic organisms isolated from the female genital tract infections (Tables 19.1 and 19.2).

(3) *Chlamydial* due to infections with *Chlamydia trachomatis*. By survey, using a variety of cultural techniques of women with a vaginal discharge, Schachter, et al. concluded that chlamydial infections were the most prevalent of the venereal diseases. This particular investigation concerned itself only with the lower genital tract and there was no implication at that time that chlamydia were responsible for acute salpingitis. However, Mardh et al., using the laparoscope, were able to recover *C. trachomatis* from the fimbria in several cases of acute salpingitis. Specifically,

Table 19.1

Anaerobic Bacteria Isolated From 200 Patients With Female Genital Tract Infections[a]

Organism	No. of Isolates		% of Total
Bacteroides	137		38
Bacteroides fragilis		47	13
Bacteroides melaninogenicus		34	10
Other *Bacteroides*		56	16
Fusobacterium	21		6
Peptostreptococcus	64		18
Peptostreptococcus anaerobius		29	8
Peptostreptococus intermedius		10	3
Other *Peptostreptococcus*		25	7
Peptococcus	53		15
Peptococcus prevotii		16	4
Peptococcus magnus		16	4
Other *Peptococcus*		21	6
"Anaerobic streptococci"	13		4
Veillonella/Acidaminococcus	15		4
Clostridium	18		5
Eubacterium	16		5
Other	19		5
Total	356		100

[a] From Chow et al.

Table 19.2

Aerobic Bacteria Isolated From 200 Patients With Female Genital Tract Infections[a]

Organism	No. of Isolates	% of Total
Escherichia coli	61	21
Proteus	16	6
Klebsiella-Enterobacter	13	4
Acinetobacter	7	2
Pseudomonas	4	1
Streptococcus, not A or D	53	18
Group D	30	10
Group A	9	3
Staphylococcus epidermidis	32	11
Staphylococcus aureus	16	6
Neisseria gonorrhoeae	7	2
"Diphtheroids"	22	8
Lactobacillis	10	3
Other	14	5
Total	294	100

[a] From Chow et al.

among 20 patients from whom satisfactory cultures could be obtained, 6 had chlamydia and no other organism as a cause of the acute salpingitis. Therefore, there seems to be no doubt that chlamydial infection must be considered in the differential diagnosis of pelvic inflammatory disease.

It is to be noted that the chlamydia has been identified with other types of infection of gynecological interest, for example, lymphogranuloma inguinale. It seems that the various clinical manifestations of very closely related organisms are due to differing serotypes of the chlamydia.

(4) *Mycoplasmal* due to infections with *Mycoplasma hominis* or *Ureaplasma urealyticum* (T (tiny)-strains of mycoplasma). As with the chlamydia, the mycoplasma have been considered to be associated with minor infections of the lower genital tract.

It needs to be emphasized that the above four types of infection by no means represent all venereal diseases. However, they represent those which fall under the category of pelvic inflammatory disease. Others cause systemic disease, as for example, syphilis, or diseases of the vagina and vulva, as for example, granuloma inguinale, lymphogranuloma inguinale, trichomoniasis, etc.

Contrariwise, pelvic infection which is not sexually transmitted may also occur, as for example, tuberculosis, which is considered in a separate chapter.

Pathology

Cervix

The immediate focus in most cases of infection of the upper genital tract is in the cervix. With gonorrhea, the organisms involved in pyogenic infection, the chlamydia, and the mycoplasma, the carrier state seems to exist as all of these organisms can be identified in a certain proportion of asymptomatic patients by routine culture of the cervix.

Endometrium

Endometritis is characterized grossly by edema and hyperemia of the mucosa and microscopically by edema and infiltration by large numbers of polynuclear leukocytes (Fig. 19.1). There is a tendency toward spontaneous resolution of the endometrial inflammation because of the usual good drainage of the uterine canal and even more because of the monthly desquamation by menstruation.

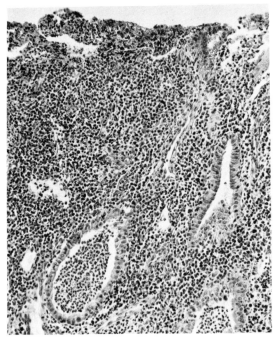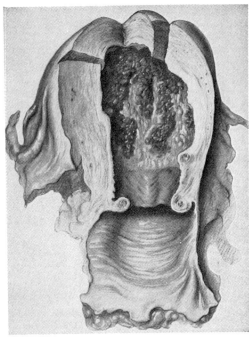

Figure 19.1. *Left*, acute endometritis. Note the purulent exudate in the glands. *Right*, acute necrotic endometritis.

Fallopian Tube

Acute salpingitis may be an almost immediate sequel of an acutely acquired infection of the lower genital tract or it may occur long afterwards, presumably being lit up from a carrier state existing in the cervix. As with the endometrium, there are few data on changes in the tube from chlamydia and mycoplasma. Except in pregnancy where the affecting organisms may reach the tubal region by direct extension through the lymphatics, it is generally thought that the organisms reach the fallopian tube by way of the mucous membrane. This becomes edematous and soon gives forth an exudate which, except in the mildest case, is purulent. If the inflammation does not promptly resolve it may become subacute. This type of involvement is unfortunate for the subsequent reproduction of the patient in that distention and later occlusion of the tube so frequently occur. The exudate and organisms may escape from the still opened end of the tube producing acute pelvic peritonitis and sometimes pelvic abscess.

The inflammatory process is rarely limited in the end of the salpinx alone, the whole tube being swollen, hyperemic, and reddened. Occlusion of the fimbriated orifice or other parts of the lumen may occur with the pro-

duction of a pyosalpinx (Fig. 19.2). Pelvic abscess may result from bacterial invasion or escape of purulent material into the pelvis. Finally, the most frequent end result of acute infection leaves a residue of chronic salpingitis in one form or another.

Ovary

The ovary not infrequently participates in acute pelvic inflammatory processes because of its proximity to the tube. However, only rarely does one observe oophoritis; it is a perioophoritis.

Peritoneum

In various types of pelvic inflammatory disease, the pelvic peritoneum is often involved. This manifests itself most frequently in the form of serous or fibrinous exudates with early development of adhesions between any of the adjoining reproductive structures or between these and the small intestines, sigmoid, or rectum.

As a result of exudation of infected material from the tube or perhaps through the lymphatics on to the peritoneal surface, pelvic abscess frequently results.

In acute gonorrheal peritonitis, spread of infection is often up the right lateral gutter

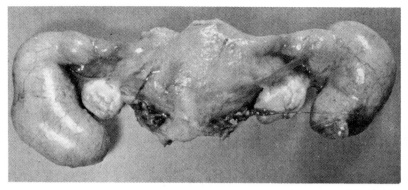

Figure 19.2. Large bilateral pyosalpinx (cervix removed separately).

lateral to the large intestine and on to the dome of the liver between the liver and the diaphragm. Thus, right upper abdominal signs may occur, sometimes just prior to a general peritonitis in the severe case.

Signs and Symptoms

In many cases, the acute symptoms appear during or immediately after a menstrual period, presumably due to the greater vulnerability of the uterine cavity to bacterial invasion at the time of menstrual desquamation.

Severe pain in the pelvis and lower abdominal region, muscular rigidity and tenderness, and, in the more severe and widespread cases, abdominal distention, nausea and vomiting, high fever, leukocytosis, and rapid pulse with considerable prostration are the common symptoms. The fever may reach as high as 103° or even higher with a marked leukocytosis. An increased pulse rate is impressive if the disease is accompanied by widespread peritoneal involvement.

Pelvic Examination

The pelvic examination should always begin with a speculum examination of the cervix. The purpose of this is to obtain a direct smear from the cervix for immediate staining and examination and to obtain aerobic and anaerobic cultures and a culture in a suitable carrying medium for the gonococcus.

The digital pelvic examination may be difficult and indeed unsatisfactory because of the patient's pain, tenderness, and rigidity. When the uterus can be outlined, it is apt to be rather fixed, and efforts to move it by manipulation of the cervix cause much pain. There is extreme bilateral tenderness, and often no definite mass or enlargement of the

adnexa can be made out. However, if the pelvic examination is satisfactory and a mass can be felt, this is very helpful in making the diagnosis.

Postpartum and Postabortive Types

In these cases the patient is often very weak and septic, with evidence of local trauma in the perineum and vagina, so that much gentleness is necessary in the examination, ideally performed with sterile technique. The cervix is apt to be lacerated and infected, especially if the pelvic infection follows full-term delivery. The uterus is large and incompletely involuted, whereas in early criminal abortions, it is only slightly enlarged. Even gentle manipulation of the uterus may be quite painful. One must always be cognizant of the possibility of uterine perforation and other trauma associated with criminal abortion.

Diagnosis

While the diagnosis of pelvic inflammatory disease can be suspected on the basis of the history and physical examination as just outlined, various alternative diagnoses need to be considered. A positive diagnosis is greatly strengthened by positive smear findings or cultural findings. The smear from the cervix obtained before digital examination and stained with gram stain is exceedingly helpful if one can identify intracellular gram-negative diplococci. A smear stained by methylene blue may be satisfactory (Fig. 19.3). This will surely indicate that the pelvic inflammatory disease is due to an acute gonococcal infection. However, this is not always positive even when the culture subsequently grows gonococci. Contrariwise, if a smear from the cervix

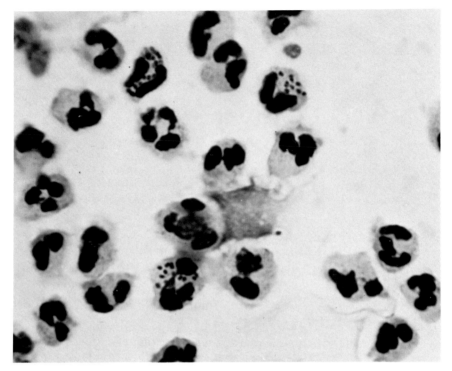

Figure 19.3. A smear from a patient with vaginal discharge. Note the large number of WBC and cells containing intracellular diplococci. These are gonococci (methylene blue ×1500).

shows very few or no pus cells and the smear consists entirely of normal desquamated epithelial cells, the probability is that the patient is not suffering from acute pelvic inflammatory disease but rather from some condition which mimics this.

Cultures take a few days but the diagnosis can be confirmed by a positive culture for the gonococcus, chlamydia, or mycoplasma; however, the usual pyogenic organisms are so common in the vagina normally that positive cultures for these organisms are only relatively helpful.

In some clinical investigative centers, especially in Scandinavia, laparoscopy has been used in patients with suspected acute pelvic inflammatory disease in order to obtain cultures from the fimbriated end of the tubes and in order to determine whether the patient was, in fact, suffering from pelvic inflammatory disease or some other disorder. This clinical investigative effort has resulted in clarifying the role of chlamydia and mycoplasma in the upper generative tract infections and could eventually be more generally used. However, at the present time, the laparoscopic investigation of patients suspected

of having acute pelvic inflammatory disease is probably indicated only where the differential diagnosis from some other life-threatening condition is encountered.

Differential Diagnosis

Nonsexually Transmitted Pelvic Inflammatory Diseases

Severe pelvic infection may follow delivery or abortion. Signs and symptoms are very similar to those for the venereally transmitted diseases. Differential diagnosis is particularly troublesome in postabortal patients, more so formerly than now when such patients were reluctant to admit the possibility of pregnancy, particularly if it had been illegally terminated. With the availability of abortion on demand, this type of patient is rapidly disappearing although occasionally is seen.

The symptoms may manifest themselves within a very short period of time after termination of pregnancy but on other occasions may simmer along for several days before flaring up into a full-blown clinical emergency.

Ectopic Pregnancy

On occasion, an ectopic pregnancy can be confused with acute pelvic inflammatory disease.

Pelvic Inflammatory Disease Associated With An IUD

A special situation exists in the presence of pelvic infection when an intrauterine device (IUD) is present. To be sure, an ordinary acute gonococcal or pyogenic infection or an infection with any of the organisms which are sexually transmitted can occur in patients with an IUD in place. In fact, there are some data to suggest that such infections are somewhat more common among IUD users than otherwise.

The special situation here referred to, however, is an infection which is often unilateral and not venereally transmitted. The onset of symptoms may be more gradual than with acute pelvic inflammatory disease, the fever of a lower grade, and the pelvic examination less tender. The last situation is fortunate because this often makes it possible to feel a unilateral mass.

Patients with a unilateral abscess often do not respond to chemotherapy very well and need to be treated by unilateral salpingo-oophorectomy. In the occasional case where the abscess is confined to the ovary, a unilateral oophorectomy might be suitable.

One of the surprise findings in these unilateral abscesses with intrauterine devices has been the presence of *Actinomyces israelii*. Lomax et al. reported two such cases and studied a total of 16 IUD wearers with serious pelvic infections due to actinomycosis. However, it is not to be assumed that actinomycosis is always present in this particular situation. Niebyl et al. reported four cases of primary ovarian abscess associated with an IUD, but anaerobic organisms were found in this group of patients.

Ruptured Tuboovarian Abscess

The rupture of a tuboovarian abscess with dissemination of the purulent material throughout the peritoneal cavity is a serious complication and needs to be recognized immediately and distinguished from ordinary uncomplicated acute pelvic inflammatory disease. Patients to whom this has occurred can usually identify the event by sudden onset of generalized abdominal pain after previously experiencing pain or discomfort which was localized to the lower pelvis. Furthermore, various degrees of shock with tachycardia and hypotension may be encountered. This is an acute emergency and prior to aggressive surgical treatment there was a very high mortality.

With an aggressive and immediate surgical attack which consists of the removal of the ruptured abscess together with a hysterectomy and removal of the adnexa on the opposite side, the mortality rate from this serious complication has been reduced to less than 5%. However, vigorous supportive measures for combating shock and infection are necessary concomitants to the surgical attack on this problem.

Acute Appendicitis

One of the most troublesome differential diagnoses in suspected pelvic inflammatory disease is acute appendicitis. Typically in acute appendicitis, the initial pain may be diffuse but later tends to localize in the lower right quadrant at McBurney's point. This is in contrast to pelvic inflammatory disease, where the pain begins in the lower abdomen and later becomes diffuse if generalized peritonitis accompanies the pelvic inflammatory disease. Appendicitis often has a lower fever than PID and the leukocytosis may be in proportion to the fever. The problem of distinction becomes much more difficult and sometimes quite impossible in the case of a perforated appendicitis with peritonitis. It is acute appendicitis which must be suspected when the smear taken from the cervix fails to show any leukocytes. As generalized peritonitis from a perforated appendix is also an exceedingly serious complication, in some circumstances an exploratory laparotomy may be necessary to make a precise diagnosis.

Acute Pyelonephritis

Although the kidneys are situated far above the pelvic level, the fact remains that severe acute pyelonephritis can at times produce a clinical picture not unlike that of acute pelvic inflammatory disease. The pain of pyelitis usually involves chiefly the upper abdominal zone although sometimes it is generally over the entire abdomen. Palpation or percussion over the kidney region may show marked tenderness in the costovertebral angle. With pyelonephritis there is usually high fever, but patients do not appear as ill or distressed as with salpingitis or appendicitis.

Adnexal Torsion

The symptomatology and clinical picture of a twisted adnexum with or without an ovarian cyst and with or without infection can mimic ordinary pelvic inflammatory disease and indeed can sometimes simulate a ruptured tuboovarian abscess. If the adnexa are diseased, as with a small ovarian cyst or with a hydrosalpinx, torsion can cause necrosis and rupture. Torsion of intrinsically normal adnexa is more common in prepubertal or teenage individuals, although this may occur at any time in life. The etiology is obscure. Considerable care should be exercised in the operative management of such cases, as simple untwisting of the adnexa might conceivably release thrombi with a potentially disastrous outcome.

TREATMENT

Bedrest, adequate fluids, intravenously, if necessary, and analgesics are obviously basic necessities in the treatment of acute pelvic inflammatory disease.

The most important aspect of therapy, however, is the selection of a suitable antibiotic administered in adequate doses.

If a diagnosis of an acute gonococcal infection can be made, specific treatment with penicillin or tetracycline, according to the regime recommended by the Center for Disease Control, is indicated (Table 19.3).

In the great majority of cases of acute pelvic inflammatory disease, rapid improvement in 24 or 48 hours is to be expected with the use of the regime just mentioned. However, in a certain residual of cases, clinical response is delayed. In this circumstance, serious consideration must be given to the presence of a pelvic abscess of one variety or another. Even though these abscesses may harbor organisms which in in vitro examination are susceptible to the antibiotic being used, clinical response is not obtained, presumably by virtue of the inaccessibility of the organisms to the antibiotic because of circulatory problems at the level of the abscess. One of the most difficult clinical decisions is the timing of an operative approach to a woman with an unresponsive pelvic infection. The traditional gynecological approach has been to avoid acute-phase operations, and there is every reason to continue this approach because in a certain residual of cases with acute pelvic inflammatory disease, the response to antibiotic therapy will be prompt and adequate and complete enough to maintain the patient's fertility.

For the unresponsive or unavailable tuboovarian inflammatory mass, which is usually an abscess, laparotomy with excisional surgery confined to the tuboovarian mass or, if the disease is bilateral as is often the case, to a bilateral salpingoophorectory and hysterectomy, subtotal if necessary, is the treatment of choice. Such a procedure is especially indicated in patients with postabortal infections, as mentioned in the section on differential diagnosis.

As also mentioned in the section on differential diagnosis, a ruptured tuboovarian abscess is an urgent indication for surgery to remove the source of the infection in the pelvis and to wash out the general peritoneal cavity.

With serious pelvic inflammatory disease which is unresponsive for patients who have had surgical removal of infected pelvic organs and in whom unexplained fever continues, the possibility of a complicating pelvic thrombophlebitis should be suspected. If this is a serious consideration, its treatment by heparin should be instituted as well, of course, as continuing suitable antibiotic therapy.

Generally speaking, acute pelvic inflammatory disease due to the chlamydia or mycoplasma seems to be self-limited, but these organisms fortunately respond to tetracycline.

In considering the treatment of venereally acquired infections, it needs to be emphasized that many times more than one venereal disease is contracted at the same time. In considering the therapy of acute pelvic inflammatory disease, it is therefore necessary to give consideration to other diseases that might be contracted simultaneously. Syphilis, of course, comes immediately to mind. Other venereal diseases which affect the vagina and vulva may also be encountered.

CHRONIC PELVIC INFLAMMATORY DISEASE

Orientation

Even a single attack of acute pelvic inflammatory disease might be expected to leave

Table 19.3
CDC Recommended Treatment Schedules, 1978[a]

UNCOMPLICATED GONOCOCCAL INFECTIONS IN MEN AND WOMEN

A. Drug Regimens of Choice

Aqueous procaine penicillin G (APPG) 4.8 million units injected intramuscularly at two sites, with 1.0 gm of probenecid by mouth.

or

Tetracycline hydrochloride[b] 0.5 gm by mouth 4 times a day for 5 days (total dosage 10.0 gm). Other tetracyclines are not more effective than tetracycline hydrochloride. All tetracyclines are ineffective as a single-dose therapy.

or

Ampicillin 3.5 gm, or amoxicillin 3.0 g, either with 1 gm probenecid by mouth. Evidence shows that these regimens are slightly less effective than the other recommended regimens.

Patients who are allergic to the penicillins or probenecid should be treated with oral tetracycline as above. Patients who cannot tolerate tetracycline may be treated with spectinomycin hydrocholoride 2.0 gm in one intramuscular injection.

B. Special Considerations

1. Single-dose treatment is preferred in patients who are unlikely to complete the multiple-dose tetracycline regimen.
2. The APPG regimen is preferred in men with anorectal infection.
3. Pharyngeal infection is difficult to treat; high failure rates have been reported with ampicillin and spectinomycin.
4. Tetracycline treatment results in fewer cases of postgonococcal urethritis in men.
5. Tetracycline may eliminate coexisting chlamydial infections in men and women.
6. Patients with incubating syphilis (seronegative, without clinical signs of syphilis) are likely to be cured by all the above regimens except spectinomycin. All patients should have a serologic test for syphilis at the time of diagnosis.
7. Patients with gonorrhea who also have syphilis or are established contacts to syphilis should be given additional treatment appropriate to the stage of syphilis.

C. Treatment of Sexual Partners

Men and women exposed to gonorrhea should be examined, cultured, and treated at once with one of the regimens above.

D. Follow-up

Follow up cultures should be obtained from the infected site(s) 3–7 days after completion of treatment. Cultures should be obtained from the anal canal of all women who have been treated for gonorrhea.

E. Treatment Failures

The patient who fails therapy with penicillin, ampicillin, amoxicillin, or tetracycline should be treated with 2.0 gm of spectinomycin intramuscularly.

Most recurrent infections after treatment with the recommended schedules are due to reinfection and indicate a need for improved contact tracing and patient education. Since infection by penicillinase (β-lactamase)-producing *Neisseria gonorrhoeae* is a cause of treatment failure, posttreatment isolates should be tested for penicillinase production.

F. Not Recommended

Although long-acting forms of penicillin (such as benzathine penicillin G) are effective in syphilotherapy, they have NO place in the treatment of gonorrhea. Oral penicillin preparations such as penicillin V are not recommended for the treatment of gonococcal infection.

PENICILLINASE-PRODUCING *NEISSERIA GONORRHOEAE* (PPNG)

Patients with uncomplicated PPNG infections and their sexual contacts should receive spectinomycin 2.0 gm intramuscularly in a single injection. Because gonococci are very rarely resistant to spectinomycin and reinfection is the most common cause of treatment failure, patients with positive cultures after spectinomycin therapy should be retreated with the same dose.

A PPNG isolate that is resistant to spectinomycin may be treated with cefoxitin 2.0 gm in a single intramuscular injection, with probenecid 1.0 gm by mouth.

Table 19.3, *Continued*

TREATMENT IN PREGNANCY

All pregnant women should have endocervical cultures for gonococci as an integral part of the prenatal care at the time of the first visit. A second culture late in the third trimester should be obtained from women at high risk for gonococcal infection.

Drug regimens of choice are APPG, ampicillin or amoxicillin, each with probenecid as described above. Women who are allergic to penicillin or probenecid should be treated with spectinomycin.

Tetracycline should not be used in pregnant women because of potential toxic effects for mother and fetus.

ACUTE SALPINGITIS (PELVIC INFLAMMATORY DISEASE)

There are no reliable clinical criteria on which to distinguish gonococcal from nongonococcal salpingitis. Endocervical cultures for *N. gonorrhoeae* are essential.

A. Hospitalization should be strongly considered in these situations:
1. Uncertain diagnosis, in which surgical emergencies such as appendicitis and ectopic pregnancy must be excluded.
2. Suspicion of pelvic abscess.
3. Severely ill patients.
4. Pregnancy.
5. Inability of the patient to follow or tolerate an outpatient regimen.
6. Failure to respond to outpatient therapy.

B. Antimicrobial Agents
1. Outpatients

Tetracycline[b] 0.5 gm taken orally 4 times a day for 10 days. This regimen should not be used for pregnant patients.

or

APPG 4.8 million units intramuscularly, ampicillin 3.5 gm or amoxicillin 3.0 gm each with probenecid 1.0 gm. Either regimen is followed by ampicillin 0.5 gm or amoxicillin 0.5 gm orally 4 times a day for 10 days.

2. Hospitalized patients

Aqueous crystalline penicillin G 20 million units given intravenously each day until improvement occurs, followed by ampicillin 0.5 gm orally 4 times a day to complete 10 days of therapy.

or

Tetracycline[b] 0.25 gm given intravenously 4 times a day until improvement occurs, followed by 0.5 g orally 4 times a day to complete 10 days of therapy. This regimen should not be used for pregnant women. The dosage may have to be adjusted if renal function is depressed. Since optimal therapy for hospitalized patients has not been established, other antibiotics in addition to penicillin are frequently used.

C. Special Considerations
1. Failure of the patient to improve on the recommended regimens does not indicate the need for stepwise additional antibiotics but requires clinical reassessment.
2. The intrauterine device is a risk factor for the development of pelvic inflammatory disease. The effect of removing an intrauterine device on the response of acute salpingitis to antimicrobial therapy and on the risk of recurrent salpingitis is unknown.
3. Adequate treatment of women with acute salpingitis must include examination and appropriate treatment of their sex partners because of their high prevalence of nonsymptomatic urethral infection. Failure to treat sex partners is a major cause of recurrent gonococcal salpingitis.
4. Follow-up of patients should be recultured for *N. gonorrhoeae* after treatment.

---

[a] *Note:* Physicians are cautioned to use no less than the recommended dosages of antibiotics.

[b] Food and some dairy products interfere with absorption. Oral forms of tetracycline should be given 1 hour before or 2 hours after meals.

behind some residual evidence of infection. This may be merely in the form of pelvic adhesions which bind the tubes to surrounding structures. More often, it is likely that the fimbriated ends of the tubes may be completely obstructed or at least partially obstructed. These residual disorders may or may not be extensive enough to interfere with subsequent pregnancy but, generally speaking, even a single attack of well treated acute pelvic inflammatory disease can be expected to have serious consequences for future fertility.

Pathology

The microscopic characteristics of chronic endometritis and salpingitis are similar to those of chronic inflammation elsewhere. The chief feature is more or less extensive infiltration with round or plasma cells.

A late result of tubal obstruction is the development of a hydrosalpinx caused by obstruction at both ends of the tube with the accumulation of clear fluid between. These may sometimes become 4 or 5 cm in diameter.

The microscopic appearance of hydrosalpinx shows a clear cystic central cavity with a flattened tubal mucosa whose folds have been ironed out and are almost entirely obliterated, although usually an occasional small fold can be seen here and there (Fig. 19.4).

An interesting special variety of chronic salpingitis is the so-called salpingitis isthmica nodosa in which the residue of a sustained chronic inflammatory process is limited chiefly to the isthmic portion of the tube. In such cases, nodulation of the tubal isthmus is seen, the nodules being sometimes large enough to simulate small cornual fibroid tumors. The remainder of the tube may seem fairly normal and the fimbriated end may be open (Fig. 19.5). While chronic inflammation presumably is responsible for some examples of salpingitis isthmica nodosa, others are probably nothing more than congenital abnormalities in which there has been a failure of the lumen to develop embryologically so that the lesion is not inflammatory at all. Microscopic examinations in such cases present a curious picture in that there may appear many small lumina instead of one (Fig. 19.6. These cases may be mistaken for adenomyosis of the tube or endosalpingosis of the

tube, which on the external surface can give the nodular appearance of inflammatory salpingitis isthmica nodosa.

The ovaries may be extensively involved in chronic pelvic inflammatory disease but the involvement is confined almost entirely to the external surface so that the disorder can more properly be labeled chronic perioophoritis. The surface involvement is expressed by the presence of adhesions of light or dense fibrous nature. The so-called germinal epithelium often extends under the adhesions producing slit-like or glandular spaces which may resemble endometriosis.

Signs and Symptoms

Chronic pelvic inflammatory disease is encountered in patients who complain either of pain or of infertility. Low-grade fever with an afternoon rise of 99.4° may be the only febrile manifestation. On the other hand, an increased sedimentation rate may be the only indication of an inflammatory residue.

A physical examination may or may not be helpful. Pelvic tenderness may be encountered, and indeed one might feel thickening in the parametrial areas. In cases with moderately extensive disease, the ovaries, although palpable, may be limited in motion. Sometimes, however, a fairly extensive chronic inflammatory process can exist in the pelvis without there being recognizable abnormality in the pelvic examination.

Diagnosis

The history and physical examinations, if positive, are important leads in suspecting chronic inflammatory disease in the pelvis. Infertility, of course, is often explained by this disorder. To make a definitive diagnosis, diagnostic laparoscopy has become a standard procedure.

Laboratory work is generally not helpful in this condition, although low-grade fever, leukocytosis, and elevated sedimentation rate are often present if there is any activity to the chronic inflammatory process.

Treatment

Treatment of the woman with chronic pelvic inflammatory disease is often taxing to the patient and to the physician. Of course, if there is any evidence of active infection as

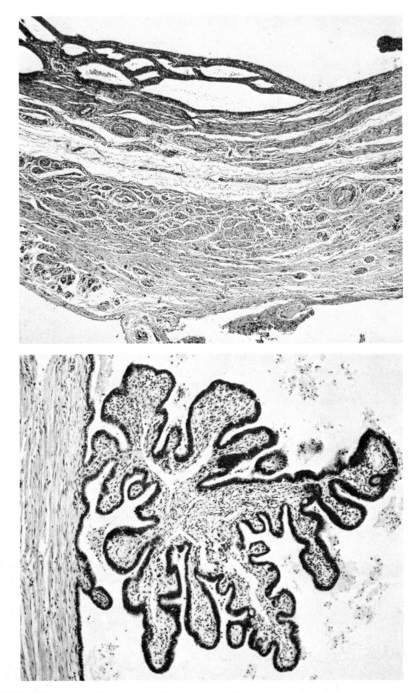

Figure 19.4. *Top,* hydrosalpinx simplex (microscopic). *Bottom,* wall of large hydrosalpinx simplex showing persistence of stunted tubal folds.

indicated by slight temperature rise or by elevated sedimentation rates or leukocytosis, the use of antibiotics might be expected to be helpful. Generally speaking, however, active infection is minimal or absent and the prob-

lem is to relieve the patient of pain or infertility. It is important to procrastinate as long as possible before advising surgical therapy because in many women with the passage of time pain slowly disappears, presumably due

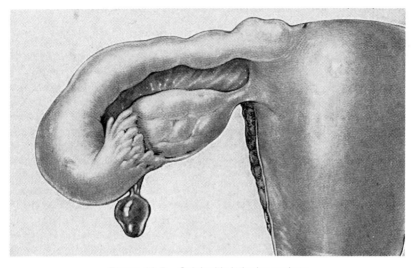

Figure 19.5. Salpingitis isthmica nodosa.

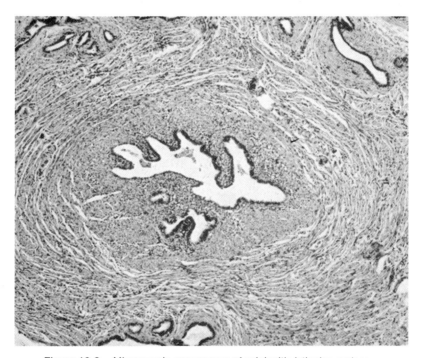

Figure 19.6. Microscopic appearance of salpingitis isthmica nodosa.

to internal adjustments which relieve the stress on the adhesions which are the source of the pain in the first instance.

However, there is a residue of patients who have prolonged pain over a sufficient period of time and of such severity that their daily activities are greatly compromised. In this circumstance, there is no alternative to offering surgical therapy. When operating for chronic pelvic inflammatory disease for pain, the operation usually consists of bilateral salpingooophorectomy and hysterectomy as conservative operations in chronic pelvic inflammatory disease and often are unsatisfactory in the long run. In some circumstances, it may be possible to save one or both ovaries but the occurrence of a postoperative ovarian or tuboovarian cyst after conservative operations for inflammatory disease is a well known problem.

When chronic pelvic inflammatory disease is encountered in women who are relatively free of pain but whose complaint is infertility, the results depend entirely on the severity and location of the pelvic adhesion. The matter of the surgical therapy of infertility due to tubal obstruction is considered at some length in the chapter on infertility (Chapter 29).

References and Additional Readings

Chow, A. W., Marshall, J. R., and Guze, L. B.: Anaerobic infections of the female generative tract: Prospects and perspectives. Obstet. Gynecol. Surv., *30:* 477, 1975.

Forslin, L., Falk, V., and Danielsson, D.: Changes in the incidence of acute gonococcal and non-gonococcal salpingitis. Br. J. Venereal Dis., *54:* 247, 1978.

Lomax, C. W., Harbert, G. M., Jr., and Thornton, W. N., Jr.: Actinomycosis of female genital tract. Obstet. Gynecol., *48:* 341, 1976.

Mardh, P. A., Ripa, T., Svenson, L., and Westrom, L.: Chlamydia trachomatis infection in patients with acute salpingitis. N. Engl. J. Med., *296:* 1377, 1977.

Mardh, P. A., and Westrom, L.: Tubal and cervical cultures and acute salpingitis with special reference to mycoplasma hominis and T-strain mycoplasmas. Br. J. Venereal Dis., *46:* 179, 1970.

McCormack, W. M., Rosner, B., and Lee, Y-H: Colonization with genital mycoplasmas in women. Am. J. Epidemiol., *240:* 97, 1973.

Niebyl, J. R., Parmley, T. H., Spence, M. R., and Woodruff, J. D.: Unilateral ovarian abscess associated with the intrauterine device. Obstet. Gynecol., *52:* 165, 1978.

Schachter, J., Hanna, L., Hill, E. C., Massad, S., Sheppard, C. W., Conte, J. E., Cohen, S. N., and Meyer, K. F.: Are chlamydial infections the most prevalent venereal diseases. JAMA, *231:* 1252, 1975.

Vermeeren, J., and TeLinde, R. W.: Intra-abdominal rupture of pelvic abscess. Am. J. Obstet. Gynecol., *68:* 402, 1954.

CHAPTER 20

Genital Tuberculosis

Although uncommon in the United States, pelvic tuberculosis is not rare in many other areas of the world. Since this text is translated into many languages, it would seem a full chapter is warranted on this problem.

With pelvic tuberculosis, there is almost uniformly initial pelvic involvement of the tubes, although there are rare cases of primary cervical tuberculosis in which the sexual partner has been thought to be the source of infection. Tubal involvement is almost 100% in the woman with pelvic tuberculosis (Table 20.1). The tubes seem to be the only logical focus for pelvic tuberculosis, at least in the United States.

Modes of Infection

In almost all cases tuberculous involvement of the female genitalia is secondary to extragenital tuberculosis, although it is rare to find this lesion currently active. Occasionally pelvic tuberculosis may be a part of a generalized miliary tuberculous disease, but the association of urinary and genital tuberculosis is rare.

However, *pulmonary disease* is the usual *primary site* and the probable route of dissemination is almost certainly hematogenous. Why the tubes usually receive the primary impact of this blood stream involvement is uncertain.

TUBERCULOSIS OF TUBES

Tuberculous salpingitis is frequent and comprises approximately 5% of all cases of salpingitis in some areas of the world where disease and malnutrition are present, although it is much less common in this country. In earlier studies Schaefer noted an 8%

incidence of genital disease in women dying of pulmonary tuberculosis. In certain areas of the United States where there is a migrant population, pelvic tuberculosis is not rare, as noted by Klein et al. in Los Angeles.

Pathology

The *gross* appearance of the tuberculous tube varies in different cases but as a rule is no different from that of the various forms of chronic gonorrheal salpingitis. The tube may resemble a pyosalpinx, occasionally hydrosalpinx, or salpingitis isthmica nodosa. In the form associated with miliary tuberculous peritonitis, numerous tubercles may stud the surface as well as the pelvic peritoneal cavity. More frequently, however, no tubercles are visible externally, although they may be present in advanced stages of the hematogenous variety. The diagnosis of tuberculous salpingitis is often not made until microscopic examination has been carried out.

Microscopic

The microscopic diagnosis is easy in the frank, advanced case, but it may be difficult in the early phases of the disease or in the late reparative phase. Many blocks may have to be taken from various parts of the tube

Table 20.1[a]
Frequency of Tuberculosis in Genital Organs

Organ	Percentage
Tubes	90–100
Uterus	50–60
Ovaries	20–30
Cervix	5–15
Vagina	1

[a] Courtesy of Dr. Geo. Schaefer, New York.

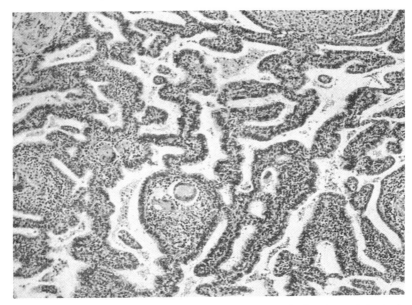

Figure 20.1. Microscopic appearance of tubal tuberculosis with typical tubercles and giant cells and marked proliferation of tubal folds.

before the telltale evidence, in the form of tubercles and giant cells, can be demonstrated (Fig. 20.1). Acid-fast stains are more specific; even when these are negative, a positive culture may be obtained.

In the early stages one often finds a markedly proliferative, adenomatous-looking pattern in the folds. This should always excite suspicion, and it *should not be mistaken for adenocarcinoma*, as it has often been. In the more outspoken cases, one finds numerous tubercles, many with giant cells, and chronic inflammation. The tubercles may be limited to the mucosa, or they may be scattered throughout the muscularis and on the peritoneal coat. In advanced stages, extensive caseation is common.

The histological criteria noted above should suggest a tuberculous infection, but it must be realized that other diseases may produce a similar granulomatous process. The final diagnosis lies in the demonstration of the acid-fast bacillus by means of an appropriate stain or culture, but, practically speaking, most cases of granulomatous disease are tuberculous.

TUBERCULOSIS OF THE ENDOMETRIUM

As noted by Greenberg, this is always secondary to tubal involvement.

The *pathology* of tuberculous endometritis is characterized by the presence of typical tubercles with epithelioid and giant cells, involving the endometrium and occasionally the myometrium. In late stages there are extensive tubercles with many giant cells and varying degrees of caseation, but even in advanced disease there are no specific gross findings. Acid-fast culture of the endometrium is positive in less than 50% of all cases, and acid-fast stains are often unsuccessful. As a rule, pelvic tuberculosis behaves like tuberculosis anywhere. While more common in the younger woman, tuberculous endometritis has been noted in postmenopausal patients by Schaefer et al. Bleeding was the presenting complaint.

TUBERCULOSIS OF THE OVARIES

This practically never occurs in the absence of tubal involvement, and, when present, it generally consists of a rather marked perioophoritis rather than a real ovarian involvement.

TUBERCULOSIS OF THE CERVIX

This has already been discussed in Chapter 11.

TUBERCULOSIS OF THE VAGINA AND THE VULVA

As a rule, tuberculosis of the vulva or the vagina presents as a shaggy ulcerative lesion which may be difficult to distinguish from a luetic ulcer. On occasion it may assume a hypertrophic character which, as with tuberculous cervicitis, may be mistaken for a genuine carcinoma. Biopsy is generally decisive.

CLINICAL FEATURES OF PELVIC TUBERCULOSIS

There is nothing pathognomonic about *tuberculous salpingitis* to distinguish it from the much more common chronic salpingitis, and, as a result of this similarity, preoperative diagnosis is rarely made. There are, however, a few features which should arouse suspicion that the adnexal involvement may be of acid-fast origin. Sutherland points out that a history of pulmonary, osseous, or miliary tuberculosis should be suggestive, although gonorrhea may, of course, coexist. The finding of adnexal inflammatory masses in virgins or women in whom other types of tubal infection can reasonably be excluded may likewise lead to a suspicion of tuberculous salpingitis, especially if there is a tendency towards a persistent slight evening elevation of temperature, slight anemia, or tachycardia. Salpingitis which is refractory to the usual means of therapy should suggest tuberculosis, although this may not prove to be the case.

SILENT PELVIC TUBERCULOSIS

In recent years there have been a considerable number of publications concerning the chance finding of endometrial tuberculosis in women with no other symptom or complaint than infertility, and Schaefer terms this *minimal* disease.

As noted previously, belief is rather uniform that endometrial involvement is nearly always secondary to diseased tubes; although the tubes are the primary pelvic focus, there is nevertheless often insufficient disease to produce symptoms. In certain instances the tubes may be patent, and ovulation is the rule.

TUBERCULOUS PERITONITIS

Tuberculous peritonitis is associated with tubal disease, generally of extensive nature, and tends to behave like other adnexal disease with the addition of ascites. Usually the pelvic peritoneum alone shows tuberculous seeding (along with that of the tubes), although the extrapelvic peritoneum is not involved.

Tuberculous peritonitis may present in several different forms. The wet variety may show extensive tubercle formation involving all visceral and parietal surfaces of the peritoneum but most marked in the pelvis. The omentum may be studded with nodules and be greatly thickened and indurated in a board like fashion. Ascites is the rule. It is frequently not generalized but is likely to be composed of multiple sacs of ascitic fluid enclosed in loops of agglutinated intestine and omentum. Various types of masses and pseudomasses may be produced by these encysted fluid sacs, but there is generally additional free fluid.

The *dry* type of peritonitis is perhaps a later stage of the ascitic form, after there have been varying amounts of resorption of the fluid. This fibroplastic form is characterized by only minor degrees of ascites, but there may be extensive adhesions and induration, with literal welding of pelvic and intestinal surfaces. Caseation, necrosis, and fistulas may occur.

All gradations between the ascitic (wet) and the adhesive (dry) types of peritoneal involvement may occur, and all types of confusing differential diagnoses may be simulated. Ascites of renal or cardiac origin must be distinguished, as must hepatic cirrhosis. Ovarian carcinomatosis is frequently suspected, especially where there is tuberculous adnexitis and abscess formation.

Clinical Course

Patients with tuberculous peritonitis may evidence no other symptom than abdominal swelling due to ascitic fluid. On the other hand, there may be profound systemic symptoms with high spiking fever, tachycardia, anorexia, and weight loss. In the fibroplastic form one may observe symptoms suggesting partial intestinal obstruction, such as obstipation, bloating, etc. If there is miliary or pulmonary tuberculosis, other symptoms may be added, so that diagnosis may be difficult.

The finding of ascites, however, in a young woman with no history of cardiorenal or hepatic difficulties, should make one suspect tuberculous peritonitis, especially if there is systemic and laboratory evidence of an inflammatory process. Palpation of tubal masses and the finding of a fixed uterus are often noted and, if this adnexal disease does not respond to the usual antibiotics and chemotherapy, a tuberculous etiology may be suspected.

DIAGNOSIS OF PELVIC TUBERCULOSIS

Many cases with acid-fast disease of the female generative organs are asymptomatic, and many more show only the diverse symptoms associated with any nonspecific inflammatory disease. Schaefer rightfully emphasizes the importance of being always suspicious of the possibility of the disease, particularly where there is a family history of tuberculosis or some proved extragenital manifestation. Infertility for which no other cause can be found, pelvic pain, general malaise, adnexal masses in virgins, and chronic refractory adnexal disease are by no means pathognomonic but might alert the wary examiner. Chest x-ray and tuberculin testing should not be neglected though of dubious value.

Where there is suspicion of the disease, we do not hesitate to perform a curettage, with full cognizance of the fact that only about 50% of those women having tubal disease also have tuberculous endometritis. In other words, the finding of endometrial tuberculosis clinches the diagnosis; failure to find the characteristic histological pattern in no way excludes the acid-fast bacillus. Bacteriological culture of menstrual blood or aspiration culture of the endometrial cavity may be obtained, but even more effective is direct culture and guinea pig inoculation with removed endometrium.

Sarcoidosis may involve the female genitalia and produce granulomatous lesions similar to tuberculosis, although there is not, of course, bacteriological evidence of the tubercle bacillus. In addition, sarcoid frequently involves many other organs, as indicated by Winslow and Funkhowsen. Various diseases such as actinomycosis as well as schistosomiasis may produce a granulomatous appearance, as noted by Fathalla.

TREATMENT

In past years the treatment of diagnosed pelvic tuberculosis was almost entirely surgical plus the usual regimen of rest, fresh air, good nutrition, etc. Recent advances in the fields of antibiotics and chemotherapy in the last 25 years have equipped us with a number of effective antituberculous drugs.

Chemotherapy alone is used only in those patients who have patent tubes, who are desirous of further pregnancy, and who have little or no discomfort. Persistent, painful adnexal masses, continued fever, and elevated sedimentation rate, ascites, and failure to respond to medical treatment are indications for surgical rather than medical treatment.

Medical Treatment

Schaefer suggests the following medical treatment for tuberculosis. Where the disease is minimal, 300 mgm of isoniazid with about 1000 mgm of ethambutol is utilized. After 1 year the ethambutol may be discontinued and patients maintained on isoniazid alone, sometimes for years, with periodic evaluation as to patency of the tubes.

With advanced disease and pelvic masses the same initial therapy is utilized, but if the masses persist or grow larger, plans are made for surgery. Prior to this, however, streptomycin therapy is instituted for at least a week and continued for several weeks postoperative. If drug therapy alone is utilized it is suggested that it be maintained for as long as 2 years.

Following diagnosis and medical treatment, the patient must be kept under close observation. Pelvic tuberculosis is still a potentially serious disease, and miliary or various forms of extragenital tuberculosis can arise. If a patient has been treated because of a curettage-proved tuberculous endometritis, repeat curettage is in order every 6 months for several years. Should the endometritis persist or recur later, surgery is indicated.

Surgical Treatment

Persistent or recurrent endometritis is only one of several indications for surgical intervention. Prime indications are continuous or recurrent pain persistent or developing adnexal masses, and recurring endometritis. We are in complete accord with Zummo et al., who feel that patients with the more advanced forms of pelvic disease are candidates for surgery. Indications consist of adnexal masses, abscesses, prominent thickenings, and ascites.

PREGNANCY AND TUBERCULOSIS

An excellent review of the subject is that of Halbrecht, who reported his material from Israel, where constant warfare with resultant poor nutrition and hygiene have made pelvic tuberculosis unusually common. Halbrecht states that "any pregnancy occurring after antibiotic treatment of genital tuberculosis demands watchful supervision, considering the fact that such a pregnancy has a four to one chance to be a tubal pregnancy or to end in miscarriage. This is especially true if the disease has reached the endometrial stage before the treatment was started." We would be somewhat skeptical of cortisone therapy with tubal occlusion following healed genital tract tuberculosis, as noted by Halbrecht and various other authors.

Thus, the changes of a normal child following medical treatment of tuberculosis are really minimal. The tendency is to treat young sterile patients conservatively, and with this policy we are in complete agreement, providing the tubes are patent. The knowledge that successful pregnancies have occurred (although few) following antituberculous treatment can frequently be a great morale builder for young brides.

Tubal plastic surgery is not to be considered for tubes obstructed by tuberculosis. It not only is not effective, but Ballon et al. have recorded a case of silent pelvic tuberculosis which was activated by tuboplasty.

References and Additional Readings

Ballon, S. C. et al: Reactivation of silent pelvic tuberculosis by reconstructive tubal surgery. Am. J. Obstet. Gynecol. *122:* 991, 1975.

Fathalla, M. S.: Assuit Univ., Cairo, Egypt. Personal communication.

Francis, W. J. A.: Female genital tuberculosis. J. Obstet. Gynaecol. Br. Common., *71:* 418, 1964.

Greenberg, J. P.: Tuberculous salpingitis; a clinical study of 200 cases. Johns Hopkins Hosp. Rep., *21:* 97, 1921.

Halbrecht, I.: Healed genital tuberculosis. Obstet. Gynecol. *10:* 73, 1957.

Halbrecht, I.: Latent genital tuberculosis in women; its early diagnosis and treatment. Tuberkulosearzt, *12:* 712, 1958.

Halbrecht, I.: Cortisone in the treatment of tubal occlusion caused by healed genital tuberculosis. Fertil. Steril., *13:* 371, 1962.

Klein, T. A., et al.: Pelvic tuberculosis. Obstet. Gynecol., *78:* 99, 1976.

Knauss, H. H.: Surgical treatment of genital and peritoneal tuberculosis in the female. Am. J. Obstet. Gynecol., *83:* 73, 1962.

Schaefer, G.: Full term pregnancy following genital tuberculosis. Obstet. Gynecol. Surv., *19:* 81, 1964.

Schaefer, G.: Diagnosis and treatment of female genital tuberculosis. Int. Surg., *48:* 240, 1967.

Schaefer, G.: Tuberculosis of the female genital tract. Clin. Obstet. Gynecol., *13:* 965, 1970.

Schaefer, G.: Genital tuberculosis. Clin. Obstet. Gynecol., *19:* 223, 1976.

Schaefer, G., Douglas, R. G., and Silverman, F.: A reevaluation of the management of pregnancy and tuberculosis. J. Obstet. Gynaecol. Br. Comm., *66:* 990, 1959.

Schaefer, G., Marcus, R. S., and Kramer, E. E.: Postmenopausal endometrial tuberculosis. Amer. J. Obstet. Gynecol., *112:* 681, 1972.

Sutherland, A. M.: Tuberculosis of the genital organs. Am. J. Obstet. Gynecol., *91:* 717, 1965.

Sutherland, A. M.: Genital tuberculosis in women. Bull. Sloane Hosp., *13:* 127, 1967.

Sutherland, A. M.: Pelvic tuberculosis. Br. J. Obstet. Gynaecol., *84:* 881, 1977.

Winslow, R. C., and Funkhowsen, J. W.: Sarcoidosis of the female reproductive organs. Obstet. Gynecol., *32:* 285, 1968.

Zummo, B. P., Sered, H., and Falls, F. H.: Diagnosis and prognosis of female genital tuberculosis. Am. J. Obstet. Gynecol., *70:* 34, 1955.

CHAPTER 21

Tumors of the Tube, Paraovarium, and Uterine Ligaments

CARCINOMA OF FALLOPIAN TUBE

Primary

The most important tumor of the tube is carcinoma, but it is extremely rare. The incidence in collected hospital series varies between 1% (Hayden and Potter) and 0.1% (Green and Scully) of all genital malignancies; obviously many cases are not reported. The disease occurs usually in middle life but may occur also in very old women.

Pathology

Grossly the tube is enlarged, sometimes enormously. It may resemble a huge pyosalpinx, which often is almost entirely free of adhesions to surrounding structures and, unlike pelvic inflammatory disease, the contralateral tube is usually normal. Although Sedlis found bilateral tumors in 26% of those patients he studied, most other series report bilateral tumors in the neighborhood of 7–10%. In most cases the carcinoma arises in the outer or middle portion of the tube, and in the occasional very early case there may be only a small nodular enlargement at the involved area. Extension out the fimbriated end of the tube or penetration of the thin tubal wall leads to dissemination of intraperitoneal tumor, much as in ovarian carcinoma (Fig. 21.1).

Microscopically the typical pattern is of a *papillary* adenocarcinoma pushing concentrically toward the lumen (Figs. 21.2 and 21.3). A less common form of the papillary type is the *alveolar* variety, in which a gland pattern is simulated by the fusion of the papillary folds.

Clinical Characteristics

The symptoms are not distinctive and in most cases they are so slight that the disease is well advanced before the patient seeks advice. *Postmenopausal bleeding* is the most common presenting complaint and the possibility of a tubal carcinoma should be entertained if routine evaluation, including dilatation and curettage, fails to delineate the cause. *Abnormal discharge* and *pelvic pain*, often cramping in nature, are also common symptoms.

Occasionally a profuse but sporadic serosanguineous vaginal discharge may occur, and if heed is given to this symptom of *hemohydrops tubae profluens*, an occasional preoperative diagnosis may be possible.

A palpable adnexal mass is occasionally noted in the asymptomatic patient, but this is usually attributed to an ovarian tumor since the latter is far more common.

Treatment

The treatment consists of hysterectomy with bilateral removal of the adnexa. Postoperative pelvic radiation is ordinarily employed, but there is some question as to its value. In early cases with no microscopic residual tumor, Benedet et al. recommended

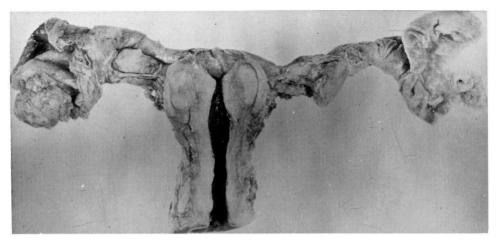

Figure 21.1.   Carcinoma, *left*; note fungoid lesion extruding from fimbria. Hydrosalpinx, *right*. (Courtesy of Dr. Albert Brown, Wilmingon, North Carolina.)

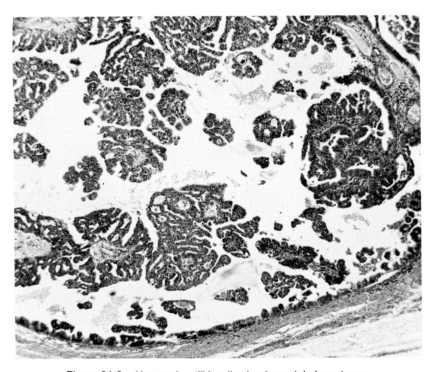

Figure 21.2.   Very early, still localized, primary tubal carcinoma.

intraperitoneal instillation of radioactive chromic phosphate.

The 5-year survival rate for all stages is generally reported to be between 34% (Sedlis) and 45% (Hanton et al.), but Benedet found eight of nine patients with Stage I disease alive and well at 5 years. In a large review of 76 cases, Schiller and Silverberg noted a 5-year survival of 91% for patients with intramural lesions, 53% with tubal involvement not reaching the serosa, and 25% or less with more advanced lesions. Boronow suggests that chemotherapy may be helpful in patients with metastatic disease.

Secondary Carcinoma

Secondary carcinoma (Figs. 21.4) of the tube is far more frequent than the primary

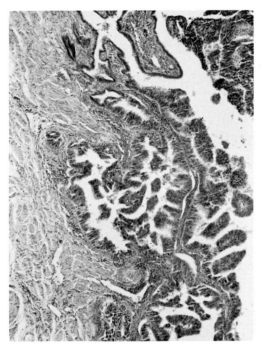

Figure 21.3.   Early lesion showing origin from "normal" tubal epithelium above and adenomatous pattern in center.

form, as might be expected from the position of the tube between the uterus and ovary. Pelvic tumors of the ovary, uterus or colon may involve the tube by means of directed extension, surface implantation, or lymphatic spread.

OTHER TUMORS OF THE TUBE

Other tumors of the tube are rare, some exceedingly so. Malignant mixed mesodermal tumors, primary choriocarcinoma following tubal pregnancy, sarcoma, fibroma, fibromyoma, and dermoid cysts have all been reported. Endometriosis, although not a true neoplasm, not infrequently involves the tubes and may simulate malignancy. Metastatic tumor from many different primary locations, especially the ovary, uterus, and bowel, often involves the tube.

PARAOVARIAN CYSTS

Paraovarian cysts may arise from vestigal portions of the Wolffian duct, from tubal epithelium, or from peritoneal inclusions. In a series of 132 cysts, Genandry et al. found that 68% arose from the mesothelial epithelium of peritoneal inclusions, 30% from tubal epithelium with a thin layer of surrounding

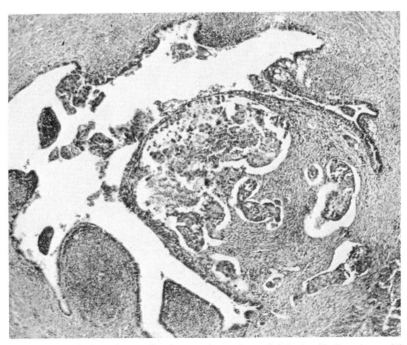

Figure 21.4.   Secondary tubal carcinoma showing carcinoma beneath intact epithelium. Loss of the epithelium would give the impression of implantation of cancer on the surface instead of spread by lymphatics.

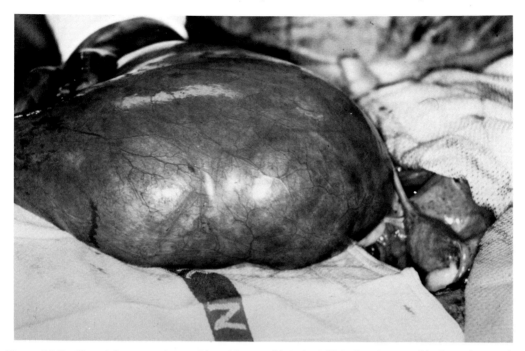

Figure 21.5. Huge left paraovarian cyst in a 19 year old student. Note the uterus and both ovaries can be seen in the lower right. The left ovary was not involved.

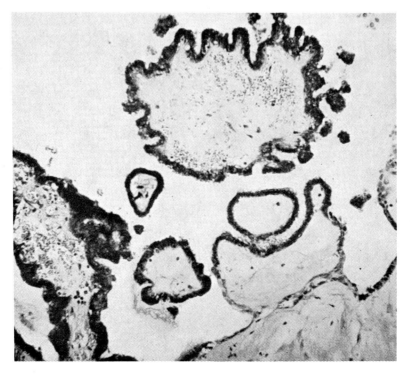

Figure 21.6. Microscopic appearance of wall of paraovarian cyst showing a low columnar epithelium and often, as in this case, a papillary tendency.

muscles, and only 2% were derived from Wolffian remnants.

Paraovarian cysts are usually small but on occasion very large cysts can be seen (Fig. 21.5). They are easily recognizable as of paraovarian origin by their position, the ovary being intact and separate from the tumor, and the tube being stretched across the upper circumference of the cyst. The walls are very thin and the cavity contains a clear fluid. *Microscopically*, cysts of peritoneal origin are lined by a single layer of cuboidal or flat epithelium surrounded by a fibrous, fatty capsule (Fig. 21.6). Cysts of tubal derivation usually have secretory epithelium, occasionally ciliated with a thin surrounding muscular layer. The rare Wolffian cysts have a thicker muscular wall.

TUMORS OF UTERINE LIGAMENTS

Like the uterus, the associated ligaments are made up of smooth muscle and leiomyomas are the most common tumor. Large intraligamentous myomas may develop between the leaves of the broad ligament presenting a challenging surgical problem. Cysts or adenocarcinomas arising from a remnant of the Wolffian duct may rarely be encountered. The pelvic ligaments are also frequent sites of endometriosis. The uterosacral ligaments are commonly involved when endometriosis is present and often give rise to low sacral or coccygeal pain.

References and Additional Readings

Benedet, J. L., White, G. W., Fairey, R. N., and Boyes, D. A.: Adenocarcinoma of the fallopian tube. Obstet. Gynecol., *50:* 654, 1977.

Boronow, R. C.: Chemotherapy for disseminated tubal carcinoma. Obstet. Gynecol., *42:* 62, 1973.

Boutselis, J. G., and Thompson, J. N.: Clinical aspects of primary tubal carcinoma. Am. J. Obstet. Gynecol., *111:* 98, 1971.

Dodson, M. G., Ford, J. M., Jr., and Avenette, H. E.: Clinical aspects of fallopian tube carcinoma. Obstet. Gynecol., *36:* 935, 1970.

Genandry, R., Parmley, T., and Woodruff, J. D.: The origin and clinical behavior of the parovarian tumor. Am. J. Obstet. Gynecol., *129:* 873, 1977.

Goldman, J. A., Gans, B., and Eckerling, B.: Hydrops tubae profluens—a symptom of tubal carcinoma. Obstet. Gynecol., *18:* 631, 1961.

Green, T. H., Jr., and Scully, R. E.: Tumors of the fallopian tube. Clin. Obstet. Gynecol., *5:* 886, 1962.

Hanton, E. M., Malkasian, G. D., Dahlin, D. C., and Pratt, J. H.: Primary carcinoma of the fallopian tube (27 cases). Am. J. Obstet. Gynecol., *94:* 832, 1966.

Hayden, G. E., and Potter, E. L.: Primary carcinoma of the fallopian tube. Am. J. Obstet. Gynecol., *79:* 24, 1960.

Janovski, N. A., and Paramanandhan, T. L.: *Ovarian Tumors, Tumorous and Tumorlike Conditions of the Ovaries, Fallopian Tubes, and Ligaments of the Uterus.* W. B. Saunders Co., Philadelphia, 1973.

Kinzel, G. E.: Primary carcinoma of the fallopian tube. Am. J. Obstet. Gynecol., *125:* 816, 1976.

Larsson, E., and Schooby, J. L.: Positive vaginal cytology in primary carcinoma of the fallopian tube. Am. J. Obstet. Gynecol., *22:* 1369, 1956.

Schiller, H. M., and Silverberg, S. G.: Staging and prognosis in primary carcinoma of the fallopian tube. Cancer, *28:* 389, 1971.

Sedlis, A.: Carcinoma of the fallopian tube. Surg. Clin. North Am., *58:* 121, 1978.

Woodruff, J. D., and Pauerstein, C. J.: *The Fallopian Tube.* Williams & Wilkins, Baltimore, 1969.

CHAPTER 22

Epithelial Tumors of the Ovary

CLASSIFICATION OF OVARIAN TUMORS—EPITHELIAL TUMORS

The ovary is unique in the range and variety of tumors that may arise from it and the numbers of malignant tumors from other primary sites that can metastasize to it. The spectrum of neoplasia that develops from this organ is continuous and infinite. All attempts at simplistic taxonomy leave much to "fall between the cracks." Efforts to achieve the ultimate in classification lead to a system that is cumbersome and unwieldy. Such is the case with the World Health Organization Histologic Classification that appears below. "This classification is based primarily on the microscopic characteristics of the tumors and thus reflects the nature of morphologically identifiable cell types and patterns."

WORLD HEALTH ORGANIZATION CLASSIFICATION OF OVARIAN TUMORS

I. Common "epithelial" tumors
  A. Serous tumors
    1. Benign
      a. Cystadenoma and papillary cystadenoma
      b. Surface papilloma
      c. Adenofibroma and cystadenofibroma
    2. Of borderline malignancy (carcinomas of low malignant potential)
      a. Cystadenoma and papillary cystadenoma
      b. Surface papilloma
      c. Adenofibroma and cystadenofibroma
    3. Malignant
      a. Adenocarcinoma, papillary adenocarcinoma, and papillary cystadenocarcinoma
      b. Surface papillary carcinoma
      c. Malignant adenofibroma and cystadenofibroma
  B. Mucinous tumors
    1. Benign
      a. Cystadenoma
      b. Adenofibroma and cystadenofibroma
    2. Of borderline malignancy (carcinomas of low malignant potential)
      a. Cystadenoma
      b. Adenofibroma and cystadenofibroma
    3. Malignant
      a. Adenocarcinoma and cystadenocarcinoma
      b. Malignant adenofibroma and cystadenofibroma
  C. Endometrioid tumors
    1. Benign
      a. Adenoma and cystadenoma
      b. Adenofibroma and cystadenofibroma
    2. Of borderline malignancy (carcinomas of low malignant potential)
      a. Adenoma and cystadenoma
      b. Adenofibroma and cystadenofibroma
    3. Malignant
      a. Carcinoma
        (1) Adenocarcinoma
        (2) Adenoacanthoma
        (3) Malignant adenofibroma and cystadenofibroma
      b. Endometrioid stromal sarcomas

c. Mesodermal (mullerian) mixed tumors, homologous and heterologous
D. Clear cell (mesonephroid) tumors
1. Benign: adenofibroma
2. Of borderline malignancy (carcinomas of low malignant potential)
3. Malignant: carcinoma and adenocarcinoma
E. Brenner tumors
1. Benign
2. Of borderline malignancy (proliferating)
3. Malignant
F. Mixed epithelial tumors
1. Benign
2. Of borderline malignancy
3. Malignant
G. Undifferentiated carcinoma
H. Unclassified epithelial tumors
II. Sex cord stromal tumors
A. Granulosa-stromal cell tumors
1. Granulosa cell tumor
2. Tumors in the thecoma-fibroma group
a. Thecoma
b. Fibroma
c. Unclassified
B. Androblastomas; Sertoli-Leydig cell tumors
1. Well differentiated
a. Tubular androblastoma; Sertoli cell tumor (tubular adenoma of Pick)
b. Tubular androblastoma with lipid storage; Sertoli cell tumor with lipid storage (folliculome lipidique of Lecene)
c. Sertoli-Leydig cell tumor (tubular adenoma with Leydig cells)
d. Leydig cell tumor; hilus cell tumor
2. Of intermediate differentiation
3. Poorly differentiated (sarcomatoid)
4. With heterologous elements
C. Gynandroblastoma
D. Unclassified
III. Lipid (lipoid) cell tumors
IV. Germ cell tumors
A. Dysgerminoma
B. Endodermal sinus tumor
C. Embryonal carcinoma
D. Polyembryoma
E. Choriocarcinoma
F. Teratomas
1. Immature
2. Mature
a. Solid
b. Cystic
(1) Dermoid cyst (mature cystic teratoma)
(2) Dermoid cyst with malignant transformation
3. Monodermal and highly specialized
a. Struma ovarii
b. Carcinoid
c. Struma ovarii and carcinoid
d. Others
G. Mixed forms
V. Gonadoblastoma
A. Pure
B. Mixed with dysgerminoma or other form of germ cell tumor
VI. Soft tissue tumors not specific to ovary
VII. Unclassified tumors
VIII. Secondary (metastatic) tumors
IX. Tumor-like conditions
A. Pregnancy luteoma
B. Hyperplasia of ovarian stroma and hyperthecosis
C. Massive edema
D. Solitary follicle cyst and corpus luteum cyst
E. Multiple follicle cysts (polycystic ovaries)
F. Multiple luteinized follicle cysts and/or corpora lutea
G. Endometriosis
H. Surface-epithelial inclusion cysts (germinal inclusion cysts)
I. Simple cysts
J. Inflammatory lesions
K. Paraovarian cysts

Before going on to simplify this classification, it is important to make several statements that will facilitate its comprehension. (1) The "so-called" germinal epithelium that overlies the ovary is modified peritoneum. The term "germinal" refers to the fact that it was originally felt to be the source of the germ cells. It is now common knowledge that this is not the case and authors prefer to classify those tumors that arise from this epithelium as "epithelial tumors of the ovary." It is to be recalled from the discussion of the development of the Müllerian system in Chapter 6 that the Müllerian duct arises as a bilateral structure in embryos of about 11 mm. The mesenchyme of the ovary and the mesenchymal structure of the adult Müllerian system are also similarly related. It is not at all surprising, then, to find that when this epithelium undergoes neoplastic change it frequently resembles, to a greater or lesser degree, the adult tissues of the tube, uterus, and vagina. Nor is it unreasonable to imagine that tumors of the ovary might appear similar to, or identical to, other spontaneous neoplasms of the Müllerian system. For this reason, epithelial tumors of the ovary are classified so that they keep this resemblance in mind. Those that resemble the tube are called serous, those that mimic the endometrium, endometrial tumors, and those that appear similar to the endocervix are classified as mucinous tumors. Clear cell carcinomas, Brenner tumors, and mixed mesodermal tumors are also felt to arise from this epithelial origin and can arise primarily along the Müllerian system. (2) The sex cord stromal tumor grouping listed above is designated as gonadal stromal or mesenchymal tumors in many classifications. The reason for this is that they were originally felt to arise from the ovarian stroma. There is considerable debate as to whether the epithelial element in this group of tumors arise from the ovarian stroma, hence the hesitation by some to call them stromal tumors. On the other hand, there are no sex cords in the female gonad and this term is objectionable to others. Suffice it to say that this large category of tumors include those that contain granulosa cells, theca cells, collagen-producing stromal cells, Sertoli cells, Leydig cells, and cells resembling their embryonic forerunners. They may occur as a pure line of cells or in any combination. We chose to use the term gonadal stromal tumors and will carry that terminology through the remainder of the text.

HISTOLOGIC CLASSIFICATION OF
OVARIAN TUMORS

I. Common "epithelial" tumors
  A. Serous tumors
    1. Benign
    2. Borderline malignancy
    3. Malignant
  B. Mucinous tumors
    1. Benign
    2. Borderline malignancy
    3. Malignant
  C. Endometrioid tumors
  D. Clear cell (mesonephroid) tumors
  E. Brenner tumors
    1. Benign
    2. Borderline malignancy (proliferating)
    3. Malignant
  F. Mixed epithelial tumors
    1. Benign
    2. Borderline
    3. Malignant
  G. Undifferentiated carcinoma
II. Gonadal stromal tumors
  A. Granulosa-thecal cell tumor
  B. Thecoma (to include fibroma)
  C. Sertoli-Leydig cell tumor
    (arrhenoblastoma)
  D. Gynandroblastoma
  E. Nonspecific gonadal stromal tumors
III. Lipid (lipoid) cell tumors
IV. Germ cell tumors
  A. Dysgerminoma
  B. Endodermal sinus tumor
  C. Malignant (immature) teratoma
  D. Benign (mature) teratoma
  E. Struma ovarii
  F. Carcinoid
  G. Embryonal cell carcinoma
  H. Choriocarcinoma
V. Gonadoblastoma
VI. Unclassified tumors
VII. Secondary of metastic tumors

Nonneoplastic (Functional) Cysts of the Ovary

The approach toward the diagnosis and management of epithelial tumors of the ovary must contain some information about the nonneoplastic cysts. Most neoplasms of the ovary are cystic and require differentiation from the functional or nonneoplastic cysts, since the latter rarely require therapy and the former nearly always do. The following is a discussion of such cysts.

Follicle Cysts

These arise from simple cystic overdistention of follicles during the process of atresia (see Chapter 3). Every month a considerable number of follicles are blighted, with death of the oocyte, followed soon by degeneration of the follicular epithelium. Frequently, the cavity is greatly overdistended with fluid, producing cysts of clinically important size, although they only rarely exceed the size of a lemon, and are usually much smaller. Hemorrhage into the cyst cavity may take place, producing the so-called follicular hematoma.

Symptoms. The symptoms of follicle cysts are not characteristic, but distinctive effects on menstruation may be produced. When the cyst is sufficiently large, it may cause a sensation of heaviness or a dull aching discomfort in the effected side. As with any other type of ovarian cyst *torsion* of the pedicle may occur, and in rare cases, *spontaneous rupture with intraabdominal bleeding* producing a clinical picture simulating ruptured tubal pregnancy. Far more frequently, however, *spontaneous resorption* takes place, just as in the normal process of atresia folliculi.

Diagnosis. The diagnosis can be made only by palpation of the cyst, but it is not possible at one examination to be sure whether the cyst is of the nonneoplastic variety or whether it is a genuine cystic tumor such as cystadenoma. One should, therefore, avoid prompt operation for small ovarian cysts. It is a common observation that cysts are frequently evanescent, and the gynecologist who is absolutely certain at one examination that he feels a cyst as large as a lemon may find on reexamination a few weeks later that the ovary has regressed to normal size. By contrast, the neoplastic type of cyst not only persists but gradually increases in size. With younger women, expectant therapy is indicated over the course of 8–10 weeks before deciding on laparotomy; in the middle age group, evaluation should not be so prolonged, and in the postmenopausal patient, any adnexal enlargement warrants prompt laparotomy. (Barber and Graber)

Treatment. When small follicle cysts are found at operation, they are best treated by either simple puncture (needling) or excision, depending upon their size. When the cyst is larger, it can be shelled out, often intact, with conservation of the normal ovarian tissue.

Lutein Cysts

The term "lutein cyst" is generally used collectively, although it is important clinically to consider the possibility of pregnancy lest removal of the cyst increase the chances of abortion, especially in the first trimester of pregnancy. Lutein cysts (Figs. 22.1 and 22.2) may, of course, occur in the absence of pregnancy.

The origin of the true lutein cyst is usually from a corpus luteum hematoma. The latter, in turn, is brought about by an exaggeration of the hemorrhage which normally takes place into the corpus cavity in the so-called stage of vascularization. When the bleeding is excessive, a large *corpus luteum hematoma* is produced, characterized chiefly by a thinned out, bright yellow lutein wall about the blood-filled central cavity. Gradually, however, there is a resorption of the blood elements, leaving a clear or slightly bloody fluid.

Symptoms. The symptoms of lutein cysts cannot always be correlated with their histological appearance. In the most interesting group, the symptoms resemble those of early tubal pregnancy. Menstruation is apt to be slightly delayed, followed by persistent scant bleeding, with often pain in one or the other of the lower quadrants, and with the presence on pelvic examination of a small tender swelling in the corresponding side of the pelvis. This represents the characteristic symptoma-

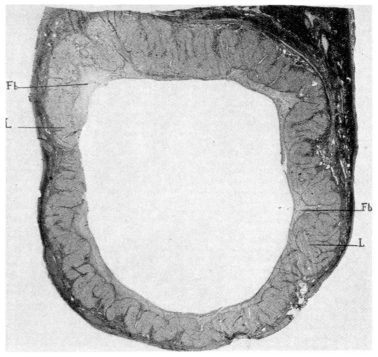

Figure 22.1. Cystic but functionally normal corpus luteum.

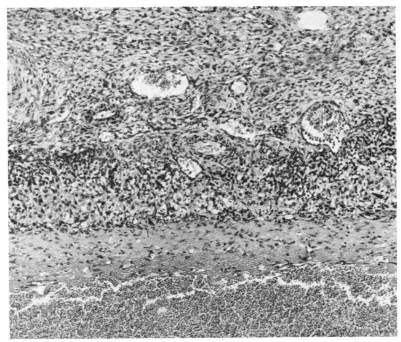

Figure 22.2.   Wall of lutein cyst.

tology of early tubal pregnancy, and yet not infrequently one may find at operation a lutein cyst instead.

There is some belief that such cases represent very early abortion of a fertilized but as yet unimplanted egg, although there is no direct evidence to substantiate this view. Others look upon the syndrome as identical with that of the so-called *corpus luteum persistens*, in which the normal regression of the corpus is deferred, with persistence of the progestational phase in the endometrium, through a mechanism which may be similar to the pseudopregnancy observed in some of the lower animals.

A rare type of lutein cyst is that found in some cases of hydatidiform mole and choriocarcinoma. In some cases of this sort, the wall of the cyst is formed by luteinized granulosal cells, but usually the cyst is composed of paralutein (*theca-lutein*) cells of connective tissue rather than epithelial origin. A review by Caspi et al. records 29 cases not associated with molar pregnancy. These cystic changes may be produced by administration of human chorionic gonadotropin (hCG).

Diagnosis. The diagnosis of lutein cysts is obviously difficult and, in the majority of cases, their presence is not suspected before operation. When of considerable size they can of course be palpated. In a small group of cases the presence of a cyst of this character can be at least suspected when a symptom complex like that of tubal pregnancy is produced. When such a problem arises, pregnancy tests may be of service, for they are often positive in tubal gestation, and negative in the corpus luteum cysts. Culdoscopy or laparoscopy is more conclusive.

Treatment. The treatment of lutein cysts or hematomas consists of observation, for most of them undergo spontaneous disappearance. In the case of hemorrhagic cysts of considerable size, or where there is evidence of intraperitoneal bleeding, excision is the proper treatment, for massive hemoperitoneum may occur. At times, the yellowish shimmer of the wall gives a clue to the lutein character of the cyst, and in such cases the surgeon should, before removal of the cyst, consider the possibility of very early gestation. In a large proportion of cases the lutein character of the cyst is not suspected before laboratory examination.

It has been noted that functional cysts are relatively uncommon in women taking birth control pills as a result of suppression of the pituitary. This may be of assistance clinically—if a cyst persists after 2 months of pill therapy, it is more likely neoplastic rather than functional.

Germinal Inclusion Cysts

Germinal inclusion cysts (Fig. 22.3) have been given a relatively low priority in previous editions of this text. To be sure, they are a very frequent incidental finding, microscopic in size, and asymptomatic. They are most frequent in women late in their reproductive career and probably arise secondary to entrapment of surface ovarian epithelium within the stroma of the ovary following ovulation. Subsequent to this sequestration, the epithelial lining of the cysts becomes taller and, frequently, more differentiated. At times, the cells are low and cuboidal with rounded nuclei but on other occasions they resemble ciliated and secretory epithelium of the fallopian tube, a single layer of mucinous epithelium, or multiple layers of squamous epithelium. It is now widely accepted that they represent the forerunners of frank epithelial neoplasms but there is general confusion as to when they cease to be just an inclusion and finally become a cystadenoma. Other queries surround the role that the ovarian stroma plays in the induction of these preneoplastic changes. It is interesting to remember that the embryonic mesenchyme of the urogenital ridge induces proliferation of the Müllerian plate epithelium when it folds into it to form the Müllerian tubal system. It is a general embryologic precept that the mesenchyme is the determining factor in the proliferation and differentiation of the contiguous epithelia. It is also of some interest that the pelvic peritoneum retains its capability to recapitulate Müllerian epithelium by way of metaplasia but that this propensity decreases at increasing distance from the ovary.

EPITHELIAL TUMORS

These tumors are frequently cystic and in the past have been classified as such. They make up approximately 60–70% of all primary neoplasms of the ovary and account for an astounding 90% of all ovarian malignancies. As noted in the prior segment of this chapter discussing germinal inclusion cysts, they are thought to arise from the coelomic epithelium or modified peritoneum overlying the ovary. The World Health Organization has applied the word "Common" to this group of tumors to underline their numerical importance in the general scheme of ovarian neoplasia. Both this organization and the International Federation of Gynecology and Obstetrics (FIGO) recognize a benign, malignant, and borderline category for each epithelial variety. The borderline tumor is de-

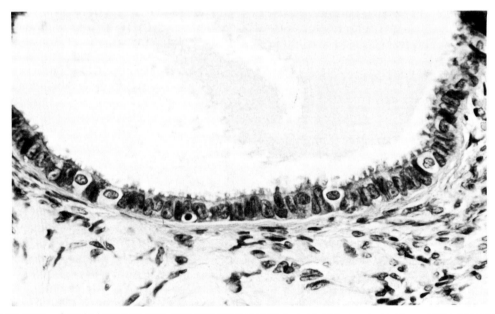

Figure 22.3. Germinal inclusion cyst. Note typical tubal epithelium of ciliated and secretory variety. Note also ''indifferent'' cell at *center* of field.

fined as one that has "some, but not all, of the morphologic features of malignancy." These include varying combinations and degrees of: mitotic activity, cellular stratification, detached cellular clusters, and nuclear atypia. All of these are intermediate between overt malignancy and tumors that are unquestionably benign. It is, again, worth noting that only taxonomists, pathologists, and clinicians herd these tumors into groups. Nature provides a panoramic spectrum of neoplasia and they pass imperceptably from benign all the way to exceedingly malignant. The virtue of classification and subdivision is that it gives the clinician a rough frame of reference as to their biologic behavior and, perhaps, response to treatment. Although the borderline category of tumors have been reasonably well defined in the serous, mucinous, and Brenner categories, this is not true of the remainder of the epithelial categories.

When reviewing any number of these tumors with the light microscope, one cannot help but be struck by the fact that although the majority are characterized by a predominence of one cell type it is quite common to see other epithelial variants present in varying degrees. These findings are confirmed by electron microscopic studies. When this is pronounced, the tumors are categorized as "mixed."

In the course of malignant transformation, cells frequently lose their capability to function as, or resemble, mature epithelium. When this occurs, the tumor is said to be relatively undifferentiated. At times, the lack of differentiation is such that it is impossible to state in which category the tumor belongs. Most of these are probably poorly differentiated variants of serous or endometrioid carcinoma.

Clinical Staging

For the purposes of future discussions regarding the borderline and malignant epithelial tumors, it is mandatory to adopt a widely accepted staging system. This allows clinicians and pathologists to compare tumors in terms of their biologic behavior and response to therapy. The following is that proposed by the Cancer Committee of FIGO. Although not perfect, it is a very usable staging system. It is to be noted that this particular staging system differs from the FIGO staging for uterine carcinoma. The latter is a clinical system that does not allow information

gleaned from laparotomy. For ovarian carcinoma, all information—clinical, operative, and pathologic—is usable for staging purposes.

FIGO CLASSIFICATION OF CLINICAL STAGING

Stage I	Growth limited to the ovaries
Stage Ia	Growth limited to one ovary; no ascites
(i)	No tumor on the external surface; capsule intact
(ii)	Tumor present on the external surface or/and capsule ruptured
Stage Ib	Growth limited to both ovaries; no ascites
(i)	No tumor on the external surface; capsules intact
(ii)	Tumor present on the external surface or/and capsule(s) ruptured
Stage Ic	Tumor either Stage Ia or Stage Ib, but with ascites[1] present or positive peritoneal washings
Stage II	Growth involving one or both ovaries with pelvic extension
Stage IIa	Extension and/or metastases to the uterus and/or tubes
Stage IIb	Extension to other pelvic tissues
Stage IIc	Tumor either Stage IIa or Stage IIb, but with ascites present or positive peritoneal washings
Stage III	Growth involving one or both ovaries with intraperitoneal metastases outside the pelvis and/or positive retroperitoneal nodes. Tumor limited to the true pelvis with histologically proven malignant extension to small bowel or omentum
Stage IV	Growth involving one or both ovaries with distant metastases. If pleural effusion is present there must be positive cytology to allot a case to Stage IV. Parenchymal liver metastases equals Stage IV
Special category	Unexplored cases which are thought to be ovarian carcinoma

Serous Tumors

Benign

Although serous cysts may reach a size of many pounds, they do not as a group attain

---

[1] Ascites is peritoneal effusion which in the opinion of the surgeon is pathologic and/or clearly exceed normal amounts.

the enormous proportions of some cases of the mucinous variety.

Grossly, the external appearance may be similar to that of the mucinous cysts but, in other cases, the surface presents papillomatous outgrowths which may in some instances resemble a cauliflower pattern. In fact, if one notes this papillary external growth, it is reasonably certain that the cyst is of serous type.

The content is generally a thin watery fluid, but may be hemorrhagic or brownish in color. The inner wall of the cyst may be entirely smooth, so that, with the smaller growths, it is difficult to distinguish the cyst from one of simple follicular variety. More characteristically, one finds warty excrescences, sometimes small and discrete, in other cases filling the cyst cavities. Unlike the mucinous cystadenoma, this *papillomatous tendency* is very characteristic of the serous growths.

Microscopically (Fig. 22.4), the epithelium of serous cysts is quite different from that of the mucinous tumors, and it presents much more variation in the individual cases. In general it is of much lower columnar type, with ciliation of many of the cells, so that there is a striking resemblance to tubal epithelium, which likewise is made up of ciliated and nonciliated columnar cells. In other tumors, or in other parts of the same cyst wall, the epithelium may be cuboidal or peg-

shaped. The stroma is fibrous, with often hydropic degeneration. Rather characteristic of this variety of cyst is the frequent presence of small calcareous granules, the so-called *psammoma bodies*, an end product of the tumor implants (Fig. 22.5).

When the epithelium is of the above type, and arranged in a single layer, there is no doubt of the benign nature of the cyst, at least from a histological standpoint.

Histogenesis. Although there may be differences of opinion about the origins of mucinous cysts, there is little doubt that the origin of the serous type is from the surface epithelium of the ovary.

Fibroadenoma and Cystadenofibroma

These tumors are properly considered here because their histogenesis is so closely allied to that of serous cystadenoma. Like the latter, they arise from the surface epithelium of the ovary, which undergoes invagination, with the formation of long, cleftlike tubules surrounded by hyperplastic fibrous tissue, similar to the ordinary fibroadenoma of the breast. Such lesions are therefore disignated as *fibroadenoma of the ovary*. They are usually of small size, and may be found only on microscopic examination (Figs. 22.6 and 22.7).

On the other hand, the invaginations often

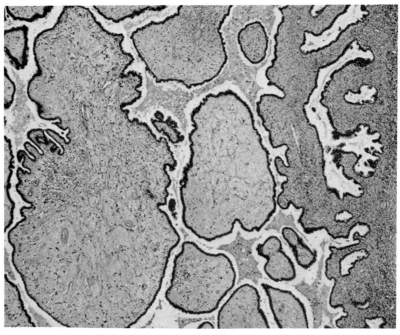

Figure 22.4. Benign serous papillomatous cystadenoma.

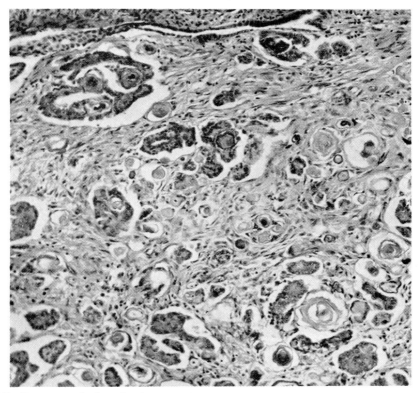

Figure 22.5. Psammoma bodies showing transition between recognizable papillae and acellular calcified bodies.

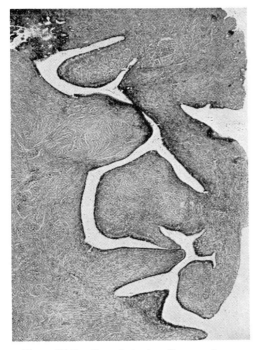

Figure 22.6. So-called adenofibroma of ovary.

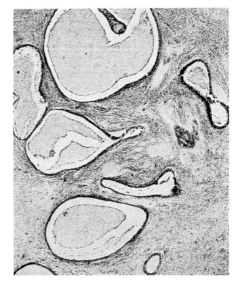

Figure 22.7. Section of cystadenofibroma.

become cystic and may attain large size. Such tumors, designated as *cystadenofibroma*, are usually partly cystic and partly solid, in varying proportions. When small, they form dense whitish, partly cystic nodules near the surface, but when large they may replace all or nearly all the ovarian substance. They are benign, but in rare cases may become malignant.

Borderline Malignancy

For many years there have been described by clinicians and pathologists a group of proliferative serous tumors of the ovary, associated with multiple peritoneal "implants" that appear clinically malignant but are histologically benign. A number of investigators in the last decade have reported that patients with these lesions have a very favorable prognosis. Conversely, their overtly malignant counterparts are associated with an extremely poor survival rate. Among epithelial tumors of the ovary, it is not uncommon, as noted above, to have a mixture of cell types and nonhomogenous differentiation. A careful analysis of each tumor with multiple sections is mandatory. Nevertheless, if the cell type remains uniform throughout the tumor, the clinical course can be predicted quite accurately. More importantly, that clinical course differs considerably from the traditional serous cystadenocarcinomas. Also of significant consequence is the fact that a considerable percentage of nonbenign serous tumors fall into this category.

Pathology. The tumors are largely cystic and characterized by one major cavity with smaller cavities within the larger one. Microscopically the cells of this tumor are those seen in the common germinal inclusions of the ovarian cortex, i.e. the ciliated secretory and mesothelial varieties (Figs. 22.6–22.8). The latter may be flattened or ovoid with abundant eosinophilic cytoplasm and a more or less centrally placed nucleus with finely granular chromatin. Mitoses are rare, 1 or less/hpf; however, small cells with hyperchromatic nuclei, similar to the indifferent cell of the uterine tube are prominent. The key to the proliferative tendencies is the formation of the "true papillus," a definable demonstration of atypical epithelial activity. The epithelium covering the papillae is frequently piled up into several layers. Loose cellular clusters are often found freely suspended in the cyst fluid. Those tumors that have external papillation undoubtedly shed cells into the peritoneal cavity. Psammoma bodies are exceedingly common and numerous. The proliferating epithelium may have mild or moderate atypicality of the nucleii. Necessary to the definition of borderline tumors is the

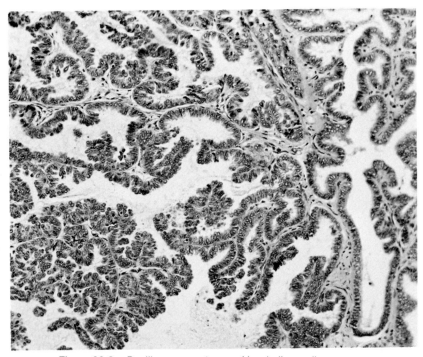

Figure 22.8. Papillary serous tumor of borderline malignancy.

absence of stromal infiltration with epithelial cells. At times, tangential sectioning makes this difficult to interpret.

Clinical Features. Among overtly malignant papillary serous tumors the borderline lesions differ significantly from the overtly malignant tumors in the extent of disease at the time of diagnosis. Over 50% of the tumors are apparently confined to one or both ovaries at the time of operative diagnosis. As a general rule, over three quarters of the malignant variant are beyond the ovaries at the time of diagnosis.

For the most part, the patients are asymptomatic at the time of diagnosis.

Surgical management is the keystone of treatment in all ovarian malignancy but its role is of even greater significance here. There is no objective evidence that the tumor responds in a significant fashion either to radiotherapy or chemotherapy, and sometimes repeated partial excision of recurrences can keep the patient alive and well for many years. Since many of the patients are quite young at the time of diagnosis (nearly 20% in the same series under the age of 30) the question of preservation of childbearing capacity arises when the tumor appears to be confined to one ovary. When the tumor has no external papillations and careful staging fails to reveal any evidence of disease elsewhere, this is probably a reasonable approach. A note of caution should be introduced here, since this tumor has a great propensity for widespread intraperitoneal extension even when not perceptible by gross examination.

Malignant

Serous Cystadenocarcinoma

This represents the overtly malignant form of serous cystadenoma. It is much more common than the mucinous variety, and is almost always characterized by a papillary architecture. The papillary growth is not infrequently present on the surface as well as within the cavity (Fig. 22.9). All grades of transition may be seen between the picture of serous tumors of borderline malignancy and that characterized by almost solid papillary masses. Woodruff and Julian have stressed the importance of microscopic grading of these lesions and their relationship to prognosis (Fig. 22.10). Many pathologists have emphasized the importance of numerous pathological sections from many areas of the lesion, for an ovarian tumor can show a highly variegated appearance, from the extremely benign to the highly malignant.

The *microscopic examination* often presents considerable difficulty, especially in the cases in which the gross appearance is much like that of the benign or borderline lesions. The number of mitotic figures/hpf has been of considerable value in gauging prognosis and this has led us to utilize this in grading this variety of tumor (Table 22.1).

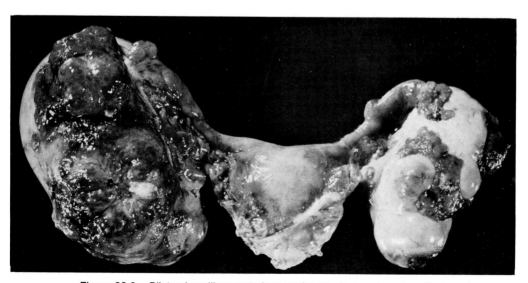

Figure 22.9. Bilateral papillary cystadenocarcinomas (note external papillae).

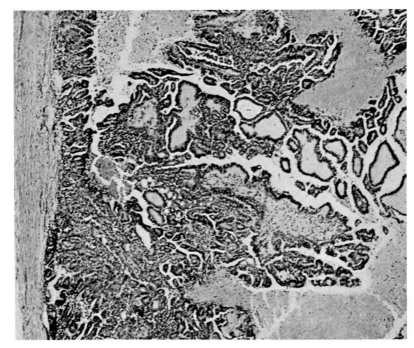

Figure 22.10. Histologically malignant papillary vegetations lining interior of serous cystadenocarcinoma although capsule is smooth (6-year-old girl). (Courtesy of Dr. Don. Walcott, San Jose, California.)

Table 22.1

Mitoses	Number of Cases	Living	Dead	5-Year Salvage
Borderline (0–1)	14	12	2	85
Grade 1 (2–5)	21	9	12	41
Grade 2 (6–15)	29	3	26	10
Grade 3 (16+)	16	0	16	0
Total	80	24	56	30

Mucinous Tumors

Benign

Mucinous Cystadenoma

This variety may reach huge size and, as a matter of fact, many of the largest human tumors belong to this group.

Grossly these tumors appear as rounded, ovoid, or irregularly lobulated growths, with a smooth outer surface of whitish or bluish white hue. The wall may in many areas be so thin as to be translucent (Fig. 22.11). Although adhesions to surrounding organs may be present, they usually represent inflamma-tory adhesions and do not connote malignant extension. The attachment to the broad ligament is by a pedicle which may be quite narrow, but in some cases rather broad, with a markedly increased blood supply.

The *content* of the cyst is generally a clear, viscid fluid, sometimes very thick, at other times thin. Admixture of blood elements may give it a chocolate or brownish hue. The *cut surface* shows the cavity to be divided by septa into a varying number of compartments or locules.

Microscopically, the distinctive feature of mucinous cysts is the characteristic single layer, often of undulating outline, of tall, pale-staining, secretory epithelium, with nuclei placed at the basal poles of the cells (Fig. 22.12). Goblet cells are often seen. On occasion even Paneth and argentaffin cells are noted. In large cyst cavities, the epithelium may be more or less flattened, with patches of immature epithelium lower than the more characteristic picket cells that line most of the cyst.

Histogenesis. It would appear that a simple metaplasia of the lining germinal epithelium (mesothelium) of the ovary into a mucinous type of cell is the initial step in the evolution of this form of cyst. Thus it should cause no surprise to note that this lining cell of the ovary may reduplicate tumors seen in the tube, endometrium, or endocervix, for the mucinous ovarian tumor is histologically closely allied to certain mucinous tumors of the endocervix.

There are two relatively common observations that make it difficult to accept the surface epithelium as the source of all mucinous tumors of the ovary. The first is that 5% of them are noted in association with dermoid cysts. The second is the fact that at least 20% have a gastric or intestinal type epithelium rather than endocervical. These suggest that a significant number evolve as a consequence of unilateral progression of germ cell tumors.

Borderline Malignancy

Borderline mucinous tumors of the ovary are a less clearly defined category than the serous lesions. Nevertheless, they comprise a significant portion of those mucinous tumors that are not clearly benign. Of great significance in regard to preservation of the opposite ovary is the finding that only 10% are bilateral. Conversely, it would seem wise to remove the opposite ovary and the uterus if future childbearing was not desired.

Pathology. Grossly, the tumors are indistinguishable from both the benign and malignant tumors without extracapsular extension. Growth on the external surface of the tumor as well as extraovarian extension is uncom-

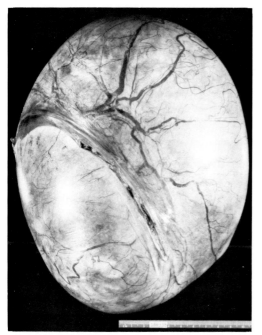

Figure 22.11. Mucinous cyst; note smooth, translucent wall.

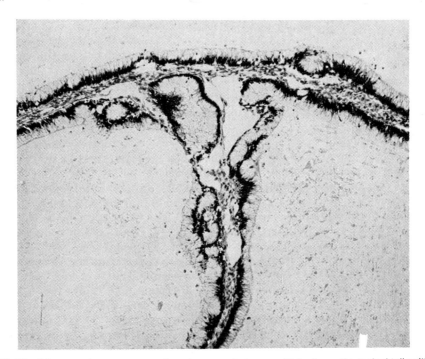

Figure 22.12. Microscopic appearance of mucinous cystadenoma. This shows the typical tall epithelium with nuclei at the base.

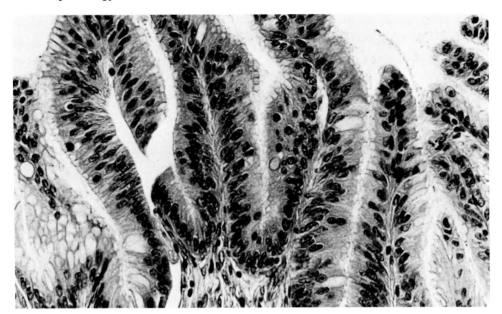

Figure 22.13. Mucinous carcinoma of ovary. Borderline malignancy. Note some "piling up" of epithelium and mild nuclear atypia.

mon, in marked contrast to the serous variant. Microscopically, the picture is not unlike that of an adenomatous polyp of the colon (Fig. 22.13). The tumor consists of cysts of varying size lined by multiple, short, papillary fronds. Secondary cyst formation and multiple, small, well defined mucin-secreting acini can be noted throughout the stroma. These parvilocular cysts make it difficult, at times, to ascertain stromal invasion. Lack of stromal invasion is a prerequisite of inclusion in this category. The cells lining the small cysts and covering the short, delicate papillary fronds are stratified into several layers (not more than three). There is some slight nuclear pleomorphism and loss of polarity as well as an occasional mitotic figure. The amount of intracellular mucin varies and is diminished in the more atypical cells. Mucinous tumors have a great propensity to vary in differentiation from field to field and the ultimate prognosis is related to the area of least differentiation. It is consequently very important that multiple sections be analyzed.

Pseudomyxoma peritoneii is a relatively uncommon and puzzling clinical situation in which there is found widespread peritoneal seeding with mucinous epithelium that is quite benign in appearance. There is often a massive accumulation within the peritoneal cavity of thick mucinous material that is almost impossible to extract through an ordinary paracentesis trocar. It is often associated with mucinous tumors of the ovary, mucocele of the appendix, and carcinoma of the large bowel. Although the etiology of this condition remains an enigma, it is to be looked upon as a widespread, low grade malignant change with an indolent but relentless course. Attempts at treatment with chemotherapy or radiotherapy have been uniformly unsuccessful. Repeated surgical attempts at removing portions of the tumor sometimes delays the progression of disease. Some have suggested the use of intraperitoneal radioactive phosphorus. This would be of value only if there were not significant bulk to the remaining tumor and if most of the mucinous material could be removed.

Malignant

Mucinous Cystadenocarcinoma

This is the malignant prototype of mucinous cystadenoma, or arises from the same tissue elements which give rise to the latter. Only about 5–10% of these undergo malignant degeneration; this occurrence is much less common than with the serous. The malignant disease may affect only a localized area of the cyst, but in most cases the latter is replaced by solid tumor (Fig. 22.14).

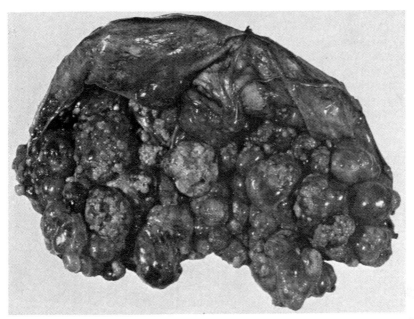

Figure 22.14. Typical gelatinous appearance of opened mucinous cystadenocarcinoma, multilocular and nonpapillary.

The *microscopic examination* shows the typical picture of adenocarcinoma, but all degrees of differentiation are possible. The cells usually retain their mucoid tendencies to a greater or less extent and, hence, one often finds large or small cavities filled with gelatinous material. Stromal invasion occurs along with stratification of the lining epithelium.

Endometrioid Tumors

Endometrioid Carcinoma

The concept originated with Sampson who, in 1925, suggested that certain cases of adenocarcinoma of the ovary arose in foci of benign ovarian endometriosis. In 1961, FIGO incorporated into their classification the group of tumors that resembled either the endometrium or tumors of the endometrium more than any other Müllerian epithelium. This was later adopted by the World Health Organization and included into their classification.

Pathology. The tumor, for the most part, appears to arise from the surface epithelium of the ovary and develop into neoplasms that are frequently cystic. Consequently, the microscopic growth characteristics are a bit different from those tumors that arise in the endometrium. They more frequently have a somewhat papillary architecture in some areas and are more commonly associated with other variants of neoplasia found in the Müllerian system, such as clear cell, mucinous, and serous carcinomas. The incidence of bilaterality is significant, comprising nearly one-third of the cases (Fig. 22.15).

Clinical features. The prognosis, as with the serous and mucinous tumors, is related to stage and differentiation. The overall prognosis, however, is better than that for the serous and mucinous variants and approximates 45% (5-year salvage).

A peculiarity that initiates a great deal of interest is the finding that there is an associated endometrial carcinoma in about 20% of the cases. The question always arises as to whether the tumor in the endometrium is the primary with subsequent metastases to the ovaries.

Mixed mesodermal tumors of the ovary are a very rare occurrence and probably rightfully belong as a variant of endometrioid carcinoma. The tumor, as with its endometrial counterpart, is a mixed malignancy of both epithelium and stroma and consequently is technically a carcinosarcoma. At times, other malignant mesodermal elements are present (Fig. 22.16) such as chondrosarcoma, liposarcoma, rhabdomyosarcoma, etc.

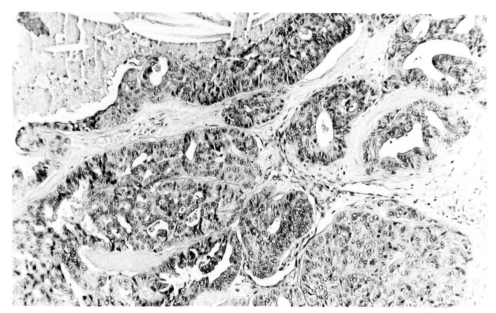

Figure 22.15. Typical endometrioid carcinoma of the ovary. Solid areas in *lower field*. Glandular arrangement typical of endometrial carcinoma—*upper right*.

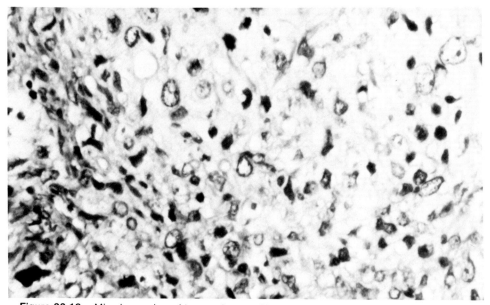

Figure 22.16. Mixed mesodermal tumor of ovary. Chondrosarcoma in *right upper corner* of figure.

When this is the case, the tumors are referred to as heterologous and, when absent, as homologous. Since it is identical to the similar lesion that arises primarily in the endometrium, it is suggested that the pathogenesis is similar. Because of the common embryonic origin of the surface epithelium of the ovary and the lining of the Müllerian system, these are commonly thought of as being of "epithelial" origin.

In a clinical sense, the disease is catastrophic. Unfortunately, patients usually do not present at an early stage of disease and it is far more common to make the diagnosis when the disease is quite advanced. The manner of extension is very much like that of other epithelial tumors of the ovary.

Clear Cell (Mesonephroid) Tumors of the Ovary

For years, differences of opinion over the origin of this particular tumor raged in the literature until, finally, the evidence is now nearly overwhelming. What we recognize as the so-called clear cell carcinoma of the genital tract, including the ovary, arises either from Müllerian epithelium or the embryologically similar epithelium that covers the surface of the ovary. Scully and Barlow present convincing evidence that at least some of these arise from the mature Müllerian epithelium in ovarian endometriosis; however, the majority of cases probably arise from neoplastic change in the surface ovarian epithelium. Clear cell carcinoma of the ovary comprises approximately 5% of all epithelial malignancies and differs enough from the remainder of the nonbenign group to earn a special taxonomic niche.

Pathology. In a large series presented by Rogers et al., the tumors were described as "cystic, solid, and semi-solid", and were usually freely movable although many authors point out that they are sometimes adherent (Fig. 22.17). In a series of 15 cases presented by Doshi and Tobon, 8 of 15 tumors ruptured during removal, and this is not an uncommon occurrence.

Clinical features. Among 78 patients in the series of Rogers et al., most patients were in the age group between 40 and 60 (58%), though there was a wide distribution with 14 patients under the age of 40. Fifty-one per cent were nulliparous.

As with most ovarian tumors, the patients were either asymptomatic or complained of vague abdominal discomfort and distention. Only 2 of 65 Stage I patients in the Rogers et al. series were bilateral and this is the lowest incidence to be noted in any of the nonbenign variants of epithelial tumors discussed so far.

Prognosis is related, for the most part, to stage; and attempts to correlate it with cellular architecture or cell type have not been fruitful for most investigators.

Brenner Tumors of the Ovary

It is only in recent years that this interesting tumor form has been recognized, largely through the investigations of Robert Meyer. Its *gross* (Fig. 22.18) characteristics are not unlike those of fibroma, and the *microscopic* (Fig. 22.19) structure of these tumors is characterized by the presence of *epithelial cell* nests or columns in a *fibromatous matrix*. The distribution of these cell nests throughout the stroma may at first suggest malignancy, but the cells show a remarkable uniformity, with not the slightest suggestion of anaplastic activity. The epithelioid cells often show a rather characteristic longitudinal "coffee-bean" grooving.

The characteristic cell nests often show a tendency to central cystic degeneration, the cavity often containing a cytoplasmic mass which superficially resembles an oocyte

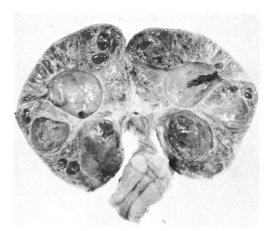

Figure 22.17. Gross appearance of cut surface of large clear cell carcinoma of the ovary (other ovary previously removed).

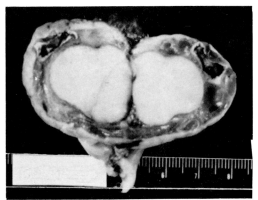

Figure 22.18. Brenner tumor arising from medullary or hilar area. Note intact cortex.

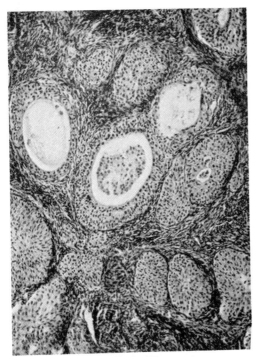

Figure 22.19. Typical Brenner tumor.

within a follicle. This indeed was the original interpretation, which led to the earlier designation of these tumors as "oophoroma folliculare."

Another interesting characteristic of some of these tumors is a tendency for *mucinous transformation*, so the cyst may contain areas resembling mucinous cystadenoma. Large cysts of the latter type may thus arise from Brenner tumors, although this is not the common origin of this type of cystadenoma, as described previously.

A close relationship between Brenner tumors and other tumors of the surface epithelium have been well documented in most large series.

Symptoms. Brenner tumors are rather rare, and they occur usually in older women, the majority of patients being beyond 50. They produce no characteristic symptoms, and the smaller ones are usually accidental findings in operations for other indications.

Malignancy

In past years it had always been stressed that Brenner tumors are to be regarded as benign, and this is still the general rule; but in the last decade numerous cases of malignant Brenner tumors have been reported in the review by Idelson.

Hormonal Activity

Although it had previously been believed that most of these tumors have been inert, it is increasingly apparent that some do appear hormonally active. A number of these neoplasms have been observed to be associated with postmenopausal endometrial hyperplasia, and adenocarcinoma as noted by Eton and Parker, as well as others. A review by Farrar and co-workers would appear to afford considerable circumstantial evidence of estrogen effect.

Mixed Epithelial Tumors

If one looks closely enough with the light microscope, there can be found some mixture of epithelial types within nearly all epithelial tumors. Ultrastructure as demonstrated by transmission electron microscopy confirms and underlines these findings, all of which aids in the incrimination of the multipotentiality of the surface epithelium and its role as the origin of most ovarian carcinomas. From a practical standpoint, it seems reasonable to insist on at least 10% involvement by another cell type to include it in this category.

Undifferentiated Carcinomas

This group represents those tumors in which there is no focus where differentiation is sufficient to classify them as any of the above variants.

SECONDARY OR METASTATIC CARCINOMA OF OVARY

Carcinoma of almost any type may occur in the ovary as a result of metastasis from primary sites in other parts of the body, especially in the latter stages of such malignant processes. A not infrequent variety of secondary ovarian cancer is that seen in association with carcinoma of the gastrointestinal tract or breast. This may present the same histological pattern in the ovary as in the primary tumor, this usually being adenocarcinoma.

With the exception of endometrial carcinoma, malignancy of the genitalia are uncommonly metastatic to the ovary.

Krukenberg Tumor

There is one particular variety of secondary ovarian carcinoma, however, which assumes special characteristics, and to which the designation of Krukenberg tumor is applied. This may be an accompaniment of primary carcinoma elswhere, but especially in any portion of the gastrointestinal tract, most frequently the pylorus, but not infrequently the colon, rectum, small intestine, liver, or gall bladder. It should be emphasized that the term "Krukenberg tumor" should not be applied to any ovarian tumor secondary to a gastrointestinal lesion. The designation is made purely on a histological basis.

Although it is generally believed that Krukenberg tumors are almost always metastatic, Woodruff and Novak have pointed out that about 20% *seem primary* in nature. An origin from teratoma, mucinous cyst, or mucoid degeneration in a Brenner tumor would seem to furnish the proper ovarian environment for a Krukenberg pattern to evolve. There has been considerable discussion as to the route by which carcinoma cells make their way to the ovary from such primary sites as the pylorus. Most students believe that retrograde lymphatic transplantation is the important factor, whereas in some cases the hematogenous route plays the important role.

The tumors are generally bilateral (over 50%). They are solid and they have a tendency to retain the original ovarian contour, so that they are ovoid or kidney-shaped. The surface is smooth, although often nodular, and the cut surface of variegated appearance, with frequently areas of gelatinous consistency.

Microscopically, the pattern of the Krukenberg tumor is quite distinctive, and the diagnosis is dependent only on the histological pattern, not on an associated or prior gastrointestinal lesion. Small nests or acini of epithelial cells are distributed throughout a fibrous or myxomatous stroma, and especially characteristic are the so-called *signet cells* (Fig. 22.20), in which the mucoid accumulation in the cytoplasm displaces the flattened nucleus to one side of the cell. A marked stromal hyperplasia mimicking sarcoma may be present, and this stromal (thecal) reaction may lead to bleeding from a hyperplastic endometrium as noted by some authors. Indeed, the striking stromal proliferation led to the original description as *sarcoma ovarii mucocellulare carcinomatodes.*

Endocrine Activity

The *estrogenic* capabilities of Krukenberg tumors have been noted by several authors.

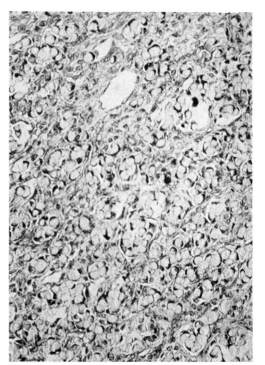

Figure 22.20. Characteristic signet cells in a Krukenberg tumor.

The presumed feminizing agent is the ovarian stroma or the stroma of the tumor matrix which is converted into a theca-like type of cell. More recently, an androgenic role has been ascribed to the same cells presumably due to conversion into a cell whose behavior parallels that of the interstitial cell.

GENERAL CONCEPTS AND CHARACTERISTICS OF OVARIAN CARCINOMA

Epidemiology

Ovarian cancer is a common malignancy with 17,000 new cases in 1978 in this country. At the present time, cancer of the ovary comprises approximately 25% of all malignancies of the female genital canal. Although there have been many advances in the management of the disease, the overall cure for ovarian cancer remains at approximately 20–30%. This is primarily a reflection of the advanced stage of the disease when detected. At present, there are approximately 11,000 deaths from this tumor each year in the United States, making ovarian cancer the fourth leading cause of cancer death in women. This represents a death rate that is greater than that from cervical and corpus uteri malignancies combined.

The effect of marital status and parity have been elegantly demonstrated in a study by Joly et al. who noted that while the risk was higher in single women it was higher still among married women who had not borne children. Compared to controls, patients with ovarian cancer included more women who attempted pregnancy but failed and more who had become pregnant only once or twice. How pregnancy protects against ovarian cancer is unclear but there is significant appeal to the thesis that suppression of ovulation is a most important factor. Newhouse et al. noted that fewer patients with ovarian cancer reported using oral contraceptives. These thoughts are in keeping with the previous discussion of germinal inclusion cysts and their relationship to epithelial ovarian neoplasia.

Studies involving women with multiple primary neoplasms suggest that ovarian and breast carcinoma share some common etiologic denominator. Women who have had carcinoma of the breast have twice the expected risk of subsequently developing a separate primary of the ovary, and women who have had ovarian carcinoma are three to four times as likely, as those without, to develop a separate breast carcinoma.

There has been considerable thought given to environmental factors. Certainly, the incidence of the disease is higher in more industrialized nations.

For most patients with epithelial malignancy of the ovary, there is no clear cut genetic predisposition but there are a few families in which the risk of cancer of the ovary in female members is so high that it appears to be transmitted as an autosomal dominant. In this unusual high risk situation special attention must be paid to prophylactic oophorectomy following the completion of childbearing. The tumors in these "susceptible" families have been mostly papillary serous variants.

NATURAL HISTORY AND CLINICAL APPROACH TO OVARIAN CARCINOMA

The most important symptoms of ovarian carcinoma are unfortunately rather late ones,

as the onset of this disease is almost always very insidious and "silent" in nature. The presence of a *mass* in the lower abdomen is the first indication of the disease in a considerable proportion of cases, and unfortunately by this time other organs are often involved. Moderate *heaviness* or occasional *pain* may be noted, but are more apt to be absent. Irregular or postmenopausal *bleeding* is an infrequent finding. *Thrombophlebitis*, otherwise unexplained, may be due to silent tumor in proximity to the large veins. It has been amply demonstrated that the finding of tumor cells in the blood does not necessarily imply metastases.

Ascites is a relatively common accompaniment of ovarian cancer, especially of the papillary varieties. It is all too frequently indicative of peritoneal extension of the growth, but may be due merely to venous obstruction caused by partial torsion of the tumor, as in any other ovarian neoplasm. The ascites may be so extreme as to make palpation of the tumor impossible, and paracentesis is often needed to palpate the lower abdominal or pelvic masses. Exudative ascites (specific gravity greater than 1.016) should be considered to represent ovarian carcinoma until proven otherwise.

For some reason, various ovarian tumors may be associated with *hypercalcemia* even when there is no osteolytic lesion. Ferenczy et al. note that this is disproportionately common with clear cell carcinoma.

Diagnosis

In a large proportion of cases the malignant nature of the tumors is not suspected before operation, and often not until pathological examination. In many, however, a strongly presumptive diagnosis is possible, chiefly on palpatory findings. Vaginal smear rarely demonstrates exfoliated tumor cells, but Rubin and Frost note a frequent estrogenic effect in the maturation index. Preoperative culdocentesis may be helpful if the removed fluid is studied cytologically.

If pelvic examination reveals a mass occupying the position of the ovary, and if the mass is hard, fixed, and firm, ovarian carcinoma should be suspected, especially if the patient is in the cancer age. Benign solid tumors of the ovary, such as fibroma, give somewhat the same feeling but are less common. Benign cystic tumors, on the other hand, give a softer, elastic sensation to the examining hands, and are usually smoother in contour, as compared to the more nodular contour of most cancers. Laparoscopy may be decisive when there is uncertainty if an adnexal mass is uterine or ovarian in origin.

When such a tumor is associated with ascites, there can be little doubt as to its malignant nature. When the ascites is extreme, the tumor may be impalpable, and other causes of ascites, such as hepatic and cardiorenal disease or tuberculous peritonitis, may have to be eliminated. Occasionally, paracentesis may be necessary to permit proper palpation of the pelvic organs, and a definite mass may be felt for the first time. Microscopic examination of the centrifuged ascitic fluid may show typically malignant cells (Fig. 22.21).

Peritoneal washing at laparotomy has been suggested by some as being of prognostic value, if performed before operative manipulation and immediately after entry into the abdomen. This should be done, but the surgeon should be mindful of the vagarious nature of ovarian tumors. Sometimes an apparently localized lesion is followed by massive recurrence. In other instances extensive disease seems compatible with longevity.

Even at the time of surgery, the exact nature of an ovarian tumor may be uncertain, and in such instances a *frozen section* may be helpful. It is perhaps preferable to remove the whole adnexal mass, and allow the pathologist to select likely areas for section rather than remove blindly one or two areas for evaluation. Although this may minimize errors, permanent sections will on occasion show malignancy that had not been noted on frozen section, so that the trained gynecologist will also strongly consider the gross appearance of the lesion at surgery.

Epithelial tumors of the ovary, because of their mode of extension, defy the usual "en bloc" approach that is traditional for the

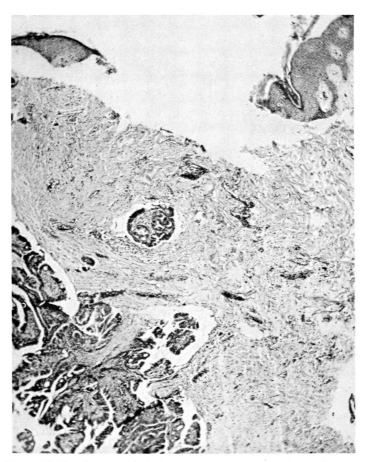

Figure 22.21.   Carcinoma cells in ascitic fluid in case of ovarian carcinoma.

management of cervical and uterine fundus tumors. Once outside the ovary, the tumor is frequently widespread throughout the peritoneal cavity. In fact, at the time of diagnosis, approximately 65% of all of the epithelial malignancies have progressed to Stage III or greater. Multiple attempts to facilitate early diagnosis have not been fruitful. It is presumed that this extension is by implantation or by subperitoneal lymphatic extension and, more probably, is a combination of both.

Although the tumor does seem to extend primarily along peritoneal surfaces, it is not uncommon for Stage I and Stage II disease to have extension to the para-aortic lymph chain at the level of the renal vessels. Recently, more attention has been paid to the role of the lymphatic drainage of the entire peritoneal cavity and the part that it plays in the spread of ovarian cancer. The true incidence of subdiaphragmatic metastases is only now becoming apparent with this understanding of the lymphatic drainage of the peritoneal cavity. It is not uncommon to find, on exploration of what appears to be relatively early disease, that the patient indeed has early macroscopic or microscopic disease up under the hemidiaphragms.

At present, there is no established staging procedure for the assessment of metastasis in the subpleural diaphragmatic nodes except for visualization and surgical biopsy, a procedure neither easily nor routinely performed (especially repetitively during the patient's course). It has been noted that attempts to study the distribution of gamma-emitting particles injected into the peritoneal cavity frequently show positive imaging in the area of the substernal nodes at an interval of a few hours from the time of injection. This might be of prognostic significance, since we know that those patients who have malignant ascites almost routinely have these efferent channels obstructed with resultant nonimaging of these nodes. Therefore, we have included this potentially important staging procedure in our approach to the disease.

Until a little over 10 years ago, little attention was paid to the grade of the tumor in relationship to survival. Since that time, a number of authors have emphasized the importance of tumor grade, suggesting that it is impossible to compare treatment modalities without including this variable in the classification. When tumors are so graded, it becomes apparent within each histologic subclassification that the salvage is related to both the stage and the grade and, perhaps more importantly, to grade than to stage.

The concept of grade is particularly important for low grade or borderline ovarian malignancies. With very low grade or borderline malignancies, even with advanced stage, conservative therapy is appropriate since prolonged survival is the rule. Another variable that one must consider in evaluating the usefulness of adjunctive therapy, whether chemotherapeutic or radiotherapeutic, is the amount and location of residual disease remaining after the initial maximal surgical effort.

In summary then, all adnexal masses ought to be approached as if they have ovarian carcinoma. Once the diagnosis of ovarian carcinoma is made, adequate operative staging should begin. This should include the following: (1) the sending of free peritoneal fluid or peritoneal washings to the cytopathology laboratory for analysis prior to manipulation of the tumor; (2) careful palpation of all abdominal and pelvic viscera; (3) palpation and visualization (with a laparoscope if necessary) of the hemidiaphragms with biopsies taken where indicated; and (4) sampling, by biopsy, of multiple peritoneal areas including the cul-de-sac, both paracolonic gutters, and a wide sample of dependent omentum. This will be followed in most cases by total abdominal hysterectomy and bilateral salpingo-oophorectomy. Conservative surgery in those patients with epithelial malignancies, with removal of only one adnexa, is reserved for those who wish to preserve further childbearing and who have a Stage Ia borderline serous tumor, borderline mucinous tumor, or clear cell carcinoma. When this is considered, wedge biopsy of the opposite ovary is mandatory. Even then, the pathologic specimens may yield information that advances the stage leading to the necessity for repeat surgery with more complete resection.

Prognosis

The outlook for the patient with ovarian carcinoma is very grave, especially if one omits from consideration the gonadal stroma group (granulosa-theca cell tumor, arrhenoblastoma, and dysgerminoma) in which the results are far better.

A suitable caveat to be injected at this time relates to the comparison of recent data on treatment with past survival figures. All forms of therapy will appear to have a more favorable prognosis in the earlier stages of disease because more effective staging techniques will remove previously inapparent Stage III patients from the earlier categories.

Treatment (Postsurgical)

Radiotherapy

The usefulness of radiotherapy as an adjuvant to the surgical treatment of ovarian cancer is difficult to evaluate. Clearly it is impossible to document any value for external therapy in Stage I disease, in spite of the fact that it had been used quite extensively for this reason in decades past. We are readily aware of the fact that Stage I ovarian cancer has a failure rate of approximately 40% when surgery alone is utilized. Putting this another way, 40% of patients with apparent Stage I disease have tumor beyond the ovary at the time of surgical intervention. Since most epithelial tumors extend mainly along peritoneal surfaces and through lymphatic pathways that drain the peritoneal cavity, it has always seemed appealing to assume that colloids or suspensions of radioactive beta-emitting isotopes might be useful as a surgical adjunct in those cases with no gross residual disease.

Adjuvant external radiotherapy does seem to be of some value in Stage II disease where in a number of series (including those of, Clark et al., Barr et al., and Van Orden et al.) the 5-year survival seemed to be improved. The numbers in each series, however, are quite small and the results must be accepted with great skepticism. It is even a bit naive to assume that Stage II is a legitimate stage. Ovarian cancer has little anatomic or biologic reason to hesitate at the pelvic brim once extension is beyond the ovary. This situation usually represents our own inadequacy at detecting extrapelvic extension and with improved attention to operative staging it should nearly disappear. It is important to note that most series employed pelvic irradiation only for Stage II tumor.

It is yet to be proven by randomized study that the use of this modality in any way alters the salvage with Stage III disease and the technique is rapidly losing popularity throughout the country.

Adjunctive Chemotherapy

Historically, chemotherapeutic agents have been employed since the 1950s for the treatment of ovarian carcinoma. For most of that time the group of drugs known as alkylating agents have been the mainstay of therapy.

The following is a classification of chemotherapeutics sometimes used in the management of ovarian carcinoma.

1. Alkylating agents
   a. Nitrogen mustard compounds
      Mustargen (mechlorethamine)
      Leukeran (chlorambucil)
      Cytoxan (endoxan, cyclophosphamide)
      Alkeran (L-sarcolysin, melphalan)
   b. Ethylenimines
      Thiotepa (triethylenethiophosphoramide)
   c. Alkyl sulfonates
      Myleran (busulfan)
2. Antimetabolites
   a. Folic acid analogs
      Methotrexate (amethopterin)
   b. Pyrimidine analogs
      Fluorouracil (5-FU)
      Cytosar (cytosine arabinoside)
   c. Purine analogs
      Purinethol (6-mercaptopurine)
      Imidazole carboxamide
3. Antibiotics
   Cosmegen (actinomycin D)
   Blenoxane (bleomycin)
   Adriamycin
4. Vinca alkaloids (periwinkle drugs)
   Velban (vinblastine)
   Oncovin (vincristine sulfate)
5. Progestogens
   Provera (medroxyprogesterone acetate)
   Delalutin (hydroxyprogesterone caproate)
   Megace (megestrol acetate)
6. Miscellaneous
   Hexamethylmelamine
   cis-Platinum

It is clear that to improve the low cure rate for early stage ovarian carcinoma, as well as for the effective therapy of advanced ovarian carcinoma, we must employ adjunctive therapy in addition to surgery. Although external radiotherapy is an important palliative tool in the treatment of ovarian carcinoma in selected cases, the weight of evidence currently suggests that it has only a minor role in the combination approach to ovarian carcinoma. Multiple effective drugs are available and the opportunities to treat ovarian carcinoma with combination chemotherapy seem

Table 22.2
Single Agent Chemotherapy in Advanced Ovarian Cancer[a]

Agents	Patients	Response
	No.	%
Melphalan	494	47
Chlorambucil	280	50
Thiotepa	144	64
Cyclosphosphamide	126	49
5-FU	81	32
Adriamycin	51	32
Hexamethylmelamine	53	41
cis-Platinum	25	16

[a] Adapted from the review of R. C. Young: *Seminars in Oncology 2:* 267, 1975.

more promising than the continued use of postoperative radiation therapy.

It is well known that several single chemotherapeutic agents have some efficacy in the treatment of advanced ovarian carcinoma. Table 22.2 lists several of these agents and response rates as summarized in the literature.

"Second Look" Operation

In 1951, Wagenstein introduced the concept of the "second look" operation for patients suffering with cancer of the colon. In the early 1960s, the group at M. D. Anderson Hospital introduced this procedure as a planned systematic approach for evaluating the therapy of extensive ovarian carcinoma. The second look operation for ovarian cancer is more than a casual exploration of the peritoneal cavity. It is a well designed operation with clear-cut goals: to establish the efficacy of previous therapy; to define the current extent of disease; to establish current histology; to remove residual tumor; and ultimately to assist in planning future therapy for the patients. A crucial and debatable question is timing of the second look procedure. Investigators agree that this should be following maximal response from chemotherapy but it is difficult to establish when this maximum response occurs. One of the disadvantages of the second look is that it is a major operative procedure and yields a window into the extent of the disease at only one moment in time. It would be ideal if one could periodically examine the peritoneal cavity to evaluate the status of disease with little risk or discomfort to the patient. This has been done to some extent with laparoscopy.

On the other hand, laparoscopy itself has significant disadvantages. After the extensive operative procedures that are traditionally performed for ovarian carcinoma, and after removal of all or large portions of the omentum, the peritoneum is compartmentalized by multiple adhesions located against the anterior abdominal wall. Under these conditions there is significant risk of injuring adherent bowel with the trocar used to introduce the laparoscope. Even if this does not occur, there is difficulty in visualizing the true extent of the peritoneal cavity. Adhesive disease also leads to difficulty in achieving distribution of radioactive phosphorus in the treatment of microscopic residual disease, if this is deemed advisable following second look procedure. Any technique that could effectively diminish the degree of adhesion formation following this variety of surgery would facilitate its sequential evaluation.

Immunology

At the present time, there is significant confusion concerning the reality of a tumor-specific antigen but definite host responsiveness to tumor-associated antigens can be demonstrated in the laboratory in a number of ways. Attempts to treat patients with ovarian carcinoma by augmentation of delayed hypersensitivity have met with little, if any, convincing success but, for the most part, these studies were performed on patients with a huge tumor load or with patients who had possibly been cured by other treatment modalities (surgical adjuvant studies).

In summary, the final chapter has not been written on this topic and much work is needed in the future to elucidate the role of immunotherapy in this disease.

ROLE AND LIMITATIONS OF NEW DIAGNOSTIC TECHNIQUES

It would seem unwise to complete a chapter on epithelial tumors of the ovary without some reference to the value of ultrasound (US) and computerized axial tomography (CAT) in the evaluation of benign and malignant tumors of the ovary (Figs. 22.22–22.24). Both of these relatively new diagnostic modalities have very definite advantages and limitations. They are, in no way, a substitute for an adequate pelvic examination and, although neither study is invasive, they are of

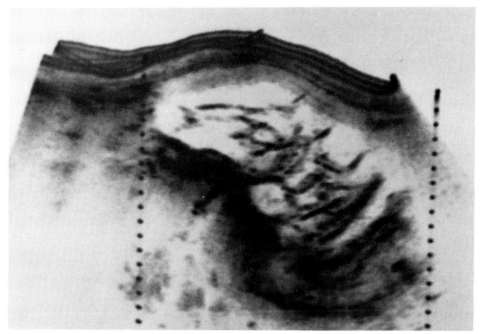

Figure 22.22.   Sagital ultrasound of benign mucinous cystadenoma of the ovary. Note prominent septation of tumor that is characteristic of this pathological entity. *Dotted line* at left indicates level of umbilicus at right level of symphysis.

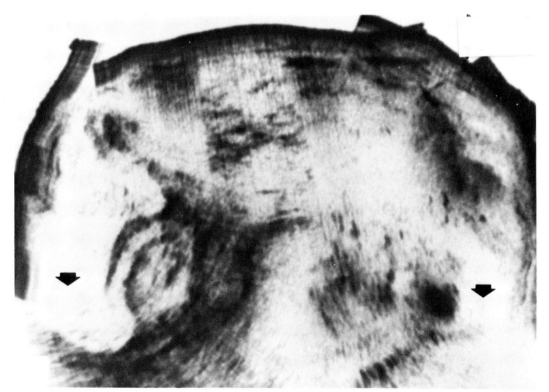

Figure 22.23.   Transverse abdominal ultrasound at level of kidneys. Note ascites in the paracolic gutters. Patient had papillary serous cystadeno carcinoma Stage III with ascites. *Arrows* indicate paracolic fluid accumulation.

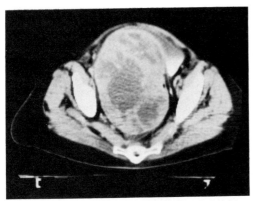

Figure 22.24. Transverse computerized axial tomography (CAT) within pelvis. Note large, clearly defined septate mass. Contrast material is seen collecting in the bladder. This tumor is a low grade mucinous cystadenocarcinoma of the ovary.

considerable expense to the patient, and the CAT does subject her to a small amount of irradiation. We ask each of these modalities to assess a number of parameters concerning a suspected or palpable pelvic mass and these include:

1. The ability to confirm or deny the presence of a mass detected on physical examination
2. Evaluation of the size, consistency, and contour of a mass
3. Definition of the origin and anatomic relation of the mass to surrounding organs
4. Definition of involvement or invasion of surrounding structures by a mass
5. Determination of the presence or absence of ascites and/or other metastatic lesions
6. Give objective changes in tumor size following or during treatment

Both modalities provide some information regarding all of the above factors but while the CAT is clearly superior and highly accurate in delineating retroperitoneal disease such as positive para-aortic nodes, it has definite limitations in assessing intraperitoneal tumor that is not of considerable size. Lesions on the parietal and visceral peritoneum of less than 3 cm are regularly missed and sometimes even omental lesions of considerable size are difficult to define. Subdiaphragmatic disease is regularly missed by both modalities unless very pronounced. Ascites, on the other hand, can be easily noted by both techniques even when well below the amount detectable by physical examination. US is especially adept at displaying cystic lesions because of the echogenic quality of the interphase be-

tween liquid and tissue. Consequently, US is of more value in the diagnosis of cystic epithelial lesions of the ovary.

The greatest number of diagnostic errors occurring in CAT studies were the results of misinterpretation of bowel loops for a pelvic mass. This problem can be minimized by having the patient ingest oral contrast media 2–3 hours prior to scanning.

Although both US and CAT can be used to follow tumors under chemotherapy, they have not been all that valuable over and above the information available from both abdominal and pelvic examination. Many times, in fact, the information was less valuable and less complete.

References and Additional Readings

American Cancer Society: Cancer Facts and Figures, 1978.
"*Annual Report*", Vol. 15. International Federation of Gynecology and Obstetrics (FIGO), Stockholm, 1976.
Ansfield, F. J., Schroeder, J. M., and Curreri, A. R.: Five years clinical experience with 5-fluorouracil. J.A.M.A., *181:* 295, 1962.
Aure, J. C., Hoeg, K., and Kolstadt, P.: Carcinoma of the ovary and endometriosis. Acta Obstet. Gynecol. Scand., *50:* 63, 1971.
Aure, J. C., Hoeg, K., and Kolstadt, P.: Clinical and histologic studies of ovarian carcinoma: long-term follow-up of 990 cases. Obstet. Gynecol., *37:* 1, 1971.
Aure, J. C., Hoeg, K., and Kolstadt, P.: Mesonephroid tumors of the ovary. Obstet. Gynecol., *37:* 860, 1971.
Aure, J. C., Hoeg, K., and Kolstadt, P.: Psammoma bodies in serous carcinoma of the ovary. Am. J. Obstet. Gynecol., *109:* 113, 1971.
Bagley, C. M., Jr., Young, R. C., Schein P. S., et al.: Ovarian carcinoma metastatic to the diaphragm—frequently undiagnosed at laparotomy: a preliminary report. Am. J. Obstet. Gynecol., *116:* 397, 1973.
Balasa, R. W., Adeoels, L. L., Prem, K. A., and Dehuer, L. P.: The Brewer tumor: a clinical pathological review. Obstet. Gynecol., *50:* 120, 1977.
Barber, H. R. K., and Graber, E. A.: The P.M.P.O. Syndrome: (The post-menopausal palpable ovary syndrome). Obstet. Gynecol., *38:* 921, 1971.
Barber, H. R. K., and Graber, E. A.: Gynecological tumors in childhood and infancy. Obstet. Gynec. Surv., *28:* 357, 1973.
Barlow, J. J., and Piver, M. S.: Single agent vs. combination chemotherapy in the treatment of ovarian cancer. Obstet. Gynecol., *49:* 609, 1977.
Barr, W., Cowell, M. A. C., and Chatfield, W. R.: The management of ovarian carcinoma: a review of 420 cases. Scott. Med. J., *15:* 250, 1970.
Bateman, J. C., and Winship, T.: Palliation of ovarian carcinoma with phosphoramide drugs. Surg. Gynecol. Obstet., *102:* 347, 1956.
Berg, J. W., and Baylor, S. M.: The epidemiologic pathology of ovarian cancer. Hum. Pathol., *4:* 537, 1973.
Bhattacharya, M., and Barlow, J. J.: Immunologic studies of human serous cystadenocarcinoma of ovary: demonstration of tumor-associated antigens. Cancer, *31:* 588, 1973.
Bhattacharya, M., and Barlow, J. J.: Immunologic study of carcinoma of the ovary. Am. J. Obstet. Gynecol., *117:* 849, 1973.
Brenner, F.: Das Oophoroma folliculare. Frankfurt. Z. Pathol., *1:* 150, 1907.
Brenner, W. E., and Scott, R. B.: Meigs-like syndrome secondary to Krukenberg tumor. Obstet. Gynecol., *31:* 40, 1968.
Broders, A. C.: Carcinoma: Grading and practical application. Arch. Pathol., *2:* 376, 1926.

Buell, P., and Dunn J. E.: Cancer mortality among Japanese Issei and Nisei of California. Cancer, *18:* 656, 1965.

Burns, B. C., Jr., Rutledge, F. N., Smith, J. P., et al.: Management of ovarian carcinoma. Surgery, Irradiation, and chemotherapy. Am. J. Obstet. Gynecol., *98:* 374, 1967.

Campbell, J. G.: The epidemiology of tumors in intensively reared chicken. In *Racial and Geographical Factors in Tumor Incidence,* edited by A. A. Shivas, p. 241. Edinburgh University Press, Edinburgh, 1967.

Campbell, J. G.: Some unusual gonadal tumors of the fowl. Br. J. Cancer, *5:* 69, 1951.

Campbell, J. S., Lou, P., Ferguson, J. P., et al.: Pseudomyxoma peritonei et ovarii with occult neoplasm of the appendix. Obstet. Gynecol., *42:* 897, 1973.

Cancer Facts and Figures. New York, American Cancer Society, 1975.

Casagrande, J. T., Pike, M. C., Ross, R. K., et al.: "Incessant ovulation" and ovarian cancer. Lancet, *2:* 170, 1979.

Caspi, E., Schreyer, P., and Bukovsky, J.: Ovarian lutein cysts in pregnancy. Obstet. Gynecol., *42:* 388, 1973.

Chang, S. H., Roberts, J. M., and Homesley, H. D.: Proliferating Brenner tumor. Obstet. Gynecol., *49:* 489, 1977.

Clark, D. G. C., Hilaris, B., Roussis, C., et al.: The role of radiation therapy (including isotopes) in the treatment of cancer of the ovary: results of 614 patients treated at Memorial Hospital, New York, N.Y. Prog. Clin. Cancer, *5:* 227, 1973.

Coonrad, E. V., and Rundles, R. W.: Mustard chemotherapy in ovarian carcinoma. Ann. Intern. Med., *50:* 1449, 1959.

Cooper, P.: Mixed mesodermal tumor and clear cell carcinoma arising in ovarian endometriosis. Cancer, *42:* 2827, 1978.

Coulam, C. M., Julian, C. G., and Fleischer, A. C.: Clinical efficacy of computed tomography and ultrasound in the evaluation of gynecologic tumors. AJR in press, 1980.

Cramer, D. W., and Cutler, S. J.: Incidence and histopathology of malignancies of the female genital organs in the United States. Am. J. Obstet. Gynecol., *118:* 443, 1974.

Creasman, W. P., and Rutledge, F.: The value of peritoneal cytology. Am. J. Obstet. Gynecol., *110:* 773, 1971.

Cutler, S. J., Myers, M. H., and Green, S. B.: Trends in survival rates of patients with cancer. N. Engl. J. Med., *293:* 122, 1975.

Decker, D. G., Mussey, E., Williams, T. J., et al.: Grading of gynecologic malignancy: epithelial ovarian cancer, Seventh National Cancer Conference Proceedings, Los Angeles, Calif., September 27–29, 1972, p. 223. J. B. Lippincott Company, Philadelphia, 1973.

Decker, D. G., Webb, W. J., and Holbrook, M. A.: Radiogold treatment of epithelial cancer of the ovary: late results. Am. J. Obstet. Gynecol., *115:* 751, 1973.

Delclos, L., and Quinlan, E. J.: Malignant tumors of the ovary managed with postoperative megavoltage irradiation. Radiology, *93:* 659, 1969.

DeSanto, D. A., Bullock, W. K., and Moore, F. J.: Ovarian cystomas. Arch. Surg., *78:* 98, 1959.

DeVita, V. T., and Schein, P. S.: The use of drugs in combination for the treatment of cancer: rationale and results. N. Engl. J. Med., *288:* 998, 1973.

DiSaia, P. J., Nalick, R. H., and Townsend, D. E.: Antibody cytotoxicity studies in ovarian and cervical malignancies. Obstet. Gynecol., *42:* 644, 1973.

DiSaia, P. J., Sinkovics, J. G., Rutledge, F. N., et al.: Cell-mediated immunity to human malignant cells. Am. J. Obstet. Gynecol., *114:* 979, 1972.

Doshi, N., and Tobon, H.: Primary clear cell carcinoma of the ovary. Cancer, *39:* 2658, 1977.

Drye, J. C.: Intraperitoneal pressure in the human. Surg. Gynecol. Obstet., *87:* 472, 1948.

Ehrlich, C. E., and Roth, L. M.: The Brenner tumor. Cancer, *27:* 32, 1971.

Esposito, J. M.: An unusual theca-lutein cyst. Obstet. Gynecol., *30:* 260, 1967.

Eton, B., and Parker, R. A.: Endometrial abnormalities including carcinoma associated with ovarian Brenner tumors. J. Obstet. Gynaec. Br. Commonw., *65:* 95, 1958.

Farrar, H. K., Jr., Elesh, R., and Libretti, J.: Brenner tumors and estrogen production. Obstet. Gynecol. Surv., *15:* 1, 1960.

Farrar, H. K., and Greene, R. R.: Bilateral Brenner tumors of the ovary. Am. J. Obstet. Gynecol., *80:* 1089, 1960.

Fathalla, M. F.: Factors in the causation and incidence of ovarian cancer. Obstet. Gynecol. Surv., *27:* 751, 1972.

Fenoglio, C. M., Ferenczy, A., and Richart, R. M.: Mucinous tumors of the ovary: ultrastructural studies of mucinous cystadenomas with histogenetic considerations. Cancer, *36:* 1709, 1975.

Ferenczy, A., Okagaki, T., and Richart, R. M.: Paraendocrine hypercalcemia in ovarian neoplasms. Cancer, *27:* 427, 1971.

Finkle, H. I., Goldman, R. L., and Sung, M.: A proliferating Brenner tumor. Obstet. Gynecol., *40:* 39, 1973.

Foda, M. S., and Shafeek, M. A.: Malignant Brenner tumor. Obstet. Gynecol., *13:* 226, 1959.

Fox, H., Kazzaz, B., and Langley, F. A.: Argyrophil and argentaffin cells in the female genital tract and in ovarian mucinous cysts. J. Pathol. Bacteriol., *88:* 479, 1964.

French, J. E., Florey, H. W., and Morris, B.: The absorption of particles by the lymphatics of the diaphragm. Q. J. Exp. Physiol., *45:* 88, 1960.

Gall, S. A., Walling, J., and Pearl, J.: Tumor associated antigens. Am. J. Obstet. Gynecol., *115:* 387, 1973.

Graham, R. M., Schueller, E. F., and Graham, J. B.: Detection of ovarian cancer at an early stage—routine culdocentesis. Obstet. Gynecol., *26:* 151, 1965.

Green, T. H., Jr.: Hemisulphur mustard in the palliation of patients with metastatic ovarian carcinoma. Obstet. Gynecol., *13:* 383, 1959.

Griffiths, C. T., Grogan, R. H., and Hall, T. C.: Advanced ovarian cancer: Primary treatment with surgery, radiotherapy, and chemotherapy. Cancer, *29:* 1, 1972.

Griffiths, C. T.: Surgical resection of tumor bulk in the primary treatment of ovarian carcinoma. Natl. Cancer Inst. Monogr., *42:* 101, 1975.

Haenszel, W., and Kurihara, M.: Studies of Japanese migrants. I. Mortality from cancer and other diseases among Japanese in the United States. J. Natl. Cancer Inst., *40:* 43, 1968.

Hale, R. W.: Krukenberg tumors of the ovary. Obstet. Gynecol., *68:* 221, 1968.

Hannemann, J. H.: Radiation therapy in selected ovarian cancers: A negative report. Rocky Mt. Med. J., *69(2):* 57, 1972.

Hart, W. R., and Norris, H. J.: Borderline and malignant mucinous tumors of the ovary: histologic criteria and clinical behavior. Cancer, *31:* 1031, 1973.

Harvald, B., and Hauge, M.: Heredity of cancer elucidated by a study of unselected twins. J.A.M.A., *186:* 749, 1963.

Hernandez, W., DiSaia, P. J., Morrow, F. C. P., et al.: Mixed mesodermal sarcoma of the ovary. Obstet. Gynecol., *49(Suppl.):* 59s, 1977.

Hester, L. L., and White, L.: Radioactive colloidal chromic phosphate in the treatment of ovarian malignancies. Am. J. Obstet. Gynecol., *103:* 911, 1969.

Hilaris, B. S., and Clark, D. G. C.: Postoperative intraperitoneal radio colloids in early carcinoma ovary. AJR, *112:* 749, 1971.

Hull, M. G. R., and Campbell, G. R.: Malignant Brenner tumor. Obstet. Gynecol., *42:* 527, 1973.

Idelson, M. G.: Malignancy in Brenner tumors of the ovary, with comments on histogenesis and possible estrogen production. Obstet. Gynec. Surv., *18:* 246, 1963.

International Federation of Gynaecology and Obstetrics: Classification and staging of malignant tumors in the female pelvis. Acta Obstet. Gynecol. Scand., *50:* 1, 1971.

Jackson, S. M.: Ovarian dysgerminoma in three generations? J. Med. Genet., *4:* 112, 1967.

Jolles, B.: Progesterone in the treatment of advanced malignant tumors of breast, ovary, and uterus. Br. J. Cancer, *16:* 209, 1962.

Joly, D. J., Lilienfeld, A. M., Diamond, E. L., et al.: An epidemiologic study of the relationship of reproductive experience to cancer of the ovary. Am. J. Epidemiol., *99:* 190, 1974.

Jorgensen, E. O., Dockerty, M. B., Wilson, R. B., et al.: Clinicopathological study of 53 Brenner tumors. Am. J. Obstet. Gynecol., *108:* 122, 1970.

Julian, C. G., Goss, J., Blanchard, K., et al.: Biologic behavior of primary ovarian malignancy. Obstet. Gynecol., *44:* 873, 1974.

Julian, C. G., and Woodruff, J. D.: Multiple anaplasias in the lower genital canal. Am. J. Obstet. Gynecol., 95: 681, 1966.

Julian, C. G., and Woodruff, J. D.: The role of chemotherapy in the treatment of primary ovarian malignancy. Obstet. Gynecol. Surv., 24: 1307, 1969.

Julian, C. G., and Woodruff, J. D.: Biologic behavior of low grade papillary serous carcinoma of the ovary. Obstet. Gynecol. 40: 860, 1972.

Keettel, W. C., Fox, M. R., Longnecker, D. S., et al.: Prophylactic use of radioactive gold in the treatment of primary ovarian cancer. Am. J. Obstet. Gynecol., 94: 766, 1966.

Kent, S. W., and McKay, D. G.: Primary cancer of the ovary: An analysis of 349 cases. Am. J. Obstet. Gynecol., 80: 430, 1960.

Kimbrough, R. A., Jr.: Coincident carcinoma of the ovary in twins. Am. J. Obstet. Gynecol., 18: 148, 1929.

Knapp, R. C., and Friedman, E. A.: Aortic lymph node metastases in early ovarian cancer. Am. J. Obstet. Gynecol., 119: 1013, 1974.

Kottmeier, H. L.: Ovarian cancer with special regard to radiotherapy. AJR, 111: 417, 1971.

Kottmeier, H. L.: Surgical management—conservative surgery: indications according to the type of the tumour. Clin. Obstet. Gynaecol 11: 157, 1968.

Kottmeier, H. L.: Treatment of ovarian cancer with Thiotepa. Clin. Obstet. Gynaecol., 11: 428, 1968.

Krukenberg, F.: Uber das Fibrosarcoma ovarii mucocellulare carcinomatodes. Arch. Gynaekol., 50: 287, 1896.

Kurman, R. J., and Craig, J. M.: Endometrioid and clear cell carcinoma of the ovary. Cancer, 29: 1653, 1972.

Kurman, R. J., and Scully, R. E.: Clear cell carcinoma of the endometrium: an analysis of 21 cases. Cancer, 37: 872, 1976.

Langley, F. A., Cummins, P. A., and Fox, H.: An ultrastructural study of mucin secreting epithelia in ovarian neoplasms. Acta Pathol. Microbiol. Scand (A), 233: 76, 1972.

Lawrence, W. D., Larson, P. N., and Hauge, E. T.: Primary Krukenberg tumor of the ovary in pregnancy. Obstet. Gynecol., 10: 54, 1957.

Lewis, A. C., and Davison, B. C.: Familial ovarian cancer. Lancet, 2: 235, 1969.

Li, F. P., Rapoport, A. H., Fraumeni, J. F., Jr., et al.: Familial ovarian carcinoma. J.A.M.A., 214: 1559, 1970.

Liber, A. F.: Ovarian cancer in mother and five daughters. Arch. Pathol., 49: 280, 1950.

Lingeman, C. H.: Etiology of cancer of the human ovary: a review. J. Natl. Cancer Inst., 53: 1603, 1974.

Long, R. T. L., Johnson, R. E., and Sala, J. M.: Variations in survival among patients with carcinoma of the ovary: analysis of 253 cases according to histologic type, anatomical stage and method of treatment. Cancer, 20: 1195, 1967.

Malkasian, G. D., Jr., Decker, D. G., Jorgensen, E. O., et al.: 6-Dehydro-6,17-dimethylprogesterone (NSC-123018) for the treatment of metastatic and recurrent ovarian carcinoma. Cancer Chemother. Rep(I), 57: 241, 1973.

Malpas, P.: Pseudomyxoma peritonei. J. Obstet. Gynaec. Br. Commonw., 66: 247, 1959.

Masterson, J. G., and Nelson, J. H., Jr.: The role of chemotherapy in the treatment of gynecologic malignancy. Am. J. Obstet. Gynecol., 93: 1102, 1965.

McCrann, D. J., Marchant, D. J., and Bardawil, W. A.: Ovarian carcinoma in three teen-age siblings. Obstet. Gynecol., 43: 132, 1974.

McGowan, L., Stein, D. B., and Miller, W.: Cul-de-sac aspiration for diagnostic cytologic study. Am. J. Obstet. Gynecol., 96: 413, 1966.

McKay, D. G.: The origin of ovarian tumors. Clin. Obstet. Gynaecol., 5: 1181, 1962.

Meyers, M. A.: The spread and localization of acute intraperitoneal effusions. Radiology, 95: 547, 1970.

Molloy, W. B.: Identical ovarian malignant disease in two sisters. Aust. N.Z. J. Obstet. Gynaecol., 10: 256, 1970.

Moore, D. W., and Langley, I. I.: Routine use of radio-gold following operation for ovarian cancer. Am. J. Obstet. Gynecol., 98: 624, 1967.

Muller, J. H.: Curative aim and results of routine intraperitoneal radiocolloid administration in the treatment of ovarian cancer. AJR, 89: 533, 1963.

Munnell, E. W.: Ovarian carcinoma: A review of 200 primary and 51 secondary cases. Am. J. Obstet. Gynecol., 58: 943, 1949.

Munnell, E. W.: The changing prognosis and treatment in cancer of the ovary: a report of 235 patients with primary ovarian carcinoma 1952–1961. Am. J. Obstet. Gynecol., 100: 790, 1968.

Munnell, E. W.: Is conservative therapy ever justified in Stage I(IA) cancer of the ovary? Am. J. Obstet. Gynecol., 103: 641, 1969.

Newhouse, M. L., Pearson, R. M., Fullerton, J. M., et al.: Br. J. Prev. Soc. Med., 31: 148, 1977.

Norris, H. J., and Robinowitz, M.: Ovarian adenocarcinoma of mesonephric type. Cancer, 28: 1074, 1971.

Ober, W. B., Pollak, A., Gerstman, K. E., and Kupperman, H. S.: Krukenberg tumor with androgenic and progestational activity. Am. J. Obstet. Gynecol., 84: 739, 1962.

Overholt, P. H.: Intraperitoneal pressure. Arch. Surg., 22: 691, 1931.

Parker, J. M., Dockerty, M. B., and Randall, L. M.: Mesonephric clear cell carcinoma of the ovary: a clinical and pathologic study. Am. J. Obstet. Gynecol., 80: 417, 1960.

Parker, L. M., Lokich, J. J., Griffiths, C. T., et al.: Adriamycin-cyclophosphamide therapy in ovarian cancer. Proc. Am. Assoc. Cancer Res. Am. Soc. Clin. Oncol., 16: 263, 1975.

Parker, R. T., Parker, C. H., and Wilbanks, G. D.: Cancer of the ovary: survival studies based upon operative therapy, chemotherapy, and radiotherapy. Am. J. Obstet. Gynecol., 108: 878, 1970.

Piver, M. S.: Management of patients with ovarian carcinoma. Obstet. Gynecol., 40: 411, 1972.

Piver, M. S., Barlow, J. J., Lee, F. T., et al.: Sequential therapy for advanced ovarian adenocarcinoma: operation, chemotherapy, second-look laparotomy, and radiation therapy. Am. J. Obstet. Gynecol., 122: 355, 1975.

Pomerance, W., and Moltz, A.: Ten-year survival in carcinoma of the ovary. Obstet. Gynecol., 37: 560, 1971.

Randall, C. L., Hall, D. W., and Armenia, C. S.: Pathology of the preserved ovary after unilateral oophorectomy. Am. J. Obstet. Gynecol., 84: 1233, 1962.

Registrar General of England and Wales. Statistical review for 1940–45. Her Majesty's Stationary Office, London, 1949.

Robert, D. K., Marshall, R. B., and Wharton, J. T.: Ultrastructure of ovarian tumors. I. Papillary serous cystadenocarcinoma. Cancer, 25: 947, 1970.

Rogers, L. W., Julian, C. G., and Woodruff, J. D.: Mesonephroid carcinoma of the ovary. A study of 95 cases from the Emil Novak Ovarian Tumor Registry. Gynecol. Oncol., 1: 76, 1972.

Rosenoff, S. H., Young, R. C., Anderson, T., et al.: Peritoneoscopy: a valuable staging tool in ovarian carcinoma. Ann. Intern. Med., 83: 37, 1975.

Rosenoff, S. H., Young, R. C., Chabner, B., et al.: Use of peritoneoscopy for initial staging and post-therapy evaluation of patients with ovarian carcinoma. Symposium on Ovarian Carcinoma, National Cancer Institute Monograph 42., edited by R. C. Young and J. P. Smith, p. 81. U.S. Government Printing Office, Washington, D.C., 1975.

Rubin, D. K., and Frost, J. K.: The cytologic detection of ovarian cancer. Acta Cytologica, 7: 191, 1963.

Sagerman, R. H., Hanks, G. E., and Bagshaw, M. A.: Supervoltage radiation therapy: Use of the linear accelerator for treating ovarian adenocarcinoma. Calif. Med., 102: 118, 1965.

Sampson, J. A.: Endometrial carcinoma of the ovary, arising in endometrial tissue in that organ. Arch. Surg., 10: 1, 1925.

Sampson, J. A.: Carcinoma of tubes and ovaries secondary to carcinoma to body of uterus. Am. J. Pathol., 10: 1, 1934.

Santesson, L.: Cited by F. T. Kraus. Gynecological Pathology, C. V. Mosby Company, St. Louis, 1967.

Santesson, L., and Lottmeier, H. L.: General classification of ovarian tumors. In Ovarian Cancer, edited by F. Gentil, and A. C. Junqueira, UICC Monograph Series, Vol. II. p. 1. Springer-Verlag, New York, 1968.

Saphir, O., and Lackner, J. E.: Adenocarcinoma with clear cells (hypernephroid) of ovary. Surg. Gynecol. Obstet., 79: 439, 1944.

Schiller, W.: Mesonephroma ovarii. Am. J. Cancer, *35:* 1, 1939.

Schoenberg, B. S., Greenberg, R. A., and Eisenberg, H.: Occurrence of certain multiple primary cancers in females. J. Natl. Cancer Inst., *43:* 15, 1969.

Schottenfeld, D., and Berg, J.: Incidence of multiple primary cancers. IV. Cancers of the female breast and genital organs. J. Natl. Cancer Inst., *46:* 161, 1971.

Scully, R. E.: Recent progress in ovarian cancer. Hum. Pathol., *1:* 73, 1970.

Scully, R. E.: The need for uniform terminology. Hum. Pathol., *4:* 602, 1973.

Scully, R. E., and Barlow, J. F.: "Mesonephroma" of the ovary. Tumor of mullerian nature related to the endometrioid carcinoma. Cancer, *20:* 1405, 1967.

Scully, R. E., Richardson, G. S., and Barlow, J. F.: The development of malignancy in endometriosis. Clin. Obstet. Gynaecol., *9:* 384, 1966.

Smith, J. P., and Rutledge, F.: Chemotherapy in the treatment of cancer of the ovary. Am. J. Obstet. Gynecol., *107:* 691, 1970.

Silverberg, S. G.: Clear cell carcinoma ovary. Am. J. Obstet. Gynecol., *115:* 394, 1973.

Silverberg, S. G.: Ultrastructure and histogenesis of clear cell carcinoma of the ovary. Am. J. Obstet. Gynecol., *115:* 394, 1973.

Simer, P. H.: The drainage of particular matter from the peritoneal cavity by lymphatics. Anat. Rec., *88:* 175, 1944.

Spadoni, L. R., Lindberg, N. C., Moffet, N. K., et al.: Virilization coexisting with Krukenberg tumor during pregnancy. Am. J. Obstet. Gynecol., *92:* 981, 1965.

Spohn, W.: Cited by Lynch, F. W., in *Pelvic Neoplasms*, edited by F. W. Lynch and A. Maxwell. Appleton-Century-Crofts, Inc., New York, 1922.

Stewart, H. L., Dunham, L., Casper, J. J., et al.: Epidemiology of cancers of uterine cervix and corpus, breast and ovary in Israel and New York City. J. Natl. Cancer Inst., *37:* 1, 1966.

Stone, M. L., Weingold, A. B., Sall, S., et al.: Factors affecting survival of patients with ovarian carcinoma. Surg. Gynecol. Obstet., *116:* 351, 1963.

Symmonds, R. E., Spraitz, A. F., and Koelsche, G. A.: Large ovarian tumor. Obstet. Gynecol., *22:* 473, 1963.

Teilum, G.: Endodermal sinus tumors of the ovary and testis. Cancer, *12:* 1092, 1959.

Tepper, E., Sanfilippo, L. J., Gray, J., et al.: Second look surgery after radiation therapy for advanced stages of cancer of the ovary. AJR, *112:* 755, 1971.

Thompson, J. D.: Primary ovarian adenocanthoma. Obstet. Gynecol., *9:* 403, 1957.

Timm, J.: Ovarian carcinoma: a ten-year series from a provincial hospital. Acta Obstet. Gynecol. Scand., *52:* 103, 1973.

Tobias, J. S., and Griffiths, C. T.: Management of ovarian carcinoma: Current concepts and future prospects. N. Engl. J. Med., *294:* 818, and 877, 1976.

Towers, R. P.: A note on the origin of pseudomucinous cystadenoma of the ovary. J. Obstet. Gynaec. Br. Commonw., *63:* 253, 1956.

Van Orden, D. E., McAllister, W. B., Zerne, S. R. M., et al.: Ovarian carcinoma: the problems of staging and grading. Am. J. Obstet. Gynecol., *94:* 195, 1966.

Wampler, G. L., Mellette, S. J., Kuperminc, M., et al.: Hexamethylmelamine (NSC-13875) in the treatment of advanced cancer. Cancer Chemother. Rep., *56:* 505, 1972.

Wangensteen, O. H., Lewis, F. J., and Tongen, L. A.: The "second look" in cancer surgery. Lancet, *71:* 303, 1951.

Webb, M. J., Decker, D. G., Mussey, E., et al.: Factors influencing survival in Stage I ovarian cancer. Am. J. Obstet. Gynecol., *116:* 222, 1973.

Willis, R. A.: *The Pathology of Tumors*, Ed. 4, p. 517, Appleton-Century-Crofts, New York, 1967.

Wilson, W. L., Bisel, H. F., Cole, D., et al.: Prolonged low-dosage administration of hexamethylmelamine. Cancer, *25:* 568, 1970.

Wiltshaw, E., and Carr, B.: *Cis*-platinum (II)diamine dichloride. Recent Results Cancer Res., *48:* 178, 1974.

Woodruff, J. D., and Julian, C. G.: Histologic grading and morphologic changes of significance in the treatment of semimalignant and malignant ovarian tumors. *Proceedings of the Sixth National Conference*, p. 347 J. B. Lippincott, Philadelphia, 1968.

Woodruff, J. D., and Julian, C. G.: Multiple malignancy in the upper genital canal. Am. J. Obstet Gynecol., *103:* 810, 1969.

Woodruff, J. D., and Julian, C. G.: Explorations into the genesis of ovarian malignancy. Int. J. Gynaecol. Obstet., *8:* 587, 1970.

Woodruff, J. D., and Novak, E. R.: Papillary serous tumors of the ovary. Am. J. Obstet. Gynecol., *67:* 1112, 1954.

Woodruff, J. D., and Novak, E. R.: Krukenberg tumors of the ovary. Obstet. Gynecol., *15:* 351, 1960.

Woodruff, J. D., Perry, F. H., Genadry, R., et al.: Mucinous cystadenocarcinoma of the ovary. Obstet. Gynecol., *51:* 483, 1978.

Young, R. C., Chabner, B. A., Hubbard, S. P., et al.: Advanced ovarian adenocarcinoma. N. Engl. J. Med., *299:* 1261, 1978.

CHAPTER 23

Germ Cell Tumors of the Ovary

INTRODUCTION

The previously hotly debated topic of the origin of the primordial germ cell is now nearly settled. Witschi in 1948 demonstrated that, in the human, these cells separate from stem cells during the embryologic cleavage stages. They are first recognized as a distinct entity, however, in the 4-week embryo. Here they appear as large distinctive cells differentiated and lodged in a localized area of the wall of the yolk sac in close proximity to the allantoic diverticulum. During the ensuing week they migrate from the yolk sac to the wall of the hindgut and from here along its dorsal mesentery to the gonadal ridge where they become concentrated in their final location. Because of their intense alkaline phosphatase reaction, the germ cells are relatively easy to spot and trace in their journey to the gonadal ridge. The fact that they arise in an extragonadal location and travel to a more distant permanent home helps to explain the myriad locations occupied by germ cells tumors.

Soon after their arrival at the gonadal ridge, the germ cells begin prophase of meiosis I. This is in marked contrast to the male in whom meiosis does not commence until puberty. The term "oogenesis" refers to the transformation of oogonia, which multiply in the ovary by mitotic division. The primary oocytes must undergo reductive division (meiosis) to yield a secondary oocyte, which is haploid in chromosomal number, and the first polar body. A second, nonreductive division, of the secondary oocyte leads to the formation of the definitive gamete (the haploid ovum) and a second polar body. During the reductive division from primary to secondary oocyte, there occurs, on occasion, an exchange of chromosomal material between homologous chromatids. The statistical likelihood of this exchange at any one locus is directly related to the distance from the centromere. This "crossing over" of chromosomal material that occurs in the reductive division of meiosis (meiosis I) produces some biologic information that is valuable in giving us a clue as to when the transformation from germ cell to neoplasm takes place.

The onset of meiosis I has already occurred in embryonic life. The secondary oocyte remains frozen in prophase meiosis I until ovulation. It then proceeds to metaphase meiosis II, and no further, unless fertilization takes place.

CLASSIFICATION

The classification of germ cell tumors of the ovary has been documented in Chapter 22 but for the sake of completeness within this chapter we would like to record it again below.

GERM CELL TUMORS

A. Dysgerminoma
B. Endodermal sinus tumor
C. Malignant (immature) teratoma
D. Benign (mature) teratoma
E. Struma ovarii
F. Carcinoid
G. Embryonal cell carcinoma
H. Polyembryoma
I. Choriocarcinoma

BENIGN MATURE TERATOMA
(Dermoid Cyst)

The dermoid cyst is, quite simply, a benign cystic teratoma. Germ cell tumors are either benign or malignant on the basis of whether the tissue is mature or not. Conversely, malignant germ cell tumors contain immature tissue that either resembles a portion or portions of the embryo or extraembryonic tissue. The "dermoids" were so named, originally, because of their predominant composition of skin and skin-like structures. If carefully analyzed, however, all three germ layers usually become apparent.

The dermoid cyst is the most common ovarian germ cell neoplasm and comprises approximately 10% of all ovarian tumors. They are the most frequently encountered type of ovarian tumor in the young woman less than 20 years of age.

The benign cystic teratoma is characterized by a thick, well formed capsule that is lined completely, or nearly completely, by squamous epithelium of varying thickness. Beneath this epithelium, a variety of the skin appendages are usually to be found. They may include ordinary sweat glands, apocrine glands and, very frequently, sebaceous glands. The cavity lined by squamous epithe-lium becomes filled with the resultant debris of both the epithelium and its appendages (Fig. 23.1) and is consequently among the most offensive of all tumors for the pathologist to open. When opened, a thick greasy pale yellow material, frequently containing hair, oozes forth. At times, choroid plexus formation is prominant enough to form a cystic structure filled with cerebrospinal fluid and this variety of dermoid can easily be mistaken, grossly, either for a cystic epithelial tumor, or a large functional cyst. The average dermoid will frequently contain a localized nubbin of tissue situated somewhere inside the wall, and this structure has a very colorful historical past. It was thought of, in the middle ages, as the "embryoid body" and was the area where baptismal waters were applied. This nubbin also has been known as Rokitansky's nodule, the nipple, focal insular protuberance, etc. The importance of the nodule is the fact that it frequently contains the other elements that make it a three-germ cell layer tumor.

Perhaps the most dramatic of all gross and radiographic findings are those of teeth, and all varieties of teeth may be found although incisors are less frequently noted. The radiographic discovery of teeth in the pelvis essentially makes the diagnosis of a dermoid cyst.

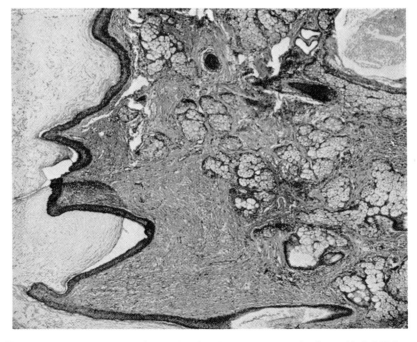

Figure 23.1. Wall of dermoid cyst showing skin, sebaceous glands, and hair follicles.

Also often found microscopically is cartilage, the latter not infrequently in the wall of small ducts lined by ciliated epithelium, and resembling the trachea in structure. Neural tissue, as noted above, is common. Endodermal elements, such as gastrointestinal mucous membrane, may also occasionally be found. A characteristic finding in the vicinity of the wall is the presence of sievelike areas in which are scattered large *giant cells*, often polynuclear. These are of foreign body type, resulting from the penetration of the cyst wall by lipoid material. The wall of the cyst is sometimes devoid of epithelium, and may show numerous endothelial leukocytes (*pseudoxanthoma cells*) as well as foreign body giant cells and cholesterol crystals. Considerable amounts of thyroid tissue (*struma ovarii*) may occur which can be thyrotoxic or undergo characteristic thyroid malignant degeneration.

Carcinoid tumors may arise from argentaffine cells of the gastrointestinal tract, and metastasize to the ovary. However, these occur primarily with the dermoid cyst, and sometimes produce characteristic symptoms primarily due to *serotonin*. Cutaneous flushing, diarrhea, and various cardiovascular symptoms may be manifest, and these symptoms in conjunction with a palpable ovarian tumor might suggest a carcinoid syndrome. A rather rare complication associated with dermoid cysts is *hemolytic anemia*, and some 15 cases have been noted in a review by Adcock. Abnormal antibodies may be noted, but the anemia is completely reversible following removal of the ovarian tumor. Should *rupture* of a dermoid cyst occur, a profound peritonitis with fistula formation may result.

Malignant change can occur in primarily benign dermoid cysts. This sequence can be assumed when the unquestionably malignant lesion occurs in a definitely localized area of a dermoid which is otherwise entirely benign. Carcinoma of the *epidermoid* type is seen in a small proportion of cases (1–3%). *Sarcoma* and malignant melanoma may also be seen, but are less frequent. Prognosis in this unusual situation is related to the intact nature of the capsule and absence of extraovarian extension. If the capsule is intact and there is no evidence of extraovarian involvement, the prognosis is excellent (approximately 80% 5-year salvage) and no further therapy need be considered. If there is extracapsular exten-

sion, the prognosis is relatively poor. Among those rare tumors with malignant change in a benign dermoid, 80% are squamous, 7% are adenocarcinoma, and the remainder include sarcomas of various types, thyroid carcinomas, carcinoids, and melanomas!

Even when a dermoid is quite benign, recurrent intraperitoneal lesions may occur, presumably because of intermittent leakage and subsequent growth.

A presumed intermediate form should be recognized, a *benign solid teratoma*, as noted by Peterson. This is made up of tissues derived from all the fetal layers, but all very mature. Some of these have been extremely large, and some have occurred in children, so that one might at first suspect such tumors to be the malignant types of teratoma seen chiefly in children and usually fatal. The particular group we are describing, however, have all been benign clinically.

Complications of Dermoids

Torsion of the Pedicle

The most frequent complication of any benign ovarian cyst is torsion or twisting of the pedicle, and the acute symptoms thus precipitated are occasionally the first indication of the presence of an ovarian tumor. This complication is more common with tumors of small or moderate size than with the very large ones. The incidence of torsion varies from one series to the next but Peterson's large series yielded a 16% incidence. The twisting of the pedicle is generally in a clockwise fashion, and it may be slight or so extreme that several complete twists of the pedicle are demonstrable (Fig. 23.2).

The occurrence of torsion of the pedicle is associated with *pain* which may be sharp and persistent, but which in other cases may be only moderately severe and transitory. The latter is true when the twisting of the pedicle corrects itself, as it not infrequently does. A common history in cases of ovarian cyst of moderate size is that from time to time the patient has experienced attacks of sharp pain, with spontaneous disappearance after a short time.

In a considerable proportion of cases, however, the symptoms produced by torsion of the pedicle are much more urgent with sudden excruciating pain. Surgery is often performed by a general surgeon who may, with

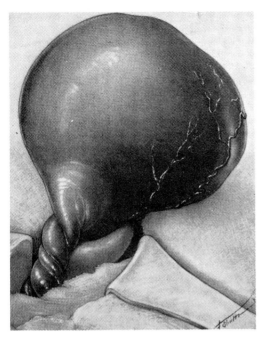

Figure 23.2. Torsion of pedicle of dermoid cyst seen at operation.

all respect, have no concept of the potential lethal nature of certain ovarian lesions so that inadequate operation is common.

Rupture of Cyst

Rupture or perforation of dermoid cysts is rare, mainly because of their thick tough capsule, but with torsion and engorgement this can become softened with resultant perforation into the peritoneal cavity. When this occurs, generalized peritonitis ensues because of marked irritation from the contents of the cyst.

Factors of Surgical and Clinical Interest

It is usually possible, with a little bit of surgical care, to resect a dermoid cyst from the ovary without removing the entire ovary. One can usually find, at one side of the tumor, what represents most of the ovarian structure compressed against it. Careful technique will allow this to be shelled out with resultant conservation of the remaining ovarian structure. This is of particular importance when one considers the fact that the patients are frequently young women and desirous of preservation of child bearing. It is of even

greater consequence since the risk of bilaterality with these tumors approximates 15%. One must look critically at that figure since it represents all patients who have bilateral dermoids. Most of these are obvious at the operating table and can be treated accordingly. The likelihood of bilateral involvement when the opposite ovary is absolutely normal at operation is much less and most clinicians have abandoned its routine bisection.

Dermoid cysts are exceedingly free and often on an elongated ovarian pedicle. It has been noted that they are not infrequently discovered to occupy a position anterior to the broad ligament on pelvic examination. Such a finding in a young woman is highly suggestive of benign cystic teratoma.

DYSGERMINOMA

The dysgerminoma is a tumor purely of germ cells without any attempt to form teratomatous elements. It is the most common of all malignant germ cell tumors of the ovary and comprises nearly 50% of all such tumors. It has the best prognosis of all ovarian cancers except for the borderline epithelial lesions and is probably the most radiosensitive solid tumor known.

Incidence

Morris and Scully note that dysgerminoma comprises 3–5% of all malignant ovarian tumors. Less than 2000 cases have been reported, three-fourths of them occurring in the second or third decade of life. There is a not infrequent association with other types of germ cell neoplasm.

Origin

This interesting tumor type is believed to arise from cells which date back to the early undifferentiated phase of gonadal development. In this stage the *germ cells* have not as yet acquired either male or female characteristics so that, as might be expected, dysgerminoma has no effect on the sex characteristics of the patient. Such an origin, first suggested by Meyer, is given much support by the fact that an identical tumor occurs in the testis, where it is commonly designated as *seminoma*.

The probable correctness of this theory is

further indicated by the fact that in a considerable proportion of the reported cases the tumor has occurred in individuals showing some degree of gonadal dysgenesis. Barr et al. stress the frequency with which these germ cell tumors occur in phenotypic females with an XY sex chromosome complement and "streak" gonads. Manuel et al. likewise indicate the importance of karyotype study.

Pathology

Grossly, these tumors are of solid type, although when large, they often show degeneration and cystic cavities (Fig. 23.3). They may be very small, measuring only a few centimeters in diameter, or they may reach such large size as to fill most of the abdominal cavity. They are, when small, surrounded by a rather dense capsule which, however, is often broken through as the tumor grows, with later infiltration of surrounding organs. The cut surface of the tumor is grayish pink with areas of hemorrhagic degeneration. The consistency is doughy but at times firm and rubbery. The growth is usually unilateral, although bilateral tumors have been noted less frequently (Chauser et al., and Williamson et al.).

Microscopically, there are few tumors of the ovary which present such a distinctive picture, so that the diagnosis in most cases is easy, once one is familiar with this picture. The tumor is made up of rather large round or ovoid cells, arranged characteristically in alveoli separated by septa of partially hyalinized connective tissue which shows a characteristic infiltration with lymphocytes (Fig.

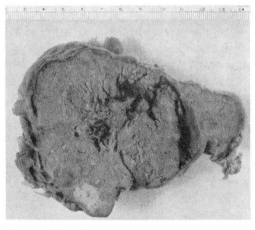

Figure 23.3. Dysgerminoma—gross appearance.

23.4). The nuclei of the epithelial cells are large and rather deeply staining, and a varying number of mitoses are to be seen, although usually they are not numerous.

Malignancy

This tumor undoubtedly belongs in the malignant group, but there is much variation in individual cases. Certainly the degree of malignancy is not to be compared to that of the common types of primary ovarian cancer, and cure has in many cases followed simple removal of the adnexa on the involved side. When the tumor is well encapsulated, the prognosis is in general good, but in the infiltrating variety, associated as it is with involvement of adjoining viscera and sometimes distant metastases, the outlook is very unfavorable. The prognosis worsens if (1) there are bilateral tumors, (2) the capsule is not intact, (3) there is spillage at operation, or (4) there are associated teratomatous or trophoblastic elements. Actually where the capsule is intact and the disease is unilateral, de Lima notes an 80% salvage. Malkasian and Symmonds record an 80.9% 5-year survival following conservative surgery as compared to 87.5% when treatment was more extensive, and the Armed Forces Institute of Pathology (AFIP) figures (Asadourian and Taylor) are even more favorable.

Clinical Characteristics

The incidence of these tumors appears to be about one-third of granulosa cell tumors which, in turn, makes up something like 10% of all primary malignant ovarian tumors. Dysgerminoma is characteristically a *tumor of early life* ("carcinoma puellarum"). It occurs not infrequently in very early childhood, and is common in the second and third decades.

Symptoms

As with so many other types of ovarian tumor, the first evidence of its presence is often the detection of a *mass* in the lower abdomen. There is *no characteristic effect on menstruation,* although it must be remembered that dysgerminoma often occurs in women who have had amenorrhea as a result of gonadal deficiency. Where other marked sex abnormalities such as (pseudo-) hermaphroditism are present, the strong possibility

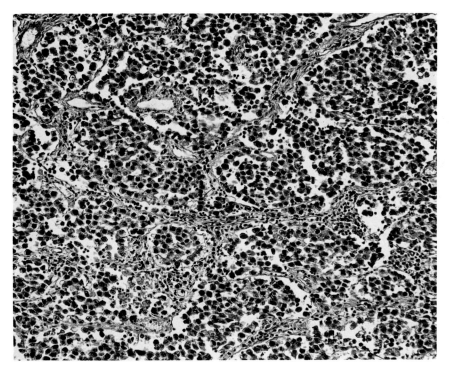

Figure 23.4.   Large clear cells with dark nucleus separated by connective tissue matrix in a typical dysgerminoma. Characteristic lymphocytic infiltration.

of dysgerminoma should be considered when a gonadal tumor is diagnosed. On the other hand, the majority of cases have occurred in ostensibly normal women with often one or more pregnancies before the development of the tumor, and it may concur with pregnancy. *Ascites* has been observed with these tumors, as with other solid ovarian growths.

Treatment

Localized Tumors

Although there is no difference of opinion as to the advisability of surgical treatment, there is still some uncertainty as to the extent of the operation in the individual case. Most of these patients are very young, so that there is a natural tendency to avoid extensive surgery if possible. In the case of young patients with *well encapsulated unilateral tumors,* conservative operation, consisting commonly of unilateral salpingo-oophorectomy, appears fully justified by the good results obtained in many reported cases. Rationalization suggests that if the tumor has exceeded the confines of the ovary, cure is unlikely. If the tumor is confined to the ovary, complete

surgery is not necessary, although some 10% of patients will have metastases despite an intact capsule.

Since approximately three-quarters of all cases of dysgerminoma are Stage I tumors and since many of the patients are so young at the time of diagnosis, we should dwell for a while on the decisions to be made at the time of initial exploration. In those patients with disease that is Stage II, III, or IV, the decision is clear-cut and total abdominal hysterectomy bilateral salpingo-oophorectomy is indicated followed fairly promptly with radiotherapy. The choices are not so easy with a young patient with Stage Ia disease, and fully two-thirds of all patients have apparent Ia disease at the time of operative diagnosis.

There is no question but that hysterectomy with bilateral adnexectomy is the proper procedure where there are no further procreative desires, irrespective of age. Thoeny et al. have noted that patients undergoing conservative salpingo-oophorectomy have a higher incidence of recurrence (43% of 14 patients) even with no apparent extension of the disease at the original operation.

The *optimal* treatment seems to be complete operation with additional irradiation if there is any evidence of local or lymphatic extension. *Conservative* surgery, however, should be reserved for the young individual with a slight calculated risk. It does not seem that women treated conservatively should be subjected to routine radiotherapy (even with the remaining ovary shielded), as suggested by Brody. If this approach seems too conservative it is because of our belief that the tumor is generally of rather low grade malignancy, which frequently involves an extremely youthful patient very anxious for further pregnancy.

Infiltrative Tumor

When, on the other hand, the tumor is infiltrative or extensive, complete removal of the pelvic organs is indicated, and this should be followed by various forms of *irradiation therapy*. Today there is general agreement that dysgerminoma is usually quite radiosensitive, and studies by Brody and by Thoeny et al. seem convincing, but we would not advocate irradiation therapy if only conservative unilateral adnexectomy is done.

ENDODERMAL SINUS TUMOR

Unlike the dysgerminoma, which is only low grade in its malignant potential, the endodermal sinus tumor (EST) is an exceedingly virulent ovarian tumor. It is the second most common malignant germ cell tumor of the ovary, comprising 22% of all malignant germ cell neoplasms in the Armed Forces Institute of Pathology (AFIP) series.

For the most part, the endodermal sinus tumor is a germ cell tumor composed of extraembryonic structures. In contrast to the dysgerminoma, it is almost never bilateral. In the series from the AFIP, ages ranged from 14 months to 45 years with a median of 19 years. A mass was palpable by the clinician in 74% of the cases. Pain was the most common presenting symptom occurring in 77% of the patients. Seventy-one per cent of the neoplasms were Stage I in this 71-patient series and none were bilateral.

The tumors frequently present as very large masses with a great deal of necrosis and hemorrhage. Approximately one-third will rupture prior to or during surgery. In the AFIP series reported by Kurman and Norris, the diameter ranged from 7 to 28 cm with a median of 15 cm.

Microscopically, the tumor displays a variety of interrelated patterns. It is characterized chiefly by a loose network of spaces and channels lined by flattened or cuboidal cells with indistinct cell outlines. The supporting stroma is very loose, immature mesenchymal

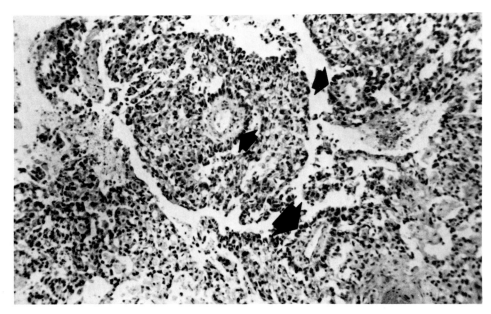

Figure 23.5. Endodermal sinus tumor demonstrating mantling of capillaries by yolk sac endoderm. *See arrows.*

tissue. In some areas, the neoplasms contain pseudopapillary structures in which small blood vessels are mantled by irregular cuboidal epithelial cells (Fig. 23.5). A sinus or free space surrounds this arrangement. Another microscopic feature that characterizes the neoplasm is the presence of hyaline bodies which occur both intracellularly and extracellularly. If one does immunofluorescent staining on these, alpha fetoprotein (AFP) can be identified. This is a characteristic product of yolk sac endoderm and helps to confirm the nature of the tumor. The clinical corollary to this is that all of these patients have elevated serum AFP and one can utilize this as a "handle" to gauge the progress of the disease.

The diagnosis of endodermal sinus tumor carries with it a very grave prognosis, in spite of the fact that the majority are confined to one ovary at the time of diagnosis. Investigators have reported a 93% mortality rate in 2 years following diagnosis, irrespective of staging. Radiation therapy has been of no obvious benefit. In the past few years, chemotherapy has been found to be a valuable surgical adjuvant.

MALIGNANT (IMMATURE) TERATOMA

In a series of 191 cases of malignant Stage I ovarian germ cell tumors reported out of the AFIP, 40 were characterized as immature or malignant teratoma. The immature teratoma is composed of varying quantities of immature tissue differentiating toward any one or all three germ layers (Figs. 23.6–23.7). For the most part, these tumors are solid and have been referred to by other authors as solid teratomatas. This terminology is confusing and the tumors frequently have cystic areas because of degeneration and hemorrhage. As with the endodermal sinus tumor, they are routinely unilateral if Stage I; consequently, removal of the opposite ovary in the course of surgical treatment achieves nothing of therapeutic value. Since these neoplasms are generally more common in children and young adults this is an important therapeutic consideration.

The degree of malignancy is quite clearly related to the degree of differentiation. Those tumors with very immature tissue are more

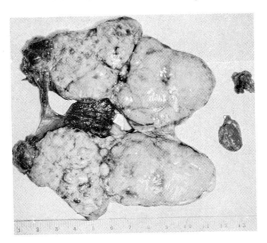

Figure 23.6. Malignant teratoma of ovary.

foreboding than those with mature elements. Robboy and Scully, and Norris et al., have arrived at a tumor grading system that allows us to predict with some degree of certainty the fate of the patient. In those cases where the tumor is confined to the ovary, the grading of the primary sets the prognostic stage. When it is metastatic, grading of the metastases is of greater significance. Because of its more quantitative precision, we would like to present the method of Norris et al. A histologic grade of 1 is given to neoplasms with some immaturity and mitotic activity but with neuroepithelium absent or limited to one × 40 field /slide. A grade of 2 indicates a greater degree of immaturity and neuroepithelium not exceeding three × 40 fields on one slide. Grade 3 is given when the immaturity and neuroepithelium are prominent, the latter occupying four or more × 40 fields on any one slide. When there is no immaturity, the teratoma is grade 0 and has an excellent prognosis.

This particular tumor accounts for 15% of all malignant germ cell tumors in the AFIP series and approximately 70% of all patients who have the neoplasm will have a Stage Ia tumor.

As far as treatment is concerned, radiotherapy appears to play no positive role. Grade 0 lesions require no further therapy following unilateral adnexal removal. Tumors that are more immature probably indicate the use of adjunctive chemotherapy, such as VAC, following unilateral ovarian removal.

The use of tumor markers is sometimes of value in following these tumors. They are,

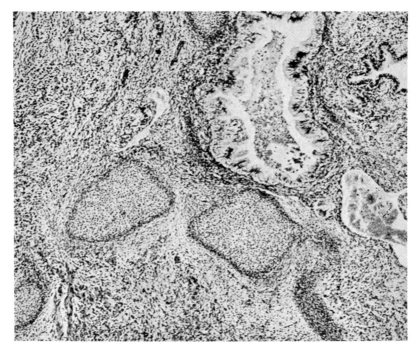

Figure 23.7. Malignant teratoma of ovary showing cartilage plates and a cavity lined by endodermic epithelium like that seen in mucinous cystadenoma.

however, not nearly so useful as with the endodermal sinus tumor. All young women with a pelvic mass should have a chorionic gonadotropin (B subunit), AFP, and carcinoembryonic antigen drawn.

EMBRYONAL CARCINOMA

This is a relatively uncommon ovarian germ cell tumor, comprising only 4% of all germ cell tumors in the AFIP series. It is remarkable for its similiarity to the common testicular embryonal carcinoma. The nomenclature is a bit misleading and it has been used for other germ cell tumors in the past. This group of neoplasms was reported as a distinct entity for the first time in 1976 by Kurman and Norris. In the original series, they presented 15 cases of this tumor variant. The patients' age ranged from 4 to 28 years with a median age of 14. An abdominal or pelvic mass was noted in 12, or 80%. Abdominal pain was a common complaint and was present in 53% of the cases. The most remarkable clinical aspect of this tumor was that 60% of the patients expressed some variety of abnormal hormonal milieu. This occurred in 9 of the 15 patients. Three of seven

prepubertal girls underwent precocious puberty. All patients (10 of 10) who had a determination for hCG were found to be positive. Seven of ten were positive for AFP.

Sixty per cent of the tumors were Stage I at initial surgery and none were bilateral. Like many of the other malignant germ cell tumors, these usually had a smooth external capsule and multiple areas where the tumors were softened and somewhat cystic because of hemorrhage and necrosis. Microscopically, it is quite distinct in appearance from the endodermal sinus tumor. There is no characteristic network of spaces lined by immature epithelial cells nor are there any of the classic papillary structures that make up the typical Schiller-Duval bodies. The tumor seems to grow more like solid cords of immature epithelial cells with papillary tendencies in some areas. There are foci made up of very primitive cells that resemble those of the embryonic disc phase of embryogenesis. In addition, there are areas of scattered syncytiotrophoblastic cells (Fig. 23.8). These can be demonstrated by immunohistochemical reaction to contain hCG. They do not represent true areas of choriocarcinoma in that both populations of cells are not present. In

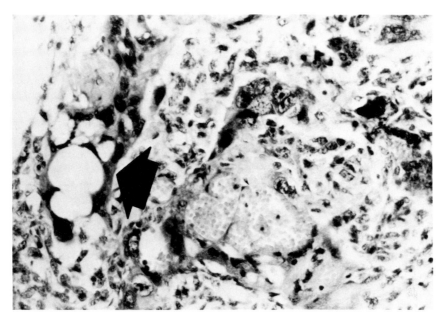

Figure 23.8. Embryonal carcinoma. Note syncytiotrophoblastic cells near *arrow*.

7 of the 10 cases examined for the presence of AFP, this protein was noted to be present. The characteristic hyaline droplets that we now know represent AFP were also present.

In terms of survival, only 6 of the 15 cases survived their therapy. The therapy varied considerably and no case included modern triple chemotherapy as adjuvant management. At this time, the regimen outlined by Einhorn and Donohue for embryonal carcinoma of the testes would be indicated for this disease, when more advanced than Stage I. VAC probably would be the postoperative therapy of choice in Stage I disease. Obviously, unilateral adnexal removal is adequate surgical treatment when the tumor appears to be confined to one ovary.

Although the terminology is misleading in that this "embryonal" carcinoma has significant *extra*embryonic features, it clearly deserves a taxonomic niche that is distinct.

POLYEMBRYOMA

This is an exceedingly uncommon malignant germ cell tumor that contains a large number of embryoid bodies similiar to presomite embryos. They are included here mainly to present the entire spectrum of tumors in this category.

CHORIOCARCINOMA

Most ovarian choriocarcinoma of the ovary is related to gestational trophoblastic disease. Although choriocarcinoma is occasionally noted as part of a mixed germ cell tumor, it is most rare to have a pure nongestational choriocarcinoma. There are only two cases recorded in the registry at the AFIP and only a few more cases in the literature. It is true that nongestational choriocarcinoma of the ovary is not as responsive to chemotherapy as is the gestational form. It is unclear as to whether this is related to the fact that it is so frequently associated with other mixed germ cell elements or that it is not an allograft such as with the gestational trophoblast.

MIXED GERM CELL TUMORS

This category is added for more than the sake of completeness. Many malignant germ cell tumors of the ovary are a composite of the pure forms discussed above. Their behavior depends on the portion of the tumor that is the most immature.

In the series from the AFIP, approximately 8% of the malignant ovarian germ cell tumors belonged in this category. Among the 30 patients presented in this series, the age ranged from 5 to 33 years with a median of 16. Forty per cent of the patients were prepubertal and one-third had isosexual precocity. Two-thirds of the patients had Stage I disease and the actuarial survival in this group was 40%. The most important prognostic features were the degree of immaturity of the tissue and the size of the lesion. Those patients with a tumor size less than 10 cm did considerably better than those patients with larger lesions. A number of patients had positive pregnancy tests in the absence of pregnancy and positive serum levels of AFP. This always reflected the presence of synctiotrophoblastic cells or yolk sac endoderm, respectively.

Surgical therapy includes unilateral removal of the affected adnexa since they are very rarely bilateral. Completion of therapy should include triple chemotherapy (VAC) for a period of 6 months to 1 year.

GONADOBLASTOMA

One of the most common tumors associated with the dysgenetic gonad is the gonadoblastoma. Most frequently, this is noted in the phenotypic female with a Y chromosome. Although not truly a germ cell tumor, the germ cells contained within the neoplasm seem to be at great risk of undergoing malignant change. In one-half of the cases, a seminoma or dysgerminoma develops. Less frequently, a more malignant germ cell tumor such as embryonal carcinoma or choriocarcinoma may arise.

As Patel and Prentice indicate, it seems there is no one consistent karyotype pattern with these neoplasms. Indeed, a calcified ovarian tumor in conjunction with ambiguous sex characteristics might suggest the possibility of gonadoblastoma, irrespective of the karyotype.

Scully has reported 74 cases of gonadoblastoma, most of which arose in gonads of "unknown nature." The largest lesion was 8 cm, and the clinical course and histological pattern seemed generally benign, although various other malignant germ cell tumors such as dysgerminoma or teratoma may be superimposed. On occasion, all combinations of germ cell and stromal tumors may occur. Talerman has noted combined dysgerminoma and gonadoblastoma in siblings with dysgenetic gonads, and has recorded two other similar cases.

OVARIAN TUMORS IN CHILDREN

There is no absolutely appropriate place to insert this section, but it seems least objectionable here, since the differential diagnosis of ovarian neoplasia in the child is so heavily involved with germ cell tumors.

Although many young teen-age females are quite mature, it seems expedient to utilize the age of 15 years as the upper limit of childhood. Ovarian tumors represent a rather infrequent neoplasm in the youthful female. If such functional cysts as follicle or lutein are excluded, the most common gonadal neoplasm would appear to be the dermoid cyst (benign cystic teratoma), which represents approximately one-third to one-half of tumors in the young female. In a review of 992 cases reported in the literature (1935–1961) Huffman reports 298 teratoma (benign or malignant) as well as 97 other germ cell tumors; 115 gonadal stromal tumors are noted along with 177 carcinomas of all types. In his own series of 75 cases, Ein has indicated that an ovarian tumor in the child has a nearly 85% chance of being benign even if functional cysts are included. Nevertheless Norris and Jensen record 67 patients less than 20 years of age with primary epithelial tumors, of which 8 were malignant or borderline malignant with at least 2 deaths. A considerable proportion (one-third) of these tumors occurred in conjunction with pregnancy.

Symptoms, Diagnosis and Treatment

The symptoms of ovarian tumors in children are quite similar to those in the adult, but many parents may assume that the young female complaining only of vague abdominal discomfort is simply "coming of age," and it is frequently not until there is a protuberant abdominal mass that the girl is presented to the gynecologist, unless a hormone-producing tumor leads to endocrine stigmata. Rupture, hemorrhage, or torsion of the pedicle may produce acute abdominal symptoms similar to appendicitis.

Treatment in young females obviously should be directed toward the conservative approach if circumstances permit. The surgeon must be guided by frozen section and pathological consultation, but his own pathological expertise is important. As a general rule, the gonadal stromal and germ cell tumors (barring teratocarcinoma and endodermal sinus tumor) are of low grade malignancy and warrant lesser degrees of surgery as noted in the appropriate chapters of this text. In separate studies, Barber and Graber, and Smith et al., indicate the disproportionate frequency of germ cell tumors which may grow rapidly in the child. Where malignancy has occurred, there have been occasional favorable responses to triple drug therapy.

OVARIAN TUMORS AND PREGNANCY

When small benign cysts are discovered in early pregnancy, most gynecologists are inclined to postpone their removal, for fear that the corpus luteum may be located in the ovary with the tumor, and that its removal might predispose to abortion, as Fraenkel found to be true in his early experiments on rabbits. Although it has been clearly established that the risk of abortion is far less in humans, it is still considered wise to defer operation until after the first trimester unless some more urgent indication should arise, such as torsion of the pedicle. By the same token, many gynecologists try to minimize the hazard of operations of this type by the substitutional administration of progesterone although, even without this, the pregnancy will not usually be disturbed. Another cyst seen early in pregnancy is the theca lutein cyst. This usually disappears late in the first trimester as the relatively high chorionic gonadotropin levels fall normally.

Whether or not an ovarian cyst should be removed promptly if discovered late in pregnancy should be decided on the basis of its size, its position, its rate of growth, and the stage of gestation. If it is of moderate size, and riding high, its removal can often be deferred until after delivery. If the consistency of the tumor suggests that it may possibly be malignant, its prompt removal is indicated. Only recently, we have examined sections of a highly malignant papillary cystadenoma which had been treated expectantly until acute symptoms arose at the 6th month of pregnancy. It is evident, therefore, that each case must be judged on its individual merits, and mistakes can easily occur.

The association of ovarian tumor and pregnancy is quite rare. Beischer was able to report only 164 such cases in a 23-year span at the Royal Womens Hospital, and in over one-half of the cases the tumors concerned were either benign dermoid cysts or mucinous cystadenoma; the incidence of malignancy in their series was only 2.5%.

Chung and Birnbaum suggest that the number of cases of malignant tumors of the ovary in pregnancy is probably less than 50. It is their feeling that laparotomy should be performed during pregnancy when an ovarian tumor is large enough or symptomatic enough "to require laparotomy," irrespective of the stage of the pregnancy. With a borderline epithelial tumor confined to the ovary (International Federation of Gynecology and Obstetrics (FIGO) Stage Ia) unilateral adnexectomy may be carried out, and surgery is most opportunely carried out in the midtrimester of pregnancy. If a solid or suspicious ovarian tumor is found, laparotomy with frozen section should be carried out and definitive surgery be performed. The clinician should always be cognizant of the possibility of a luteoma of pregnancy. The prevailing concept is that this represents merely a physiological enlargement of the ovary rather than a true neoplasm, and as such requires only confirmatory diagnosis rather than ablation.

References and Additional Readings

Abell, M. R.: The nature and classification of ovarian neoplasms. Can. Med. Assoc. J., *94:* 1102, 1966.

Abell, M. R., and Holtz, F.: Ovarian neoplasms in childhood and adolescence. II. Tumors of non-germ cell origin. Am. J. Obstet. Gynecol., *93:* 850, 1965.

Abell, M. R., Johnson, V. J., and Holtz, F.: Ovarian neoplasms in childhood and adolescence. I. Tumors of germ cell origin. Am. J. Obstet. Gynecol., *92:* 1059, 1965.

Abitbol, M. M., Pomerance, W., and Mackles, A.: Spontaneous intraperitoneal rupture of benign teratomas. Obstet. Gynecol. *13:* 198, 1959.

Adcock, L. L.: Unusual manifestation of benign cystic teratoma. Obstet. Gynecol. Surv., *27:* 476, 1972.

Asadourian, L. A., and Taylor, H. B.: Dysgerminoma. Obstet. Gynecol., *33:* 370, 1969.

Azoury, R. S., Jubayli, N. W., and Barakat, B. Y.: Dermoid cyst of ovary containing fetus-like structure. Obstet. Gynecol., *42:* 887, 1973.

Barber, H. R. K., and Graber, E. A.: Gynecological tumors in childhood and infancy. Obstet. Gynecol. Surv., *28:* 357, 1973.

Barr, M. L., Carr, D. H., Plunkett, E. R., Soltan, H. C., and Wiens, R. G.: Male pseudohermaphroditism and pure gonadal dysgenesis in sisters. Am. J. Obstet. Gynecol., *99:* 1074, 1967.

Beischer, N. A.: Ovarian tumors in pregnancy. Obstet. Gynec. Surv., *27:* 429, 1972.

Blackwell, W. J.: Dermoid cysts of the ovary. Their clinical and pathologic significance. Am. J. Obstet. Gynecol., *51:* 151, 1946.

Block, J., and Hall, F. J.: A case of dermoid of the female urinary bladder. Am. J. Med. Sci., *129:* 651, 1905.

Bonney, V.: An ovarian dermoid cyst expelled through the rectum during labor. Proc. R. Soc. Med. Obstet. Gynaecol., *Sect. 7:* 226, 1914.

Brody, S.: Clinical aspects of dysgerminoma of the ovary. Acta Radiol., *56:* 209, 1961.

Caruso, P. A., Marsh, M. R., and Minkowitz, S., et al: An intense clinicopathologic study of 305 teratomas of the ovary. Cancer, *27:* 343, 1971.

Chauser, B. J., Green, J. P., and Klein, H. Z.: Bilateral metachronous dysgerminoma with 15-year interval. Cancer, *27:* 939, 1971.

Chung, A., and Birnbaum, S. J.: Ovarian cancer with pregnancy. Obstet. Gynecol., *41:* 211, 1973.

de Lima, F. O. A.: Disgerminoma do ovario, contribucao para o seu estudo anatomo-clinico. São Paulo, Brazil, 1966.

Ein, S. H.: Cystic and solid tumors in children. J. Pediatr. Surg., *5:* 148, 1970.

Einhorn, L. H., and Donohue, J. P.: Combination chemotherapy in disseminated testicular cancer. Semin. Oncol. 6: 87, 1979.

El-Minaw, M. F., and Hori, J. M.: Malignant melanoma in bilateral dermoid cysts. Int. J. Gynaecol. Obstet., *11:* 218, 1973.

Fraenkel, L.: Die funkton des corpus leteum. Arch. Gynaek., *68;* 438, 1903.

Friedman, N. B.: The comparative morphogenesis of extragenital and gonadal teratoid tumors. Cancer, *4:* 265, 1951.

Garvin, A. J., Pratt-Thomas, H. R., Spector M., et al: Gonadoblastoma: histologic, ultrastructural, and histochemical observations in five cases. J. Obstet. Gynecol., *125:* 459, 1976.

Groeber, W. R.: Ovarian tumors during infancy and childhood. Am. J. Obstet. Gynecol., *86:* 1027, 1963.

Hall, J. E., Caband, P. G., and Sullivan, T.: Squamous carcinoma in previously benign cystic teratoma. Obstet. Gynecol., *6:* 93, 1955.

Huffman, J. W.: *The Gynecology of Childhood and Adolescence.* W. B. Saunders Co., Philadelphia, 1968.

Hunter, W. F., Lennox, B., and Durh, M. D.: The sex of teratomata. Lancet, *2:* 633, 1954.

Huntington, R. W., Jr., and Bullock, W. K.: Yolk sac tumors of the ovary. Cancer, *25:* 1357, 1970.

Jakobovits, A.: Hormone production by miscellaneous ovarian tumors. Am. J. Obstet. Gynecol., *85:* 90, 1963.

Jubb, E. D.: Primary ovarian carcinoma in pregnancy. Am. J. Obstet. Gynecol., *85:* 345, 1963.

Kistner, R. W.: Intraperitoneal rupture of benign cystic teratomas. Review of the literature with a report of two cases. Obstet. Gynecol. Surv., *7:* 603, 1952.

Klionsky, B. L., Nickers, O. J., and Amontegui, A. J.: Squamous cell carcinoma in situ in adult cystic teratoma. Arch. Pathol., *93:* 161, 1972.

Kurman, R. J., and Norris, H. J.: Embryonal carcinoma of the ovary: A clinicopathologic entity distinct from endodermal sinus tumor resembling embryonal carcinoma of the adult testis. Cancer, *38:* 2420, 1976.

Kurman, R. J., and Norris, H. J.: Malignant mixed germ cell tumors of the ovary: a clinical and pathologic analysis of 30 cases. Obstet. Gynecol., *48:* 579, 1976.

Leo, S., Robat, E., and Parekh, M.: Malignant melanoma in dermoid cyst. Obstet. Gynecol., *41:* 205, 1973.

Linder, D., McCaw, B. K., and Hecht, F.: Parthenogenetic origin of benign ovarian teratomas. N. Engl. J. Med., *292:* 63, 1975.

Malkasian, G. D., Jr., and Symmonds, R. E.: Treatment of unilateral encapsulated ovarian dysgerminoma. Am. J. Obstet. Gynecol., *90:* 379, 1964.

Manuel, M., Katayama, K. P., and Jones, H. W., Jr.: The age of occurrence of gonadal tumors in intersex patients with a Y chromosome. Am. J. Obstet. Gynecol., *124:* 293, 1976.

McKay, D. G., Hertig, A. T., Adams, E. C., et al: Histochemical observations on the germ cells of human embryos. Anat. Rec., *117:* 201, 1953.

Morris, J. M., and Scully, R. E.: *Endocrine Pathology of the Ovary.* C. V. Mosby Company, St. Louis, 1958.

Neubecker, R. D., and Breen, J. L.: Embryonal carcinoma of the ovary. Cancer, *15:* 546, 1962.

Nissen, E. D.: Consideration of the malignant carcinoid syndrome. Obstet. Gynecol. Surv., *14:* 459, 1959.

Nogales, F. F., Jr., and Oliva, H. A.: Peritoneal gliomatosis produced by ovarian teratomas. Obstet. Gynecol., *43:* 915, 1974.

Norris, H. J., and Jensen, R. D.: Relative frequency of ovarian neoplasms in children and adolescents. Cancer, *30:* 713, 1972.

Norris, H. J., Zirkin, H.J., and Benson, W. L.: Immature (malignant) teratoma of the ovary: A clinical and pathologic study of 58 cases. Cancer, *37:* 2359, 1976.

Pantoja, E., Noy, M. A., Axtmayer, R. W., et al: Ovarian dermoids and their complications: comprehensive historical review. Obstet. Gynecol. Surv., *30:* 1, 1975.

Patel, S. K., and Prentice, R. S. A.: Gonadoblastoma. Arch. Pathol., *94:* 165, 1972.

Pedowitz, P., Felmus, L. B., and Grayzel, D. M.: Dysgerminoma of the ovary; prognosis and treatment. Am. J. Obstet. Gynecol., *70:* 1284, 1955.

Peterson, W. F.: Malignant degeneration of benign cystic teratomas of the ovary. A collective review of the literature. Obstet. Gynecol. Surv., *12:* 793, 1957.

Peterson, W. F.: Solid, histologically benign teratomas of ovary; report of four cases and review of literature. Am. J. Obstet. Gynecol., *72:* 1094, 1956.

Peterson, W. F., Prevost, E. C., Edmunds, F. T., et al: Benign cystic teratoma of ovary. Am. J. Obstet. Gynecol., *70:* 368, 1955.

Peterson, W. F., Prevost, E. C., Edmunds, F. T., et al: Epidermoid carcinoma arising in a benign cystic teratoma. A report of 15 cases. Am. J. Obstet. Gynecol., *71:* 173, 1956.

Robboy, S. J., Norris, H. J., and Scully, R. E.: Insular carcinoid primary in the ovary: a clinicopathologic analysis of 48 cases. Cancer, *36:* 404, 1975.

Robboy, S. J., and Scully, R. E.: Ovarian teratoma with glial implants on the peritoneum: An analysis of 12 cases. Hum. Pathol., *1:* 643, 1970.

Sawai, M. M., and Sirsat, M. V.: Ovarian tumors in children and adolescence. Indian J. Cancer, *10:* 302, 1973.

Schellhas, H. F.: Malignant potential of the dysgenetic gonad. Part I. Obstet. Gynecol., *44:* 298, 1974.

Scheullhas, H. F.: Malignant potential of the dysgenetic gonad. Part II. Obstet. Gynecol., *44:* 455, 1974.

Schiller, W.: Mesonephroma ovarii. Am. J. Cancer *35:* 1, 1939.

Scully, R. E.: Gonadoblastoma: a review of 74. Cancer, *25:* 1340, 1970.

Scully, R. E.: Ovarian tumors of germ cell origin. In *Progress in Gynecology,* edited by Sturgis and Taymor, Vol. 5. Grune & Stratton, New York, 1970.

Scully, R. E.: Recent progress in ovarian cancer. Hum. Pathol. *1:* 73, 1970.

Smith, A. H., and Ward, S. V.: Dysgerminoma in pregnancy. Obstet. Gynecol., *28:* 502, 1966.

Smith, J. P., Rutledge, F., and Sutow, W.: Malignant gynecologic tumors in children. Am. J. Obstet. Gynecol., *116:* 261, 1973.

Talerman, A.: Gonadoblastoma associated with embryonal carcinoma. Obstet. Gynecol., *43:* 138, 1974.

Tancer, M. L., Orron, A., Baker, J. D., et al: Spontaneous rupture 1 164of ovarian teratoid tumor (dermoid cyst) into the urinary of ovarian teratoid tumor (dermoid cyst) into the urinary bladder. Review of eleven cases and report of one new case. Obstet. Gynecol., *6:* 668, 1955.

Teilum, G.: Classification of endodermal sinus tumour (mesoblastoma vitellinum) and so-called "embryonal carcinoma" of the ovary. Acta Pathol. Microbiol. Scand., *64:* 407, 1946.

Teilum, G: Endodermal sinus tumors of the ovary and testis: Comparative morphogenesis of the so-called mesonephroma ovarii (schiller) and extraembryonic (yolk sac-allantoic) structures of the rat's placenta. Cancer, *12:* 1092, 1959.

Teilum, G. Albrechtsen, R., and Norgaard-Pedersen, B.: Immunofluorescent localization of alpha-fetoprotein synthesis in endodermal sinus tumor (yolk sac tumor). Acta Pathol. Microbiol. Scand., *82A:* 586, 1974.

Teter, J.: Germ cell tumor in dysgenetic gonads. Am. J. Obstet. Gynecol., *108:* 894, 1970.

Thoeny, R. H., Dockerty, M. B., Hunt, A. B., and Childs, D. S.: Study of ovarian dysgerminoma with emphasis on role of radiation therapy. Surg. Gynecol. Obstet., *113:* 692, 1961.

Thurlbeck, W. M., and Scully, R. E.: Solid teratoma of the ovary: A clinicopathological analysis of 9 cases. Cancer, *13:* 804, 1960.

Usizama, H.: Ovarian dysgerminoma associated with masculinization. Cancer, *9:* 736, 1956

White, K. C.: Ovarian tumors in pregnancy. Am. J. Obstet.

Gynecol., *116:* 544, 1973.

Witschi, E.: Migration of the germ cells of human embryos from the yolk sac to the primitive gonadal folds. Contrib. Embryol. *32:* 69, 1948.

Wilkinson, E. J., Friederich, E. G., and Hasty, T. A.: Alpha fetoprotein and endodermal sinus tumor. Am. J. Obstet. Gynecol., *116:* 711, 1973.

Williamson, H. O., and Pratt-Thomas, H. R.: Bilateral gonadoblastoma with dysgerminoma. Obstet. Gynecol., *39:* 263, 1972.

Williamson, H., Underwood, P. B., Jr., Kreutner, A., Jr., et al: Gonadoblastoma: Clinicopathologic correlation in six patients. Am. J. Obstet. Gynecol., *126:* 579, 1976.

Woodruff, J. D., Protos, P., and Peterson, W. F.: Ovarian teratomas. Am. J. Obstet. Gynecol., *102:* 702, 1968.

CHAPTER 24

Gonadal Stromal and Special Tumors of the Ovary

INTRODUCTION

The category of gonadal stromal tumors has existed under a variety of designations and labels.

We have chosen to employ the overall term *gonadal stromal tumors*, which suggests that this group of neoplasms originates from the ovarian stroma. It makes no claim as to exact cell of embryonic origin, for this is a confusing and still debated topic. In terms of sub-classification, we have elected to use histologic resemblance to ovarian or testicular structure.

By definition, tumors in this category are composed of cells that resemble one or any combination of cells of the female and/or male gonadal endocrine system. Those that resemble the female gonad have elements that mimic granulosa cells, theca cells, and their luteinized derivatives. Those that echo the male gonad are composed of what appear to be Sertoli cells and Leydig cells. For the most part, function follows form, and those tumors resembling the female endocrine system are feminizing and those appearing as testicular endocrine tissue are virilizing. As noted above, such might not always be the case. The reverse may be true, and at least 15% of these tumors have *no* apparent clinical effect. The vast majority of the tumors are in the granulosa theca cell category and a smaller number in the Sertoli-Leydig cell group but there is an even smaller number of mixed tumors.

To further clarify what must seem to be a very confusing situation for the student, the term *gonadal stromal tumors* refers to the origin of these neoplasms from mesenchyme (primitive stroma). It does not suggest that the tumor has no epithelial elements for, clearly, the granulosa and Sertoli cells fulfill the criteria for epithelia in that they line a cavity, have some secretory function, and have no blood supply of their own.

FIBROMA-THECOMA GROUP OF TUMORS

These are primarily benign tumors arising from the ovarian stroma (theca). They have no epithelial or sex-cord element. That is, they contain no granulosa or Sertoli cell elements. In the past, the fibromas and thecomas were classified separately but, in point of fact, this group of neoplasms is a continuous spectrum. At one end are those tumors in which the stromal cells differentiate in such a fashion that the formation of collagen-producing fibroblasts predominates and at the other end are those tumors in which the formation of steroid producing theca cells predominate. One cannot make a clear separation between the two either with the light or electron microscope. Only histochemical studies can give one a valid clue in many cases.

Fibroma

The fibroma is a not uncommon tumor of the ovary, appearing sometimes as a small nodule on the surface or in the substance of the ovary, while in some cases it may attain huge size, filling most of the abdominal cavity and weighing many pounds. The tumors are generally solid, but in the larger ones cavities may form as a result of cystic degeneration. The cut surface is whitish or yellowish white, and is of either homogeneous or of trabeculated appearance (Fig. 24.1).

Microscopic. Microscopically (Fig. 24.2), the structure is that of fibrous tissue of varying morphology. In some areas, the cells are stellate or fusiform but, in other areas, the cells are rather closely packed and spindle-shaped, and may show an admixture of muscle cells (*fibromyoma*). In other tumors, areas of cartilage or bone may be found (*fibrochondroma* or *fibroosteoma*), suggesting a teratomatous origin. Admixtures of *theca* cells are common if routine fat stains are performed.

The small growths produce no *symptoms.* With those of larger size, the patient herself notices the tumor sooner or later, and there is likely to be pain and heaviness in the affected side. There are no characteristic effects on menstruation, but menorrhagia and dysmenorrhea may be noted. Because of the heaviness of the growths, partial twisting or angulation of the pedicle may occur, with venous obstruction and eventual infarction.

Meigs' Syndrome

Meigs called attention to a peculiar syndrome which may occur with these tumors, characterized by *hydrothorax* as well as *ascites*, and a considerable group of such cases has been described. The mechanism of this syndrome is not completely understood, but various lymphatics through the diaphragm seem the likely route for ascitic fluid into the chest. Contrary to an earlier belief, it is not distinctive of fibromas, as it has been noted with Brenner tumors, granulosal and thecomatous growths, and carcinoma, even in the absence of pleural metastasis.

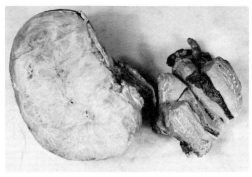

Figure 24.1. Fibroma of ovary.

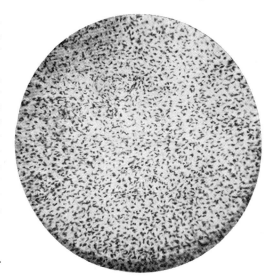

Figure 24.2. Microscopic appearance of fibroma of ovary.

The *treatment* of fibroma is surgical, and this results in complete disappearance of chest and peritoneal fluid where there is a *Meigs' syndrome.* As a matter of fact, operation is indicated in any solid tumor of the ovary, although distinction from a pedunculated fibroid is not easy.

Thecoma

Gross. In a certain proportion of cases, a fibroma-like character may be given to the histological picture by the presence of large numbers of connective tissue elements. The term of fibrothecoma seems appropriate, although the general term, thecoma, is most commonly employed. Such tumors are commonly firm and fibrous in appearance and consistency and are less likely to show a tendency to cystic degeneration. The contralateral ovary may show evidence of profound overgrowth of stromal cells, the so-called "*diffuse thecomatosis,*" and this is a frequent finding with many ovarian tumors, especially where there is apparent endocrine activity.

Microscopic. Microscopically, they are distinguished especially by the presence of bundles of broad spindle cells distributed in an irregular interlacing manner throughout the tumor (Fig. 24.3), separated by varying sized bands of connective tissue and often hyaline plaques. Stress is laid also upon the presence of doubly refractile fat in large amounts

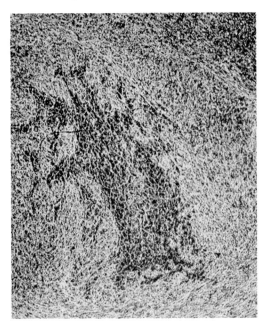

Figure 24.3. Thecoma with lutein-like transformation in certain areas.

within the cells and, to a lesser extent, in the surrounding connective tissue.

Malignancy. Unlike the granulosa cell tumor which represents a low grade malignancy, the thecoma is an essentially benign tumor. It probably evolves from mature ovarian stroma and is similar in some ways to non-neoplastic ovarian stromal changes such as those associated with follicular development and nodular stromal hyperplasia.

GRANULOSA-THECA CELL TUMORS

These neoplasms are properly discussed together, since it seems probable that they have a common origin and biological effect. They are given their special designations chiefly because of the different morphological patterns which they may assume. Not all authors, however, are convinced of the wisdom of any sharp separation, especially since mixed forms are not infrequent; indeed some admixture is the rule. For convention, however, we shall allude to granulosa and theca cell lesions as if they are discrete tumors.

Histogenesis

The exact histogenesis is far from certain, but the prevailing concept of the origin of

granulosa cell tumors has been that they arise from cells of the early ovarian mesenchyme or gonadal stroma.

Pathology of Granulosa Cell Tumors

Gross. Grossly, these tumors vary in size from only a few millimeters in diameter to tumors filling a large part of the abdominal cavity and weighing over 150 pounds (Robertson). The larger tumors often show one or many cystic cavities. The intervening solid tissue is of friable or granular consistency, and of grayish-yellowish hue.

Microscopic. Microscopically, the diagnosis of granulosa cell tumor is based upon the *granulosal character of the constituent cells* and upon the *growth characteristics* of these cells, which are quite like those of normal granulosa. Many different patterns may be found in a single tumor.

Luteinization of Granulosa-Theca Cell Tumors

An interesting histological characteristic of the granulosa-theca cell tumors (Figs. 24.4) is that the constituent granulosa or theca cells may at times undergo transformation into what are typical lutein cells. We have seen a considerable group in which such a transition is in progress, so that parts of the tumor have a lutein appearance, whereas others are still typically granulosal in character. It seems desirable to call these simply *"luteinized granulosa-theca tumors."* Although the term "luteoma" was formerly utilized, we feel it is misleading and reserve it exclusively for the *luteoma* of *pregnancy*. The term *"folliculoma lipidique"* is often applied to markedly luteinized granulosa cell tumors, often tubular, although Teilum has indicated that the origin is the Sertoli cell.

Association of cell type and endocrine effect is inconstant.

Peutz-Jeghers Syndrome

Scully has described certain lipid sex-cord tumors with associated *intestinal polyps* and *melanin spots* on the aural mucosa and skin; the so-called *Peutz-Jeghers syndrome.* Actually, this syndrome may occur with many varieties of ovarian tumors. Christian has suggested that granulosa cells may evolve from certain endodermal sources.

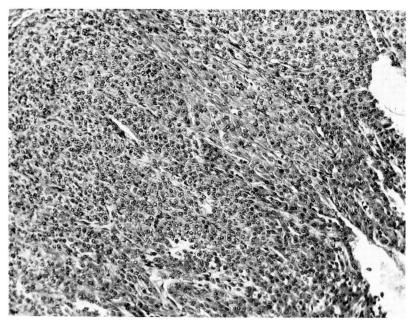

Figure 24.4. Most areas show only a typical granulosa-thecal pattern with beginning luteinization in *right central area.*

Pregnancy Luteoma

Sternberg describes a "pregnancy luteoma" as an ovarian enlargement (up to 12 cm), which is generally solid, composed of eosinophilic, polyhedral cells, which are not a part of the corpus luteum of pregnancy and may, on occasion, be bilateral. It was not certain whether this is a true neoplasm or merely a physiological response to pregnancy, similar to the theca lutein cysts so frequently seen in trophoblastic disease, and occasionally with normal pregnancy.

Most of these cases of ovarian enlargement regress spontaneously despite no other treatment than biopsy, which would further indicate a physiological rather than a neoplastic origin. However, Sternberg and Barclay report a case where lutein enlargement persisted and necessitated surgery (Fig. 24.5). Whether a true neoplasm followed this physiological advent must be left open for speculation. Focal stromal luteinization is common in the ovary removed during pregnancy, and this would seem a logical beginning to the luteoma of pregnancy.

Clinical Characteristics of Granulosa-Theca Tumors

The granulosa cell neoplasms of the ovary may be considered a fairly common tumor,

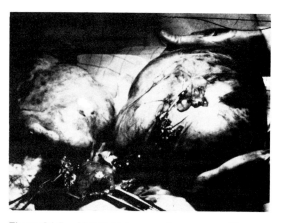

Figure 24.5. Massive luteomas of pregnancy. (Courtesy of Dr. D. L. Barclay, New Orleans, La.)

comprising probably nearly 10% of all solid malignant ovarian neoplasms. The thecoma is much less frequent, although admixture is nearly the rule. These tumors may occur at any age—before puberty, during the reproductive epoch, or after the menopause. Although the larger tumors, like other ovarian neoplasms, may cause such symptoms as pain or discomfort, the more distinctive symptomatology is dependent upon the capability of the tumor cells to produce the estrogenic hormone. However, perforation of the tumor with intraperitoneal hemorrhage may lead to acute symptoms simulating those associated with a ruptured ectopic pregnancy (French, and Gondos and Monroe). Bilaterality is rare (approximately 5%).

When the tumor occurs *during reproductive life*, as it does in a large proportion of cases, the clinical syndrome is not so striking as when it occurs against the background of the prepubertal or postmenopausal phase, during which there is normally little or no estrogenic hormone in the circulation.

During the reproductive years, the tumor merely adds quantitatively to the cyclical hormonal content of the blood. No change would be expected in the secondary sex characters, for example, because these have long since been developed, whereas the effect upon menstruation would be merely a quantitative one, not unlike that which characterizes the relative hyperestrogenism which is associated with most cases of functional bleeding.

When, on the other hand, such tumors occur in *young children*, long before the in-auguration of the normal estrogenic function of the ovary, the clinical manifestations of precocious puberty are evoked, viz., precocious menstruation and the premature appearance of secondary sex characters, such as hypertrophy of the breasts, the appearance of axillary and pubic hair, pubertal development of the external genitalia (Figs. 24.6), and also hypertrophy of the uterus. With the removal of the tumor, these manifestations promptly regress, constituting a crucial biological demonstration of the direct causal role of the tumor in the production of the symptoms.

In the *postmenopausal* group of cases occurring at a life phase at which little or no estrogenic hormone is found in the blood, the tumors may produce a re-establishment of periodic menstruation-like bleeding, an estrogenic type of cytological specimen, and hypertrophy of the uterus, with cases noted up to 84 years of age. No effect is seen upon secondary sex characters, presumably be-

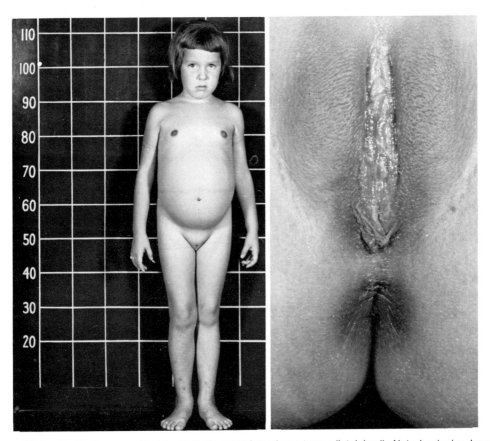

Figure 24.6. (*Left*), five-year-old girl with large granulosa-theca tumor (luteinized). Note beginning breast development, prominent labia, and abdominal distention. (*Right*), adult labia in same child.

cause of the higher threshold or unreceptivity of these at this phase of life. With the removal of tumors at this age, the abnormal menstruation of course ceases and, interestingly enough, the patient may experience a second menopause from the standpoint of the characteristic vasomotor phenomena.

Malignancy

Like Flick and Banfield we found that thecoma is considerably less malignant than the predominantly granulosa cell tumors.

Fox et al. feel that the usual 5-year salvage quoted for granulosa cell tumors is not valid because of the frequent late recurrence. They estimate a 50%, 20-year salvage and describe various factors leading to poor prognosis. As in all low grade or borderline malignancy, 5-year salvage can be misleading.

Association of Endometrial Carcinoma with Feminizing Tumors

Various investigators have found that from 15 to 25% of postmenopausal women with feminizing tumors of the ovary develop endometrial carcinoma. In our review of OTR material, adenocarcinoma was encountered in 23% and hyperplasia in an additional 68%. This association emphasizes the predisposing role of postmenopausal stimulation of the endometrium by estrogen in the development of cancer.

Treatment

Little need be said on the subject of treatment, which is, of course, surgical. When the tumors are small and unilateral, as they have been in practically all the prepuberal cases, unilateral salpingo-oophorectomy has frequently resulted in permanent cure. Preferable to random *frozen section* is removal of the total tumor so that the pathologist can select the most suspicious areas for microscopic evaluation; on the basis of this, the clinician is in a better position to make a decision as to the extent of the operation, although the degree of differentiation and mitotic activity of these "special" tumors does not always parallel their malignant potential.

In any case, one must realize that conservative operation is attended by some slight risk and periodic postoperative examinations are of obvious importance. Considerable individ-

ualization should be practiced, according to age, parity, extent of the tumor, whether encapsulated, etc.

Irradiation has a very limited role in the treatment. Multiple drug therapy has been suggested by some. At present, all we can say about this tumor is that it can be quite responsive to chemotherapy.

SERTOLI-LEYDIG CELL TUMORS
(Androblastomas, Arrhenoblastomas)

This group of tumors, which is frequently masculinizing, is far less common than the granulosa cell variant tumor. They constitute less than 0.4% of ovarian neoplasms. The terms in most common usage are *Sertoli-Leydig cell tumor* and *androblastoma*. The term *androblastoma* suggests that the tumor attempts to recapitulate testicular development. The nomenclature *Sertoli-Leydig cell tumor* dwells on the direction of differentiation of the neoplastic cells. The term *arrhenoblastoma*, referring to the clinically virilizing effect, was originally coined by Meyer and was applied by him to a group of ovarian tumors whose common characteristic seemed to be an origin from male gonadogenic structures at one place or another of development.

Pathology

Gross. These tumors, as encountered at operation, are usually of moderate size, and may be very small, although in a number of reported instances they have reached large proportions, up to 26 pounds in our study. Characteristically, especially when small, they are solid tumors, although they not infrequently exhibit cystic areas, and in the larger tumors the cysts may be of considerable size. The color and consistency are variable, depending upon their widely differing histological structure. They may be grayish, frequently with areas of definitely yellowish hue, but in some the cut surface is bluish or reddish blue. The consistency may be quite firm in some cases, but degenerative changes with hemorrhage are common.

Microscopic. A description of the microscopic characteristics of Sertoli-Leydig cell tumor is not easy, because of the extreme variations which may be encountered in certain cases, and in different parts of the same tumor. At one extreme is the highly *differen-*

tiated variety corresponding to the *testicular adenoma* described by Pick in 1905, and characterized by a very definite tubular structure, reproducing more or less perfectly the structure of normal testicular tubules. At the other extreme is the very *undifferentiated* variety which, at first sight, may be considered a typical sarcoma, and in which only very careful study of many blocks may reveal the presence of structures like sex-cords, imperfect tubules (Fig. 24.7), or lipoid-containing cells corresponding to *interstitial cells* identical to those of the testis and the presumed source of the androgenic stimulation. Finally, in the group designated by Meyer as the *intermediate*, one usually finds a varying number and distribution of definite tubular structures, interstitial cells, and of cell columns arranged in rather zig-zag fashion, quite like the sex-cords seen in the early development of the gonads.

It is clear, therefore, that the microscopic recognition of these tumors presupposes some familiarity with the various phases of development of the seminiferous apparatus.

Malignancy

Although Sertoli-Leydig cell tumor is properly classified as a malignant tumor,

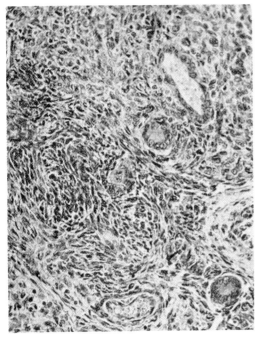

Figure 24.7. Microscopic appearance of an intermediate variety of Sertoli-Leydig cell tumor showing imperfect efforts at testicular tubule formation.

there is no doubt that its degree of malignancy like that of granulosa cell carcinoma, is much less than that of ovarian cancer in general. On the other hand, it must be remembered that many of the reports of this interesting tumor type have been made very soon after treatment so that one cannot always be certain whether or not later recurrence had occurred.

Clinical Features

Sertoli-Leydig cell tumor of the ovary occurs most frequently in relatively young patients, the decade between age 20 and 30 showing the largest incidence.

The clinical course of these patients is characteristically divisible into two phases. There is first a stage of *defeminization* in which certain typical feminine characteristics are subtracted from the patient, and this is followed, with possible overlapping, by a stage of *masculinization*, in which certain positive masculine stigmata are added. Chief among the defeminization symptoms are amenorrhea, atrophy of the breasts, and loss of the subcutaneous fatty deposits which are responsible for the rounding of the feminine figure. The masculinization signs include hypertrophy of the clitoris, hirsutism, and deepening of the voice.

The first symptom noted by most patients is *amenorrhea* which may come on abruptly. *Regression of the mammary glands* soon occurs. *Changes in body contour* may not be conspicuous and are often not noticed by the patient herself, or not at least until *hirsutism* has developed.

A *change in the patient's voice* is often very noticeable, she herself often attributing this to a persistent "cold" or laryngitis. A normally soft, high-pitched feminine voice may be changed to a baritone or even to a basso, with often hoarseness or roughening of the voice. These vocal changes are due to lengthening of the vocal cords, while in marked cases there is overgrowth of the laryngeal cartilages with the development of a prominent "Adam's apple."

With reference to the *hypertrophy of the clitoris*, here again there are marked individual variations. In some cases, it is only slight; in others the clitoris may assume the proportions of a miniature penis. As noted earlier eight cases of concomitant pregnancy with Sertoli-Leydig cell tumor have been recorded.

Transient virilism of a female child was noted occasionally.

Hormone Studies. In these days of serum and urine hormone studies, elevated values of serum testosterone or urinary 17-ketosteroid are diagnostically helpful.

In suspected cases of virilizing ovarian tumors of this or other types, retrograde venous catheterization with serum hormone analysis to determine the site (adrenal vs ovary) and the side is sometimes helpful.

Effects of Tumor Removal on Symptoms. The ultimate clinical test in the substantiation of a diagnosis of arrhenoblastoma is the regression of the abnormal masculinization symptoms after the removal of the tumor. Although this regression may not be complete in every case, it is usually striking in most cases of arrhenoblastoma. The return of menstruation is the first manifestation of returning femininity, and in general the symptoms disappear in the order of their appearance. The positive manifestations of masculinization, however, disappear much more slowly than those of defeminization, and often incompletely. Some degree of hirsutism and enlarged clitoris has persisted for over 20 years in the patient shown in Figures 24.8 and 24.9.

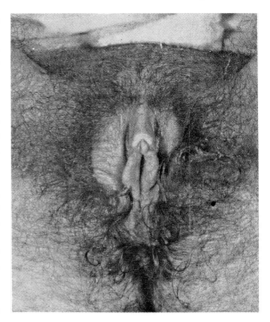

Figure 24.9.   Hypertrophy of clitoris in same patient.

Treatment

Therapy of the Sertoli-Leydig group of tumors is obviously surgery. In view of the usual low grade of malignancy and infrequent incidence of bilateral tumors, unilateral oophorectomy is indicated in the patient who desires preservation of childbearing capacity. All of the usual precautions concerning staging of ovarian neoplasms need to be observed as outlined in Chapter 23. With those patients who have extra ovarian extension, Schwartz and Smith suggest actinomycin D, cyclophosphamide, and vincristine.

GYNANDROBLASTOMA

The name gynandroblastoma was applied by Meyer (1930) to a rare type of ovarian tumor which histologically shows components of both granulosa cell carcinoma and arrhenoblastoma.

We suspect that increasing awareness of the bisexual potential of normal and neoplastic cells, confirmed by histochemical techniques, may reveal that many tumors secrete both androgenic and estrogenic substances. If these be considered gynandroblastomas, the number will certainly increase.

The approach toward this tumor clinically is identical to that for the Sertoli-Leydig cell tumor.

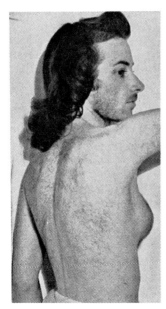

Figure 24.8.   Appearance of patient with arrhenoblastoma showing extensive hirsutism with moderate flattening of breasts; she had not menstruated for 3 years.

LIPID (LIPOID) CELL TUMOR
(Adrenal Rest Tumor, Adrenal Tumor of the Ovary)

This is an unfortunate designation for a very small group of tumors composed of cells of endocrine nature that resemble cells of the adrenal cortex, luteinized cells, or Leydig cells but do not have sufficient histologically identifying criteria to make an absolute diagnosis.

Microscopically, the picture is one of sheets and cords of large round or polyhedral clear- or pale-staining cells separated by delicate vascular septae (Fig. 24.10). Histologically, the differential diagnosis to be made is among hilus cell tumors, stromal luteoma, luteoma of pregnancy, etc. This tumor should be distinguished where possible from the hilus cell tumor. Some taxonomists include these in the category of lipid cell tumors. It also should be separated from the so-called "folliculoma lipidque" which, according to Teilum, is a tumor entirely composed of Sertoli cells in a tubular arrangement. The cells in this tumor are large, pale and appear to contain lipid. These tumors are usually feminizing in contrast to the lipid cell tumors which are usually virilizing.

The tumors may occur in any age category and may achieve considerable size but are much more commonly quite small and frequently nonpalpable on pelvic examination. They are nearly always unilateral and grossly appear as solid tumors that are yellowish in color when cut. They appear grossly and microscopically like adrenal tumors and are also functionally similar to these, leading a number of investigators to classify them as adrenal rest tumors. How many arise from adrenal rests is unknown. Teilum considered the majority of these tumors to arise as a selective differentiation of Leydig cells from ovarian mesenchyme.

HILUS CELL TUMORS
(Ovarian Leydig Cell Tumors)

Hilus cell tumors of the ovary may arise as an overgrowth of mature hilar cells or from ovarian mesenchyme. The neoplasm is composed of uniform, closely packed, polyhedral cells with granular eosinophilic cytoplasm, lipoid vacuoles, and occasionally rod-shaped "Reinke" crystalloids.

A very scant group of cases, estimated at 50 by Dunniho et al., has been regarded as true hilus cell tumors. Because all these tumors have shown masculinization effects, support is given to the prevailing view that the hilus cells are the homologues of the interstitial or Leydig cells of the testis, especially as the tumor cells have been found to show the Reinke albuminoid crystals (Fig. 24.11) so characteristic of the Leydig cells in some but by no means all cases.

Tumors with Functioning Stroma

It is becoming increasingly apparent to all pathologists that a certain number of ovarian tumors, not morphologically of the endocrinologically productive variety, possess hormonal activity. Indeed, these tumors may be of many types, both benign or malignant, and may produce either estrogenic or androgenic features.

It would appear that the *ovarian stroma* is capable of steroid synthesis similar to a theca (lutein) or Leydig cell, apparently as a result of stimulation or irritation by adjacent tumor. Consequently, a great many supposedly inert tumors such as Brenner, Krukenberg, and various carcinomas have seemed to exert a *feminizing* influence. Fewer androgenic tumors have been reported, but a review by

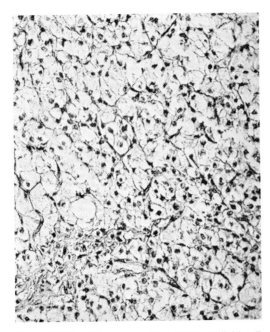

Figure 24.10. Microscopic appearance of lipid cell tumor of ovary characterized by a syndrome identical with that of Sertoli-Leydig cell tumor.

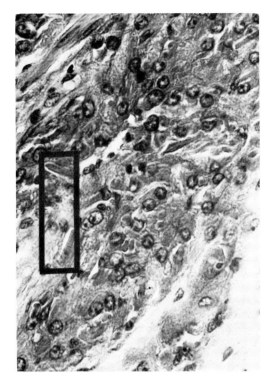

Figure 24.11. Reinke crystalloids apparent in hilus cell tumor. Though pathognomonic, they are not mandatory for diagnosis. (Courtesy of W. Peterson, Washington, D.C.)

Scully notes 11 diverse tumors with virilizing tendencies. Scully has observed a virilized patient whose endometrium showed a frank decidual reaction in association with a metastatic ovarian tumor secondary to a gastric cancer. A progestational pattern is a rare finding in the endometrium and should always raise the question of exogenous hormones.

The question of what supplies the stimulation to the stroma to transform it into a tissue actively involved in steroid synthesis is a perplexing one. To assume it is purely mechanical seems unlikely in view of the fact that certain tumors are more likely than others to achieve this in the face of what appears to be similar patterns of tumor involvement. Luteinization of the stroma accompanies steroid production in these situations as it does in the normal ovary.

Although we think of tumors with a functioning matrix as an unusual situation, it is only uncommon in the sense that steroid synthesis is insufficient to have grossly recognizable clinical effects.

SARCOMA OF OVARY

It is probably appropriate to include these tumors in this section since at least most of the primary sarcomas of the ovary (excluding the mixed mesodermal tumors) are probably of gonadal stromal origin.

Sarcoma of the ovary is far less common than carcinoma, its *incidence* as compared with carcinoma being about 1:40. It *may occur at any age*. Most authors emphasize that it is frequent in children, but this is open to doubt, as so many ovarian tumors in children which were formerly diagnosed as sarcoma are now recognized as either gonadal stromal carcinoma, dysgerminoma, or lymphomas.

Various types of sarcoma are found in the ovary, the spindle variety being more common than the round cell, although mixed forms often occur. The lymphomas, occasionally primary, and angiosarcoma are also described, but it appears that, in the latter, the perivascular arrangement of the cells is due to the fact that extensive degeneration has occurred except where the cells are near to their blood supply. Endometrial or mixed mesodermal sarcomas seem probable sequelae of endometriosis. Symptoms are identical to those of carcinoma.

Azoury and Woodruff have recently reviewed 43 cases of primary ovarian sarcomas from the Emil Novak Ovarian Tumor Registry. They felt it was possible to divide these into three different categories (excluding lymphomas) as follows:

1. Teratoid sarcomas—most common in youthful patients with a very poor prognosis
2. Mesenchymal or stromal—occurring at any age with malignancy definitely comparable to the degree of histologic malignancy
3. Para mesonephric sarcomas—occurring at any age, not infrequently in association with endometriosis and with a poor prognosis

We would doubt that the third category is truly of paramesonephric origin, and would favor looking upon this as a subset of mixed mesodermal tumor.

References and Additional Readings

Amin, H. K., Okagaki, T., and Richart, R. M.: Classification of fibroma and thecoma of the ovary: an ultrastructural study. Cancer, *27:* 438, 1971.
Amin, H., Richart, R. M., and Brinson, A. O.: Preovulatory granulosa cells and steroidogenesis: an ultrastructural study in the rhesus monkey. Obstet. Gynecol., *47:* 562, 1976.

Azoury, R., and Woodruff, J. D.: Primary ovarian sarcoma. Obstet. Gynecol., *37:* 920, 1971.

Berendsen, P. B., Smith, E. B., Abell, M. R., et al.: Fine structure of Leydig cells from an arrhenoblastoma of the ovary. Am. J. Obstet. Gynecol., *103:* 192, 1969.

Berger, L.: La glande sympathicotrope due hile de l'ovaire; ses homologies avec la gland interstitielle du testicule. Les rapports nerveuses des deux glandes. Arch. Anat., *2:* 255, 1923.

Boivin, Y., and Richart, R. M.: Hilus cell tumors of the ovary. Cancer, *18:* 231, 1965.

Braunstein, G. D., Vaitukaitis, J. L., Carbone, P. P., et al.: Ectopic production of human chorionic gonadotropin by neoplasms. Ann. Intern. Med., *78:* 39, 1973.

Busby, T., and Anderson, G. W.: Feminizing mesenchymomas of ovary. Am. J. Obstet. Gynecol., *68:* 1391, 1954.

Chan, L. K. C., and Prathrop, K.: Virilization in pregnancy with mucinous cystadenoma. Am. J. Obstet. Gynecol., *108:* 946, 1970.

Christian, C. D.: Ovarian tumors and Peutz-Jeghers syndrome. Am. J. Obstet. Gynecol., *111:* 529, 1971.

Connor, T. B., Gavin, F. M., Levin, H. S., et al.: Gonadotropin-dependent Krukenberg tumor causing virilization during pregnancy. J. Clin. Endocrinol. Metab., *28:* 198, 1968.

Diddle, A. W., and Devereux, W. P.: Ovarian mesenchymomas. Obstet. Gynecol., *13:* 294, 1959.

Diddle, A. W., and O'Connor, K. A.: Feminizing ovarian tumors and pregnancy. Am. J. Obstet. Gynecol., *62:* 1071, 1951.

DiSaia, P., Saltz, A., Kagan, A., et al.: A temporary response of recurrent granulosa cell tumor to adria mycin. Obstet. Gynecol., *52:* 355, 1978.

Dorrington, J. H., and Armstrong, D. T.: Follicle-stimulating hormone stimulates estradiol-17 synthesis in cultured Sertoli cells. Proc. Natl. Acad. Sci. U.S.A., *72:* 2677, 1975.

Dunniho, D. R., Grieme, D. L., and Wolfe, R. J.: Hilus cell tumors of the ovary. Obstet. Gynecol., *27:* 703, 1966.

Echt, C. R., and Hadd, H. E.: Androgen excretion patterns in a patient with metastic hilus cell tumor of the ovary. Am. J. Obstet. Gynecol., *100:* 1055, 1968.

Falck, B.: Site of production of estrogen in rat ovary as studied in micro-transplants. Acta Physiol. Scand., (Suppl. 163), *47:* 5, 1959.

Falls, J. L.: Accessory adrenal cortex in the broad ligament: incidence and functional significance. Cancer, *8:* 143, 1955.

Fathalla, M. F.: The occurrence of granulosa and theca tumors in clinically normal ovaries. J. Obstet. Gynaecol. Br. Commonw., *71:* 279, 1967.

Fathalla, M. F.: The role of the ovarian stroma in hormone production by ovarian tumors. J. Obstet. Gynaecol. Br. Commonw., *75:* 32, 1968.

Flick, F. H., and Banfield, R. S., Jr.: Theca and granulosa cell tumors. Bull. Sloane Hosp. Wom., *2:* 31, 1956.

Fox, H., Agrawal, K., and Langley, F. A.: A clinicopathologic study of 92 cases of granulosa cell tumor of the ovary with special reference to the factors influencing prognosis. Cancer, *35:* 231, 1975.

Francis, H. H.: Granulosa cell tumor of the ovary at the age of 85 years. J. Obstet. Gynaecol. Br. Commonw., *64:* 274, 1957.

French, W. G.: Clinical behavior of granulosa-cell tumor of ovary. Am. J. Obstet. Gynecol., *62:* 75, 1951.

Furth, J., and Butterworth, J. S.: Neoplastic diseases occurring among mice subjected to general irradiation with X-ray. Am. J. Cancer, *28:* 666, 1936.

Gabrilove, J. L., Nicolis, G. L., Mitty, H. A., et al.: Feminizing interstitial cell tumor of the testis: personal observations and a review of the literature. Cancer, *35:* 1184, 1975.

Gillibrand, P. N.: Granulosa-theca tumors of the ovary associated with pregnancy. Am. J. Obstet. Gynecol., *94:* 1108, 1966.

Giuntoli, R. L., Celebre, J. A., Wu, C. H., et al.: Androgenic function of a granulosa cell tumor. Obstet. Gynecol., *47:* 77, 1976.

Goldberg, B., Jones, S. E. S., and Woodruff, J. D.: A histochemical study of steroid 3β-ol dehydrogenase activity in some steroid-producing tumors. Am. J. Obstet. Gynecol., *86:* 1003, 1963.

Goldstein, D. P., and Lamb, E. J.: Arrhenoblastoma in first cousins. Obstet. Gynecol., *35:* 444, 1970.

Goldston, W. R., Johnston, W. W., Fetter, B. F., et al.: Clinico-pathological studies in feminizing tumors of the ovary. Am. J. Obstet. Gynecol., *112:* 422, 1972.

Gondos, B., and Monroe, S. A.: Cystic granulosa cell tumor with massive hemoperitoneum: light and electron microscopic study. Obstet. Gynecol., *38:* 683, 1971.

Graber, E. A., O'Rourke, J. J., and Sturman, M.: Arrhenoblastoma of the ovary. Am. J. Obstet. Gynecol., *81:* 783, 1961.

Greene, J. W., Jr.: Feminizing mesenchymomas (granulosa and theca-cell tumors) with associated endometrial carcinoma. Am. J. Obstet. Gynecol., *74:* 31, 1957.

Greene, R. R., Holzwarth, D., and Roddick, J. W., Jr.: Luteomas of pregnancy. Am. J. Obstet. Gynecol., *88:* 1001, 1964.

Guraya, S. S.: Histochemical study of granulosa and theca interna during follicular development, ovulation, and corpus luteum formation and regression in the human ovary. Am. J. Obstet. Gynecol., *101:* 448, 1968.

Gusberg, S. B., and Karden, P.: Endometrial response to theca-granulosal cell tumors. Am. J. Obstet. Gynecol., *111:* 633, 1971.

Huggins, C., and Moulder, P. V.: Estrogen production by Sertoli cell tumors of the testis. Cancer Res., *5:* 510, 1945.

Hughesdon, P. E.: The structure and origin of theca-granulosa tumors. J. Obstet. Gynaecol. Br. Commonw., *65:* 540, 1958.

Ireland, K., and Woodruff, J. D.: Masculinizing ovarian tumors. Obstet. Gynecol. Surv., *31:* 83, 1976.

Jakobovits, A.: Hormone production by miscellaneous ovarian tumors. Am. J. Obstet. Gynecol., *85:* 90, 1963.

Janko, A. B., and Sandberg, E. C.: The Reinke crystalloid. Obstet. Gynecol., *35:* 493, 1970.

Jeffcoate, S. L., and Prunty, F. T. G.: Steroid synthesis in vitro by a hilar cell tumor. Am. J. Obstet. Gynecol., *101:* 684, 1968.

Jenson, A. B., and Fechner, R. E.: Ultrastructure of an intermediate Sertoli-Leydig cell tumor: a histogenetic misnomer. Lab. Invest., *21:* 527, 1969.

Jones, G. S., Goldberg, B., and Woodruff, J. D.: Enzyme histochemistry of a masculinizing arrhenoblastoma. Obstet. Gynecol., *9:* 328, 1967.

Judd, H. L., Spore, W. W., Talner, L. B., et al.: Preoperative localization of a testosterone-secreting ovarian tumor by retrograde venous catheterization and selective sampling. Am. J. Obstet. Gynecol., *120:* 91, 1974.

Kase, N., and Conrad, S. H.: Steroid synthesis in abnormal ovaries. I. Arrhenoblastoma. II. Granulosa cell tumor. Am. J. Obstet. Gynecol., *90:* 1251, 1964.

Kempson, R. L.: Ultrastructure of ovarian stromal cell tumors: Sertoli-Leydig cell tumor and lipid cell tumor. Arch. Pathol. Lab. Med., *86:* 492, 1968.

Koudstall, J., Bossenbroek, B., and Hardonk, M. J.: Ovarian tumors investigated by histochemical and enzyme histochemical methods. Am. J. Obstet. Gynecol., *102:* 1004, 1969.

Krause, D. E., and Stembridge, V. A.: Luteomas of pregnancy. Am. J. Obstet. Gynecol., *95:* 192, 1966.

Kurman, R. J., and Norris, H. J.: Malignant mixed germ cell tumors of the ovary: a clinical and pathologic analysis of 30 cases. Obstet. Gynecol., *48:* 579, 1976.

Lewis, P. D., and Percival, R. C.: Combined thecoma and teratoma. J. Obstet. Gynaecol. Br. Commonw., *72:* 447, 1965.

Lusch, C. J., Mercurio, T., and Runyeon, W.: Delayed recurrence and chemotherapy of a granulosa cell tumor. Obstet. Gynecol., *51:* 505, 1978.

Lynn, J. A., Varon, H. H., Kingsley, W. B., et al.: Ultrastructural and biochemical studies of estrogen secretory capacity of a "nonfunctional" ovarian neoplasm (dysgerminoma). Am. J. Pathol., *51:* 639, 1967.

Mahesh, V. B., McDonough, P. G., and Deleo, C. A.: Endocrine studies in arrhenoblastoma. Am. J. Obstet. Gynecol., *107:* 183, 1970.

MacDonald, P. C., Rombaut, R. P., and Siiteri, P. K.: Plasma precursors of estrogen. I. Extent of conversion of plasma ^{4}-androstenedione to estrone in normal males and nonpregnant normal, castrated and adrenalectomized females. J. Clin. Endocrinol. Metab., *27:* 1103, 1967.

Meyer, R.: Pathology of some special ovarian tumors and their relation to sex characteristics. Am. J. Obstet. Gynecol., *26:* 505, 1933.

Morris, J. M., and Scully, R. E.: *Endocrine Pathology of the Ovary.* C. V. Mosby Company, St. Louis, 1958.

Murad, T. M., Mancini, R., and George, J.: Ultrastructure of a virilizing ovarian Sertoli-Leydig cell: Tumor with familial incidence. Cancer, *31:* 1440, 1973.

Nokes, J. M., Claiborne, H. A., and Reingold, W. N.: Thecoma with associated virilization. Am. J. Obstet. Gynecol., *78:* 722, 1958.

Norris, H. J., Garner, F. M., and Taylor, H. B.: Comparative pathology of ovarian neoplasms. IV. Gonadal stromal tumors of canine species. J. Comp. Pathol., *80:* 399, 1970.

Norris, H. J., and Taylor, H. B.: Luteoma of pregnancy. Am. J. Clin. Pathol., *47:* 557, 1967.

Norris, H. J., and Taylor, H. B.: Virilization associated with cystic granulosa tumors. Obstet. Gynecol., *34:* 629, 1969.

Novak, E. R., and Long, J. H.: Arrhenoblastoma of the ovary. A review of the Ovarian Tumor Registry. Am. J. Obstet. Gynecol., *92:* 1082, 1965.

Novak, E. R., and Mattingly, R. F.: Hilus cell tumors of the ovary (with a review of 18 cases). Obstet. Gynecol., *15:* 425, 1960.

Novak, E. R., Woodruff, J. D., and Linthicum, J. M.: Evaluation of the unclassified tumors of the Ovarian Tumor Registry 1942–1962. Am. J. Obstet. Gynecol., *87:* 999, 1963.

Novak, E. R., Kutchmeshgi, J., Mupas, R. S., et al.: Feminizing gonadal stromal tumors. Obstet. Gynecol., *38:* 701, 1971.

Pedowitz, P., and O'Brien, F. B.: Arrhenoblastoma of the ovary. Obstet. Gynecol., *16:* 62, 1960.

Pedowitz, P., and Pomerance, W.: Adrenal-like tumors of the ovary. Obstet. Gynecol., *19:* 183, 1962.

Persaud, V., Patterson, A. W., and Pathak, U. N.: Theca cell tumor associated with pregnancy. Int. Surg., *53:* 48, 1970.

Pfleideren, A., and Teufely, G.: Incidence and histochemical investigation of enzymatically active cells in stroma of ovarian tumors. Am. J. Obstet. Gynecol., *102:* 907, 1968.

Pick, L.: Uber Adenome der mannlichen und weiblichen Keim-druse. Klin. Wochenschr., *42:* 502, 1905.

Robertson, M. G., and Miller, R. E. C.: Massive cystic granulosa-theca cell tumor. Am. J. Obstet. Gynecol., *109:* 407, 1971.

Roth, L. M., and Sternberg, W. H.: Ovarian stromal tumors containing Leydig cells. II. Pure Leydig cell tumor, non-hilar type. Cancer, *32:* 952, 1973.

Rubin, D. K., and Frost, J. K.: The cytologic detection of ovarian cancer. Acta. Cytol., *7:* 191, 1963.

Ryan, K. J., Petro, Z., and Kaiser, J.: Steroid formation by isolated and recombined ovarian granulosa and thecal cells. J. Clin. Endocrinol., *28:* 355, 1968.

Sandberg, E. C.: The virilizing ovary. Obstet. Gynecol. Surv., *17:* 165, 1962.

Schwartz, P. E., and Smith, J. P.: Treatment of ovarian stromal tumors. Am. J. Obstet. Gynecol., *125:* 402, 1976.

Scully, R. E.: Androgenic lesions of the ovary. In *The Ovary, International Academy of Pathology Monograph No. 3,* edited by H. G. Grady and D. E. Smith, p. 143. Williams & Wilkins, Baltimore, 1963.

Scully, R. E.: The need for uniform terminology. Hum. Pathol., *4:* 602, 1973.

Scully, R. E.: Sex cord tumor with annular tubules: A distinctive ovarian tumor of the Peutz-Jeghers syndrome. Cancer, *25:* 1107, 1970.

Scully, R. E.: Stromal luteoma of the ovary: a distinctive type of lipoid cell tumor. Cancer, *17:* 769, 1964.

Scully, R. E., and Richardson, G. S.: Luteinization of the stroma of metastatic cancer involving the ovary and its endocrine significance. Cancer, *14:* 827, 1961.

Shippel, S.: Ovarian theca cell. J. Obstet. Gynaecol. Br. Com-monw., *57:* 362, 1950.

Simmons, R. L., and Sciarra, J. J.: Treatment of late recurrent granulosa cell tumors of the ovary. Surg. Gynecol. Obstet., *124:* 65, 1967.

Sobrinho, L. G., and Kase, N. G.: Adrenal rest cell tumor of the ovary. Obstet. Gynecol., *36:* 895, 1970.

Sommers, S. C., Gates, O., and Goodof, I. I.: Late recurrence of granulosa cell tumors. Obstet. Gynecol., *6:* 395, 1955.

Spadoni, L. R., Lindberg, M. C., Mottet, N. K., et al.: Virilization coexisting with Krukenberg tumor during pregnancy. Am. J. Obstet. Gynecol., *92:* 981, 1965.

Steenstrup, E. K.: Ovarian tumors and Peutz-Jeghers syndrome. Acta Obstet. Gynecol. Scand., *51:* 237, 1972.

Sternberg, W. H.: The morphology, androgenic function, hyper-plasia and tumors of the human ovarian hilus cells. Am. J. Pathol., *25:* 493, 1949.

Sternberg, W. H.: Nonfunctioning ovarian neoplasms. In *The Ovary, International Academy of Pathologists Monograph No. 3,* edited by H. G. Grady and D. E. Smith, p. 209. Williams & Wilkins, Baltimore, 1963.

Sternberg, W. H., and Barclay, D. L.: Luteoma of pregnancy. Am. J. Obstet. Gynecol., *95:* 165, 1966.

Sternberg, W. H., and Roth, L. M.: Ovarian stromal tumors containing Leydig cells. I. Stromal Leydig cell tumor and non-neoplastic transformation of ovarian stroma to Leydig cells. Cancer, *32:* 940, 1973.

Stewart, R. S., and Woodard, D. E.: Malignant ovarian hilus cell tumor. Arch. Pathol. Lab. Med., *73:* 91, 1962.

Taylor, H. B., and Norris, H. J.: Lipid cell tumors of the ovary. Cancer, *20:* 1953, 1967.

Teilum, G.: Classification of testicular and ovarian androblas-toma and Sertoli cell tumors. Cancer, *11:* 769, 1958.

Teilum, G.: *Special Tumors of the Ovary and Testis.* J. B. Lippin-cott, Philadelphia, 1971.

Thompson, J. P., Dockerty, M. B., and Symmonds, R. E.: Gran-ulosa cell carcinoma arising in a cystic teratoma of the ovary. Obstet. Gynecol., *28:* 549, 1966.

Verhoeven, A. T. M., Mastboom, J. L., Van Lousden, H. A. I. M.: Virilization in pregnancy coexisting with an (ovarian) mucinous cystadenoma: A case report and review of the viril-izing ovarian tumors in pregnancy. Obstet. Gynecol. Surv., *28:* 597, 1973.

Waisman, J., Lischke, J. H., Mwasi, L. M., et al.: The ultrastruc-ture of a feminizing granulosa-theca tumor. Am. J. Obstet. Gynecol., *123:* 147, 1975.

Warren, J. C., Erkman, B., and Cheatum, S.: Hilus-cell adenoma in a dysgenetic gonad with XX/XO mosaicism. Lancet, *1:* 141, 1964.

Woodruff, J. D., Williams, T. J., and Goldberg, B.: Hormone activity of the common ovarian neoplasm. Am. J. Obstet. Gynecol., *87:* 679, 1963.

Younglai, E. V., Richmond, H., Atyed, R., and Johnson, F. L.: Arrhenoblastoma: *in vivo* and *in vitro* studies. Am. J. Obstet. Gynecol. *34:* 861–866, 1973.

Zander, J., Mickan, H., Holzman, K., et al.: Androluteoma syndrome of pregnancy. Am. J. Obstet. Gynecol., *130:* 170, 1978.

CHAPTER 25

Endometriosis

One of the most interesting lesions encountered in gynecological practice is pelvic endometriosis, a clinical and pathological entity publicized primarily by the classic contributions of Sampson in 1921. It may be defined as the condition in which tissue resembling endometrium is found in various extrauterine locations, but chiefly in the pelvic cavity.

SITES OF ENDOMETRIOSIS

The endometrial islands may be found in many possible locations, of which the following are the most common: (1) ovaries; (2) uterine ligaments (round, broad, uterosacral); (3) rectovaginal septum; (4) pelvic peritoneum covering the uterus, tubes, rectum, sigmoid, or bladder; (5) umbilicus; (6) laparotomy scars; (7) hernial sacs; (8) appendix; (9) vagina; (10) vulva; (11) cervix; (12) tubal stumps; (13) lymph glands. In rare cases, still other locations, such as the arm, thigh, or pleural and pericardial cavity, have been reported.

HISTOGENESIS

Since Sampson's paper in 1921, there has been much discussion as to the origin of the aberrant endometrium in cases of pelvic endometriosis. There are various theories on this point.

(1) Sampson's original concept of *transtubal regurgitation of menstrual blood* and endometrial particles at the time of menstruation, with their subsequent implantation and growth on the ovaries and elsewhere in the pelvis.

(2) The so-called *celomic metaplasia doctrine*, according to which the aberrant endometrium develops as a result of abnormal differentiation changes in the germinal epithelium and various parts of the pelvic peritoneum which are embryologically derived from the celomic epithelium.

(3) The *lymphatic dissemination* theory which states that the aberrant tissue was derived from endometrium entering the uterine lymphatic vessels of the uterus at the time of menstruation, being thus disseminated throughout the pelvis.

(4) *Hematogenous* spread of endometrium, as an explanation for certain rare cases of endometriosis which would be difficult to explain on any other basis.

Indeed, *most critical gynecologists believe that there is more than one mode of origin for endometriosis, and that no single theory explains all cases.* The implantation doctrine seems a likely one for the majority of cases of endometriosis. Plantation of endometrium into the abdominal wall of patient subsequently scheduled for laparotomy by Ridley has suggested growth of the implanted tissue in a few, but by no means a majority of women.

PATHOLOGY

Gross

The gross picture in cases of endometriosis is extremely variable. On opening the abdomen and exposing the pelvic organs, the surgeon may find a small adherent mass in one or both sides of the pelvis, usually attached to the posterior surface of the uterus quite low down. On loosening these adhesions to rotate the adnexa into the field of operation, there is a gush of chocolate-colored or dark, rusty-looking fluid, and this should at once make the surgeon think of endometriosis. Examination of the ovary may disclose a cyst with a dark hemorrhagic lining which has been opened in bringing up the adherent adnexa.

The cyst may be only a centimeter or so in diameter, and is rarely larger than a grapefruit. The tube is usually quite normal, with a patent fimbriated extremity, although it may be surrounded by peritoneal adhesions with a number of rather puckered hemorrhagic areas of dark bluish color, in one or both uterosacral ligaments. Similar areas may be seen on the anterior surface of the sigmoid or rectum or elsewhere in the pelvis.

This, then, is the typical picure, but it may present all sorts of degrees and variations. In a few mild cases the adnexa may initially seem quite normal, but close inspection of the ovaries may reveal a number of reddish-blue, fibrin-like areas representing tiny endometrial islands or "implants" with occasional bloody ascites (Fig. 25.1).

At the other extreme are cases in which the pelvis may be filled with a "frozen" mass, consisting of a uterus with adenomyosis, firmly adherent adnexa, bilateral endometrial cysts, and extensive endometrial invasion of the rectal or sigmoidal wall. In fact, the bowel may be so enormously infiltrated as to simulate malignancy or to produce complete obstruction, and Davis and Truehart have thoroughly discussed surgical management of co-

lonic endometriosis. At times the invading endometrium may push far down into the rectovaginal septum. Like Cavanagh, we are inclined to believe that endometriosis may progress rapidly in the youthful (less than 30 years) patient. Endometrial cysts may enlarge enormously within a few months as a result of extensive intracystic hemorrhage.

Microscopic

From a microscopic standpoint, there is considerable variation, the essential criterion being the presence of endometrial tissue in the wall of the cyst, preferably stroma as well as glands. It should be remembered that the aberrant tissue resembles the uterine mucosa not only histologically but also physiologically, so that it may sometimes, but not by any means always, show evidence of response to menstrual and pregnancy stimuli (Figs. 25.2 and 25.3). Because of the constant recurrence of menstrual desquamation, with perhaps the pressure of the retained menstrual blood in the cyst cavities, the endometrial lining of the latter may be almost completely absent, and in its place one may see only reactive connective tissue elements, with usually a large number of endothelial leukocytes heavily laden with blood pigment (*pseudoxanthoma cells*) (Fig. 25.4). Indeed, in about

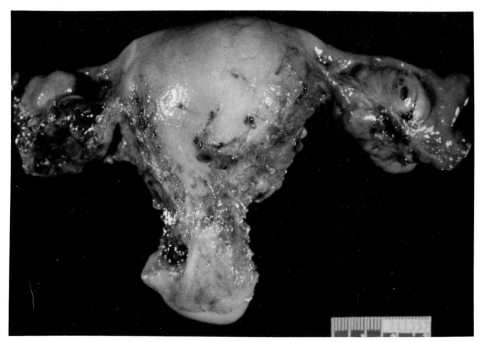

Figure 25.1. Multiple small implants over serosal surfaces.

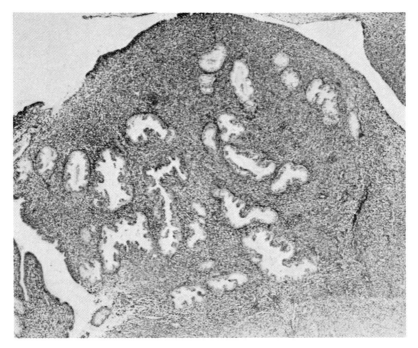

Figure 25.2.   Marked premenstrual reaction in the lining of an endometrial cyst.

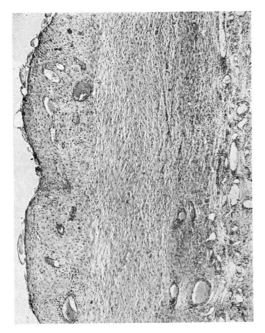

Figure 25.3.   Decidual changes in wall of endometrial cyst in pregnancy. Pseudodecidual changes may occur in the nonpregnant ovary in the absence of endometriosis.

one-third of all cases of typical, even extensive, "clinical" endometriosis as seen at operation, there may be no histological proof of its existence, even if many pathological sec-

tions are made. Tissue committees should be aware of this fact.

The term "*chocolate cyst*" of the ovary has come into general vogue as synonymous with "endometrial cyst." The latter term, however, is a much better one, in spite of the expressiveness of the former. There are some surgeons who forget that other types of ovarian cyst may have a chocolate-colored content—e.g., follicle or corpus luteum hematoma, cystadenoma, etc.—so that when a cyst discharges such a fluid, it should not categorically be concluded that endometriosis is present.

Malignant degeneration of an endometrial cyst may occur, but it is so rare that it does not influence the handling of the patient. The usual lesion is adenoacanthoma, a relatively low-grade type of malignancy (Fig. 25.5), and acanthosis is a frequent finding with uterine adenocarcinoma.

The most recent FIGO annual report indicated that serous lesions are nearly four times as common as mucinous lesions and more than twice as common as endometrioid malignancies.

"Endometrioid carcinoma" was accepted as one of the tumors of epithelial origin, and it has been popularized in this country by Long and Taylor as a suggested diagnosis for certain ovarian tumors which have a histological similarity to endometrial adenocarcinoma. This would include most adenoacanthomas, which are often observed to occur in conjunction with pelvic endometriosis, although it is on occasion impossible to demonstrate a frank transition between benign and malignant ovarian endometrium, which Sampson insisted should be mandatory in indicating an endometrial origin.

Although endometriosis can give rise to malignant tumors, it is not to be inferred that "endometrioid tumors" of the ovary arise from endometriosis. The word "endometrioid" in this context is merely descriptive and indicates that the tumors so labeled resemble endometrium. Such tumors are epithelial and arise from the ovarian covering mesothelium. Their resemblance to endometrium is by virtue of metaplasia.

OTHER SITES OF ENDOMETRIOSIS

Uterosacral Ligaments

This location is very common, and this is one of the arguments by those who favor Sampson's theory, inasmuch as endometrial particles regurgitating through the tube might be expected to gravitate toward the cul-de-sac and implant themselves on the uterosacral ligaments. In this region the endometriosis occurs in the form of bluish, somewhat puckered nodules, which may be minute or the size of a walnut so that they may be easily palpable through the vaginal vault. There is the usual perforative tendency of endometriosis, with peritoneal irritation and the formation of dense adhesions to the rectum or adnexa.

Rectovaginal Septum

As an extension of uterosacral endometriosis, one may find endometrial tissue extending downward along the rectovaginal septum, with sometimes enormous infiltration of the rectum and cyclic rectal bleeding. In other cases such growths may penetrate into the vagina (Fig. 25.6), producing *vaginal endometrial polyps* which may bleed with each menstrual period or after such contact as intercourse or douche.

Round Ligaments

These may be involved in the form of small superficial endometrial "implants" or in the form of nodules of adenomyosis, in which both endometrium and muscle are to be found.

Umbilicus

Many cases of umbilical endometriosis have been reported (Fig. 25.7). This group is

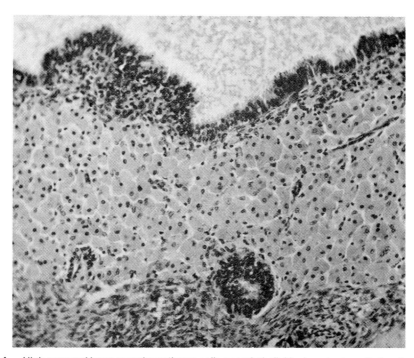

Figure 25.4.   High power of large pseudoxanthoma cells or endothelial leukocytes in wall of endometrial cyst.

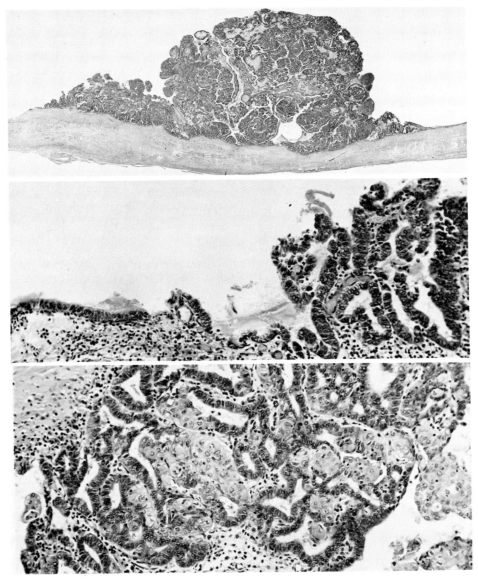

Figure 25.5.   *Top,* lesion arising from the wall of endometrial cyst. *Middle,* transition zone between benign and malignant. *Bottom,* full-fledged adenoacanthoma. (Courtesy of Dr. Dan Thompson, Atlanta, Georgia.)

of interest, as it seems impossible to rationalize by Sampson's theory, although it is explainable by the metaplasia theory, inasmuch as remnants of celomic epithelium are normally found at the umbilicus. Scott and TeLinde described Cullen's sign occurring with endometriosis due to transplantation of blood and menstrual debris from the peritoneal cavity via certain umbilical lymphatics.

Umbilical endometriosis presents in the form of small nodules which may, when they approach the surface, be of bluish hue. They increase in size at the menstrual periods,

when they become tender, painful, and sometimes break through the skin, with periodic external bleeding.

Laparotomy Scars

This interesting group likewise has evoked much discussion by the proponents of the two principal theories of histogenesis. The postoperative development of endometrial nodules in laparotomy scars, sometimes long after the original operation, may be noted after any type of laparotomy and not, as was originally suggested by some, only in those in which direct implantation of endometrial tissue seemed mechanically possible. As a matter of fact, it is uncommon after cesarean section, although a small group of such cases has been observed. Indeed, endometriosis has been noted in McBurney scars long after appendectomy in the prepubertal female. The endometrial nodules in laparotomy scars may reach considerable size, and they show the same characteristic cyclic menstrual swelling, pain, tenderness, and sometimes external bleeding described for the umbilical form.

Other Sites

The chief locations have already been enumerated, and it should again be emphasized that any portion of the *pelvic peritoneum* may be involved. In some instances only a single tiny island may be observed, without involvement of the ovaries and without clinical significance. At the other extreme one may find extensive pelvic dissemination, usually including the ovaries. The appendix, small intestines, rectum, sigmoid, bladder, lymph glands, hernial sacs—any of these may show endometriosis.

In discussing the urological location of endometriosis Ball and Platt note such complications as intravesical endometrioma, endometriosis of the ureter, etc., with operative damage to the urinary tract in 0.5% of all cases, although minor degrees of the disease are common. Simon et al. discuss the possibility of complete ureteral obstruction in their report of 10 cases, including an apparent case of bilateral disease, necessitating reimplantation into the bladder. Endometriosis of the kidney has been observed and would seem to

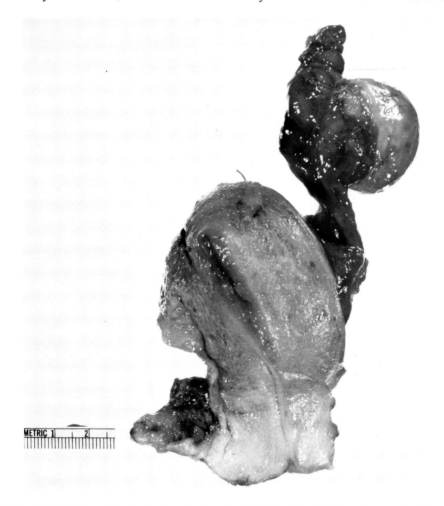

Figure 25.6.   Typical endometriosis of rectovaginal septum (just at ruler) which had also extended into vagina. Small endometrial cyst of ovary is also present.

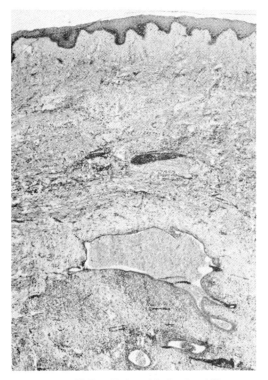

Figure 25.7.   Endometriosis of umbilicus.

arise from a hematogenous or lymphatic basis (Hajdu and Koss).

The cervix, the vagina, and even the vulva will occasionally harbor endometriosis, as may the perineum, especially in the region of episiotomy scars. In reporting 35 cases, Williams and Richardson enlarged on cervical endometriosis, and Novak and Hoge discussed the occurrence of lower genital tract endometriosis.

Finally, there are a number of reported instances of what is apparently unquestionable endometriosis of both the upper and lower extremities. One would be inclined to invoke the hematogenous route in the explanation of these bizarre cases except for the difficulty of explaining how the endometrium could get through the pulmonary capillaries if it were transported from the uterus. A mechanism which might possibly be invoked would be the pathway along the vertebral veins or by the lung "shunts" which have apparently been demonstrated between pulmonary arteries and veins, bypassing the capillaries.

Similarly, there have been a few cases in which the pleural cavity or lung was involved.

Shearin et al. and others have called attention to chronic recurrent pneumothorax often at the time of menses due to endometriosis of the diaphragm.

CLINICAL CHARACTERISTICS OF ENDOMETRIOSIS

In most series 75% of the patients with endometriosis are between the ages of 25 and 45. However, Fallon reported a considerable group below the age of 20, and Schiffrain also commented on teenage endometriosis.

Early or frequent pregnancy with interruption of cyclic menstruation is suggested as having some kind of guarding effect against the disease, and there is general agreement that pregnancy may incur some regression of endometriosis, although McArthur and Ulfelder have reported 24 cases which do not conform to this thesis.

Although there are no characteristic symptoms, and although in a large proportion of cases none whatsoever are referable to the endometriosis, *disturbances of menstruation* are often present. *Dysmenorrhea* is a frequent symptom, being noted in about one-third of all series studied. It may be moderate or very severe, and there is no correlation with extent of disease. When the rectovaginal septum or uterosacral region is involved, as is so often the case, the dysmenorrhea is often referred to the rectum or to the lower sacral or coccygeal regions. This is due to the premenstrual and menstrual swelling of the endometrium in the uterosacral islands.

In cases of moderate or slight degree, there is ordinarily no *pelvic* or *abdominal pain* or discomfort, but in the more extensive cases these may be present, resembling the symptoms of chronic pelvic inflammatory disease. *Dyspareunia* is often complained of, especially in the cases of uterosacral involvement or vaginal extension. In the same group of cases *constipation* and *pain on defecation* may be noted. However, there is no correlation between the amount of endometriosis and the symptoms. On occasion *minor degrees of the disease lead to severe pain; however, massive amounts of endometriosis are compatible with no symptoms.* Indeed, the clinician is often struck by this disparity, which may be difficult to justify to the pathologist.

An endometrial cyst can leak blood, causing considerable pain; perforation may occur and produce a clinical picture much like a ruptured ectopic pregnancy or appendicitis. Golditch indicates that nearly 10% of patients with endometriosis present with acute symptoms which may require exploration for diagnosis and treatment. Ranney made similar observations, and his contributions on the behavior of endometriosis are recommended for all readers.

Infertility is present in the majority of cases. If pregnancy should occur, the woman may be reassured that, despite her endometriosis, the gestation will not be complicated by the disease, and that, if anything, her symptoms will be improved.

Among patients whose chief complaint is *infertility,* endometriosis is a major cause. Katayama et al., based on the series from Johns Hopkins, reported that 25% of infertile couples were found to have endometriosis in the female; this figure may be taken as representative of the experience of many others.

The precise mechanism by which endometriosis causes infertility escapes identification. The tubes are generally open and the fimbria free, many times not even disturbed by peritubal adhesions. Of course, at other times, the tubes are partially inhibited in their motion by peritubal endometriosis and adhesions, but it is very rare for endometriosis to obstruct a fallopian tube mechanically. No consistent ovulatory or other problems have been identified in patients with endometriosis. In spite of the inability to specify the cause, there seems little doubt that endometriosis is the problem in these cases, because therapy directed against the endometriosis will be rewarded with pregnancy in many cases; this will be detailed in the section on therapy.

DIAGNOSIS

It can be seen that no characteristic symptoms are to be expected in endometriosis. This fact, together with the complete absence of symptoms in many cases and the further fact that endometriosis so often coexists with other lesions that obscure it symptomatically, explains why diagnosis is often difficult. There are, however, certain helps in diagnosis which may be yielded by history and pelvic examination. The most distinctive of the

symptoms, although it is present in only a fraction of the cases, is *menstrual pain referred to the rectum, the lower sacral, or coccygeal regions,* as described above.

In many intances the findings on bimanual examination may be exactly the same as in chronic adnexitis, there being palpable in one or both sides of the pelvis a tender, irregular mass, consisting of the adherent tube and ovary.

In a certain proportion of cases, however, the internal examining finger reveals *nodular thickening in the uterosacral ligaments,* corresponding to endometrial islands in this location. Sometimes the nodules are small and shotlike, but they may reach the size of a hickory nut and be single or multiple. Such a finding, when noted in a patient who otherwise exhibits the symptoms and signs of chronic pelvic inflammatory disease, should suggest the probability of endometriosis, and usually this suspicion is verified by operation. A fixed retroflexion of the uterus is present in cases of this description, but there are exceptions to this. *It is hazardous to make a diagnosis of endometriosis on the basis of symptoms alone, in the complete absence of palpatory findings.*

In patients with unexplained lower abdominal pain or in patients who otherwise are suspected of having endometriosis, it may be necessary to utilize diagnostic laparoscopy. This is especially true if endocrinological management is contemplated (Fig. 25.8).

In patients with infertility, diagnostic laparoscopy is a necessary part of the work-up, and in a residue of cases—7% in the Johns Hopkins series—previously unsuspected asymptomatic endometriosis can be identified at this examination (Fig. 25.9).

CLASSIFICATION

The evaluation of treatment of patients with endometriosis has been handicapped by the heterogeneity of the clinical material. Although most authors have traditionally described their material according to the extent of disease, a generally agreed upon workable clinical classification would greatly facilitate not only evaluation of therapy but the selection of appropriate treatment for an individual patient. The ability to develop a useful

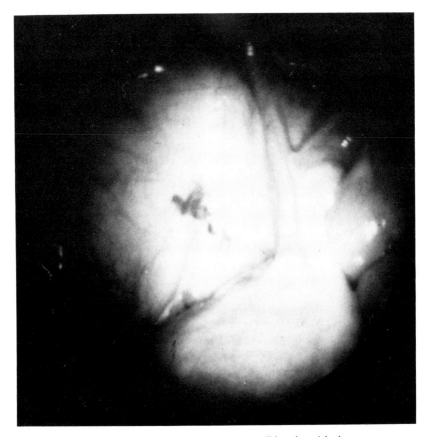

Figure 25.8.   Laparoscopic view of mild endometriosis.

classification has been greatly facilitated by the widespread use of the laparoscope.

Although several classifications have been proposed, it is probably fair to say that, up to the present time, there is no general agreement on this matter.

TREATMENT

Although endometriosis causes a variety of symptoms, in general, therapy is undertaken either because of pain in some form or because of infertility. These two indications are sometimes combined, but it is amazing how frequently patients with infertility due to endometriosis have relatively little discomfort.

Treatment may be either endocrinological or surgical.

Endocrinological

Most authors have stated that endocrinological therapy can be advocated only for patients with mild or moderate extent of dis-

ease as defined in one or another of the various classifications. For extensive disease, surgical therapy is generally recommended as the primary approach.

Progestogens

Kistner deserves the credit for introducing and popularizing the concept of pseudopregnancy. This concept was based on the observation that pregnancy tended to cause atrophy in preexisting endometriosis. It is to be noted, however, that McArthur and Ulfelder presented evidence that tended to question this old observation. In any event, pseudopregnancy utilizing a progestogen such as Enovid in increasing doses up to 40 mg a day will give relief of pain in well over 85% of patients and of infertility in up to 40%, at least in Kistner's experience. This therapy suppresses menstruation for the duration of therapy, which usually extends for about 9 months. Other progestational agents have been used with approximately equal success

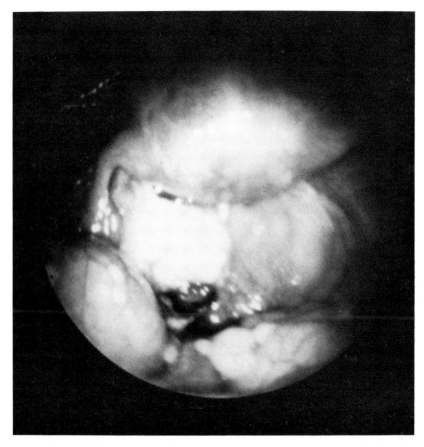

Figure 25.9.   Laparoscopic view of moderately extensive endometriosis.

Table 25.1
Conception Rates in Patients after Endocrine Therapy

Author	Drug	No. of Patients	Conception Rate
			%
Preston and Campbell	Methyltestosterone	80	60
Kistner	Norethynodrel Mestranol	110	47
Kourides and Kistner	Norethindrone Acetate Ethinyl estradiol	11	63
Andrews and Larsen	Norethynodrel Mestranol	8	43
Greenblatt et al.	Danazol	21	43
Hammond et al.	Norethynodrel Mestranol	23	30
Katayama et al.	Methyltestosterone	64	28
Dmowski and Cohen	Danazol	84	46

in pain relief. However, authors other than Kistner often report less enthusiastic results in the treatment of infertility (Table 25.1). Although pseudopregnancy enjoyed a considerable vogue in the early 1970's, it is used less frequently at the present time.

Androgens

That androgen will cause atrophy of endometriosis is an old observation. It is still a useful form of therapy. It will relieve pain in a very high proportion of cases, just as high as the progestogens. If a patient is relieved of pain by a therapeutic trial of 5 mg of methyltestosterone a day for 100 days, it is presumptive evidence that she is suffering from endometriosis. Menstruation is not inhibited by this dose. About 10% of patients experience some mild form of virilization, such as acne or slight increase in hirsutism. In the event pregnancy occurs, the prompt discontinuation of methyltestosterone is obviously indicated to prevent masculinization of a female child.

Danazol

Danazol was introduced on an experimental basis into clinical medicine for the treatment of endometriosis in the early 1970s. It became available for general use in 1977. Danazol is an isoxazol derivative of 17-ethyltestosterone. This synthetic steroid has an interesting action. It suppresses the ovulatory gonadotropin peak and is mildly androgenic in the standard dose of 800 mg per day. Like the progestogens, it induces amenorrhea during the course of its therapy. Pain relief has been reported to occur in almost all patients, and the pregnancy rate has been encouraging (Table 25.1).

Surgical

Surgery is indicated for pain, infertility, or other symptoms in patients with extensive degrees of pelvic endometriosis or in the face of failure of endocrinological manipulation to relieve symptoms in patients with lesser degrees of pelvic endometriosis.

Surgery is successful in relieving pain in a very high percentage of cases and offers a better prognosis for pregnancy than endocrine therapy (Table 25.2). The goal of infertility surgery for endometriosis is to relieve by excision or fulgeration any or all endo-

Table 25.2

Conception Rates in Patients after Surgical Therapy

Author	No. of Patients	Conception Rate
		%
Ranney	48	87.5
Spangler et al.	73	58
Andrews and Larsen	45	59
Hammond et al.	12	50
Jones (unpublished)	147	60

metrial tissue, whether it be peritoneal or intraovarian or otherwise, and to restore the condition of the pelvis to as normal a condition as possible (Fig. 25.10). After conservative surgery, pregnancy may not occur for some months after operation so that it is important that neither patient nor surgeon be impatient (Fig. 25.11).

When pregnancy is not a consideration, the goal of surgery is to relieve the patient's symptoms. These usually include pain. Under such circumstances, hysterectomy and bilateral salpingo-oophorectomy may be the most suitable operation. On the other hand, if the patient is still relatively young, consideration might be given to sparing one ovary. Indeed hysterectomy alone may often incur prolonged relief of symptoms up to and through the menopause, despite conservation of one adnexa. All sorts of individual variations in the problem may arise, and the conservatively inclined surgeon will find that the patient's social and marital status are factors often quite as important in guiding his decision as are the pelvic findings.

In cases in which the endometriosis is really very extensive, with bilateral endometrial cysts and endometrial implants at many points in the pelvis, nothing short of hysterectomy and bilateral salpingo-oophorectomy can be expected to solve the patient's problem.

It may frequently be impossible to remove all the aberrant endometrium, as it may, for example, infiltrate the bowel wall and perhaps the rectovaginal septum. Occasionally, bowel resection is preferable to castration in the young patient.

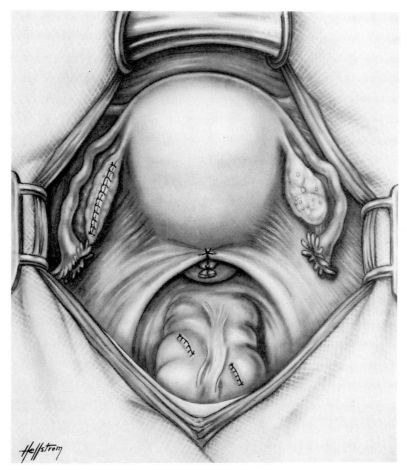

Figure 25.10.   A diagrammatic drawing of the postoperative appearance of the pelvis which has been involved in extensive pelvic endometriosis. (Courtesy of Dr. Laman A Gray.)

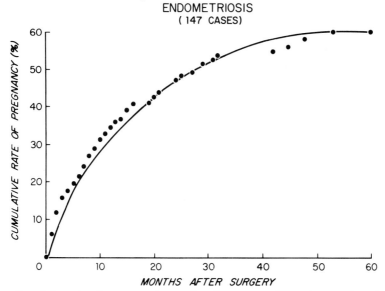

Figure 25.11.   Cumulative rate of pregnancy by months after surgery. Although approximately one-half of all patients who are going to become pregnant do so within the first year after surgery, pregnancies continue to occur for up to 5 years after the original surgery. (Unpublished series of H. W. Jones.)

Hormone Therapy Postoperative

Inasmuch as endometriosis seems dependent on estrogen stimulation, the question often arises as to whether hormone therapy is indicated in the symptomatic postcastrate woman who has had extensive endometriosis. Theoretically it might be expected to stimulate any residual endometrium not removed at surgery, and sometimes this happens. However, the small dosage of estrogen necessary to suppress vasomotor symptoms many times does not cause endometrial activation, although some gynecologists might prefer birth control (estrogen-progesterone) pills because of the antiestrogen effect of progesterone at the endometrial level.

References and Additional Readings

Acosta, A. A., Buttram, V. C., Jr., Besch, P. K., Malinak, R. L., Franklin, R. R., and Vanderheyden, J. D.: A proposed classification of endometriosis. Obstet. Gynecol., 42: 19, 1973.

Andrews, W. C., and Larsen, G. D.: Endometriosis: Treatment with hormonal pseudopregnancy and/or operation. Am. J. Obstet. Gynecol., 118: 643, 1974.

Ball, T. L., and Platt, M. A.: Urologic complications of endometriosis. Am. J. Obstet. Gynecol., 84: 1516, 1962.

Cavanagh, W. F.: Endometriosis. Bull. Sloane Hosp., 6: 115, 1960.

Davis, C., Jr., and Truehart, R.: Surgical management of endometrioma of the colon. Am. J. Obstet. Gynecol., 89: 453, 1964.

Dmowski, W. P., and Cohen, M. R.: Antigonadotropin (danazol) in the treatment of endometriosis: evaluation of posttreatment fertility and three-year follow-up data. Am. J. Obstet. Gyneol., 130: 41, 1978.

Fallon, R.: Endometriosis. Am. J. Obstet. Gynecol., 72: 557, 1956.

Fathalla, M. F.: Malignant tranformation in ovarian endometriosis. J. Obstet. Gynaecol., Br. Commonw., 74: 85, 1967.

Fenn, M. E., and Abell, M. R.: Carcinosarcoma of the ovary. Am. J. Obstet. Gynecol., 110: 1066, 1971.

Golditch, I. M.: Endometriosis presenting as an acute abdominal emergency. Obstet. Gynecol., 26: 180, 1965.

Gray, L. A., and Barnes, M. L.: Endometrioid carcinoma of the ovary. Obstet. Gynecol., 29: 694, 1967.

Greenblatt, R. B., Dmowski, W. P., Mahesh, V. B., and Scholer, H. F. L.: Clinical studies with an antigonadotropin—Danazol. Fertil. Steril., 22: 102, 1971.

Hajdu, S. I., and Koss, L. G.: Endometriosis of the kidney. Am. J. Obstet. Gynecol., 106: 314, 1970.

Hammond, C. B., Rock, J. A., and Parker, R. T.: Conservative treatment of endometriosis: the effects of limited surgery and hormonal pseudopregnancy. Fertil. Steril., 27: 756, 1976.

Hartz, P. H.: Occurrence of decidual-like tissue in the lung. Am. J. Clin. Pathol., 26: 48, 1956.

Katayama, K. P., Kap-Soon, J., May, M., Jones, G. S., and Jones, H. W., Jr.: Computer analysis of etiology and pregnancy rate in 636 cases of primary infertility. Am. J. Obstet. Gynecol., 135: 207, 1979.

Katayama, K. P., Manuel, M., Jones, H. W., Jr., and Jones, G. S.: Methyltestosterone treatment of infertility associated with pelvic endometriosis. Fertil. Steril., 27: 83, 1976.

Kistner, R. W.: Endometriosis. Fertil. Steril., 13: 237, 1962.

Kistner, R. W.: Current status of the hormonal treatment of endometriosis. Clin. Obstet. Gynecol., 9: 271, 1966.

Kistner, R. W., Siegler, A. M., and Behrman, S. J.: Suggested classification for endometriosis: relationship to infertility. Fertil. Steril., 28: 1008, 1977.

Kourides, I. A., and Kistner, R. W.: Three synthetic progestins in the treatment of endometriosis. Obstet. Gynecol., 31: 821, 1968.

Lattes, R.: A clinical and pathological study of endometriosis of the lung. Surg. Gynecol. Obstet., 103: 552, 1956.

Long, M. E., and Taylor, H. C.: Endometrioid carcinoma of the ovary. Am. J. Obstet. Gynecol., 90: 936, 1964.

McArthur, J. W., and Ulfelder, H.: The effect of pregnancy upon endometriosis. Obstet. Gynecol. Surv., 20: 709, 1965.

Mitchell, G. W., Jr., and Farber, M.: Medical versus surgical management of endometriosis. In Controversies in OB-GYN, II, edited by D. Reed and D. Christian, p. 631. W. B. Saunders, Philadelphia, 1974.

Novak, E. R., and Hoge, A. F.: Endometriosis of the lower genital tract. Obstet. Gynecol., 12: 687, 1958.

Preston, S. N., and Campbell, H. B.: Pelvic endometriosis—treatment with methyltestosterone. Obstet. Gynecol., 12: 152, 1953.

Ranney, B.: Endometriosis. I. Conservative operations. Am. J. Obstet. Gynecol., 107: 743, 1970.

Ranney, B.: Endometriosis II. Emergency operations due to hemoperitoneum. Obstet. Gynecol., 36: 437, 1970.

Ranney, B.: Endometriosis. III. Complete operations. Am. J. Obstet. Gynecol., 109: 1137, 1971.

Ranney, B.: Endometriosis. IV. Hereditary tendencies. Obstet. Gynecol., 37: 734, 1971.

Ridley, J. H.: The histogenesis of endometriosis. Obstet. Gynecol. Surv., 23: 1, 1968.

Ridley, J. H.: Primary adenocarcinoma in an implant of endometriosis. Obstet. Gynecol., 27: 261, 1966.

Sampson, J. A.: Perforating haemorrhagic (chocolate) cysts of the ovary. Arch. Surg., 3: 245, 1921.

Sampson, J. A.: Peritoneal endometriosis due to the menstrual dissemination of endometrial tissue into the peritoneal cavity. Am. J. Obstet. Gynecol., 14: 422, 1927.

Schiffrain, B. S., Erex, S., and Moore, J. G.: Teen-age endometriosis. Am. J. Obstet. Gynecol., 116: 973, 1973.

Scott, R. B., and TeLinde, R. W.: External endometriosis: scourge of the private patient. Ann. Surg., 131: 697, 1950.

Shearin, R. P. N., Hepper, N. G. G., and Payne, W. S.: Recurrent spontaneous pneumothorax concurrent with menses. Mayo Clin. Proc., 49: 98, 1974.

Simon, H. B., Zimet, R. R., Schneider, E., and Morgenstern, L. L.: Bilateral ureteral obstruction due to endometriosis. J.A.M.A., 183: 191, 1963.

Spangler, D. B., Jones, G. S., and Jones, H. W.: Infertility due to endometrosis. Am. J. Obstet. Gynecol., 109: 850, 1971.

Williams, G. A., and Richardson, A. C.: Endometriosis of cervix uteri. Obstet. Gynecol., 6: 309, 1955.

Williams, J. F., Williams, J. B., and Harper, J. W.: Thoracic endometriosis. Am. J. Obstet. Gynecol., 84: 1512, 1962.

CHAPTER 26

Ectopic Pregnancy

Definition

The term ectopic pregnancy is applied to pregnancy following implantation of the fertilized egg on any tissue other than the mucous membrane lining the uterine cavity. It is a better and more inclusive term than extra-uterine pregnancy, as a pregnancy may be ectopic and yet be situated within the uterus, as in the case of interstitial or cervical pregnancy.

TUBAL PREGNANCY

Much the most common type of ectopic pregnancy is that which occurs in the tube (Fig. 26.1). The tube is normally concerned in the transportation of the fertilized egg to the uterus, but under certain conditions the egg may plant itself on the tube wall. The latter is ill adapted for either satisfactory nidation or later continuance of the gestation, so that with rare exceptions the embryo succumbs at an early stage.

Etiology

The causes ascribed for tubal pregnancy may be placed in two chief groups:

(1) Factors Which Delay or Prevent Passage of The Fertilized Egg into The Uterine Cavity (Maternal Factors). This is probably the more important of the two groups of causes. Partial obstruction of the tube by *chronic salpingitis* is most often concerned, not only because of the mechanical factor but also because on one hand of the impairment of sperm migration and on the other of ciliary activity and muscle peristalsis, so important in the propagation of the egg. Follicular salpingitis especially is believed to be a frequent cause, because of the formation of blind gutters into which a fertilized egg may stray.

Endometriosis on the serosal surface of the tube is seldom associated with ectopic gestation. However, patches of endometrium replacing the endosalpinx may provide a nidus for implantation.

Congenital abnormalities of the tube, especially diverticula and accessory ostia, may likewise be concerned, as may *partial occlusion by adhesions or tumors* outside the tube. Persaud recorded a high incidence of diverticula and believed this to be the most frequent cause of tubal gestation.

A special situation sometimes results after tubal ligation. Metz and Mastroianni studied the circumstances when tubal pregnancies occur *distal* to complete tubal occlusion or separation. Presumably such pregnancies result from transperitoneal migration of sperm from a fistula in the proximal stump of one or another of the ligated tubes.

(2) Factors Inherent in the Embryo (Embryonic Factors). It is quite possible that embryonic abnormalities may predispose to ectopic gestation. Since the classic studies of Mall, it has been known that, just as spontaneous abortuses, ectopic pregnancies may be malformed. This has been confirmed since Mall's time by other workers.

It seems that in ectopic gestation, embryonic maldevelopment and gross chromosomal defects are common findings. Of course, the same may be said for abortuses of normally implanted embryos. The number of ectopic pregnancies carefully studied is limited so it is difficult to be certain, but it seems that embryonic abnormalities predispose to an ectopic location of the implantation and must be considered as a cause of this mallo-

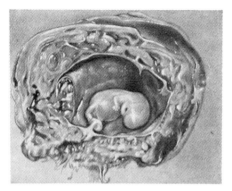

Figure 26.1. Cut surface of tubal pregnancy sac at 2½ months showing embryo alive at time of operation.

cation. It is especially likely that embryonic abnormalities could explain ectopic gestations in tubes that seem to be grossly normal with no abnormality on the opposite side. It is this type of patient who, if she has an ectopic pregnancy on one side, might have a number of normal intrauterine pregnancies through the opposite side at a subsequent date.

Incidence

Although it has been frequently quoted that 1 of 300 pregnancies is ectopic, Fontanilla and Anderson, in an excellent statistical study, indicate that the occurrence is considerably more frequent. In Baltimore, ectopic gestation occurs once in 200 pregnancies among white women and once in 120 pregnancies among black patients, nearly an 80% difference. This certainly suggests that inflammatory disease is the responsible factor, and obviously consideration of any reported incidence should include the racial percentages.

That repeat ectopic pregnancy may recur in the remaining tube in approximately 10% of cases (Schiffer) has been accepted by most gynecologists, although normal intrauterine gestation is much more common (approximately 25%).

A special situation exists with respect to the incidence of ectopic pregnancies when an intrauterine contraceptive device is in place. It is difficult to know whether the intrauterine device actually increases the incidence of ectopic pregnancies or whether their occurrence is accentuated by the absence of intrauterine pregnancies by virtue of the protection against such pregnancies afforded by the in-

trauterine device. Attempts to get at this incidence problem by ordinary demographic methods have been inconclusive.

The same question, but less pressing, is the frequency of ectopic pregnancies among low-dose progesterone oral contraceptive users. The ectopic pregnancy problem among low-dose progestogen users fits in with the failure of these drugs to inhibit ovulation as indicated by their failure to influence the date of the last menses. They presumably exert most of their action by making the endometrium unsuitable for implantation.

Pathology

Once the fertilized egg has implanted into the tubal mucosa, the early nidation changes are much like those seen in uterine pregnancy, except for an absence of the striking decidual reaction in the endometrium. The erosive action of the villous trophoblast causes penetration of the tubal wall, and this may extend through the muscularis. The invasion of blood vessels causes bleeding into the lumen, the tubal wall, or the peritoneal cavity. Therefore, the environment is a very unfavorable one, and the embryo usually succumbs within a few weeks, although a certain number of *full-term, viable tubal pregnancies* are on record and may be diagnosed by hysterogram and ultrasound.

Bleeding into the lumen of the tube converts the latter into a *hematosalpinx* (Fig. 26.2). Indeed, when hematosalpinx is found at operation or in the laboratory the first thought should always be of tubal pregnancy. When the latter is in the outer portion of the tube, the fimbriated orifice may be distended by an extruding blood clot.

Microscopically, the pathognomonic fea-

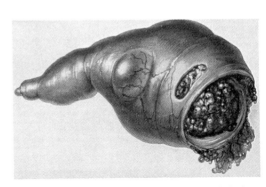

Figure 26.2. Large hematosalpinx with tubal abortion.

ture of tubal pregnancy is the *finding of chorionic villi* (Fig. 26.3) in the blood-filled lumen, sometimes penetrating the wall. The villi may be well preserved or they may show marked degeneration and hyalinization, although even then the characteristic outline is sharply preserved. However, care should be taken not to mistake for villi the organized thrombi not infrequently seen.

There has been much discussion as to the frequency of a *decidual reaction* (Fig. 26.4) in the tube. That genuine decidual response may occur is certain; for that matter, even with uterine pregnancy one may, in rare instances, find fields of typical decidual cells in the tube. On the other hand, there is also no doubt that trophoblastic cells invading the tubal wall are often mistaken for decidual cells, especially where only cytotrophoblast is evident, for this is not nearly so distinctive as the mature syncytial cell. Finally, even when a decidual response is demonstrated, as it is in a minority of cases, it is always of patchy and incomplete nature, in contrast to the massive and uniform response seen in the uterus.

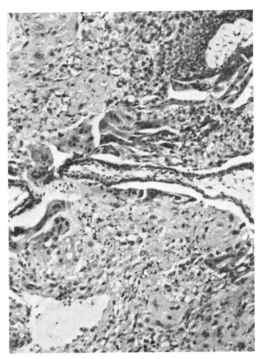

Figure 26.4. Decidual reaction in the tube, which in this section is distinguishable from trophoblastic invasion.

Possible Terminations of Tubal Pregnancy

(1) Tubal Rupture. This may occur as a result of the erosive action of the trophoblast, with bleeding into the peritoneal cavity, sometimes slight, sometimes profuse or even fatal. As a result of the rupture of the imperfectly formed capsularis, *intratubal hemorrhage* takes place. In both conditions there may be free bleeding from the fimbriated end of the tube, although tubal perforation generally produces much more massive hemoperitoneum.

(2) Tubal Abortion. This refers to an actual separation of the ovum from the tubal wall, with bleeding from the fimbriated orifice, which may be stuffed with clots. The dead embryo may be passed into the peritoneal cavity. Tubal abortion is frequently unrecognized, with only minor degrees of bleeding that ceases spontaneously.

(3) Secondary Abdominal Pregnancy. The older descriptions of secondary abdominal pregnancy would lead one to believe that when tubal rupture occurs, the product of conception may be expelled into the abdo-

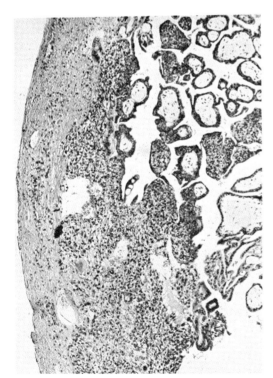

Figure 26.3. Tubal pregnancy with numerous young villi and marked trophoblastic invasion of tubal wall which is often mistaken for decidua (*lower right*).

men, and reimplant itself upon the peritoneal surface of the tube, broad ligament, or small intestine. Such a reimplantation is obviously impossible; instead more and more of the still attached placenta emerges, to grow external to the tube. Finally, the whole placenta is weaned away from the tubal lumen and continues its growth externally on the peritoneal surface, perhaps even to full term, although this is rare.

(4) Broad Ligament or Intraligamentary Pregnancy. When the tubal perforation is along the line of attachment of the mesosalpinx, the embryo escapes between the folds of the broad ligament and is gradually followed by the still attached placenta, as described in the preceding paragraph. Such pregnancies may advance to late stages, and a considerable number have progressed to full term.

(5) Spontaneous Regression. A good many tubal pregnancies undoubtedly pass unrecognized and never reach operation at the time but come to laparotomy at a later date for various reasons. On occasion there is evidence in the tubes of old hyalinized villi long after a possible pregnancy. Careful retrospective analysis of the histories of such patients often elicits the probability of a tubal gestation, perhaps many years previously. In such cases the embryo has evidently succumbed at a very early phase, with retrogression of the placenta and with symptoms not severe or acute enough to compel medical attention.

(6) Mummification of the Fetus. This may occur in unrecognized ruptured tubal pregnancies which have advanced to a later stage, whereas in other cases extensive *calcification* may convert it into a so-called *lithopedion.* On occasion, fetal bones may be passed vaginally, rectally, or through an abdominal sinus tract.

Behavior of Uterine Mucosa in Cases of Tubal Pregnancy

No matter where a pregnancy is located, the uterine mucosa responds by a decidual reaction (Fig. 26.5) to the hormonal stimuli set in motion by the implanted egg. As long as the latter is alive, this decidual reaction in the uterus is maintained. With the death of the embryo, however, the uterine decidua is cast off, generally piecemeal and in fragments, but on occasion as a single cast of the uterine cavity. When an entire cast is passed, the patient usually believes she has had a miscarriage, and the same error is frequently made by her physician.

One must remember that a decidual reaction in the endometrium is present in only about one-third of patients with a tubal pregnancy on whom a curettage is performed, because in many instances fetal death and subsequent passage of the decidua has allowed the reestablishment of ovulation and any type of endometrial pattern may be found. In addition, the finding of a decidual reaction, without villi, is not pathognomonic of a tubal pregnancy. Even in the absence of pregnancy some endometria can overrespond in an exaggerated fashion to the usual pro-

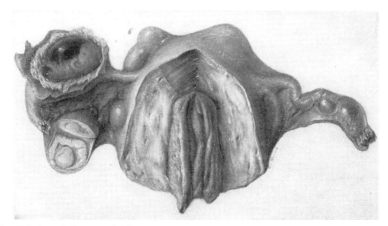

Figure 26.5. Tubal gestation sac laid open to show contained embryo in amniotic sac. The large corpus luteum of pregnancy is seen in the ovary of the same side, while the interior of the uterus shows the very thick decidua.

gestational hormones to produce a decidua-lke endometrial pattern.

Arias-Stella Reaction

In 1954 Arias-Stella described certain endometrial glandular changes supposedly pathognomonic of pregnancy, whether intra- or extrauterine, or as a result of trophoblastic disease. These changes are characterized by cellular enlargement with significant hyperchromatosis, pleomorphism, and mitotic activity, a tendency for the cellular lining to be almost decapitated so that the nucleus is exfoliated into the gland lumen, and a generalized tendency to appear neoplastic (Fig. 26.6). These changes are usually focal and associated with a stromal decidual change and a hypersecretory glandular pattern, although this is not invariably so. Indeed it has been stressed by many authors that these changes can be very helpful in making a diagnosis of an ectopic pregnancy, even though the endometrium shows no other evidence of potential pregnancy and may appear as proliferative, interval, etc.

It should be noted that Sturgis adequately described and depicted these endometrial changes long before Arias-Stella.

The incidence of the Arias-Stella Reaction (ASR) in conjunction with an ectopic or other pregnancy varies tremendously in different laboratories—from less than 5% to nearly 75%, as noted by numerous authors. It has been observed as early as 22 days after the last period. How late in pregnancy it may present or how long it may persist after fetal death seem open to considerable question. With the ever increasing frequency of elective termination of pregnancy and the occasional hysterectomy for abortion-sterilization, there is ample opportunity to study the gravid endometrium. It is our belief that the ASR is rarely apparent after 14 to 16 weeks of pregnancy, perhaps due to glandular exhaustion, and that it does not persist longer than 4 to 6 weeks after fetal death. As has been noted by many authors, it seems just as common after therapeutic abortion as after spontaneous abortion, which would imply that it represents a response to trophoblast rather than a degenerative sequel.

Expulsion of a decidual cast (Figs. 26.7 and 26.8) in cases of tubal pregnancy signifies the death of the embryo, but a considerable interval, often several days, may elapse before the cast is thrown off. Most cases of tubal

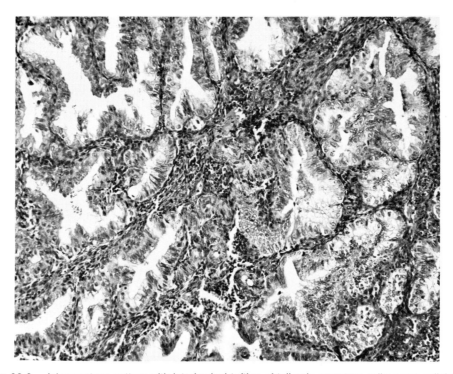

Figure 26.6. Adenomatous pattern with intraluminal tufting of tall pale secretory cells; some cellular atypia and mitotic activity present in this *Arias-Stella reaction*.

pregnancy do not come under observation until after the embryo has succumbed, sometimes not until weeks afterward. The endo-

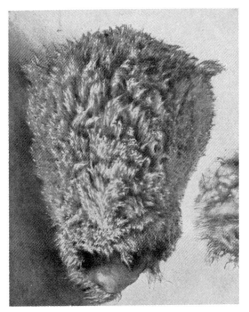

Figure 26.7. Decidual case thrown off at about 6th week of extrauterine pregnancy.

metrium in the meantime has regenerated itself, so that, if it is examined at the time of operation for tubal pregnancy, it may show little or no suggestion of decidual change. For this reason, *curettage* or *endometrial biopsy* and microscopic examination of the endometrium *are of limited value* in the diagnosis of tubal pregnancy; nevertheless, this may be helpful if the clinician is aware of the shortcomings.

If the embryo is still viable, typical decidua may be obtained on biopsy or curettage, with no villi. Often the curettage is contraindicated under such circumstances, as there is usually scant external bleeding, and the possibility of early uterine gestation cannot be eliminated. When, on the other hand, curettage is performed in patients who have been bleeding for many days or weeks, the endometrium may be entirely normal or it may still show a persistence of decidual change, depending on the time which has elapsed since embryonic death.

As already intimated, the external bleeding so common with tubal pregnancy is generally of uterine origin, but there are exceptions to this, as in the case of interstitial pregnancy

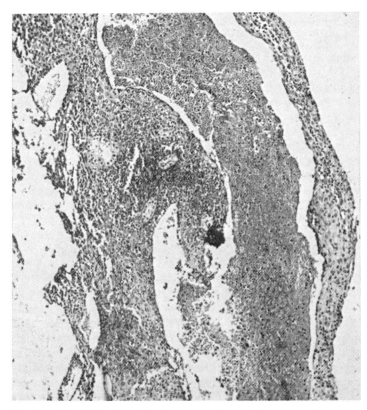

Figure 26.8. Structure of a decidual cast. In other cases the cast shows a much thicker decidual layer.

(Fig. 26.9). Even with a living embryo in the tube, slight bleeding may at times be noted, probably due to "ovular unrest" at the implantation area. There is rather general acceptance of the view that the persistent slight bleeding characterizing most cases of tubal pregnancy is of endometrial origin and that it is initiated by separation of the decidua.

Symptoms and Signs

The first symptom noted by the patient is apt to be a 7- to 14-day *delay in menstruation*, followed by slight bleeding which persists, with perhaps only a scant show of blood almost every day. Although this *spotting type of bleeding* is rather characteristic, not infrequently the bleeding may be somewhat freer, but it is rarely so profuse as with an incomplete abortion. Again, instead of the menstrual period being delayed, there may be an apparent anticipation of the flow by a few days. In still other cases, where the embryo survives sufficiently long, amenorrhea may continue for 2 or even 3 months, or in the rare cases of ectopic pregnancy which continue to term, for the full duration of the pregnancy.

Pain is an early symptom, although it is sometimes very slight. In the beginning there may be only a vague soreness in the affected side of the pelvis, but often the patient complains of sharp colicky pain occurring from time to time. When rupture or tubal abortion takes place, the pain may be very severe, and it may be associated with faintness or actual syncope and often nausea and vomiting. These symptoms are the result of the peritoneal reaction produced by the escape of blood from the tube. Pain in the right shoulder may be noted, as a result of the diaphragmatic reflex excited by free blood in the peritoneal cavity. *Expulsion of a cast* may or may not be noticed by the patient.

When the hemorrhage is slight, the pain may subside quickly, leaving only *soreness*. With recurrence of bleeding repeated attacks may occur. If the intraperitoneal bleeding is very profuse, *symptoms of shock* occur, such

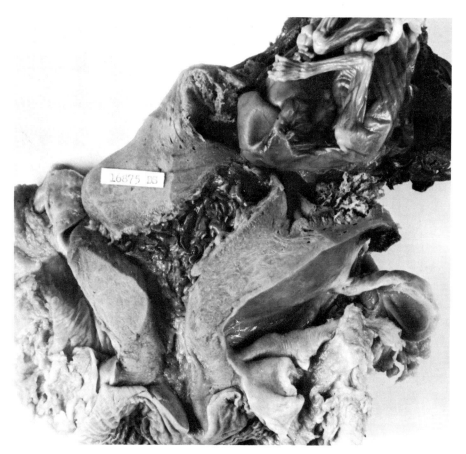

Figure 26.9. Interstitial tubal gestation (*upper right*).

as a rapid, thready pulse, extreme pallor of the skin and mucous membranes, air-hunger, a cold, clammy skin, and a subnormal temperature. In the occasional case in which prompt treatment is not instituted, death may occur in a short time. In only a small proportion of cases, about 5%, is the intraperitoneal bleeding of such cataclysmic proportions, the hemorrhage being much more often of the moderate and repeated type. For that matter, most cases are of the ambulatory type, and Parker and Parker aptly described *"chronic ectopics"* with various types of pelvic hematocele but without acute symptoms.

Subjective signs of pregnancy, such as morning nausea and enlargement of the breasts, are not often seen because of the usually early termination of the gestation, although in later cases they may be noted. *Laboratory findings* are of little value in the cases with moderate internal bleeding, with the possible exception of the pregnancy tests, to be discussed. When bleeding is free, the hemogram shows varying degrees of anemia, with a low hematocrit. Under such conditions slight leukocytosis is the rule, rarely exceeding a white cell count of 12,000. When the blood loss is great, however, the degree of leukocytosis is apt to be higher. The temperature with mild bleeding may be normal, but with more abundant hemorrhage it is slightly elevated; with extreme hemoperitoneum, it is subnormal.

Physical Signs. *Abdominal examination* may be entirely negative or there may be only slight tenderness over the lower abdomen, usually more marked on one side. When the stage of the pregnancy or the intratubal bleeding makes the tubal mass correspondingly large, it may even be felt through the lower abdominal wall, if this is very thin and lax, but this is unusual. *Percussion* comes into valuable play in cases in which free abdominal bleeding is suspected, and it frequently gives evidence, especially by dullness in the flanks, of free fluid in the abdomen.

Even *inspection* may be of value in the occasional case. Where there has been repeated bleeding into the abdomen for a considerable time, a bluish, bruise-like discoloration may be found surrounding the umbilicus (*Cullen's sign*), especially if the latter is very thin or if there is an umbilical hernia. This sign, only rarely observed, is due to deposit of blood pigment absorbed by way of the lymphatics in the umbilical region. *Tym-*

panites and *abdominal distention* are not infrequently associated with free abdominal bleeding.

Pelvic Examination. Of the greatest importance are the findings on pelvic examination. The cervix may become patulous and softened. The uterus may enlarge slightly (Fig. 26.5), even in early tubal pregnancy, but this is rarely noticeable in the average case. Where the tubal mass is large, the uterus may be pushed somewhat to one side. The distinctive finding is the presence of a *tender mass on one side of the pelvis.* The opposite side of the pelvis may show no demonstrable abnormalities, although not infrequently there may be evidence of chronic adnexitis. Where bleeding into the pelvis has been profuse, *pelvic hematocele* is produced, with a doughy consistency in the cul-de-sac.

Diagnosis

The clinical picture of tubal pregnancy is so typical in many cases that diagnosis is very easy, but many errors are made, and it may well be considered a disease of diagnostic surprises. The physician who has extrauterine pregnancy "on the brain" will rarely fail to diagnose it when it exists. On the other hand, one who is not alert to its possibility will meet with many surprises which greater care could have avoided.

When a woman presents herself with a history of slight spotting beginning a few days after an expected missed period, with pain in one side of the pelvis, and when examination in such a patient reveals a unilateral tender pelvic mass, the first thought should be of tubal pregnancy, and often this will prove to be the case.

Pelvic aspiration or puncture (culdocentesis) with a large bore needle (5-inch number 18) is of frequent value.

Several series have reported a high degree of correlation with ectopic pregnancy and the aspiration of nonclotting blood from the cul-de-sac. Clinical rupture does not have to occur to have sufficient blood in the cul-de-sac to have a positive tap. Most ectopic pregnancies leak at least a little blood.

The use of the laparoscope has taken much of the uncertainty from the resolution of the diagnosis of ectopic pregnancy in patients suspected of having this condition. Not only does visualization of the pelvis by way of the laparoscope circumvent the uncertainty of diagnosis with its potential for serious inter- peritoneal hemorrhage, but it allows the di- agnosis of an unruptured ectopic pregnancy, thereby providing the opportunity to correct the condition surgically before the opposite tube is compromised by peritoneal reaction from free blood. Therefore, a suspected ec- topic pregnancy is a clear indication for lap- aroscopy (Fig. 26.10).

Ultrasonography has come into vogue as a method of examination, and it has a certain usefulness. If a small sac can be identified within the uterus, this, of course, differen- tiates clearly between a normal intrauterine pregnancy and an ectopic one. Sometimes, a small sac can be identified in the region of the tube. Tubal localization may be expected in about half of the cases which really are tubal, but it depends in the final analysis on the health of the ectopically located gestation. Kukard and Goetzee reported a correct di- agnosis of ectopic pregnancy by ultrasonog- raphy in 12 of 22 cases (55%).

However, this more or less 50% expectancy of correctness in tubal gestation is based on cases which are, in fact, tubal in location. In practice, many other problems are among the suspect cases. A better idea of the practicality of ultrasonography may be obtained from the study of Kelly et al. These workers reported their sonographic experiences with 260 sus-

pect cases. Among these, it was determined by other means that the correct diagnosis was as follows: 136 were not pregnant at all, 99 had an intrauterine pregnancy, and only 25 really had an ectopic gestation. By sonogra- phy, 8 of the 25 ectopic gestations were not diagnosed. On the other hand, in the entire series, there were 27 ultrasonography diag- noses of ectopic gestations. This means that there were 10 false positives. It is interesting that of the 99 intrauterine pregnancies, 94 of these could be diagnosed by ultrasonography. Many times the differential diagnosis is be- tween an intrauterine pregnancy sometimes threatening to abort with a small corpus lu- teum cyst and an ectopic pregnancy. Thus, ultrasonography is helpful but, like other ex- aminations, must be considered in the light of the other findings (Fig. 26.11).

The frequency of positivity of immunolog- ical tests for pregnancy depends on one hand on the number, viability, and accessibility to the circulation of the chorionic cells, and on the other on the sensitivity of the particular test in question. The same considerations, of course, apply to the radio-receptor assay. Pos- itivity of any of these tests may be expected, but less frequently in ectopic pregnancies than in normal intrauterine pregnancies. Therefore, in a case of suspected ectopic preg- nancy, if the test is positive, the result can be very helpful in clinical management in veri- fying that the patient is pregnant, although, of course, the test does not help in determin- ing the location of that pregnancy. However, a poorly implanted, dead, or dying ectopic pregnancy may be present, in consequence of which the pregnancy test may be negative. Using a radio-receptor assay with the sensi- tivity of 200 mIU/ml for human chorionic gonadotropin (hCG) (blood serum), Berry et al. found 94% positivity among 67 patients with proven tubal pregnancy. It is interesting that only 69% of these same patients had a positive urine 2-minute latex agglutination slide pregnancy test with a sensitivity of 1,500 mIU/ml of hCG (urine).

To be preferred, however, because of its specificity is the test for the specific β subunit of hCG. The same considerations, of course, apply to this test as applied to any other, but its quantitation is often particularly helpful. When the exact duration of pregnancy is known, if the quantitative estimation of the β subunit of hCG is below the lower limit of

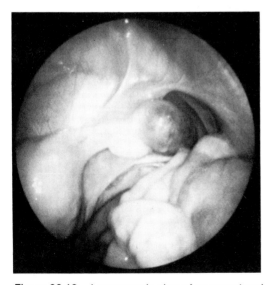

Figure 26.10. Laparoscopic view of an unruptured tubal pregnancy in the right fallopian tube. (Courtesy of Dr. Melvin R. Cohen.)

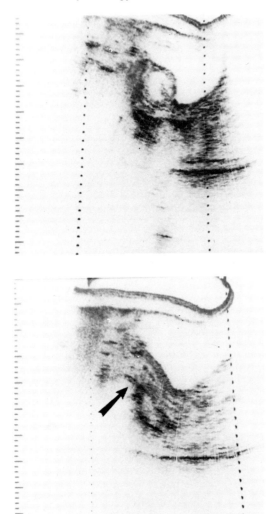

Figure 26.11. Sonogram taken on a patient with a suspected ectopic pregnancy. *Upper,* a sagittal section taken 0.5 cm to the right of the midline. The clear space in the *upper right* portion of the figure represents the bladder filled with water. Just below and to the left is a clear round area with echos within. This is the gestational sac. From this view, it can be suspected that the sac is not within the endometrial cavity because of the thinness of the echo between the bladder and the gestational sac. *Lower,* a sagittal cut 3 cm to the left of the midline. The pubis is to the right and the xyphoid to the left. The bladder may again be seen. The tip of the *arrow* is within the gestational sac; to the right of the *arrow* and below it is the echo from the uterus showing the endometrial cavity. This view clearly shows that the gestational sac is outside of the endometrial cavity. At operation an ectopic pregnancy in the left tube was found.

normal for that date, one can be quite suspicious that one is dealing with a threatened miscarriage of an intrauterine pregnancy or

a poorly implanted pregnancy, as one might expect in an ectopic situation. The difficulty, of course, is that quantitation may require more time than one has in the clinical setting, and the results may be available only after the clinical problem has been resolved.

Special alertness is required in suspecting ectopic pregnancy when a patient is wearing an intrauterine contraceptive device (IUD). As has been mentioned, the intrauterine device does not protect against ectopic pregnancies and there is some suspicion that the incidence of ectopic pregnancy may be higher among IUD users than among others. Many times the symptoms are erroneously attributed to the mere presence of the IUD, and it is interesting that often the IUD is removed in the vain hope that its removal will somehow alleviate the symptoms. For example, Hallatt reported a series of 70 ectopic pregnancies among IUD wearers. He found that in 95% of the cases the symptoms were initially attributed to the presence of the IUD, and, significantly, in 40% of the cases the IUD was removed some time prior to a definitive diagnosis of the ectopic pregnancy at surgery. All of this seems to show that the possibility of an ectopic pregnancy is not uppermost in the mind of either the patient or physician when odd symptoms occur in an IUD wearer. In this regard, it was significant in Hallatt's analysis that the symptoms and findings were basically no different from the symptoms and findings in patients with ectopic pregnancies among patients without an IUD.

The conditions with which tubal pregnancy is most easily confused are: (1) incomplete or threatened abortion of intrauterine pregnancy; (2) pelvic inflammatory disease; (3) ovarian cyst with twisted pedicle; (4) corpus luteum or follicle cyst, with or without a normal intrauterine pregnancy; and (5) torsion of adnexa. The percentage of error given by all authors is quite large, varying from 15% to as much as 35%.

Treatment

Once tubal pregnancy has been diagnosed, the indication for surgical treatment is clear. Even in patients who are ambulatory and whose symptoms are relatively mild, there should be no undue delay in recommending operation, because of the ever present possibility of life-endangering hemorrhage from tubal rupture or abortion. In the comparatively small proportion of cases in which such alarming hemorrhage has occurred, the operation should be performed at once. In such cases, transfusion before or during the operation is of prime importance.

There has been some discussion about whether oophorectomy should be carried out routinely when a fallopian tube is removed for an ectopic pregnancy. Oophorectomy might be considered theoretically desirable in that ovulation would then always occur from the residual ovary immediately adjacent to the residual tube.

Pertinent to this discussion is the finding that the corpus luteum of pregnancy has been found on the side opposite to the ectopic pregnancy in about 20% of cases. This figure is representative of several studies and exactly the figure developed by Saito et al. in a study of 130 cases. In these 20% of patients, external migration of the oocyte must have occurred, and this evidence from ectopic pregnancies is the best available on the likelihood that external migration is a normal physiological occurrence.

The over-all pregnancy rate after treatment for an ectopic pregnancy is about 50%, including an expectancy of a repeat ectopic pregnancy in about 10% (Table 26.1).

Throughout the years, there have been recurrent recommendations for the preservation when possible of the fallopian tube containing the ectopic pregnancy. If the tube has not been blown apart by rupture, preservation can be accomplished either by milking the conceptus from the fimbriated end of the tube or by making a longitudinal incision along the antimesenteric border of the tube and suturing the incision with fine material. Data to demonstrate the usefulness of this method have been difficult to come by for the simple reason that if there is also a tube

on the opposite side, it is impossible, in the event of subsequent pregnancy, to know through which tube the pregnancy occurred. One of the best studies on this point was by Jarvinen et al. who reported 10 patients who had but a single tube in which an ectopic pregnancy occurred. In each instance, the tube was preserved. Following operation, hydrotubation was used daily throughout the patient's hospital stay of 8 or 9 days. Follow-up studies showed that there were five term deliveries; however, there were three repeat ectopic pregnancies, a 30% rate in this small series, which is about 3 times the rate of repeat ectopics in the opposite tube when one tube is removed. In addition, there were also two miscarriages. On the basis of present evidence, therefore, it would seem desirable to preserve the tube only as a last resort, i.e., when there is a residual tube in which an ectopic gestation had occurred. To use this routinely would seem to expose the patient to an increased risk of ectopic pregnancy in that tube.

OTHER TYPES OF ECTOPIC PREGNANCY

Interstitial (Cornual)

In this rare form, the pregnancy is located in that portion of the tube which traverses the uterine wall. Diagnosis is difficult and is most likely mistaken for a soft myoma, with perhaps an early abortion of an intrauterine pregnancy. The symptoms are similar to those of tubal pregnancy, although the pain may not be as severe and the amenorrhea preceding any vaginal bleeding a little prolonged due to a more favorable implantation site. Should rupture occur, intraperitoneal bleeding may be very profuse.

Ovarian Pregnancy

This is extremely rare, and until recent years its occurrence was doubted. There is now, however, a considerable group of well authenticated cases; these have been reviewed by Tan and Yeo. The generally accepted criteria of diagnosis are those originally postulated by Spiegelberg. They are: (1) that the tube, including the fimbria ovarica, be intact and the former clearly separate from the ovary; (2) that the gestation sac definitely occupy the normal position of the ovary; (3) that the sac be connected with the uterus by

Table 26.1
Fertility after Treated Tubal Pregnancy

	No. of Patients	Patients Conceiving	Patients with Term Pregnancy	Patients with Ectopic Pregnancy
		%	%	%
Douglas	106	45.3	33.9	7.5
Bender	239	48.5	35.5	7.5
Timonen	743	50.2	28.7	12.5
Totals	1,088	49.4	30.7	10.9

the ovarian ligament; and (4) that unquestionable ovarian tissue be demonstrable in the walls of the sac (Figs. 26.12 and 26.13).

The rarity of ovarian pregnancy, in view of the ready accessibility of the ovary to the spermatozoa and the portals offered by ruptured follicles, is probably due to the fact that the ovum as given off from the ovary has not reached maturation, this being normally completed in its passage through the tube.

Several cases of ovarian pregnancy in association with an intrauterine contraceptive device have been noted by Piver et al. and others.

Abdominal (Peritoneal) Pregnancy

There was much skepticism as to the possibility of the fertilized egg implanting itself directly on the pelvic peritoneum, outside the genital canal, but the case reported in 1942 by Studdiford seems to establish this possibility beyond question.

Most abdominal pregnancies are secondary to a pregnancy which originally occurred in a fallopian tube or occasionally within the uterus. The pregnancy ends up in the peritoneal cavity by virtue of tubal abortion or rupture which, when the pregnancy survives

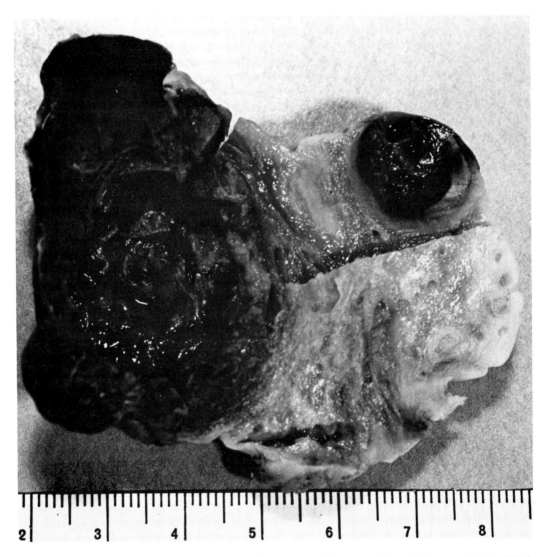

Figure 26.12. Pregnancy in ovarian substance. Tube normal. (Courtesy of Dr. J. M. Croak, Oregon, Ohio.)

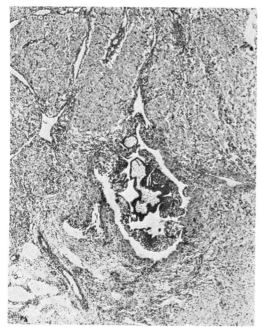

Figure 26.13. Chorionic villi in ovarian pregnancy in which the implantation may have been in the corpus luteum, which can be seen surrounding the villi in this section.

in the peritoneal cavity, must at first be partial, so that for a time the placenta is able to derive blood from the tube while it attaches to the peritoneal cavity, but finally as the placenta develops its entire attachment is outside the fallopian tube. Cases which are secondary to intrauterine pregnancy usually are secondary to a rupture of the uterus through an old scar.

The fetal prognosis is very poor in abdominal pregnancy, although Clark and Guy reported an 11% fetal salvage in their 26 cases. There were no maternal deaths.

It may be well to mention that the surgeon, in dealing with an abdominal pregnancy, should generally not attempt to remove the placenta, which may be firmly fixed to the mesentery and the abdominal viscera (Fig. 26.14). Profuse hemorrhage can occur on manipulation, and the placenta, if left in situ, resorbs without sequelae in most instances, although bowel obstruction may be a late complication. Removal of the fetus with ligation of the cord is usually the wise procedure. Hreshchyshyn et al., Lathrop and Bowles, and others have suggested the use of

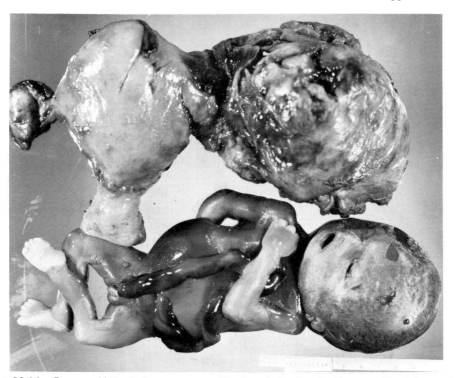

Figure 26.14. Presumed intrauterine pregnancy with attempted saline abortion was ultimately revealed to be an abdominal pregnancy. Placenta (*upper right*) with fetus in peritoneal cavity. A similar case is reported by Walton and Nikuri.

methotrexate to facilitate devascularization and absorption of any unremoved placenta.

Cervical Pregnancy

Although exceedingly rare, the possibility of cervical pregnancy does exist. Just as in placenta praevia the egg may implant itself in the region of the internal os, so it may, in rare instances, implant on the cervical mucosa. As would be expected, this bizarre type of pregnancy produces profuse bleeding in the early months of pregnancy and necessitates surgical intervention (hysterectomy), which may be of difficult and serious nature. In reporting a case, Resnick noted only some 65 instances of a true cervical pregnancy in his exhaustive review of reported cases. He pointed out the difficulties in diagnosis and the mortality (20%), primarily due to hemorrhage, understandably due to repeated pelvic examinations in an effort to establish the diagnosis (Fig. 26.15). Roth and Birnbaum, and Jauchlen and Baker likewise emphasized the frequent need for hysterectomy.

Combined Pregnancy (Intra- and Extrauterine)

There are now several hundred reported cases of combined pregnancy, one embryo being implanted normally within the uterus, the other ectopically in the tube. Interesting diagnostic problems may arise with such a combination. For example, rupture of the tubal pregnancy may cause serious intraabdominal bleeding, with none from the vagina, since the integrity of the uterine decidua is maintained by the presence of the lining intrauterine pregnancy. For a discussion of the clinical connotations of combined pregnancy, however, the reader must be referred to textbooks of obstetrics. Schaefer believed that the pathogenesis is a double-ovum twin pregnancy in which both ova are fertilized at a single coitus; he separated this (combined) form from a compound pregnancy where an intrauterine is superimposed upon a preexisting resolving ectopic gestation. In any case diagnosis is seldom made because the slightly enlarged boggy uterus is believed to represent merely a decidual reaction. In adding an additional case, Brody and Stevens brought up to 506 the cases of combined pregnancy and provided an extensive review of the literature.

Simultaneous pregnancy in both tubes may occur, and many such cases have been noted, as well as simultaneous intrauterine gestation. Less common is *unilateral twin pregnancy.* Only 84 cases were noted by Loh and Loh, who emphasized that such twins are usually monozygotic. Forbes and Natale reported a *triplet tubal pregnancy* (Fig. 26.16).

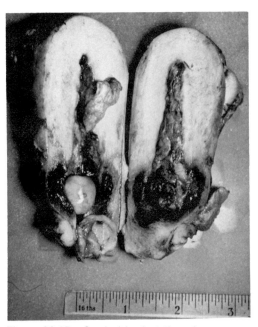

Figure 26.15.   Cervical implantation of pregnancy. (Courtesy of Dr. L. Resnick, South Africa.)

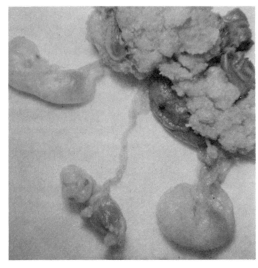

Figure 26.16.   Placenta and three fetuses from tubal pregnancy. (Courtesy of Dr. Don Forbes, Springfield, Massachusetts.)

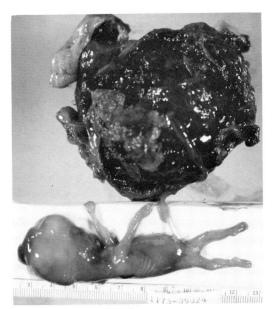

Figure 26.17. Tubal pregnancy 3 months after vaginal hysterectomy ("stormy postoperative course with low hCT—presumed pelvic hematoma").

Posthysterectomy Ectopic Pregnancy

Although we have seen a few cases of prolapsed fallopian tubes after hysterectomy where the tubal fimbria protruded through the vaginal vault, it has been our impression that an ectopic pregnancy would be unlikely. The physiology of such a prolapsed tube without an intermediate uterus would seemingly be impaired, so the possibility of pregnancy would seem minimal.

Although tubal pregnancy posthysterectomy is rare, the careful clinician cannot absolutely promise the woman that she will not become pregnant after removal of the uterus. Hanes reported 11 cases of pregnancy after abdominal or vaginal hysterectomy. In four instances the pregnancy probably antedated the operative procedure, with conception occurring before and not recognizable at the time of surgery. Perhaps this occurs much more often than realized, with subsequent anemia and pelvic induration being construed as intraabdominal bleeding incurred by the surgery itself. Often this is self-limited and does not require operative intervention, but not always (Fig. 26.17).

References and Additional Readings

Arias-Stella, J.: Atypical endometrial changes associated with the presence of chorionic tissue. Arch. Pathol. *58:* 112, 1954.

Arias-Stella, J., and Gutierrez, J.: Frequencia y signficando de las atypias endometriales en al embarazo cotopico. Rev. Lat. Am. Anat. Patol., *1:* 81, 1957.

Bender, S.: Fertility after tubal pregnancy. J. Obstet. Gynaecol. Br. Emp., *63:* 400, 1956.

Berry, C. M., Thompson, J. D., and Hatcher, R.: The radio receptor assay for HCG in ectopic pregnancy. Obstet. Gynecol. *54:* 43, 1979.

Bobrow, M. L., and Bell, H. G.: Ectopic pregnancy: a 16-year survey of 905 cases. Obstet. Gynecol., *20:* 500, 1962.

Breen, J. L.: A 21-year survey of 654 ectopic pregnancies. Am. J. Obstet. Gynecol. *106:* 1004, 1970.

Brody, S., and Stevens, F. L.: Combined intra- and extrauterine pregnancy. Obstet. Gynecol., *21:* 129, 1963.

Cavanagh, D.: Primary peritoneal pregnancy. Am. J. Obstet. Gynecol., *76:* 523, 1958.

Clark, J. F. and Guy, R. S.: Abdominal pregnancy. Am. J. Obstet. Gynecol. *96:* 511, 1966.

Douglas, C. P.: Tubal ectopic pregnancy. Br. Med. J., *2:* 838, 1963.

Douglas, E. S., Jr.: Surgical management of tubal pregnancy. South. Med. J., *62:* 954, 1969.

Erkkola, R., and Liukko, P.: Intrauterine device and ectopic pregnancy. Contraception, *16:* 569, 1977.

Erkkola, R. and Liukko, P.: Oral contraceptives and ectopic pregnancy. Contraception, *16:* 575, 1977.

Fontanilla, J., and Anderson, G. W.: Further studies on racial incidence and mortality of ectopic pregnancy. Am. J. Obstet. Gynecol., *70:* 312, 1955.

Forbes, D. A., and Natale, A.: Unilateral tubal triplet pregnancy. Obstet. Gynecol., *31:* 360, 1968.

Halbrecht, I.: Healed genital tuberculosis: new etiologic factor in ectopic pregnancy. Obstet. Gynecol., *10:* 73, 1957.

Hallatt, J. G.: Ectopic pregnancy associated with the intrauterine device: a study of seventy cases. Am. J. Obstet. Gynecol., *125:* 754, 1976.

Hanes, M. V.: Ectopic pregnancy following total hysterectomy. Obstet. Gynecol., *23:* 882, 1964.

Helde, M.D., et al.: Detection of unsuspected ovarian pregnancy by wedge resection. Can. Med. Assoc. J., *106:* 237, 1972.

Hreshchyshyn, M. M., Naples, J. D., Jr., and Randall, C. L.: Amethopterin in abdominal pregnancy. Am. J. Obstet. Gynecol., *93:* 286, 1965.

Jarvinen, P. A., Nummi, S., and Pietila, K.: Conservative operative treatment of tubal pregnancy with postoperative daily hydrotubations. Acta Obstet. Gynecol. Scand., *51:* 169, 1972.

Jauchlen, G. W., and Baker, R. L.: Cervical pregnancy. Obstet. Gynecol., *35:* 370, 1970.

Kelly, M. T., Santos-Ramos, R., and Duenhoelter, J. H.: The value of sonography in suspected ectopic pregnancy. Obstet. Gynecol., *53:* 703, 1979.

Kukard, R. F. P., and Goetzee, U.: A comparison between ultrasonic and clinical diagnostic reliability in early pregnancy complications. South Afr. Med. J., *48:* 2109, 1974.

Lathrop, J. C., and Bowles, G. E.: Methotrexate in abdominal pregnancy. Obstet. Gynecol., *32:* 81, 1968.

Lehfeldt, H., Tietze, C., and Gonstein, F.: Ovarian pregnancy and IUD. Am. J. Obstet. Gynecol., *108:* 1005, 1970.

Loh, W., and Loh, H. C.: Unilateral tubal twin pregnancy with intraperitoneal rupture. Obstet. Gynecol., *19:* 267, 1961.

Lucas, C., and Hassim, A. U.: Place of culdocentesis in the diagnoses of ectopic pregnancy. Br. Med. J., *1:* 200, 1970.

Mall, F. P.: A study of the causes underlying the origin of human monsters (3rd contribution to the study of pathology of human embryos). J. Morphol., *19:* 3, 1908.

Metz, K. G. P., and Mastroianni, L., Jr.: Tubal pregnancy subsequent to transperitoneal migration of spermatozoa. Obstet. Gynecol. Surv., *34:* 554, 1979.

Parker, S. L., and Parker. R. T.: "Chronic" ectopic tubal pregnancy. Am. J. Obstet. Gynecol., *74:* 1174, 1957.

Persaud, V.: Etiology of tubal ectopic pregnancy. Obstet. Gynecol., *36:* 257, 1970.

Piver, M. S., Baer, K. A., and Zachary, T. V.: Ovarian pregnancy intrauterine device. J.A.M.A., *201:* 107, 1967.

Poland, B. J., Dill, F. J., and Stylblo, C.: Embryonic development in ectopic human pregnancy. Teratology, *14:* 315, 1976.

Resnick, L.: Cervical pregnancy. South Afr. Med. J., *36:* 73, 1962.

Roth, D. J., and Birnbaum, S. J.: Cervical pregnancy. Obstet. Gynecol., *42:* 675: 1973.

Saito, M., Kayama, T., Yaoi, Y., Kumasaki, T., Yazawa, K., Kato, K., Nushi, N., and Ohkura, T.: Site of ovulation and ectopic pregnancy. Acta Obstet. Gynecol. Scand., *54:* 227, 1975.

Schaefer, G.: Extrauterine pregnancy with concomitant term uterine pregnancy. Clin. Obstet. Gynecol., *5:* 875, 1962.

Schiffer, M. A.: A review of 268 ectopic pregnancies. Am. J. Obstet. Gynecol., *80:* 264, 1963.

Spiegelberg, O.: Zur casuistik den ovarial-schwangenschaft. Arch. Gynaekol., *13:* 73, 1878.

Stratford, B. F.: Abnormalities in early human development. Am. J. Obstet. Gynecol., *107:* 1223, 1970.

Studdiford, W. E.: Primary peritoneal pregnancy. Am. J. Obstet. Gynecol., *44:* 487, 1942.

Sturgis, S. H.: Arias-Stella phenomenon. Am. J. Obstet. Gynecol., *116:* 589, 1973.

Tan, K., and Yeo, O.: Primary ovarian pregnancy. Am. J. Obstet. Gynecol., *100:* 240, 1968.

Timonen, S., and Niemonem, O.: Tubal pregnancy: choice of operative methods of treatment. Acta Obstet. Gynecol. Scand. *46:* 237, 1967.

Walton, L. A., and Nikrui, N.: "Salting out" an abdominal pregnancy. N.Y. State J. Med., *73:* 2782, 1973.

CHAPTER 27

Gestational Trophoblastic Disease

Gestational trophoblastic disease is the general term for a spectrum of proliferative abnormalities of the trophoblast. Hydatidiform mole represents a usually benign form of the disease, and choriocarcinoma is a very malignant, frequently metastatic lesion. These neoplasms arise from the trophoblastic elements of the developing blastocyst and retain certain characteristics of the normal placenta, such as invasive tendencies and the ability to make the polypeptide hormone *human chorionic gonadotropin.* The disease is always related to some pregnancy event and thus specifically differs from choriocarcinoma found in germ cell tumors of the ovary or testes.

Pathologic Classification. These proliferative trophoblastic abnormalities are classified as *hydatidiform mole, invasive mole*, or *choriocarcinoma* based on their histopathologic appearance (Table 27.1). Approximately 80% of patients initially diagnosed as having hydatidiform mole will follow a benign course with spontaneous resolution after dilatation and curettage, but 12 to 15% subsequently develop locally invasive disease and 5 to 8% eventually prove to have metastatic lesions. The pathologic classification of hydatidiform mole has not proven to be an accurate prognostic indicator to select those 20% of patients who will subsequently require therapy for malignant forms of trophoblastic disease. Predictability is better with the other forms of trophoblastic disease since most, although not all, patients with a pathologic diagnosis of invasive mole or choriocarcinoma will follow a malignant course and require therapy.

Clinical Classification. The development of sensitive assays for human chorionic gonad-otropin, which accurately reflect the course and prognosis of the disease, together with the use of effective chemotherapeutic agents have drastically changed the classification, management, and prognosis of this disease. As will be discussed in detail on the following pages, trophoblastic disease is clinically classified as *benign* or *malignant,* and the malignant category is further subdivided into *metastatic* and *nonmetastatic.* Patients with a pathologic diagnosis of choriocarcinoma or invasive mole are placed in the clinical classification of malignant trophoblastic disease, because these almost always act in a malignant fashion and require therapy. On the other hand, patients with a pathologic diagnosis of hydatidiform mole may wind up in either the benign (80%) or malignant (20%) trophoblastic disease category of the clinical classification based on their clinical course. The use of both pathologic and clinical classifications is often confusing to the student, but it reflects an evolution in our understanding of this fascinating disease.

Incidence

Trophoblastic disease is relatively uncommon in the United States, but its occurrence varies considerably throughout the world. Although it is clear that the incidence of trophoblastic disease varies from one country to another, the reason for this variation is not understood. Manahan and others have found that the incidence of hydatidiform mole is higher in women of low socioeconomic class. Some investigators have suggested that this is related to diet and commented that protein deficiency in the diet was associated with a

Table 27.1
Classification Schemes for Gestational
Trophoblastic Disease

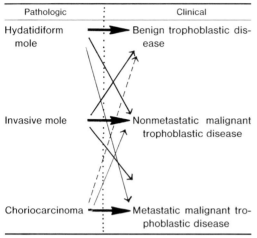

Pathologic	Clinical
Hydatidiform mole	Benign trophoblastic disease
Invasive mole	Nonmetastatic malignant trophoblastic disease
Choriocarcinoma	Metastatic malignant trophoblastic disease

high incidence of mole. Other nutritional factors, such as folic acid and iron deficiency, have also been suggested. In a careful review, Reynolds presented a theory of vascular agenesis as a result of folic acid deficiency as the cause of hydatidiform mole. The epidemiologic evidence is conflicting and inadequate to make any conclusions concerning the etiology of gestational trophoblastic disease, and, as we shall see, recent cytogenetic information suggests a chromosomal basis for the disease.

PSEUDOMALIGNANT BEHAVIOR OF THE TROPHOBLAST

To understand better the abnormal behavior of gestational trophoblastic disease, it is first necessary to review the pathologic characteristics of the placenta during normal pregnancy. Of primary interest is the ability of the placental chorionic villi to exhibit rather extensive degrees of invasion into and through the maternal decidua. Trophoblastic buds may often burrow down into the myometrium as discrete small foci of cells (syncytial myometritis), although there is often rather abrupt termination of their invasive propensities at the myometrial-decidual junction (layer of Nitabuch), presumably due to some type of local inhibition. It is by no means rare, however, to find foci of trophoblast deep in the myometrium, for example, after cesarean section hysterectomy. Hertig indicated that villi form during the 14th day

of fetal life, and added that late ovulation incurs a higher frequency of such abnormal pregnancies as abortion and mole.

Second is the frequent possibility of migration of the trophoblast to the lungs, as noted originally by Schmorl in 1893. This so-called "deportation of villi" is an accepted possibility in an occasional normal pregnancy, although probably not as frequently as documented by Schmorl. Yet this form of pulmonary "metastatis" does not behave like a malignant embolus, for there is rarely more than minor transitory difficulty, if any, as far as the mother is concerned.

HYDATIDIFORM MOLE

Hydatidiform mole is a condition in which the chorionic villi become enormously overdistended with fluid, appearing as translucent grapelike vesicles which may vary in size from a few millimeters to that of a cherry. Thus, the derivation of the name is from Latin *hydatid*, meaning *watery vesicle*, and *mole* or *mass*. The characteristic macroscopic appearance of a hydatidiform mole is that of a bunch of grapes (Fig. 27.1) due to the enormous edema of the villi. Often the whole uterine cavity is filled with vesicular molar tissue, but on other occasions only a small portion of the placenta is involved.

In the past there has been some uncertainty as to whether the disease is of *neoplastic* or *degenerative* character. However, it is now generally agreed that the chief microscopic characteristics of a *classic* or *true hydatidiform mole* are (1) marked edema and enlargement of the villi, (2) disappearance of the villous blood vessels, (3) proliferation of the lining trophoblast of the villi, and (4) absence of fetal tissue (Fig. 27.2). Of these, the last two are probably the most important. In portions of the mole within the uterine cavity or in extruded portions there may be little or no trophoblastic overgrowth seen, although in the same lesion villi still receiving a good blood supply from the uterine wall may show marked trophoblastic proliferation. Thus, it is not unusual to fail to find evidence of trophoblastic proliferation on the curettings of a patient who is subsequently found unequivocally to have hydatidiform mole. Therefore, we believe that a true hydatidiform mole is a *proliferative* or *neoplastic* lesion. In addition, recent evidence would suggest that a

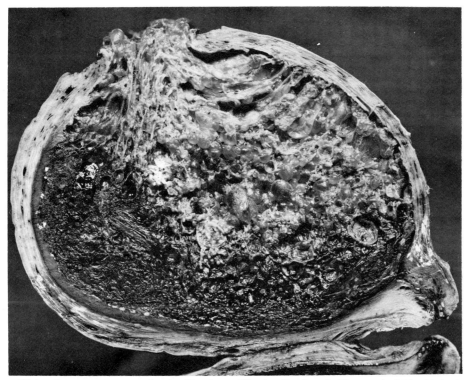

Figure 27.1.   Gross appearance of mole. (Courtesy of Dr. Jan Smalbraak, Bloemendaal, The Netherlands.)

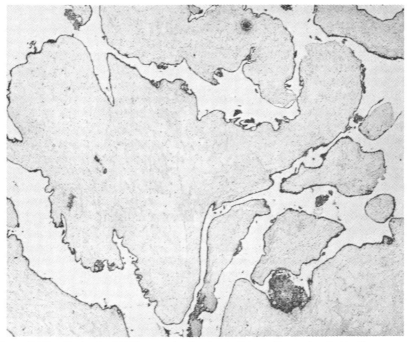

Figure 27.2.   Benign hydatidiform mole showing in this section no trophoblastic overgrowth.

true hydatidiform mole has no evidence of fetal tissue.

Occasionally, grossly edematous villi have been seen in the presence of a fetus or amnion in specimens from spontaneous or missed abortion (Fig. 27.3). These cases have often

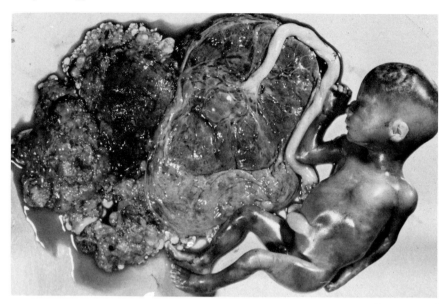

Figure 27.3. Six-month fetus in association with incomplete hydatidiform mole. (Courtesy of Dr. N. A. Beischer, Melbourne, Australia.)

been included in discussions of hydatidiform mole, and such changes have been referred to as *hydropic degeneration* or hydatidiform changes. However, Szulman and Surti have recommended that such cases be called *incomplete* or *partial mole*, inasmuch as they differ from classic hydatidiform mole in both morphologic and cytogenetic aspects. In contrast to true hydatidiform moles, these patients have identifiable fetal tissues, edematous villi with no trophoblastic proliferation, and a triploid chromosomal compliment. Many of the associated fetuses have gross congenital anomalies.

Chromosomes of Hydatidiform Mole

The pathologic criteria of trophoblastic proliferation with no evidence of fetal tissue seems to correlate fairly well with the cytogenetic findings of a 46, XX karyotype. Baggish et al. reported the presence of a chromatin body in each of 90 moles studied. More recently, Kajii and Ohama obtained karyotypes on molar tissue and both parents in seven cases of true hydatidiform mole and, with banding techniques, were able to demonstrate in 20 of 26 pairs studied that a paternal chromosome was inherited in duplicate by the mole. In none of the 26 pairs of chromosomes was the maternal chromosome transmitted to the mole. In all of the 49 pairs scored, homologous chromosomes were

homozygous for banding polymorphisms. This evidence strongly suggests that all of the genetic material of the ovocyte is lost or inactivated and the *entire chromosome complement of the mole comes from the sperm.*

Pathologic-Clinical Correlation

Hertig and Sheldon published a *pathologic classification* of hydatidiform mole in 1947 in which they attempted to correlate the histologic appearance of these lesions with their subsequent behavior. Among 32 patients with very slight or no trophoblastic proliferation, there were no malignant sequelae, whereas 17 patients with "exuberant trophoblastic growth" all developed malignancy. Although it is probably true that the more proliferative moles are followed by a higher incidence of complication, a considerable number of invasive or malignant tendencies develop after even the most innocuous-appearing mole. As will be noted subsequently, it would seem that the biological behavior of trophoblast is more important than the histological pattern.

INVASIVE MOLE

The diagnosis *invasive mole* or *chorioadenoma destruens* is applied to moles characterized by abnormal penetrativeness and *extensive local invasion* along with *excessive tropho-*

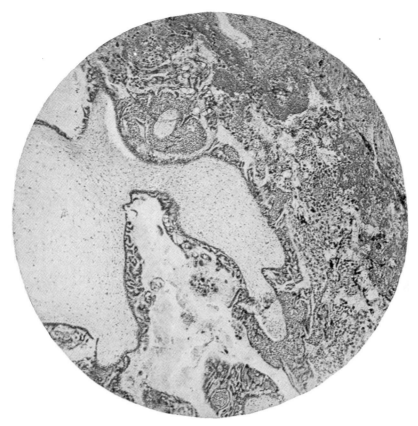

Figure 27.4. Highly proliferative mole in situ in uterine wall. This would be called chorioadenoma destruens by most pathologists.

blastic proliferation. (Figure 27.4) Microscopically, the criteria for the diagnosis are imprecise, because the degree of trophoblastic proliferation is quite variable. As a rule, there is increased trophoblastic proliferation with a preserved villous pattern. The proliferative villi may invade the parametrium or the vaginal wall, although there is rarely evidence of metastasis. It is this variety of mole which has so often wrongly been diagnosed as choriocarcinoma. It differs very crucially from the latter, not only microscopically, but in that it rarely metastasizes. Therefore, unlike choriocarcinoma, it has been usually cured by hysterectomy, although treatment of this era is often nonsurgical.

The morbidity and mortality of this disease result from penetration of the tumor through the myometrium and into the pelvic vessels, with resultant hemorrhage. Tow notes a mortality rate of up to 10%, mostly due to hemorrhage. Occasionally, metastases may occur which may be differentiated from choriocar-

cinoma by the persistence of villus structures. Such metastatic lesions probably have a more favorable prognosis than solid choriocarcinoma. In 1961, Wilson et al. reported eight patients with pulmonary metastases from invasive mole, all of whom cleared spontaneously with no therapy. These patients would undoubtedly be treated with chemotherapy today.

CHORIOCARCINOMA

Choriocarinoma or chorionepithelioma is a very malignant, frequently metastatic form of gestational trophoblastic disease. It is rather infrequent, occurring with an incidence of about 1 per 40,000 pregnancies in the United States. Gestational choriocarcinoma may follow hydatidiform mole (50%), spontaneous abortion (30%), or normal pregnancy (20%) and is clinically and prognostically different from choriocarcinoma, which occurs in germ cell tumors of the ovary. It should be noted that, although approximately one-half of all choriocarcinomas are preceded by a molar pregnancy, only about 3 to 5% of all molar pregnancies eventuate in choriocarcinoma.

Grossly, the tumor appears as a dark, hemorrhagic mass on the uterine wall, cervix, or vagina. It soon shows extensive ulceration, with increasing spread on the surface or with penetration of the musculature. Uterine perforation and hemorrhage are common. Only malignant trophoblast has the ability to invade arterial channels. Benign trophoblast may be found in the venous circulation, but is generally arrested in the lung; malignant change with tumor emboli in the pulmonic capillaries allows bypass of the lung, with passage into the arterial system, and the development of cor pulmonale due to right-sided heart failure. Cerebral accidents due to intracranial tumor with hemorrhage are a common cause of death in choriocarcinoma.

Microscopically, gestational choriocarcinoma is characterized by a disorderly growth of trophoblastic tissue, both syncytotrophoblast and cytotrophoblast, into the muscle, with destruction of the latter and extensive coagulation necrosis, as well as hemorrhage. The villous pattern is completely blotted out by the proliferating trophoblast (Fig. 27.5).

Histopathologically, the lesions most commonly misdiagnosed as choriocarcinoma are benign trophoblastic disease and syncytial endometritis or myometritis. There are two chief points of difference between benign infiltration of the myometrium by trophoblast (syncytial myometritis) and choriocarcinoma. In the benign conditions, trophoblastic cells are seen to invade singly or in small groups, and they do not produce any muscle necrosis. On the other hand, one of the chief characteristics of choriocarcinoma is the destruction of tissue by the infiltrating columns of trophoblastic tissue with associated coagulation necrosis and hemorrhage. The degrees of trophoblastic proliferation and anaplasia are important but are much more variable.

CLINICAL FEATURES

Signs and Symptoms

Gestational trophoblastic disease usually presents with vaginal bleeding and uterine cramps during the first or early second trimester. The diagnosis of threatened or incomplete abortion is frequently entertained. Passage of the classic vesicular tissue may occur, but it is usually a late sign. Nausea, vomiting, or preeclampsia may be seen on occasion, and Cave and Dunn have reviewed the mechanism of thyrotoxicosis which is occasionally seen as a presenting symptom.

With hydatidiform mole, approximately 50% of patients have a uterus which is large for dates. The uterus is normal size in about 20% of patients, and 30% have a uterus which is smaller than would be expected for the length of gestation.

Signs of a normal intrauterine pregnancy are absent. There are no fetal heart tones audible with a stethoscope or doppler, and, even if the uterus is enlarged beyond 20 weeks' gestation, no fetal skeleton can be seen on the x-ray.

In the malignant or *invasive mole* the growth may perforate the uterine wall, with sometimes severe or even fatal intraabdominal bleeding. This destructive variety may likewise invade the vascular channels, and very occasionally metastases may appear in the vagina, vulva, or lungs as in the more frankly malignant choriocarcinoma.

Metastases are frequent with choriocarcinoma, but vaginal bleeding is still the most common presenting complaint. In this rapidly growing tumor, metastases usually appear comparatively early and involve the lung, brain, liver, bone, and even skin. Not infrequently, it is these which first call attention to the probability of choriocarcinoma. The vagina and vulva are often the sites of such metastases, which appear as dark hemorrhagic nodules, resembling thrombosed varices (Fig. 27.6). *Cough* or *hemoptysis* should always lead to the suspicion of pulmonary metastases, and this is often confirmed by x-ray examination (Fig. 27.7). Occasionally, central nervous system metastases will be heralded by symptoms of a cerebral vascularaccident with weakness, paralysis, seizures, or coma.

Associated Ovarian Changes

In at least some cases of hydatidiform mole, as well as of its malignant prototype, choriocarcinoma, the ovaries exhibit an interesting change in the form of a marked polycystic enlargement, with exaggerated luteinization of predominately theca rather than

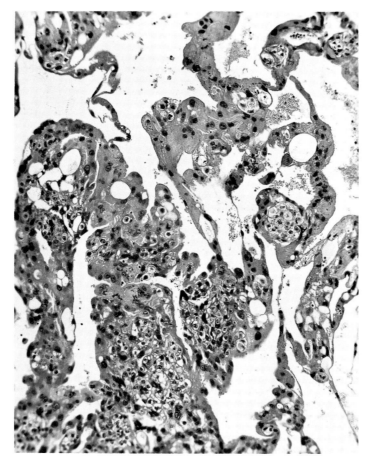

Figure 27.5. Curettings from a case of choriocarcinoma which terminated fatally 5 months later with multiple metastases.

granulosa cells. Curry et al. reported that these *theca luteincysts* occur clinically in about 20% of patients with hydatidiform mole. They are also occasionally found with normal intrauterine pregnancy. The ovarian enlargement is usually in the 5- to 10-cm range, but very large cysts have been reported. The time of appearance of such theca lutein cysts seems to be variable, and in some cases they have not appeared until after the evacuation of the mole.

These ovarian changes represent an exaggerated response of the ovarian tissue to the abnormally high levels of HCG, which is very similar in structure to luteinizing hormone (LH). With declining HCG levels after treatment, the theca lutein cysts regress spontaneously and require no therapy. Curry et al. found that ovarian enlargement accompanying hydatidiform mole was associated with a high incidence of malignant sequelae. Forty-

nine percent of the patients with ovarian enlargement accompanying hydatidiform mole subsequently required chemotherapy for trophoblastic disease, whereas only 14% of the patients without theca lutein cysts needed any therapy after evacuation of the mole.

DIAGNOSIS

Recurrence of bleeding and the disproportionately large size of the uterus should lead to the suspicion of hydatidiform mole. Once the diagnosis of hydatidiform mole has been suspected clinically, several tests are available to confirm the diagnosis. Although detection of high levels of HCG has been used in the past, this is time consuming and not consistently accurate; twin gestation may present with a large uterus and a high HCG titer.

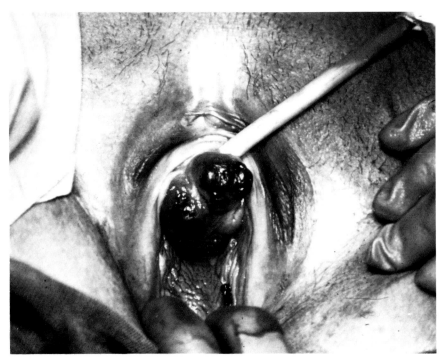

Figure 27.6. Choriocarcinoma metastatic to the suburethral area of the anterior vaginal wall. (Courtesy of Dr. Carolina Braga, San Francisco, Calif.)

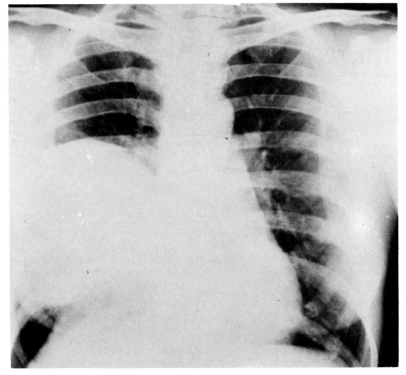

Figure 27.7. Massive pulmonary metastasis which regressed after methotrexate. (Courtesy of Dr. M. S. Baggish, Hartford, Conn.)

Ultrasound is extremely accurate for the diagnosis of hydatidiform mole and for differentiating such other conditions as threatened abortion or ectopic pregnancy which may present problems in a differential diagnosis (Fig. 27.8). This noninvasive technique is widely available, but the experience of the physician who interprets the scan is most critical for an accurate diagnosis.

An *amniogram* may also be utilized. It requires only standard x-ray equipment and readily available radiologic contrast material. An amniocentesis is done with the standard technique, and, after checking the needle po-

sition by aspiration, a small volume of radiopaque dye is injected into the uterine cavity. The presence of the hydatidiform mole will produce a typical "honeycomb" pattern (Fig. 27.9).

An *arteriogram* may be useful in localizing metastatic lesions within the pelvis or abdomen, but is usually not done for the primary diagnosis of hydatidiform mole.

Once the diagnosis has been established, a simple preoperative evaluation will rule out the most frequent areas of metastasis. A good pelvic examination looking for vulvar, vaginal, or cervical metastasis or evidence of pel-

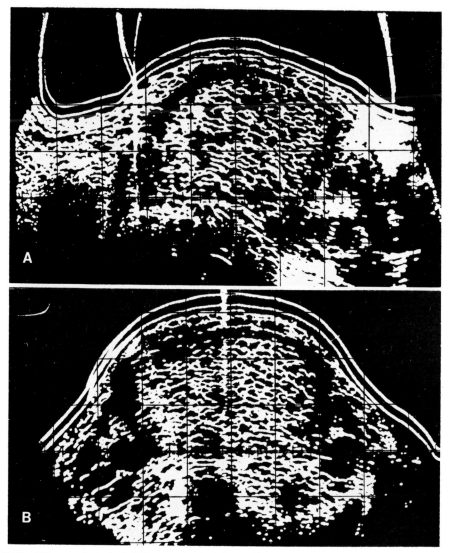

Figure 27.8.   Ultrasound of a hydatidiform mole. *A*, right marker is at pubis; *left*, umbilicus. Note characteristic honeycomb molar mass in center. Each grid 3 cm. *B*, transverse view. Note absence of fetal sac. Diffuse echoes with "snowstorm effect" (high sensitivity settings).

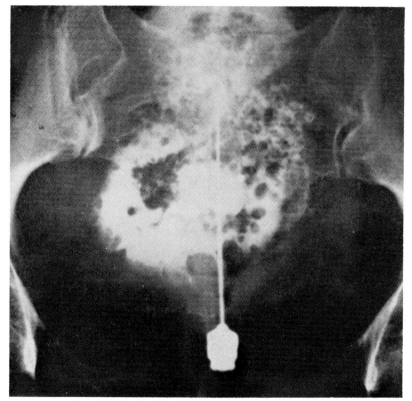

Figure 27.9. X-ray of uterine cavity in patient suspected of having a molar pregnancy taken approximately 5 minutes after injection of 20 ml of radiopaque material (Hyopaque). "Moth-eaten" or "honeycombed" pattern is diagnostic for molar pregnancy. (From D. P. Goldstein and D. E. Reid: *Clinical Obstetrics and Gynecology, 10:* 313, 1966.)

vic masses, together with a chest x-ray and routine blood studies, including blood urea nitrogen and liver function tests, are all that is usually required.

Serum is drawn for measurement of pre-evacuation HCG levels.

Human Chorionic Gonadotropin

During the early months of normal pregnancy there is a markedly elevated level of human chorionic gonadotropin. Normally during the 50th to 80th days of the average pregnancy there is peak of gonadotropin secretion. Multiple gestation may lead to an inordinately high level. In general, however, serum HCG levels of greater than 100,000 mIU/ml are associated with gestational trophoblastic disease rather than normal pregnancy.

In the past, quantitative determinations of HCG levels in urine or blood were made by bioassay of the increased weight of an im-

mature rat or mouse uterus or by the spermatozoa response in a male frog or toad. With the advent of the radioimmunoassay technique, antibodies were raised to the α-chain of purified HCG, and a radioimmunoassay for HCG was described and utilized for the management for trophoblastic disease. More recently, Vaitukaitis et al. described a specific radioimmunoassay for the β-subunit of HCG which is able to measure low levels of HCG in the presence of LH because it does not cross-react to any significant degree. This assay generally takes several days to run.

The serum assay for the β-subunit of HCG is generally used by most clinicians in the routine management of patients with gestational trophoblastic disease. It does not require troublesome and frequently inaccurate 24-hour urine collection, and it is accurate at low levels of HCG, making it extremely valuable in monitoring the clinical course of the disease.

The development of these sensitive assay

techniques, which allow the clinician to monitor carefully and to quantitate roughly the amount of residual trophoblastic tissue, together with the discovery of highly effective chemotherapy for trophoblastic disease, has resulted in a complete change in the management of gestational trophoblastic disease over the past 20 years. Today, treatment indications are based more on the course of the HCG levels and proven malignant behavior and to a much lesser degree on the histologic appearance of the trophoblast.

MANAGEMENT OF HYDATIDIFORM MOLE

Once the diagnosis of hydatidiform mole has been made by ultrasound or other means, evacuation of the uterus is in order. A preliminary metastatic work-up as previously noted, including careful examination and chest x-ray, is performed, and the patient's general physical condition is checked. Transfusions are given preoperatively if the patient is severely anemic, and blood is cross-matched for use if needed.

Evacuation

Suction curettage of the uterus is the most effective and safest method of evacuation of hydatidiform mole. The cervix is usually soft and easily dilated, but if this is a problem, laminaria can be inserted 8 to 12 hours before dilatation and curettage to provide a slow dilatation, enabling the insertion of large dilators and suction tips with little cervical trauma. It is not uncommon for the diagnosis of hydatidiform mole to be made by the pathologist following evacuation of what was presumed to be an incomplete abortion in a patient who presented with bleeding, cramping, and passage of tissue.

Hysterectomy may occasionally be utilized for removal of a molar pregnancy in a woman who has completed her family and desires sterilization. This minimizes the possibility of malignant sequelae, but the operation may be technically difficult due to the enlarged uterus and increased blood supply. Curry et al. reported that 2 of 10 patients who underwent primary hysterectomy for hydatidiform mole required subsequent chemotherapy for metastatic trophoblastic disease.

Hysterotomy and *induction of labor* with either pitocin or prostaglandins are poor alternative choices for evacuation of a mole and should be considered only if suction curettage is not available. Traumatic embolization of the trophoblast to the lungs is occasionally seen after spontaneous labor or evacuation and may be massive enough to produce hypoxia, dyspnea, cyanosis, or shock.

Following evacuation of a hydatidiform mole, approximately 80% of patients undergo spontaneous regression of any residual trophoblastic tissue and resume normal menstrual function. However, 3 to 5% develop choriocarcinoma, and another 15% have persistent mole or invasive mole. Therefore, *the importance of careful follow-up cannot be overemphasized.*

The use of *prophylactic chemotherapy* has been proposed by Goldstein and others in an attempt to decrease the incidence of malignant sequelae. Using low-dose actinomycin-D in 73 patients with hydatidiform mole, Goldstein was able to reduce the rate of malignancy to 8%. This compares with a 20% rate of persistent trophoblastic disease requiring chemotherapy in 116 patients who received no prophylactic chemotherapy. However, because 80% of patients with hydatidiform mole will undergo spontaneous remission and chemotherapy is successful in almost all of the rest, the routine use of toxic chemotherapy at the time of initial evacuation of a hydatidiform mole with no evidence of metastasis is not recommended unless follow-up will be a problem.

Follow-up

Once the mole has been evacuated by whatever means, including hysterectomy, careful follow-up utilizing serum HCG levels is absolutely essential in order to identify he 20% of patients who will require additional therapy. The β-subunit radioimmunoassay for HCG should be used. Following evacuation of a hydatidiform mole, serum HCG titers should return to undetectable levels within 8 to 12 weeks. Morrow et al. constructed a normal postmolar regression curve from the serum β-HCG levels measured by radioimmunoassay of women whose HCG levels fell spontaneously to normal following molar pregnancy (Fig. 27.10). By 60 days, 70% of the patients still had detectable serum β-HCG levels and at 10 weeks 58% still had elevated levels of HCG in the serum. Not

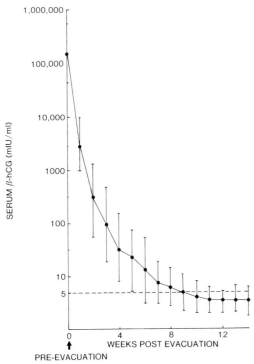

Figure 27.10. Normal regression curve of serum β-HCG after evacuation of a hydatidiform mole. The 95% confidence limits are shown for 24 patients who underwent spontaneous resolution to normal after evacuation. (Reproduced with permission from C. P. Morrow, O. A. Kletzky, P. J. DiSaia, D. E. Townsend, D. R. Mishell, and R. M. Nakamura: *American Journal of Obstetrics and Gynecology, 128:* 424, 1977.)

rare for a patient to redevelop trophoblastic disease after negative β-HCG assays for 1 year if no new pregnancy episode has occurred.

Because normal pregnancy also results in production of HCG, which cannot be differentiated from that produced by persistent or recurrent trophoblastic disease, *it is essential to avoid pregnancy during the year of follow-up.* If there are no contraindications, oral contraceptives are recommended because of their effectiveness and the fact that they suppress LH which prevents occasional, confusing, low-level cross-reactivity with the β-HCG assay.

Repeated moles in the same patient are uncommon, but they do occur, as tabulated by Hsu et al. Only one of their six cases developed malignancy. Wu reported nine recurrent moles in one patient with no progression to malignancy.

until 12 weeks had all but one of the patients dropped below the minimum detectable level. Thus, it seems apparent that with more sensitive assays for following the HCG, we must revise our criteria for diagnosis of persistent trophoblastic disease on the basis of HCG levels. They also noted that all patients who subsequently required therapy for trophoblastic disease, except one, had clearly abnormal regression curves by 4 weeks' postevacuation.

When the β-HCG level is nondetectable for 4 successive weeks, the patient is considered free of disease and is then followed with monthly β-HCG assays for the next year. Pelvic examinations and interval history should be done every 3rd month. After 1 year of normal follow-up the patient may be assumed to be disease free, and surveillance is continued only on a yearly basis. With sensitive modern assay techniques it is extremely

MALIGNANT TROPHOBLASTIC DISEASE

After evacuation of a hydatidiform mole, patients will occasionally experience a new episode of vaginal bleeding. Unless the previous curettage was unsatisfactory, this is a poor prognostic sign, and careful evaluation of the tissue and close monitoring of the serum β-HCG level are in order. Unlike most other malignancies and the previous "pathologic era" of this disease, today it is not necessary to have a tissue diagnosis of invasive mole or choriocarcinoma before starting therapy. The difficulties of making this diagnosis and the frequent lack of correlation between the histology and clinical course, together with the effectiveness of chemotherapy and the correlation between the HCG level and the clinical course, have made a tissue diagnosis unnecessary.

Chemotherapy for trophoblastic disease is indicated when (1) the histologic diagnosis of choriocarcinoma is made, (2) metastatic disease is detected, (3) the β-HCG level plateaus or rises after evacuation of a hydatidiform mole, (4) the β-HCG level has not returned to undetectable levels by 12 weeks' postevacuation, or (5) an elevated β-HCG level is detected during follow-up sometime after a negative titer was achieved (Table 27.2). As with any laboratory test it is important to use common sense in interpretation of the β-

Table 27.2
Trophoblastic Disease—Indications for Chemotherapy

1. Histologic diagnosis of choriocarcinoma
2. Evidence of metastatic disease
3. A plateaued or rising serum β-HCG level after evacuation of a hydatidiform mole
4. A β-HCG level which has not returned to normal by 12 weeks' postevacuation
5. An elevated β-HCG level detected after attainment of a normal serum level

HCG results. Treatment should rarely, if ever, be instituted on the basis of a single laboratory determination, and the clinical picture must always be correlated with the reported β-HCG level. Unless the patient is having uterine bleeding, it is not necessary to do a dilatation and curettage prior to or during the first course of therapy.

Staging

Once the decision to treat has been made the patient must be "staged" and the treatment selected. The history should be carefully reviewed and a complete physical examination performed. This is important, not only to search for evidence of metastases, but to ascertain the general condition of the patient and assess her ability to tolerate cytotoxic chemotherapy. In many cases it is also worthwhile to restudy the pathology in light of the clinical course. A chest x-ray should be repeated unless one has been done within the past week. If negative, full-lung tomograms may reveal previously undetected metastasis. The liver and brain should be evaluated for evidence of metastasis by a radioisotope or computerized tomographic scan. Blood studies should include a complete blood count with differential and platelet count, liver function tests, and blood urea nitrogen, and creatinine. Additional studies such as ultrasound, arteriogram, electroencephalogram, and lumbar puncture are necessary only when routine studies suggest further evaluation.

Once the pretreatment evaluation is completed it is possible to classify the patient according to the generally accepted scheme shown in Table 27.3. This is a clinically oriented classification which divides patients depending on whether there is metastatic disease or not. Hertz found that the level of gonadotropin prior to the start of therapy and the duration of disease prior to treatment were important prognostic characteristics. Because methotrexate and actinomycin-D do

not effectively pass the blood-brain barrier and enter the central nervous system and are quickly detoxified by the liver, metastases to these organs also put patients in the "high-risk" category. In patients who have failed previous chemotherapy, Hammond et al. reported cures in only 6 of 12 patients with metastatic disease. Miller and the group from Duke, in a separate report, found a survival rate of only 60% among 20 patients who developed choriocarcinoma after full-term pregnancy. Thus, a "high-risk" group with metastatic disease has been identified on the basis of the prognostic experience of patients with gestational trophoblastic disease.

Surgery

Prior to the introduction of chemotherapy, surgery was the treatment of choice for gestational trophoblastic disease. Hysterectomy was quite successful in the treatment of hydatidiform mole and locally invasive mole, but it was totally inadequate for the management of metastatic choriocarcinoma.

Role of Hysterectomy. Hysterectomy seems to be of decreasing importance in the management of trophoblastic disease, with certain exceptions as noted by Lewis, Ketcham, and Hertz. When hysterectomy is contemplated it should be done during a course of chemotherapy to minimize the possibility of disseminating tumor emboli. Possible indications for surgery include the following:

(1) Drug resistance or toxicity, especially in cases with the disease seemingly confined to the uterus.

(2) Such complications as vaginal hemorrhage, uterine perforation with intraperitoneal bleeding, and infection.

(3) The older multiparous patient with localized disease.

Certainly it is a tremendous advantage for the young woman desirous of more children to avoid hysterectomy, retain her uterus, and subsequently become pregnant.

Surgical excision of isolated metastatic le-

Table 27.3
Clinical Classification of Gestational Trophoblastic Disease

I. Nonmetastatic
II. Metastatic
    A. Low risk—All patients with documented metastatic disease who do not have ''high-risk'' factors
    B. High risk
        1. β-HCG level higher than 100,000 mIU/ml
        2. Associated pregnancy episode more than 4 months prior to diagnosis
        3. Following full-term pregnancy
        4. Liver or brain metastasis (? bowel)
        5. Failure of previous chemotherapy

sions in the abdomen, lung, or occasionally, brain may also be considered in patients with resistant disease.

Chemotherapy

Since the work of Li, Hertz, and Spencer, chemotherapy with methotrexate or actinomycin-D has been the mainstay of treatment for patients with gestational trophoblastic disease.

Methotrexate. Methotrexate is an antimetabolite which combines with folic acid reductase, thereby inhibiting the reduction of folic acid to tetrahydrofolic acid. Because tetrahydrofolic acid is essential in the transfer of one-carbon fragments in the synthesis of DNA, methotrexate effectively blocks DNA synthesis, inhibiting cell replication. Among chemotherapeutic agents, methotrexate is unique in that an antidote, leukovorin—a reduced folic acid derivative—is available, which can bypass the enzymatic block produced by methotrexate. When given after methotrexate, leukovorin prevents or minimizes the toxicity of methotrexate and allows higher doses of methotrexate to be used. The effectiveness of this high dose of methotrexate followed by leukovorin "rescue" has been reported by Goldstein et al.

Toxicity to methotrexate frequently involves mucous membranes, with stomatitis, esophagitis, vaginitis, and, occasionally, gastrointestinal ulcerations. Bone marrow suppression with granulocytopenia and thrombocytopenia are common, but generally not severe. Skin rashes and alopecia are uncommon, but they do occur; nephrotoxicity, hepatotoxicity, and pulmonary fibrosis are very rare.

Actinomycin-D. Actinomycin-D is an antitumor antibiotic which binds to DNA, preventing the synthesis of RNA. It is excreted by the liver and does not seem to enter the central nervous system. It is given intravenously, and extravisation into the tissues must be avoided because this leads to necrosis with skin sloughing.

Toxicity to actinomycin-D includes nausea and vomiting, bone marrow suppression with thrombocytopenia, stomatitis, alopecia, and skin reaction. Enhanced toxicity may be seen in areas of prior or current radiation therapy.

Nonmetastatic Disease

In patients with nonmetastatic gestational trophoblastic disease, single-agent chemotherapy is used initially.

Metastatic Disease

Patients with *metastatic low-risk disease* are treated exactly as patients with nonmetastatic disease. For patients with *metastatic, high-risk disease,* combination chemotherapy using three drugs is used. This "triple therapy" involves the use of methotrexate, actinomycin-D, and an alkylating agent such as cyclophosphamide or chlorambucil. High-dose methotrexate with leukovorin "rescue" and other combinations of multiple drugs also have been effective in patients who develop resistance to single-agent chemotherapy. The protocol for some of these drugs is shown in Table 27.4. Although many gynecologists who have utilized chemotherapeutic agents in their training programs may be able to manage a patient with single-agent chemotherapy, Brewer et al. have shown that the treatment success was only 34% in patients treated with chemotherapy by outside physicians, whereas a 63% cure rate was reported for patients treated by the physicians at Northwestern University. Even better results can be expected today, but the message is clear that inexperienced physicians tend to be somewhat timid in the application of these chemotherapeutic agents, and resistant disease with eventual failure is the end result. Certainly patients who require triple therapy or who fail single-agent therapy should be referred to centers where experienced gynecologic oncologists can manage their therapy.

Radiation Therapy

Trophoblastic disease is not especially sensitive to radiation therapy, but several special circumstances are indications for its use in this disease. Patients with metastases to the brain or liver may develop hemorrhage into these metastatic lesions as they undergo necrosis from chemotherapy. In such cases external radiation with 2,000 rads tumor dose is usually given over a 10- to 14-day period in conjunction with combination chemotherapy. Occasionally, continuous intravenous or arterial infusions are utilized to treat resistant liver or brain metastases.

Results

The results of treatment of gestational trophoblastic disease are shown in Table 27.5. With chemotherapy, 100% of patients with nonmetastatic disease can be cured, and a high percentage of patients with metastatic lesions are also curable. Note that the treatment results of Hammond et al. include many patients with "high-risk" metastatic disease treated prior to our understanding of the importance of starting with multiple drug chemotherapy in these patients. Today, we should expect to cure more than 80 to 90% of these "high-risk" patients, as indicated by the reports of Smith and Lewis.

Choriocarcinoma following a full-term pregnancy seems to have a poor prognosis. Miller et al. recently reported a survival rate of only 60% in a series of 20 patients who developed choriocarcinoma after full-term gestation.

Follow-up

Once a negative β-HCG level has been achieved, it is recommended that one more course of therapy be given "for good measure." This practice was instituted when measurement of HCG levels was not so sensitive as now, but it may still be useful inasmuch as there are apparently patients with negative

Table 27.4
Chemotherapy for Gestational Trophoblastic Disease

Single agent	Methotrexate: 15-25 mg intramuscularly or intravenously daily for 5 days
	Actinomycin-D: 0.015 mg/kg or 0.5 mg intravenously daily for 5 days
	Treatment courses are repeated as often as toxicity will allow.
"Triple therapy"	Methotrexate: 10-15 mg intravenously daily for 5 days
	Actinomycin-D: 0.5 mg intravenously daily for 5 days
	Chlorambucil:10 mg orally daily for 5 days.
	or
	Cytoxan: 150-250 mg intravenously daily for 5 days
Leukovorin "rescue"	Methotrexate: 1.0 mg/kg intramuscularly followed in 12–24 hours by citrovorum factor: 0.1 mg/kg intramuscularly. The methotrexate is given every other day for four doses or until toxicity develops.

Table 27.5
Results of Treatment of Gestational Trophoblastic Disease with Chemotherapy

Author	Nonmetastatic Disease		Metastatic Disease			
			Low risk		High risk	
	Patients	Survival	Patients	Survival	Patients	Survival
		%		%		%
Hertz et al. (1963)	22	100				
Brewer (1971)	80	100	71	87		
Goldstein (1972)	49	100	37	93		
Hammond et al. (1973)	57	100	89	98	17	47
Smith (1973)	18	100	18	95	14	100
Jones and Lewis (1974)	18	100	6	100	15	80

serum β-HCG levels in whom urinary concentrates have demonstrated persistent HCG. Schrieber et al. reported two such cases. Therefore, except in cases of severe toxicity to therapy, it has been our practice to give one additional course of chemotherapy after the attainment of an undetectable level of serum β-HCG. Recurrence rates of 3 to 8% are expected during the first treatment year, and rare cases have been reported to occur more than 1 year after therapy. A patient is said to be in remission after four consecutive weekly β-HCG levels are negative. She is then followed with monthly HCG assays for at least 1 year, and an interval history and physical examination, including pelvic, are done every 3 months. If the patient has had metastatic disease, it is important to follow that parameter with the appropriate tests, such as chest x-ray or scan, to be sure that resolution is complete. If chemotherapy has been extensive, follow-up evaluation of the status of the bone marrow with complete blood count and platelet count is advisable, and liver and renal function may also be checked. The patient is given good contraception, usually with birth control pills, for the first year to prevent the confusing and anxiety-producing possibility of a pregnancy with accompanying rise in HCG levels. After 1 year she is seen twice yearly until 5 years and then annually. β-HCG levels are checked at each visit.

In the younger woman treated for trophoblastic disease, chemotherapy permits retention of the uterus with the possibility of subsequent pregnancy, and a considerable number of these cases have been recorded. Hammond et al. stated that the likelihood of a second molar pregnancy is about 1 in 500. Van Thiel et al. reported a follow-up of 50 women who had been treated for both metastatic and nonmetastatic trophoblastic disease and subsequently had 88 pregnancies, with no increase in fetal wastage, congenital abnormalities, or complicated pregnancy, with the possible exception of placenta accretia.

References and Additional Readings

Acosta-Sison, H.: Changing attitudes in management of hydatidiform mole (196 cases). Am. J. Obstet. Gynecol., 88: 634, 1964.

Baggish, M. S., Tow, S. H., and Jones, H. W.: Sex chromatin pattern in hydatidiform mole. Am. J. Obstet. Gynecol., 102: 362, 1968.

Bagshawe, K. C.: Choriocarcinoma, Edward Arnold, London, 1969.

Beischer, N. A.: Hydatidiform mole with coexistant fetus. J. Abstet. Gynaecol. Br. Commonw., 68: 231, 1961.

Beischer, N. A.: Significance of chromatin pattern in cases of hydatidiform mole with associated fetus. Aust N. Z. J. Obstet. Gynaecol., 6: 127, 1966.

Birnholz, J. C., and Barnes, A. B.: Early diagnosis of hydatidiform mole by ultrasound imaging. J.A.M.A., 225: 1359, 1973.

Brandes, J., and Peretz, A.: Recurrent hydatidiform mole. Obstet. Gynecol., 25: 398, 1965.

Brandes, J., Grunstein, S., and Peretz, A.: Suction evacuation of the uterine cavity in hydatidiform mole. Obstet. Gynecol., 28: 689, 1966.

Brewer, J. L., Eckman, T. R. Dolkart, R. E., Torok, E. E., and Webster, A.: Gestational Trophoblastic Disease. Am. J. Obstet. Gynecol. 109: 335, 1971.

Brindeau, A., Hinglais, A., and Hinglais, M.:La mole hydatiform. Bull. Fed. Soc. Gynecol. Obstet. Franc., 4: 3, 1952.

Canlas, B. D.: Benign lesions of aberrant trophoblast in the lung. Obstet. Gynecol., 20: 602, 1962.

Carr, D. H.: Cytogenetics and the pathology of hydatidiform degeneration. Obstet. Gynecol., 33: 333, 1969.

Cave, W. T., and Dunn, J. T.: Choriocarcinoma with hyperthyroidism: probable identity of the thyrotropin with human chorionic gonadotropin. Ann. Intern. Med., 85: 60, 1976.

Chun, D., Braga, C., Chow, C., and Lok, L.: Clinical observations on some aspects of hydatidiform mole. J. Obstet. Gynecol. Br. Commonw., 71: 180, 1964.

Chun, D., Braga, C., Chow, C., and Lok, L.: Treatment of hydatidiform mole. J. Obstet. Gynecol. Br. Commonw., 71: 185, 1964.

Curry, S. L., et al.: Hydatidiform mole (diagnosis, management and long-term follow-up of 347 patients). Obstet. Gynecol., 45: 1, 1975.

Driscoll, S. G.: Choriocarcinoma: An "incidental finding" within a term placenta. Obstet. Gynecol., 21: 96, 1963.

Driscoll, S. G.: Gestational trophoblastic neoplasms: morphologic considerations. Hum. Pathol., 8: 529, 1977.

Goldstein, D. P., Goldstein, P. R., Bottomley, P., Osanthanondh, R., and Marean, A. R.: Methotrexate with citrovorum factor rescue for nonmetastatic gestational trophoblastic neoplasms. Obstet. Gynecol., 48: 321, 1976.

Goldstein, D. P., Winig, P., and Shirley, R. L.: Actinomycin D as initial therapy of gestational trophoblastic disease. Obstet. Gynecol., 39: 341, 1972.

Hammond, C. B., Borchert, L. G., Tyrey, L., Creasman, W. J., and Parker, R. T.: Treatment of metastatic trophoblastic disease: good and poor prognosis. Am. J. Obstet. Gynecol., 115: 451, 1973.

Hasegawa, T.: Recent trend in studies on trophoblastic neoplasia. Obstet. Gynecol., 30: 19, 1960.

Hertig, A. T.: Human trophoblast: normal and abnormal. A plea for the study of the normal so as to understand the abnormal. Am. J. Clin. Pathol., 47: 249, 1967.

Hertig, A. T., and Sheldon, W. H.: Hydatidiform mole—a pathologic-clinical correlation of 200 cases. Am. J. Obstet. Gynecol., 53: 1, 1947.

Hertz, R.: Choriocarcinoma and Related Gestational Trophoblastic Tumors in Women. Raven Press, New York, 1978.

Hertz, R., Ross, G. T., and Lipsett, M. B.: Chemotherapy in women with trophoblastic disease: choriocarcinoma, chorioadenoma destruens, and complicated hydatidiform mole. Ann. N.Y. Acad. Sci., 114: 881, 1964.

Hsu, C., Huang, L., and Chen, T.: Metastases in benign hydatidiform mole and chorioadenoma destruens. Am. J. Obstet. Gynecol., 84: 1412, 1962.

Jones, W. B.: Treatment of chorionic tumors. Clin. Obstet. Gynecol., 18: 247, 1975.

Jones, W. B. and Lewis, J. L.: Treatment of gestational trophoblastic disease. Am J. Obstet. Gynecol., 120: 14, 1974.

Kajii, T., and Ohama, K.: Androgenetic origin of hydatidiform mole. Nature, 268: 633, 1977.

Lewis, J. L., Jr.: Chemotherapy for metastatic gestational trophoblastic neoplasms. Clin. Obstet. Gynecol., 10: 330, 1967.

Lewis, J. L.: Chemotherapy and surgery in the treatment of gestational trophoblastic neoplasms. Surg. Clin. North Am., 49: 371, 1969.

Lewis, J. L., Jr., Ketcham, A. S., and Hertz, R.: Surgical intervention during chemotherapy of gestational trophoblastic disease. Cancer, *19:* 1517, 1966.

Li, M. C., Hertz, R., and Spencer, D. B.: Effect of methotrexate therapy upon choriocarcinoma and chorioadenoma. Proc. Soc. Exp. Biol. Med., *93:* 361, 1956.

Marquez-Monten, H., et al. Gestational choriocarcinoma in the General Hospital of Mexico. Cancer, *21:* 1337, 1968.

Miller, J. M., Surwit, E. A., and Hammond, C. B.: Choriocarcinoma following term pregnancy. Obstet. Gynecol., *53:* 207, 1969.

Morrow, C. P., Kletzky, O. A., DeSaia, P. J., Townsend, D. E., Mishell, D. R., and Nakamura, R. M.: Clinical and laboratory correlates of molar pregnancy and trophoblastic disease. Am. J. Obstet. Gynecol., *128:* 424, 1977.

Pai, K. N.: A study of choriocarinoma: its incidence in India and its aetiopathogenesis. *Choriocarinoma: Transactions of a Conference of the International Union Against Cancer.* p. 54. Edited by J. F. Holland and M. M. Hreshchyshyn Springer-Verlag, Berlin, 1967.

Reynolds, S. R. M.: Hydatidiform mole: a vascular congenital anomaly. Obstet. Gynecol., *47:* 244, 1976.

Ringertz, N.: Hydatidiform mole, invasive mole and choriocarcinoma in Sweden. Acta Gynecol. Scand., *49:* 195, 1970.

Saxena, B. B., Hossan, S. H., Haour, F., et al.: Radioreceptor assay of human chorionic gonadotropin. Science, *184:* 793, 1974.

Schmorl, G.: *Pathologisch-anatomische untersuching uber puerperal eclampsie.* Vogel, Leipzig, 1893.

Schreiber, J. R., Rebar, R. W., Chen, H. C., Hodgen, G. D., and

Ross, G. T.: Limitation of the specific serum radioimmunoassay for human chorionic gonadotropin in the management of trophoblastic neoplasms. Am. J. Obstet. Gynecol., *125:* 705, 1976.

Smith, J.: *Trophoblastic Disease: Diagnosis and Management. Endocrine and Nonendocrine Hormone-Producing Tumors.* Year Book Medical Publishers, Chicago, 1973.

Stevenson, A. C., Dudgeon, M. Y. and McClure, H. I.: Observations on the results of pregnancies in women residents in Belfast. II. Abortions, hydatidiform moles and ectopic pregnancies. Ann. Hum. Genet. 23: 395,1959.

Szulman, A. E., and Surti, U.: The syndromes of hydatidiform mole. I. Cytogenic and morphologic correlations. Am. J. Obstet. Gynecol., *131:* 665, 1978.

Tow, S. H.: University of Singapore, personal communication.

Vaitukaitis, J., Braunstein, G., and Ross, G.: A radioimmunoassay which specifically measures human chorionic gonadotropin in the presence of human luteinizing hormone. Am. J. Obstet. Gynecol., *113:* 751, 1972.

Van Thiel, D. H., Ross, G. T., and Lipsett, M. B.: Pregnancies after chemotherapy of trophoblastic neoplasms. Science, *169:* 132, 1970.

Vassilakos, P., Riotton, G., and Kajii, T.: Hydatidiform mole: two entities. Am. J. Obstet. Gynecol., *127:* 167, 1977.

Wei, P. Y., and Ouy ang, P. C.: Trophoblastic disease in Taiwan. Am. J. Obstet. Gynecol., *85:* 844, 1963.

Wilson, R. B., Hunter, J. S., and Dockerty, M. B.: Chorioadenoma destruens. Am. J. Obstet. Gynecol., *81:* 546, 1961.

Wu, F. Y. W.: Recurrent hydatidiform mole. Obstet. Gynecol., *41:* 200, 1973.

CHAPTER 28

Leukorrhea

Leukorrhea, the term applied to any vaginal discharge other than blood, is perhaps the most frequently encountered of gynecological symptoms. It is rarely serious, and generally is associated with simple infections of the cervix, vagina, or tube.

VULVA

Strictly speaking, vulvar secretions should not be considered in the present discussion, as the vulva is an external structure. However, vulvar secretions may contribute to the leukorrhea complained of by the patient, who cannot know the source of the discharge.

In addition to the sebaceous and sudoriferous glands in the vulva, the vulvovaginal gland, Bartholin's gland, plays the most important role in the lubrication of the vaginal introitus. It secretes a thick viscid mucus, which is increased during sexual excitement. Finally, in the periurethral region of the vestibule are situated Skene's ducts and a number of mucous crypts which, likewise, contribute to the lubrication of the vulvar structures.

In infections of Bartholin's gland, there is often a profuse purulent discharge either from the duct or from a ruptured abscess. Such discharge, or those from the periurethral structures, are apt to be interpreted by the patient as of vaginal origin. Although the most frequent cause of inflammation of the Bartholin's, Skene's, and periurethral ducts is the gonococcus, other bacterial infections can occur. Persistent or recurrent vulvovaginitis is most often due to a monilial (yeast) vaginitis. Patients with such symptoms and clinical findings should be checked for an associated diabetes.

Treatment of inflammation of the glands of the vulva should be both systemic and local. Systemic treatment is a specific antibiotic selected according to the sensitivity of the organism involved. The local treatment consists of hot sitz baths for 15 minutes 3 or 4 times a day and incision and drainage, if a fluctuant abscess has occurred. Chronically inflamed Bartholin glands frequently need to be surgically removed in a quiescent stage.

VAGINA

Although the vagina is itself devoid of glands, its surface is moistened by the secretion of the cervical glands, and to a much less extent by transudation from its own surface. Normally, the vaginal secretion is acid in reaction and is dependent upon the presence of lactic acid produced by the action of vaginal organisms, the chief among these being the large rod shaped bacillus of Döderlein, upon the glycogen content of the vaginal epithelium. The vagina undergoes constant desquamation and discharges of vaginal origin are characterized by the presence of many epithelial cells. When actual inflammation and infection of the vagina occurs, an exudate develops which is usually mucopurulent or purulent in character and associated with pruritus.

Although the usual symptomatology is a foul, smelly, irritating discharge, vaginitis can be severe enough to cause a hemorrhagic exudate which can be interpreted as metrorrhagia unless a careful examination is made.

The two most common forms of vaginitis in the mature menstruating woman are those caused by *Candida albicans* and by *trichomonas*. Yeast vaginitis, also called monilial vaginitis associated with the *C. albicans*, is characterized by a cheesy type of discharge having a sweetish odor. The vaginitis associated with the *trichomonas* infestation is characterized by a bubbly, yellowish, thin discharge sometimes having a foul odor. The diagnosis is made by microscopic examination of a saline wash from the vagina and identification of the organism. The microscopic diagnosis can be confirmed by culture on Sabouraud's media for the *C. albicans.*

Yeast vaginitis is especially prone to occur during pregnancy, in women taking oral contraception, in the diabetic patient, or after prolonged antibiotic therapy. It can be treated by an antifungicide, nystatin (Mycostatin), 500,000 units 3 times a day given with a 100,000-unit vaginal suppository every night over a 10-day period. Persistent infections can be treated by scrubbing the vagina with Zephiran to remove the colonies and then painting with 2% aqueous Gentian Violet solution. This treatment should be carried out every other day for 3 treatments only, as a chemical vaginitis can be induced due to the Gentian Violet solution if too frequent or prolonged applications are given. If recurrent yeast infections occur, a glucose tolerance test should be done to check the possibility of diabetes. The use of tight slacks or shorts, and prolonged intervals in bathing suits can cause an exacerbation of this vaginitis among women who are predisposed to monilial infections.

Trichomonas vaginitis, which must be regarded as a venereal disease, is treated by metronidazole (Flagyl) 250 mg 3 times a day for 10 days. It is advisable to prescribe a similar course of treatment for the sexual partner and request that condom protection be used during intercourse. Lang et al. have emphasized the frequency of associated trichomoniasis and candida vaginitis. It is, therefore, wise to check for both organisms when the patient returns for her final examination after completion of therapy.

Herpetic lesions of the cervix, vagina, and vulva are resistant to most treatments which are currently available. These infections are characterized by painful ulcerations with a recurrent tendency. Development of a vaccine is being attempted.

Gardnerella vaginales is the current designation of the organism once called *Haemophilus* or *Corynebacterium vaginale* and which is associated also with vaginitis. The diagnosis is made by a vaginal pH of 5.5 or above, or the microscopic identification of the "clue" or "glitter" cell, or by culture. The association

between the organism and symptomatology is not as consistent as with the organs previously described. This organism is sensitive to tetracycline and/or metronidazole (Flagyl). It is thought that anaerobic organisms may act in symbiosis with *Gardnerella* to produce the symptomatology.

Rarely one will find a **foreign body** in the vagina to account for a profuse, malodorous discharge. A forgotten tampon is by far the most common finding, although neglected pessaries are also occasionally found.

The adult vagina is resistant to the gonococcus, but that of the immature child is not, and the most common cause of **vulvovaginitis in children**, aside from a foreign body infection, is gonorrhea. The diagnosis is made by inspection and lavage to rule out the presence of a foreign body and by a Gram stain on a direct smear to identify the intracellular diplococci. The treatment is by stilbestrol vaginal suppository, 0.1 mg nightly over a period of 2 weeks. This causes maturation of the vaginal epithelium to the adult stage and makes it resistant to the gonococcal organism. It is, of course, necessary to establish the infected contacts and institute treatment both as a public health method and to avoid reinfection of the patient.

At the opposite end of the age scale, **senile vaginitis** of nonspecific origin is not uncommon. The decreased ovarian function at the menopause causes the vaginal mucosa to become atrophic and prone to secondary infection. Although usually nonspecific in type, occasionally, as in a child, it is due to the gonococcus. Tiny areas of ulceration can produce not only leukorrhea but also slight vaginal bleeding. Estrogen suppositories (stilbestrol 0.5 mg) or creams are usually curative and rarely lead to bleeding even if the uterus is still present.

CERVIX

The mucous glands of the cervix are the chief source of the secretion normally found in the vagina, and it is not strange, therefore, that they are the chief source of leukorrheal discharge. The normal secretion is a clear, viscid, alkaline mucus which varies in its amount and viscidity at different phases of the menstrual cycle, the greatest amount being at the time of ovulation.

The secretion may be merely increased in

amount without alteration in character, as a result of hyperactivity of the glands produced by hyperemic or endocrine factors. However, the histological structure of the cervix, with its numerous gland invaginations, makes it peculiarly prone to persistent infections, characterized by excessive and pathological alterations of the secretion. Cervicitis is etiologically divisible into two major groups; the gonorrheal and the nonspecific. The latter, in which puerperal lacerations often play an important causative role, is the result of infection by various organisms, chiefly of streptococcal and staphylococcal groups (see Chapter 11 under Cervicitis). The diagnosis of gonorrheal cervicitis is made by identification of the organisms from a Gram stain on a direct cervical smear. It can be suspected when a foul smelling, copious, purulent discharge has developed rapidly in the absence of a pregnancy or cervical neoplasm. The treatment is as outlined in Chapter 11 under Cervicitis and consists of specific antibiotic therapy and the usual public health measures necessary for such a communicable disease. A serological test for syphilis is indicated.

A syphilitic chancre of the cervix is only a cause of leukorrhea when secondary infection occurs and must be differentiated from a nonspecific ulceration, an herpetic lesion, or a tuberculous granuloma. An examination of a wet smear under dark-field illumination will demonstrate the spirochetes in a syphilitic chancre while a biopsy of the lesion will show giant cells and tuberculous bacilli in a tuberculous granuloma. The treatment for either of these is, of course, specific.

The treatment of nonspecific cervicitis should also be directed towards the systemic treatment of the infection and local eradication of the infected area. Specific antibiotic therapy, both orally and supplied locally, is given in conjunction with hot douches 15 minutes, two or three times a day for 2 weeks, followed by a cauterization of the lesion if it is on the portio. For more extensive involvement of the cervix, radial cauterization or cryosurgery may be indicated. Such procedures should be followed by cervical dilatation to avoid cervical stenosis.

UTERINE BODY

Although the endometrium contains innumerable glands, these are inactive until the postovulatory phases of the cycle, and even then the secretion adds little to the secretory content of the lower genital canal. However, a certain amount of serous transudation undoubtedly occurs, and this may at times be increased in amount as a result of vascular or endocrine factors or neoplasia.

Endometritis is of little importance as a cause of leukorrhea. An exception to this is the occasional case of acute septic endometritis, in which a profuse purulent discharge may be present associated with retention of placental tissue. Pyometra with cervical stenosis is also associated with a profuse, foul discharge in the postmenopausal patient.

Finally, uterine polyps, submucous myomas, carcinomas, and other tumors are not infrequently the cause of uterine discharges, particularly when complicated by infection and necrosis. A most unusual cause of copious vaginal discharge is lymphorrhea associated with anomalies and obstruction of the lymphatic ducts. This can only be cured by surgical correction of the defect and has been described by Martorell as chylous metrorrhea.

The treatment of all causes of leukorrhea, originating in the uterine body, is directed towards removal of the etiological factor associated with specific antibiotic therapy.

TUBES

Although rare, leukorrhea of tubal origin may occur, the usual example being that of the so-called profluent salpingitis (hydrosalpinx profluens), in which a hydrosalpinx may periodically expel its content through a partially patent inner orifice into the uterus and thus cause gushes of watery fluid from the vagina. In most cases of hydrosalpinx, however, the uterine end of the tubal lumen is completely closed, so that the above mentioned mechanism must be extremely uncommon.

References and Additional Readings

Anderson, F. D., Ushijima, R. N., and Larson, C. L.: Recurrent herpes genitalis; treatment with Myobacterium bovis (BCG). Obstet. Gynecol., 43: 797, 1974.

Balsdon, M. J., Taylor, G. E., Pead, L., and Maskell, R.: Cornebacterium vaginale and vaginitis: a controlled trial of treatment. Lancet 1: 501, 1980.

Brewer, J. I., Halpern, B., and Thomas, G.: Hemophilus vaginalis vaginitis. Am. J. Obstet. Gynecol., 74: 834, 1957.

Forster, S. A., Raminez, O. G., and Rapaport, A. H.: Metronidazole and trichomonal vaginitis. Am. J. Obstet. Gynecol., 87: 1013, 1963.

Gardner, H. L., Dampeer, T. K., and Dukes, C. D.: The prevalence of vaginitis. Am. J. Obstet. Gynecol., *73:* 1080, 1957.

Gray, M. S.: Trichomonas vaginalis in pregnancy: results of metronidazole therapy on mother and child. J. Obstet. Gynaecol. Br. Common., *68:* 723, 1961.

Henricksen, E.: Pyometra associated with benign lesions of the cervix and corpus. West. J. Surg., *60:* 305, 1952.

Henricksen, E.: Pyometra associated with malignant lesions of the cervix and uterus. Am. J. Obstet. Gynecol., *72:* 884, 1956.

Hesseltine, H. C.: Vulval and vaginal mycosis and trichomoniasis. Am. J. Obstet. Gynecol., *40:* 641, 1940.

Johnson, D. G.: Infections of the cervix. Clin. Obstet. Gynecol., *2:* 476, 1959.

Kauraniemi, T.: Gynecological health screening by means of questionnaire and cytology. Acta Obstet. Gynecol. Scand., *48:* Supp. 4, 1969.

Lang, W. R.: Genital infections in female children. Clin. Obstet. Gynecol., *2:* 428, 1959.

Lang, W. R.: Premenarchal vaginitis. Obstet. Gynecol., *13:* 723, 1959.

Lang, W. R., Fritz, M. A., and Menduke, H.: The bacteriological diagnosis of trichomonal candidal and combined infections. Obstet. Gynecol., *20:* 788, 1962.

Liston, W. G., and Cruickshank, L. G.: Etiology and pathogenesis of leucorrhea in pregnancy; study of 200 cases. J. Obstet. Gynaecol. Br. Common., *47:* 109, 1940.

Martorell, F.: Chylus metrorrhea. Vasc. Dis., *1:* 160, 1964.

McCoogan, L. S.: The treatment of vaginitis. Clin. Obstet. Gynecol., *2:* 450, 1959.

Reich, W. J., Nechtow, M. J., Zaworsky, B., and Adams, A. P.: Investigation and management of the patient with vaginal discharge. Clin. Obstet. Gynecol. *2:* 441, 1959.

Watt, L., and Jennison, R. F.: Metronidazole treatment of trichomoniasis in the female. Br. Med. J., *1:* 276, 1962.

CHAPTER 29

Infertility, Recurrent and Spontaneous Abortion

INFERTILITY

Definitions

Sterility is a term which can correctly be applied only to an individual who has some absolute factor preventing procreation with the implication that the condition is irreversible. **Infertility** is the inability to achieve pregnancy within a stipulated period of time, usually 1 year.

Primary infertility is a term used to designate those patients who have never conceived, whereas **secondary infertility** indicates that the patient has had a pregnancy. In this country, about one in every seven marriages, or 15% of couples, are involuntarily infertile. Not only is the problem of some magnitude, but the widespread use of effective contraception and the increasing utilization of abortion to limit unwanted pregnancies have resulted in fewer and fewer babies being available for adoption. Thus, there is increased interest in and need for improved diagnosis and management of both male and female infertility.

Medical Considerations

Medically, infertility is a unique condition in that two individuals must be considered. As the husband or wife, or both, may have factors contributing to the condition, both must cooperate in the investigation.

The Goals of an Infertility Evaluation

The goals of an infertility evaluation are to establish the diagnosis and to give a prognosis for future fertility. Ordinarily, only 50-60% of couples initiating an infertility evaluation will ultimately achieve fertility. However these statistics may be improved by careful attention to an etiologic diagnosis, as appropriate management can only be undertaken if the reason for infertility has been established. Once the diagnosis is made, then a discussion of alternative methods of therapy, and the statistical prognosis for pregnancy, can be undertaken. The goal of establishing a diagnosis is realistic for both physician and patient: certain patients will not follow through with essential studies or diagnostic procedures, or with therapy designed to treat the discovered etiology; these patients can be informed how much a particular study would contribute to the overall diagnosis, or how much a particular therapy might statistically benefit the prognosis. An infertility evaluation is, after all, entirely elective. No matter how organized, efficient, and thorough the approach to diagnosis, only if the patient understands the goals of the evaluation will a satisfactory result be achieved.

Three major areas must be considered in establishing the diagnosis and prognosis. These include (1) the age of the wife; (2) the duration of pregnancy exposure; and (3) the medical factor etiologically responsible.

Fertility in women declines after the age of 35 years. Pregnancy is rare after the age of 45 years and the maximal age for successful pregnancy is about 52 years, with only 1 out of more than 60,000 births occurring past the age of 50.

The duration of pregnancy exposure dictates when to initiate an evaluation for infertility and also gives some indication of the prognosis for fertility. Approximately 25% of women will be pregnant the 1st month of unprotected intercourse, 63% in 6 months, 75% in 9 months, 80–90% in a year, and only an additional 3–5% will achieve pregnancy in the next 6 months of exposure. Increased coital frequency may increase the percentage of couples achieving pregnancy: 83% of couples having intercourse four or more times a week were pregnant in under 6 months of exposure, whereas only 16% of couples having intercourse less than once a week conceived. Importantly, one year of unprotected intercourse without pregnancy is sufficient for an evaluation to be undertaken, as a normal couple should have conceived and an abnormality will likely be found.

Thus, both the age of the wife, and the duration of the infertility are prognostic indicators of the seriousness of the problem. Establishing the medical factor responsible is the major area of concern. This is accomplished through history, physical, and pelvic examination. In the initial interview, the development of the rapport necessary to ensure the couple's open cooperation with the investigator is of primary importance.

The Initial Interview

Investigation of the infertile couple begins with a careful history and physical examination to exclude major medical or gynecological conditions. A proper history explores the age of the couple, the duration of the marriage, previous reproductive histories of both partners, and the results of any previous studies. A past and present medical history is essential: the search for significant disease, chronic drug use, or exposure to toxins is important; normality of function of the reproductive organs must be established. The taking of such a history is time consuming, and requires a candid account of the sexual and behavioral interactions of the couple. It is appropriate to interview the wife first alone, as some confidential details may not be revealed in the presence of the partner. These relate to premarital relations or pregnancies and history of venereal disease.

Socioeconomic factors, may be of practical importance, because of the expense and considerable inconvenience of an infertility evaluation.

Religion also may be a consideration in an infertility evaluation. Clerical dispensation may be requested for a Catholic male to

obtain a semen specimen; the Orthodox Jewish woman who ovulates during the time of prescribed abstinence following menstruation can be treated by delaying ovulation with estrogens.

The physical examination seeks clues related to ovarian or hormonal dysfunction and physical or mechanical problems within the pelvis. The pelvic examination establishes the normality of the reproductive organs insofar as possible with bimanual examination and a Pap smear. The cervix may show evidence of infection, prior cryosurgery, or lacerations; the bimanual examination should seek nodularity, tenderness or thickening of the uterosacral ligaments, and scarred areas in the posterior cul-de-sac. Prior pelvic inflammatory disease is suggested by the finding of thickened adnexal areas or lack of uterine mobility.

Although an etiologic diagnosis may be impossible at the first visit, a tentative explanation is appropriate if there are suggestive factors in the history or physical examination, as these observations focus attention on important details during the subsequent examinations and tests. Involving both partners, it is wise to discuss goals and expectations, the need for a complete investigation, the time and expense involved, the statistical probability of help, and the prognostic value of the investigation. The couple should be advised that if treatment seems indicated, a year should elapse to evaluate the benefit of therapy. Educating a couple about the evaluation, the tests, and procedures is a function of the initial visit, and a definite investigative plan, with a predictable end point, should be outlined at this time. A routine screening infertility evaluation can be completed with an additional three or four office visits, and a "wait and see" attitude can only be condemned. The couple must be provided with sufficient information to make intelligent choices of alternatives and their questions, as well as their anxieties and concerns, must be conscientiously addressed.

Fundamental Areas of Investigation

The diagnosis and prognosis in infertility are established by investigating the age of the wife, the duration of the infertility, and the medical factor responsible. Ninety-five percent of couples will be found to have a reason for infertility in one or more of six clearly defined areas. Since two or more factors may be operative in fully 35% of all infertility cases, it is essential that both partners and all areas be thoroughly evaluated.

The six major factors of importance in fertilization and implantation of an ovum are:

1. Central, or ovulatory, factor—involving the physical act of ovulation and release of a mature oocyte;
2. Male factor—involving adequate production of normal sperm;
3. Mucus or cervical factor—involving the presence of adequate cervical mucus which can act as a transport medium and repository for sperm;
4. Endometrial/uterine factor—involving the development of the endometrial implantation site, which is dependent on ovarian endocrine function, and uterine end organ normality and response;
5. Tubal factor—involving patency of tubes allowing transport of sperm and oocyte; and
6. Peritoneal factor—involving the absence of any physical or mechanical barrier to fertility within the peritoneal cavity.

Less important ancillary factors might be considered. For example, in stubborn or unexplained cases of infertility indicated studies might include an evaluation of thyroid function, a glucose tolerance test, and a 17-ketosteroid assay or measure of circulating androgens to detect metabolic disease processes. Hyperprolactinemia can be associated with regular menses but luteal phase inadequacy is common. A cervical mucus culture for mycoplasma might be obtained. Under rare circumstances, psychiatric or psychologic counseling may be indicated. The blood grouping of husband and wife may have some significance, as blood group incompatibilities may suggest an immunologic basis for infertility or that a sperm-mucus incompatibility may exist.

The prognosis for the "normal infertile couple" is dismal, necessitating a diligent search for the factor causing infertility. The 10–20% incidence of unexplained infertility quoted in earlier studies is far too high, probably because of increased utilization of pelvic endoscopy for diagnostic purposes. Thus, most success in the diagnosis and management of infertility is achieved if an etiologic

reason for the infertility is found. If therapy is based on the discovered etiology, prognosis for future fertility can be made for the couple.

The Infertility Evaluation

Central or Ovulatory Factor

Using strict criteria, ovulation refers to the physical act of rupture of the follicle with extrusion of the oocyte. Definite evidence of ovulation is afforded only by diagnosing a pregnancy, or by capture of the oocyte from within the tubal or uterine lumen. Thus, when we speak of diagnosing ovulation, we are making a presumptive diagnosis which depends upon the direct or indirect measurement of progesterone or observation of its effects at other sites in the body.

A definite diagnosis of ovulation is difficult but, from a practical standpoint, any woman who is having regular menstrual cycles at 30 ± 2-day intervals can be assumed to be ovulating. Regular periods, especially if accompanied by premenstrual molimina including headaches, breast tenderness, weight gain, bloating, fatigue and/or irritability, indicate ovulatory rather than anovulatory cycles. Progesterone effects can be observed by **serial** evaluation of the cervical mucus or vaginal cytology, recording of a biphasic temperature chart, secretory endometrial histology, measurement of the urinary pregnanediol, or assay of serial plasma progesterone. These observations reflect corpus luteum function and do not necessarily mean that the physical act of ovulation has occurred.

Although we recognize the fallibility of relying upon presumptive criteria of ovulation, the clinical usefulness of these methods cannot be denied. The most helpful change observed is that of the cervical mucus under the influence of estrogen: the mucus increases in amount in the periovulatory part of the cycle; under the influence of progesterone in the luteal phase, the mucus decreases in amount, changes in character, and no longer dries in a ferning pattern (Fig. 29.1).

The basal body temperature chart is a clinically useful tool, but the real purpose of keeping a chart is not to establish that ovulation is occurring, which the chart cannot do, but rather to aid in the scheduling and interpretation of infertility studies (Fig. 29.2). Such entities as follicular shortening or late ovulation, and luteal shortening or delay, can

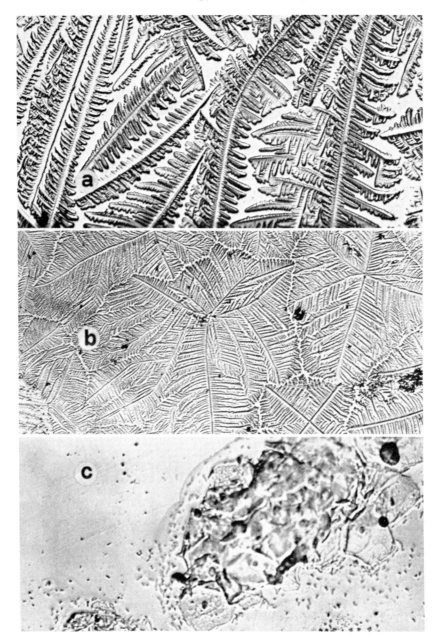

Figure 29.1. Presumptive ovulation determined by cervical mucus changes. Ovulation occurs at the time when fern formation is strongly positive (*a* and *b*); when progesterone is present the mucus shows a negative reaction or only a slight fern pattern (*c*).

be observed. Importantly, proper timing for Huhner tests and endometrial biopsies can be decided, and pregnancy easily diagnosed early. If the patient understands that the temperature chart is to be used for scheduling and interpretation and not to time intercourse, the anxiety-provoking aspects of keeping the chart are greatly lessened.

The patient should be asked to record her daily basal temperature orally, at the same time each morning, before any activity. The chart can be used as a diary of events, and such things as alcohol consumption, sickness, intercourse, and bleeding or cramping can be recorded.

Methods to detect ovulation which depend

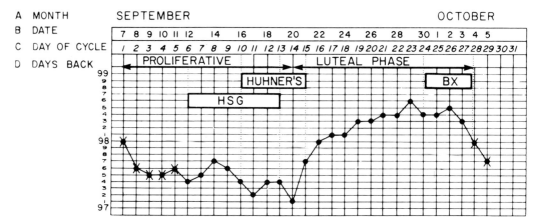

Figure 29.2. Typical ovulatory basal temperature record, showing the appropriate times during the cycle for the performance of tests to evalute fertility potential.

upon complicated hormone analyses are too expensive and too time-consuming to be clinically applicable.

Although the hormonal changes are reflected by a change in the endometrial histology from a proliferative to a secretory pattern, the endometrial biopsy should not be used to make the diagnosis of presumptive ovulation; rather, a carefully timed, late luteal specimen is used to establish luteal phase adequacy, as described later.

Treatment of Anovulation

The etiology of ovulation defects will be discussed in detail in Chapter 30, Amenorrhea, and will be simply itemized here:
1. Central Nervous System Factors: tumors or scars, heritable defects of the hypothalamus, psychogenic factors, drug-induced (oral contraceptives, phenothiazines) pituitary dysfunction, tumors or destructive lesions
2. Intermediate Factors: nutritional, chronic illness, metabolic disease including endocrine, renal, or hepatic disease
3. Gonadal Factors: premature ovarian failure, ovarian tumors, or destructive lesions including autoimmune disease of the ovary

The effective treatment of anovulation depends upon its etiology; any specific factor diagnosed may have an indicated treatment, for instance, diet, thyroid medication, or adrenal suppression. Pituitary insufficiency or neurogenic disturbances causing inadequate pituitary stimulation are satisfactorily managed with hormones extracted from meno-

pausal urine or isolated from pituitary glands. Cyclic estrogen followed by a progestational agent is more often contraceptive and antiovulatory although regular periods result. The most useful drug to treat anovulatory infertility is the antiestrogen, clomiphene citrate, which can correct dysfunction of feedback control mechanisms in patients with an intact pituitary gland and normal ovaries.

A discussion of ovulation induction is detailed in Chapter 30. A major point to be emphasized here is that clomiphene citrate, used in conjunction with hCG, will result in a cumulative 95% probability of ovulation. The addition of human menopausal gonadotropins or pituitary gonadotropins to the treatment armamentarium increases the probability of ovulation induction to 99.9%. Treatment of an ovulatory or central factor is highly satisfactory with a high incidence of ovulation and a cumulative 60–65% pregnancy rate. However, a diagnosis of why a patient is anovulatory or irregularly ovulatory should first be made and other fertility factors investigated if an appropriate result is to be obtained.

Male Factor

Initial Assessment

The sperm count is essential in the evaluation of an infertile couple and provides different information from that obtained from a postcoital test. Seventy-two to eighty-four days are required for completion of spermatogenesis, so subsequent samples should not be collected too frequently. The quantitative measurements obtained from the sperm count, including volume, count/ml and total count, percentage of normal and abnormal forms, and percentage of motility, are helpful indicators of fertility and may dictate areas requiring further evaluation of the male partner. The conditions under which the specimen is obtained should be carefully controlled to avoid errors of interpretation.

Semen samples should be collected after a period of abstinence in accord with the usual intercourse habits of the couple. It is of no clinical use to analyze a semen specimen after 3 days of abstinence when a couple has intercourse daily, or after 3 days when a couple has intercourse only once a month. Clear, written instructions concerning the collection of the seminal ejaculate should be provided for the patient. The semen is best obtained by induced ejaculation or by intercourse with withdrawal; a rubber condom must not be used because it contains substances that kill the spermatozoa but a clean wide mouth jar is adequate.

A total ejaculate must be obtained, as any loss may seriously influence the sperm count and concentration. The sample should arrive in the laboratory within 1 hour, marked with the time of collection and the date of the previous intercourse. Liquefaction of seminal fluid should occur at room temperature within 20 minutes, and failure of liquefaction may indicate a lack of proteolytic enzyme and makes evaluation of the sample difficult. Heat to body temperatures is deleterious.

Complete mixing of the specimen is essential before examination. Details of the seminal analysis are beyond the scope of this chapter; however, the sperm count should be obtained in a diluted well mixed semen specimen and counted after transfer to a standard hemocytometer chamber. The quality of the semen is judged by the numbers per milliliter, the percentage and type of abnormal forms, and the motility. Spermatozoa morphology is characterized after one of several types of staining procedures and the morphologic rating should include a count of spermatozoa that appear normal; those with abnormal heads that are either too large, too small, tapering, or amorphous; those with abnormal neck pieces; and those with tail defects. Motility should be assessed under constant temperature conditions, and both motile and immotile cells should be counted. Motility should be recorded over at least 4 hours, and

if motility falls off rapidly over 2–3 hours, a further semen sample should be analyzed, with observation every half hour.

The total volume, pH, and viscosity are also of some importance. A large volume of ejaculate may produce a low sperm concentration. More than the normal 2–5 leukocytes per high power field may suggest prostatitis or another significant infection.

Although absolute criteria of male fertility cannot be obtained with these crude methods of evaluation, the following standards may be considered as representative of the usual fertile male.

Count per milliliter
   normal fertile   above 30,000,000
   subfertile   between 20–30,000,000
   infertile   less than 10,000,000
Volume: 2.5 ml
Motility: 60% motile within 4 hours of
   collection; higher motility suggests
   higher fertility
Differential: less than 25% abnormal forms

The survival time of sperm in the human female genital tract is at least 96 hours, and 10 days may not be improbable. Sperm can fertilize for 24 up to probably 48 hours, indicating that intercourse every 2–3 days is sufficient for constant exposure to pregnancy.

After ejaculation, spermatozoa must undergo a capacitation process, which occurs in the female reproductive tract. Acrosin allows the spermatozoa to penetrate the zona, and inhibitors to acrosin prevent fertilization. At the time of ejaculation, most acrosin is present in the form of an inactive precursor, proacrosin, and becomes the active form, acrosin, during the capacitation process.

Seminal Insufficiency

Semen analysis gives information about the quantity and quality of the spermatozoa and the secretory function of the accessory genital glands. Seminal insufficiency can be due to either a defect in spermatogenesis or in sperm maturation or to an abnormality in the components or constituents of the seminal ejaculate.

The seminal plasma is a composite mixture of secretions from the various accessory genital glands. The chemical composition of the seminal plasma is strikingly different from that of any other body fluid, and the biochemistry of the seminal plasma may affect the fertilizing capacity of the spermatozoa. The pH of the seminal plasma is important, as prostatic fluid is acid and inhibitory to sperm, and the vesicular secretion is alkaline; the pH of normal semen, 7.2–7.8, may reflect the relative proportions between these two secretions. The volume of the seminal ejaculate is dependent on the proportion of secretion coming from one or another of the contributing glands. Therefore, a low-volume, highly acidic ejaculate may reflect a decreased function of the seminal vesicle. The chemical composition can also be analyzed for acid phosphatase, which originates mainly from the prostate or for fructose and prostaglandins, which are specific secretory products of the human seminal vesicles. A change in prostaglandin content in the seminal ejaculate may suggest dysfunction of the seminal vesicles and have a prognostic value in determining fertilizing capacity. Most patients with a low volume ejaculate have low fructose levels, suggestive of dysfunction of the seminal vesicles, possibly due to vesiculitis. The presence of fructose in the seminal ejaculate is evidence for patency of the ejaculatory ducts and eliminates obstruction as a cause of azospermia.

Constitutional factors such as nutritional problems, acute or chronic illness, general metabolic disease, specific poisonings or occupational exposures, competitive exercise, central defects occurring in the hypothalamic pituitary axis, genital tract infections causing blockage of the vas, or congenital defects of testicular development such as Klinefelter's syndrome will first be suggested by abnormalities in the seminal analysis. A varicocele can be responsible for abnormalities of the major parameters, decreasing sperm count and motility, and increasing the percentage of abnormal forms. A drug history is helpful as phenothiazines can cause retrograde ejaculation, furadantin may cause necrospermia, and colchicine has been reported to cause transient inhibition of spermatogenesis and even azospermia.

Evaluation of the Infertile Male

In the evaluation of male infertility, the history, physical examination, and evaluation of at least two sperm specimens is important. The husband ordinarily should be examined by a urologist interested in male infertility, and the history should explore all facets of reproductive function. The physical examination should include a careful scrotal palpation, including an evaluation for varicocele performed in the upright position with the subject performing a Valsalva maneuver. A careful seminal evaluation is performed and, if oligospermia or some other form of abnormality is diagnosed on at least two specimens, then a laboratory evaluation must be undertaken.

Evaluation of the oligospermic male begins with a measurement of serum FSH and LH, testosterone, and possibly prolactin. One helpful scheme involves segregation into pregerminal, germinal, and postgerminal pathologic categories. Azospermic male subjects with normal serum FSH levels can be anticipated to demonstrate an anatomic obstruction of the reproductive tract, classified as postgerminal hypofertility. Contrast vasography should confirm the preoperative diagnosis and may define an obstructed area suitable for repair. Testicular biopsy should be performed, and should demonstrate no abnormality for these patients to be appropriate candidates for surgical reconstruction. Primary germinal hypofertility can be suspected when the patient is either azospermic or oligospermic and the serum FSH level is elevated beyond the normal range. Exogenous hormonal stimulation is rarely effective. Increased FSH levels suggest tubular damage, and enhanced spermatogenesis is unlikely. No drug or hormone treatment has been developed to manage the patient with elevated FSH levels. Oligospermic male subjects with normal FSH levels have pregerminal hypofertility, a better prognosis following hormonal stimulation, and are optimum candidates for pharmacologic management utilizing either gonadotropin stimulation, LRH, or testosterone.

Unfortunately, in spite of concerted efforts to make an etiologic diagnosis in males, the most frequent finding is idiopathic oligospermia with spermatogenic arrest of undetermined etiology. Attempts are being made to correlate the arrest patterns with the clinical course and response to clinical therapy, but at present the results have been disappointing.

Treatment is targeted toward the specific diagnosis and the choice depends upon the findings. Low-dose testosterone has been utilized to increase sperm motility, especially when sperm counts are relatively normal, and the percentage of abnormal forms is relatively low. Impotence and psychosexual difficulties are certainly approachable but require the services of a competent sex therapist. The surgical approach to therapy of a varicocele is reported to improve the characteristics of the seminal ejaculate in well over 50% of patients so treated. Since 40% of male infertility may be due to a varicocele, and ligation may offer some benefit, a varicocele is a significant finding.

Some suggestions can be made in the office setting to improve the characteristics of the ejaculate. General hygiene is important, with limitation of smoking and excessive alcohol intake, attention to diet, adequate rest, relief of emotional tension, and treatment of any chronic illness or metabolic disease. Because heat damages testicular function, underwear which holds the testicles in contact with the body may be injurious, as are excessively hot, prolonged tub or steam baths. Specific hormone therapy occasionally has been successful. It has been estimated that only 10% of men with idiopathic oligospermia will be improved; compared to the 50% improvement shown with therapy of a varicocele, the importance of making this diagnosis is emphasized.

Techniques of Insemination

Homologous Artificial Insemination (AIH). Homologous artificial insemination is of demonstrable value when potentially normal semen does not reach the cervix, ordinarily because of some local or anatomical problem, or rarely in a psychological setting of impotence or vaginismus. In the unusual case in which hypospadias is present so that deposition of spermatozoa on the cervix is inadequate, or in which a spinal cord injury has occurred, semen may be obtained mechanically and artificial insemination attempted. Any means of delivering semen to the cervix is likely to prove successful, and the method should be one that the couple can use themselves at home. In cases of retrograde ejaculation, seen after transurethral prostatectomy, in diabetes or sometimes during phenothiazine (Thorazine, Mellaril) treatment, catheterization of the bladder or postcoital voiding can result in the recovery of motile spermatozoa; ordinarily centrifugation and alkalinization of the urine or the recovered specimen are done, with the insemination of the sediment.

Homologous artificial insemination is less useful in the presence of oligospermia and, in fact, probably offers no benefit for the couple with this problem.

A more concentrated semen sample can be obtained by collection of a split ejaculate. Since the first portion of the ejaculate usually contains the majority of sperm, this offers a simple method of concentrating specimens with total counts between 20,000,000 and 60,000,000 sperm; when followed by cervical insemination, some improvement in fertility rate has been reported. Moghissi et al. found a 21.6% pregnancy rate using the split ejaculate, but 50% of these pregnancies aborted, suggesting the pregnancy wastage might be due to male factors. Other means of mechanical concentration are centrifugation of the ejaculate or the use of a millipore filter. Pooling of multiple samples of frozen semen, and subsequent concentration, is possible where sperm banks are available; however, in normal semen, only 25–50% of the sperm may be motile when unthawed. Unfortunately, sperm from infertile men are more easily damaged by freezing process and no motile sperm may be recoverable.

Donor Artificial Insemination (AID). The procedure of donor artificial insemination is a satisfactory solution for the right couple. The entire subject of artificial insemination in the human is very adequately treated in the review by Beck.

In addition to repeated interviews with the couple, there are several rules of thumb which should be followed. (1) The husband must have been aware of his inadequacy for at least a year prior to the first serious consideration of the planning of insemination. (2) The physician must be convinced that the husband is taking the initiative and not being pushed by an overaggressive and overanxious wife. (3) There must be no religious background in either partner which would suggest that either might harbor moral scruples about the procedure. (4) Every possible medical investigation and aid must have been employed to diagnose and treat the cause of the male infertility. (5) A basal temperature chart and Rubin's test or hysterosalpingography (HSG) should indicate normal fertility in the female.

The couple should be informed that pregnancy is unlikely to occur immediately: at least 3 months, and probably more, should be anticipated, especially if frozen sperm are used. A cumulative 70% success rate has been reported although most authors achieve closer to 50–60%. Of those women who do achieve pregnancy, 50% have done so within 3 months and 90% within 6 months.

Some couples want the husband's sperm to be mixed with that of the donor, but this is complicated by the occurrence of sperm agglutination in some specimens. Intrauterine insemination of raw semen should probably never be performed because of the risk of infection, severe cramping, and low rates of success. In women with regular menstrual cycles, our figures indicate that a single insemination is as satisfactory as repeated inseminations, and this observation is substantiated by Kleegman.

The selection of a donor is, of course, of utmost importance. He should be of proven fertility, healthy, physically fit, emotionally stable, intelligent, and free of any family history of congenital hereditary defects. He should resemble the patient's husband in somatic type, skin, and hair and eye color, and his blood type should be compatible with the wife. He should have no history of venereal disease, have a negative culture for gonorrhea, and a negative Tay-Sachs test if Jewish.

Cervical Factor

The examination of the cervical mucus with reference to the amount, quality, and presence or absence of infection should be made at the first office visit. The quality of mucus is judged by the viscosity and spinnbarkeit (ability to spin a thread), as well as by the number of epithelial cells and bacteria and crystallization. A good estrogenic mucus, in the pre- and periovulatory phase, is watery, copious, and clear; is acellular; has excellent spinnbarkeit (8 cm or longer); and supports progressive motility of sperm. When the mucus is dried, ferning patterns may be seen. In the luteal phase, under progesterone influence and in the postmenstrual phase, when estrogen levels are low, the mucus is scanty, thick, cloudy, highly cellular, does not support sperm penetration, and does not exhibit ferning when dried. The changes in the mucus throughout the menstrual cycle have been described by Moghissi et al., and techniques

of mucus collection and interpretation of sperm-mucus tests have been discussed by Davajan.

A postcoital examination (The Sims-Huhner test) should be scheduled at the periovulatory phase, when the cervical mucus is well estrogenized. The patient is requested to have intercourse within 12–24 hours of her visit. It is better not to make an issue of this as some husbands do not do well with command performances and the wife might rather call for her appointment when prepared. To make this test interpretable and repeatable, the last menstrual period, date of previous intercourse, hour of the last intercourse, and hour of the examination must be recorded. Davajan and Kunitake have described a simple method for aspirating and investigating cervical mucus. A satisfactory alternative collection device is a tuberculin syringe (without needle), as described by Moghissi et al. The amount of mucus is measured and the quality and presence or absence of infection are recorded, as well as the number of actively progressive sperm per high power field and those with poor or no activity.

A successful Sims-Huhner (S-H) test implies (1) satisfactory intercourse techniques, (2) normal mucus for the transport and preservation of sperm, and (3) adequate ovarian estrogenic function, as well as (4) at least the possibility of normal male fertility. This test, however, does not substitute for a semen analysis but merely complements it. A negative S-H test has little clinical value and must be repeated, but recurrent unsuccessful tests are probably significant and may result from a variety of causes.

The causes of abnormal postcoital tests include anatomical defects of which cervical stenosis is most common. Conization of the cervix is a common cause of cervical stenosis, but congenital stenosis is an infrequent finding The diagnosis is made by history and examination, and the attempt to pass a small probe through the endocervical canal is met with resistence. The usual reason for this difficulty is failure to straighten the canal, so the diagnosis must be made with caution.

Abnormal cervical mucus is a more common finding and can include problems with quantity and quality. An inadequate quantity of cervical mucus is ordinarily due to destruction of the endocervical glands and may be treated with low dose estrogen to increase the amount of mucus. An abnormal mucus quality usually implies an **infected mucus.** Occasionally a specific vaginitis, e.g., *Candida krusei,* can secondarily infect the cervical mucus, and it is worthwhile to culture the mucus in such cases. The pH of the mucus may be tested, and should be relatively alkaline; treatment with alkaline vaginal douches may be utilized, although there are few statistically significant studies reporting improved results.

Abnormal S-H tests may also occur in the presence of **normal cervical mucus.** The differential diagnosis includes faulty coital technique, oligospermia or lack of semen volume, some type of vaginal factor, or possibly sperm immobilization or poor mucus penetration; this could be due to specific sperm defect, such as failure of normal capacitation or to a sperm-mucus incompatibility.

Faulty coital technique is ordinarily signaled by the failure to observe *any* sperm in the cervical mucus despite a history of ejaculation, and a reasonable sperm count. The diagnosis can be made by performing AIH and looking for sperm in the mucus later that day. Oligospermia is ordinarily associated with fewer-than-normal sperm within the cervical mucus, although usually these exhibit normal progressive motility. The technique of utilizing a split ejaculate and cup insemination may be appropriate with oligospermic males. Occasionally, when penetration tests are used, the inability of the sperm to penetrate the cervical mucus is observed. Although frequently due to a thick hostile mucus, this may suggest a defect in the sperm motility. Crossmatch testing, using both mucus and sperm from donors, may isolate the cause: if neither donor nor husband sperm penetrate the wife's cervical mucus, as observed under the microscope, the problem may be one intrinsic to the mucus.

The existence of **antisperm antibodies** in the cervical mucus is difficult to diagnose. Evidence of agglutinating antibody has been reported in infertile women, but may be nonspecific, also having been isolated from the mucus of both pregnant women and women of proven fertility. Sperm-agglutinating activity in the cervical mucus can therefore be a relatively nonselective and nonspecific finding, but may be responsible for some types of infertility. Of more significance appears to be the finding of immobilization antibodies. These appear to be either IgG or IgM anti-

bodies, and the antigens responsible appear to be sperm-coating antigens, as well as those found in acrosome and the midpiece. Sperm immobilization antibodies are complement-dependent, and there is a 9% correlation with female infertility. The Isojima sperm immobilization test seems clinically reliable, and its sensitivity has been increased by using washed spermatozoa and an adequate amount of complement. The major difficulty with interpreting any test of cervical mucus antibody content is the so-called "background noise," which refers to the detection of nonspecific agglutinating and immobilizing factors. Local antibody effects can appear to be associated with male and female infertility but are relatively difficult to detect. Secretory IgA is a local antibody, which is capable of embryo toxicity; it may cause sperm immobilization, and possibly prevent sperm penetration of the ovum, interfere with ovum or zygote transport, interfere with the acrosomal enzymes, prevent adherence of the ovum to the implantation site, and interfere with embryonic development. Finally, sperm antibodies can be demonstrated in blood serum, as detected by two quite different methods: the Kibrick method (gelatin agglutination test), and the Franklin-Dukes method, a tube-slide agglutination test. The immunologic story is still in its developmental phase, and is moving ahead slowly.

Potential forms of therapy for immunologic problems include the use of condom contraception, which is probably justified for up to 3 months if follow-up titers are performed on serum and cervical mucus by a competent laboratory. Antibodies are formed within the reproductive tract to infection by *Escherichia coli,* and these antibodies have been shown to cross-react with sperm. Condom contraception can reduce exposure to these *E. coli* antibodies. Corticoid administration has been shown to be without value in the female, although in the male it may have some utility.

In vitro tests of sperm mucus interaction include the capillary tube testing systems and the slide tests. The Kremer test involves the use of a capillary tube containing cervical mucus introduced into a reservoir containing semen, with observation of the penetration of sperm into the cervical mucus over time. This is a simple and very helpful test but requires reasonable care to prevent the introduction of the air bubbles into the capillary tube and careful focusing with the microscope to scan the entire thickness of the tube. Additionally, temperature should be controlled, but the test is relatively easy to perform, and can be reproduced.

Slide tests are of more practical importance for the clinician. The seminal ejaculate and the cervical mucus are immiscible liquids like oil and water, and therefore will not readily mix when placed in contiguity on a glass slide. The formation of phalanges of sperm penetrating the mucus can be observed under the microscope and the ability of the sperm to penetrate and evidence of immobilization can be detected. The method is not quantitatible, is difficult to reproduce, and can give misleading results; however, using slide tests in a so-called sperm-mucus crossmatch, with sperm from both the husband and a donor and mucus from both the wife and a donor can give valuable guidelines to clinical management. For instance, results of such clinical testing in the office can dictate whether extensive testing for serum or mucus antibodies would be important.

Endometrial-Uterine Factor

A study of the premenstrual endometrium gives information about the implantation site for the fertilized ovum and the ovarian luteal function as well as presumptive evidence concerning ovulation. In anovulatory patients endometrial hyperplasia due to a continuous estrogen stimulation should be identified and treated before ovulation induction is attempted.

The endometrial biopsy, taken with a Novak curette, should be obtained from high in the fundus and timed, according to the menstrual history and the basal temperature chart, to be within 2–3 days of menstruation. The histologic pattern then reflects the progesterone influence throughout the luteal phase. Accurate endometrial dating by the criteria of Noyes et al. (Fig. 29.3) is most satisfactory just prior to the onset of menses and the biopsy serves as a bioassay of corpus luteum progesterone output.

Luteal Phase Defect

If the histologic dating of the endometrium is 2 or more days behind the menstrual dating in two or more cycles, the diagnosis of a luteal phase defect can be made. For practical pur-

poses, the day of onset of menses is called day 28; a biopsy obtained 2 days before should have the histologic pattern of a secretory day 26 endometrium. If the pattern is no farther advanced than secretory day 24, the biopsy is said to be 2 days out of phase (Fig. 29.4). In our experience, an endometrium unresponsive to hormonal stimulation is rare, and even the fragmented lining in severe endometrial sclerosis or overlying a submucous myoma, undergoes some secretory change. The usual cause of endometrial inadequacy is insufficient progesterone production; the luteal phase defect is defined as a progesterone defect reflected by a lag in the expected endometrial pattern or by lower than normal serial progesterone levels.

Luteal phase defects are associated with several clinical entities including early recurrent miscarriages, primary infertility, and subclinical occult miscarriages. Defective progesterone output is observed frequently during the 1st year following menarche, in the first ovulatory cycles following delivery or abortion, in the over-35-year-old woman, during clomiphene-induced ovulation, in women undergoing strenuous physical conditioning, and in women with hyperprolactinemia. Although luteal phase inadequacy affects only 3% of the general population, it has been diagnosed in 35–50% of clomipheneinduced ovulations and in 35–65% of patients with recurrent miscarriages; this will be discussed later in this chapter.

Treatment of the inadequate luteal phase should be determined by the etiology diagnosed, but this is not always possible to identify. Hypothyroidism, or hyperprolactinemia should be readily diagnosed and treated, but if no specific factors are found, progesterone substitution therapy is reasonable and effective. Progesterone vaginal suppositories, 25 mg twice daily, beginning 3 or 4 days into the luteal phase and continuing until the onset of menses, is a satisfactory regimen which does not exceed progesterone levels found in the normal luteal phase. A repeat biopsy on therapy is indicated to document satisfactory endometrial repair. Alternatively, the intramuscular administration of 12.5 mg of progesterone daily does not delay menses and satisfactorily substitutes for the progesterone defect.

Synthetic progestational agents, contraindicated in pregnancy, are also ineffective therapy. The effect on the endometrium is not equivalent to that of progesterone, a glan-

DATING THE ENDOMETRIUM
APPROXIMATE RELATIONSHIP OF USEFUL MORPHOLOGICAL FACTORS

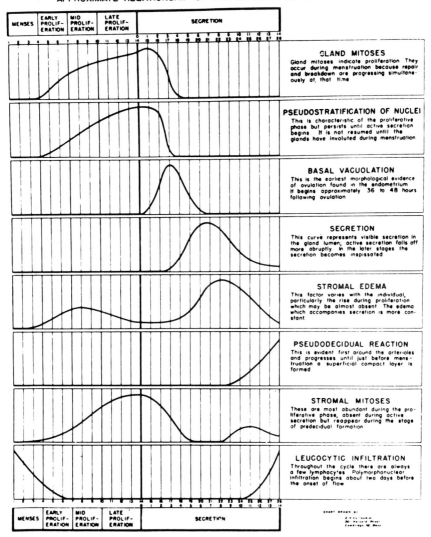

Figure 29.3. Criteria used to date the endometrium. (Reproduced with permission from R. W. Noyes, A. T. Hertig, and J. Rock: *Fertility and Sterility, 1:*3, 1950.)

dular-stromal disparity will be observed, and implantation may not occur normally.

Endometritis

Czernobilsky has recently described the acute and chronic endometrial infections associated with infertility and explained the importance of endometrial biopsy and of skilled pathologic interpretation. The finding of plasma cells is pathognomonic of chronic infection, and the observation of foci of lymphocytes and macrophages may be the sole clue of a Mycoplasma endometritis.

The diagnosis of Mycoplasma also can be made in the female, of midcycle cervical mucus and in the male of an entire seminal ejaculate. Either specimen may be frozen, as this does not appear to interfere with the ability to culture T-mycoplasma. Doxycycline (Vibramycin) 100 mg daily for 10 days is used to treat both husband and wife.

The number of patients investigated thus far is too small to provide statistical significance of Mycoplasma infection. However, recurrent abortion and infertility may be due to infection with this organism so its existence should be considered.

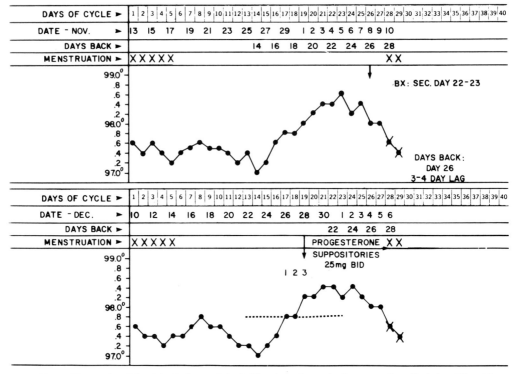

Figure 29.4. Diagnosis of the luteal phase defect. The day of onset of menses is called day 28; a biopsy obtained 2 days before should have the histologic pattern of secretory day 26. The illustration (*top*) shows the findings in a patient whose endometrium is 3–4 days out of phase. Progesterone suppositories are begun only after ovulation has occurred and are continued until menses. A rebiopsy should be obtained to document adequate support.

Tubal Factor

The Fallopian tubes must not only be patent, but must also be mobile. Tests of tubal function serve not only as diagnostic procedures but also as therapeutic ones in that they tend to overcome minor obstructions and fimbrial agglutination. There are several accepted methods for establishing the patency of the Fallopian tubes.

Gas (carbon dioxide) insufflation, described by Rubin in 1920, and known as the Rubin's test, is uncomplicated and easily accomplished in the office setting. The test is performed using a mercury manometer, and tubal patency is indicated if, using a stethoscope over the abdomen, gas is heard to pass at pressures below 180 mm Hg. Partial occlusion is probably present if pressures above 180 and below 200 mm Hg are obtained, and pressures over 200 mm Hg confirm complete tubal obstruction. A safety valve shuts off CO_2 inflow at pressures over 200 mm Hg, to prevent insufflation into the vascular system.

Although it is a helpful office diagnostic aid, the Rubin's test is nonspecific and can give misleading information about bilateral tubal patency.

In contrast, hysterosalpingography (HSG), is convenient and provides detailed information about the uterine cavity, tubal patency, intrapelvic disease and adhesion formation (Fig. 29.5). HSG performed with fluoroscopic image intensification provides more information about tubal patency, position, and mobility and about the flow and dissemination of dye. The radiation dosage to the ovaries is significant therefore the procedure must be efficiently and quickly performed.

The timing of the hysterogram is important, and HSG should be performed after menstrual bleeding has ceased, and prior to ovulation. At this stage of the menstrual cycle, the oocyte is relatively radioresistant and is resting in prophase of meiosis I. Once meiosis has resumed, the oocyte enters into a relatively radiosensitive stage and radiation should be avoided.

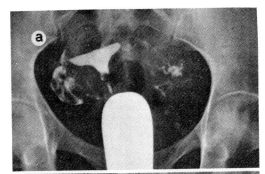

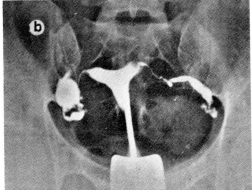

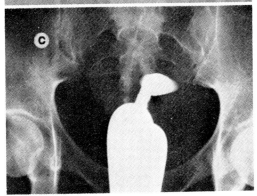

Figure 29.5. A, normal hysterosalpingogram showing the outline of a delicate tube and spill into the peritoneal cavity on the left. The right tube is obscured by massive peritoneal spill on the right. The sweeping, smeared appearance is characteristic when water soluble media are used. B, obstruction at the fimbriated ends of the tubes with bilateral hydrosalpinx. The uterus is arcuate. C, bilateral tubal occlusion at the cornu. The uterine cavity has been distorted by overdistention with a radiopaque medium.

For HSG, a Rubin's or Jarcho cannula is used through which the water-soluble contrast medium is injected, and the progress of the infused dye is followed by fluoroscopy. To outline the endometrial cavity, an initial ejection of 1–2 ml of dye, if the uterus is not enlarged, is adequate to show submucous myomata, polyps, and other intracavitary abnormalities. More dye is then injected which will extend the cavity and also demonstrate an incompetent os. The progress of the contrast medium is followed through the tubes, and the uterus can be manipulated to identify peritubal and periovarian adhesions. The thickness of the tubal lumen is observed, tubal convolutions are identified, and the pattern of contrast dispersion is noted. Carbon dioxide may be introduced to provide additional information or contrast.

Delicate tubes with slightly dilated distal ends are usually normal. Spill appears as a smear and can be followed during fluoroscopy. A collection of dye may occur in either a hydrosalpinx or in peritubal adhesions. Convolutions or corkscrewing of tubes may be suggestive of endometriosis. Nonvisualization of one or both tubes suggests cornual obstruction but spasm can be misleading. Pretreatment with atropine, 0.5 mg, may prevent this spasm.

HSG may be therapeutic. A water-soluble opaque medium is used in preference to an oil-based medium, which may carry a greater potential for serious complications such as oil embolus and granulomata. Whatever the reason, the incidence of conception increases during the 3–4 months after a hysterosalpingogram, and oil-based contrast is associated with a higher pregnancy rate than water-soluble contrast medium; a waiting period following HSG before proceeding to diagnostic laparoscopy is important. Neither a Rubin's test nor HSG is infallible and each can be technically unsatisfactory. This has led to the suggestion that three tests, preferably different types, be performed before the diagnosis of tubal occlusion is made and before considering a tubal plastic procedure. However, it is not justifiable to perform repeated tubal studies if a normal test has been obtained. If real doubt exists, a direct visual examination should be made.

Diagnosis of tubal occlusion at the cornuum may be difficult because of the possibility of tubal spasm. Usually, cornual occlusion is due to the sequelae of a severe postpartum or postabortal infection: salpingitis isthmica nodosa is also an important cause of cornual or isthmic occlusion. The treatment of tubal occlusion is usually surgical and, in the final analysis, diagnostic laparoscopy provides important prognostic information for surgical procedures.

Peritoneal Factor

The peritoneal factor includes those physical or mechanical barriers to fertility occurring within the pelvis, which ordinarily are undetected by HSG, history, or bimanual examination. These include such entities as *peritubal adhesions* and *endometriosis.*

Fully 35–60% of patients with endoscopic or operative evidence of endometriosis have a normal hysterosalpingogram. Diagnostic laparoscopy with instillation of indigo carmine or methylene blue dye through the tubes, will diagnose an additional 20% of infertility-causing problems. However, neither procedure is infallible, both are useful, and the findings are complementary. For instance, in 207 women having both HSG and laparoscopy, 17% who had HSG findings suggestive of pelvic abnormalities had a normal laparoscopy; and 18% who had normal HSG findings had unsuspected peritubal adhesions. There is complete agreement only half the time using both techniques. The hysterosalpingogram tends to miss peritubal adhesions and endometriosis, and over-diagnoses tubal occlusion. Overall, patients fully evaluated as outlined above, and in whom no reason for infertility was found on the initial screening tests, had an expectation of 20–25% of having a mechanical etiology for infertility discovered at endoscopy. Therefore, diagnostic laparoscopy or less commonly culdoscopy in competent hands (Fig. 29.6) is an essential part of the evaluation of the infertile couple.

Tubal or fimbrial occlusion may be the result of adhesions from pelvic inflammatory disease due to gonorrhea, tuberculosis, or postabortal or postpartum infection. Adhesions may be due to endometriosis or other more unusual causes of blood in the peritoneal cavity, such as an unrecognized ectopic pregnancy, ruptured corpus luteum cyst, or bleeding from the follicle at ovulation. Extrapelvic inflammatory processes, including regional enteritis or an appendiceal abscess, may also cause tubal adhesions with occlusion. Recently, some evidence has been presented that the intrauterine device may be associated with filmy peritubular adhesions, possibly because of subclinical inflammation or infection.

The treatment of tubal occlusion is ordinarily surgical in the final analysis. However, three tubal patency tests should be performed both for diagnosis and also in an effort to rupture adhesions; these simple diagnostic procedures may increase the incidence of conception in the three or four cycles following their utilization.

With the use of the microsurgery in cases without extensive tubal damage, the statistical probability of pregnancy approaches 80%. The use of the 2-0 nylon suture as a stent in reimplantation procedures has also resulted in an 80% incidence of pregnancy and over a 90% chance of reestablishing tubal patency at the cornuum.

Other Considerations

Psychogenic Aspects of Infertility

There are relatively few studies of the psychodynamics of the infertile couple. Clearly, however, infertility imposes stress and strain on any marriage or interrelationship. Patients with infertility, who are tactfully questioned, will often admit to feelings of guilt, resentment, suspicion, frustration, and anger. The patient may treat her physician with open hostility or make unreasonable demands. The self-image suffers, as the wife may see herself as barren, and the husband himself as demasculinized, or castrated. By its very nature, the infertility evaluation must probe into the most intimate parts of the anatomy for the most intimate of details; the management of infertility requires insight, sympathy, compassion, and tact because of these invasions of the patients' privacy.

Unfortunately, physicians often do much to increase the stress felt by the childless couple. Typically, a well meaning physician will suggest that a couple have intercourse daily or every other day at a certain time of the cycle, especially as guided by basal temperature or the perceived mucus flood. Sex-on-demand takes the spontaneity and pleasure out of the sexual act and substitutes compulsion and rigidity.

Counselling may have a role by breaking the vicious cycle of infertility-emotional tension-infertility and secondly, by reducing the associated symptoms that seriously impair the quality of life for childless couples, including frustration, disappointment, fear, and depression. Recognition of the importance of these factors, and the dysphoric effects of involuntary infertility, are integral to the total management of an infertile couple.

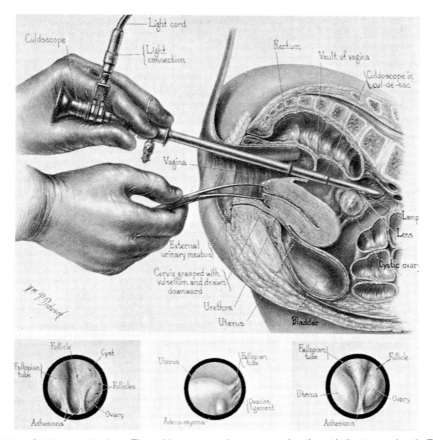

Figure 29.6. Culdoscope in place. The culdoscope can be seen passing through the trocar sheath. The trocar is introduced into the cul-de-sac through the posterior vagina, which has been "tented" by pushing the cervix forward and downward. The trocar is then withdrawn and the culdoscope inserted. (From A. Decker: *Culdoscopy*, W. B. Saunders Co., Philadelphia, 1952.)

RECURRENT ABORTION

Introduction

The incidence of spontaneous miscarriage in the general population approximates 15–20%, but the likelihood of a second or a third miscarriage remains a controversial statistic. Of women who had a single spontaneous abortion, 22% had a second abortion. After three consecutive abortions the risk of a subsequent abortion rises to 47%. However, somewhat more optimistic figures have been proposed by Warburton and Fraser: a 24% risk after one abortion, 26% after two, and a 32% risk of subsequent abortion after three early miscarriages.

Using information of this type we can arrive at guidelines for evaluations: a patient who has had one abortion should be reassured, but one who has had two consecutive early miscarriages, or a total of three miscarriages interspersed with normal pregnancies, has an increased likelihood of another pregnancy loss. Additionally, any couple with one miscarriage and a malformed fetus in another pregnancy has a 27% chance of a balanced translocation.

Etiologic Diagnosis of Recurrent Miscarriage

There are probably only three categories of importance in establishing the etiologic cause of early recurrent miscarriage: genetic, hormonal, or anatomic causes. However, less commonly, an infectious, metabolic/endocrine, immunologic, iatrogenic, or male factor may be identified; a single spontaneous abortion is more likely due to one of these causes.

Genetic Causes

Approximately 50–60% of spontaneous first trimester miscarriages are due to a chromosomal aberration, of which trisomy accounts for some 50–60%, monosomy X for 15–25%,, and polyploidy for 20–25% of these single abortions. If the index abortus has a normal karyotype, the second is also likely to have a normal karyotype; and similarly, if the initial abortus is abnormal, the second subsequent abortion is also likely to be abnormal. Thus, the second abortion has an 80% chance of being chromosomally abnormal if the index abortus was abnormal, but the risk for the mother under these circumstances is about 15% of having a second abortion. However, if the index miscarriage were chromosomally normal, the risk of a second or a third abortion is as high as 45%.

In the general population, a balanced translocation, in which there is a mutual exchange of broken-off fragments between chromosomes, occurs with an incidence of about 1.9/1000. However, of couples with two or more spontaneous abortions, almost 3% will be found to have balanced reciprocal translocations. If the couples have had both early abortion and fetal malformation, a 27% incidence of cytogenetically abnormal parents is discovered.

Because of the expense, a genetic analysis of both parents is probably unwarranted until at least three early spontaneous miscarriages have occurred. Karyotypic analysis might be attempted on any tissue passed or obtained at curettage after a second early miscarriage and should certainly be performed in a third. There is no known treatment for parental genetic defects and genetic counseling is all that can be offered to such couples.

Hormonal Causes

Adequacy of corpus luteum function, specifically **progesterone** output, is essential both to implantation and to maintenance of an early pregnancy. An inadequate corpus luteum, with a lower-than-normal progesterone production, may be etiologically responsible for recurrent miscarriage. The incidence of luteal phase inadequacy is only about 3% in the general population; however, in patients presenting with recurrent abortions, the incidence approaches 35–50%. Recent studies have shown that patients with habitual abortion had lower than normal progesterone levels during the luteal phase (Fig. 29.7); when pregnant, progesterone levels were also lower than normal, and these patients again

subsequently aborted. The use of the endometrial biopsy as a bioassay of progesterone output has proved a satisfactory alternative to serial progesterone levels. The normal luteal phase is dependent upon adquate FSH and LH stimulation to follicular development receptor synthesis and interaction with estradiol; and a defect may be caused by anything that disrupts luteal development, for example, central factors related to psychogenic, neurogenic or specific pituitary dysfunction; intermediate disturbances related to nutritional factors, drug toxicity, chronic disease processes or metabolic disease; or to a specific ovarian insufficiency.

At present, there are no studies sufficiently controlled to prove that progesterone therapy prevents subsequent miscarriage. Progesterone is essential to the maintenance of early pregnancy but whether progesterone treatment can substitute for endogenous progesterone production has not been statistically substantiated. However, progesterone therapy, if utilized, must be begun before the missed period and, since normality of the endometrium and of the implantation site appear to be important, treatment with progesterone after the first missed period is too late to be effective. It is inappropriate to institute therapy in an attempt to "rescue" a threatened abortion. All progestational agents are presently contraindicated in early pregnancy.

Uterine and Cervical Causes

The incompetent cervical os is characterized by sudden expulsion of a normal sac and fetus between the 18th and 32nd week of pregnancy without prior cramps or bleeding. The factor seems to be more prevalent in those areas of the world where abortion is frequent or obstetrical care, at delivery, poor. The traumatic type of cervical incompetence is best treated by an interval trachelorrhapy, suture must be placed before dilatation of the cervix begins, usually between 12 and 16 weeks and should be used only when other fetal and maternal endocrine findings are normal.

Recurrent abortion can be due to uterine anomalies, particularly the septate uterus, but the relative frequency of these anomalies in the general population is not ordinarily recognized. Only approximately 25% of patients with a bicornuate uterus have problems with

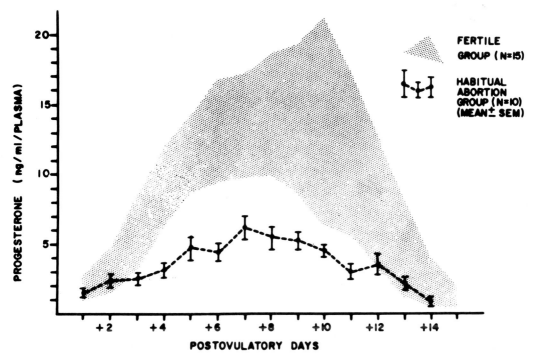

Figure 29.7.   Plasma progesterone levels (mean ± SE) during the luteal phase of the menstrual cycle. Shaded area shows range in 15 women with normal menses and proved fertility; broken line shows range in 10 women who habitually aborted. (Reproduced with permission from J. L. H. Horta, J. G. Fernandez, B. Soto de Leon, and V. Cortes-Gallegos: *Obstetrics and Gynecology, 49:*705, 1977.)

fetal wastage, and the pregnancy termination may occur in any trimester. Ordinarily, the defect is characterized by delivery of a normal fetus or premature infant usually after the 16th week of pregnancy and the patient with a bicornuate uterus who does miscarry tends to carry each pregnancy longer than the preceding one.

Submucous fibroids, endometrial polyps, or uterine synechiae which distort the endometrial cavity may also cause repeated abortion (Fig. 29.8). Failure of implantation or placentation may be responsible, although the incidence of recurrent abortion associated with endometrial sclerosis is unknown and must be relatively rare. The diagnosis of uterine defects is made by HSG and exploration of the uterine cavity by dilatation and curettage, or possibly by hysteroscopy in the nonpregnant state.

Rare causes of repeated miscarriage, mentioned for completeness, include the heritable disorders of connective tissue, particularly the Ehlers-Danlos syndrome. Pregnancy poses hazards to the mother because of the "generalized loosening" of connective tissue, and

the fetus with Ehlers-Danlos is at risk since the fetal membranes share the fragility of other connective tissues resulting in premature rupture of the membrane leading to premature delivery.

Infectious Causes

Both uterine and disseminated infections have been etiologically related to miscarriage. Among these, viral infections, herpes, rubella, and cytomegalic inclusion disease have been implicated in causing a single miscarriage. Listeria, toxoplasma, and brucella have been implicated in causing recurrent miscarriages.

The T-mycoplasma, a common finding in the vagina and cervix of fertile and infertile women, has more convincingly been associated with recurrent miscarriage. Culture for the T-mycoplasma, and possibly treatment with Doxycycline, is indicated in otherwise unexplained cases of recurrent abortion.

Metabolic/Endocrine Causes

Any chronic disease, toxic environmental exposure, and metabolic or endocrine abnor-

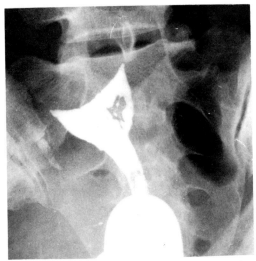

Figure 29.8. Hysterogram of uterus of patient who had repeated early miscarriages following a therapeutic abortion. There is a single area of endometrial sclerosis and scarring.

mality could be associated with frequent miscarriage. Hepatic and renal disorders more commonly result in anovulation and not recurrent abortion, but exposure to anesthetic gases and volatile fumes may cause either miscarriage or fetal anomalies.

Hypothyroidism is a rare and subtle cause of recurrent miscarriage but should be suspected clinically and diagnosed by measuring TSH. Only late-stage diabetes mellitus may be associated with recurrent miscarriage and, although diabetic patients may have an increased incidence of bacteriuria, the connection with recurrent abortion has not been established.

Collagen vascular diseases, particularly systemic lupus erythematosus (SLE), have been associated with causing miscarriage. Although, reportedly, a pregnant patient with SLE has a 40% chance of abortion, the disease is ordinarily diagnosed before repeated miscarriage occurs.

Immunologic Causes

Immunologic factors are rare causes of recurrent miscarriages. Circulating blocking antibody may protect the fetus against attack by maternal lymphocytes, and patients with habitual abortion may lack appreciable levels of this blocking factor. hCG appears to be a suppressant of lymphocytes. If the trophoblast were unable to produce sufficient hCG, possibly because of inadequate progesterone support or inadequate placentation, then possibly a failure of immunologic suppression could result in miscarriage.

Iatrogenic Causes

Iatrogenic causes of recurrent miscarriage include the administration of certain chemotherapeutic and/or cytotoxic agents including cytoxan; colchicine, used in the treatment of gout; and luteolytic agents, including progestational agents and estrogens.

Male Factors

Both hyperspermia, greater than 250,000,000 sperm/ml, and oligospermia have been associated with frequent miscarriages. This may be secondary to a decreased DNA content of the sperm, but this has not been substantiated.

PRECONCEPTIONAL EVALUATION OF COUPLES WITH HABITUAL ABORTION

The history includes a detailed list of prior miscarriages, including actual documentation of the pregnancy, its duration, pathologic description, autopsy reports, and chromosomal studies if performed; notes the presence or absence of cramping and bleeding, a description of the labor and occurrence of any physical or emotional trauma before the occurrence of the abortion; and records preceding illnesses or operations, chronic or acute infection, weight change, drug intake, or illness prior to conception or during early pregnancy. A family history of miscarriages, abortions, congenital anomalies, heritable diseases, stillbirths, and infertility should be mentioned.

The physical examination looks for evidence of acute or chronic illness, endocrinopathy, or infection, myomata or the "broad-shouldered" fundus suggestive of a double uterus. The passage of a no. 8 Hegar dilator without pain into the endometrial cavity may suggest an incompetent internal cervical os. Cervical lacerations, a double vagina, double cervix, or other congenital abnormalities suggestive of Müllerian fusion problems should be noted.

The preconceptional evaluation ordinarily will include a karyotypic analysis of both husband and wife, an evaluation of luteal phase adequacy, and the performance of a hysterosalpingogram. The *chromosomal analysis* should include routine karyotyping, plus banding studies. Although numerical aberrations are more common, structural chromosomal abnormalities, specifically translocations, are an important cause of recurrent miscarriages.

Diagnosis of *luteal phase inadequacy* is most easily made by taking an endometrial biopsy timed to be obtained within 2 or 3 days of the expected period. The histologic date must then be correlated with the next menstrual period. If the patient's next menstrual period occurs, for example, the next day after the biopsy was obtained, the histologic pattern of the endometrium should be equivalent to a secretory day 27 pattern, which reflects approximately 13 days of progesterone exposure. If, however, the endometrial biopsy is read as earlier, for instance secretory day 21–22, then the biopsy is out of phase, reflecting the histologic pattern expected from a shorter duration of progesterone exposure. Thus, the endometrial biopsy is a bioassay of progesterone output. For a valid diagnosis of luteal phase inadequacy, a biopsy out of phase by 2 or more days must be obtained in two or more cycles.

A hysterosalpingogram will diagnose Müllerian anomalies, Asherman's syndrome, polyps, or submucous myomata. Müllerian abnormalities occur in 1 of every 700 women, and about 10% of women presenting with habitual abortion will ultimately require a corrective operative procedure. The suggested surgical procedure for a bicornuate uterus is a Strassman unification and either the Tompkins or the Jones procedure for the septate uterus. Endometrial sclerosis may be approached by hysteroscopic lysis of adhesions, followed by insertion of either an IUD, or Foley catheter, with estrogenic hormonal support.

The remaining aspects of the preconceptional evaluation include diagnosing and ruling out other *less common etiologic factors.* A complete blood count, serum chemistries including liver and renal function tests, thyroid studies, and blood group and Coombs tests on husband and wife may be indicated. TORCH studies including titers for toxoplasmosis, rubella, cytomegalovirus, and herpes may be indicated. An endometrial biopsy to diagnose chronic endometritis and for culture for T-mycoplasma may be obtained, and possibly a menstrual collection will be needed to diagnose tuberculous endometritis. The cervical mucus might be collected and sent for Mycoplasma culture, and the male seminal ejaculate may also be cultured for Mycoplasma after freezing. Glucose tolerance tests are usually unnecessary, and ordinarily only an appropriate detailed drug history is necessary to identify iatrogenic factors or environmental toxins. Although of unusual occurence, a sperm count looking for hyper- or oligospermia may be indicated.

POSTCONCEPTIONAL MONITORING AND EARLY PREGNANCY MANAGEMENT

Following appropriate evaluation and indicated therapy, the patient may discontinue the barrier method of contraception necessary during the time of evaluation. The basal body temperature chart should be continued, in order that a pregnancy may be diagnosed as early as possible. The patient should be instructed to report delayed menses immediately.

The quantitative measurement of hCG is ordinarily helpful, although two or more values are needed so that the rising hCG indicative of normality can be observed. A pregnancy with low hCG titers should not be supported with progesterone to avoid masking a missed abortion or intrauterine fetal death.

Serum progesterone in very early pregnancy may decrease from the time of the missed period until approximately 6–7 weeks from the last menstrual period; even serial values may be shown to be normally decreasing at this stage of gestation. However, if values are below 10 ng/ml, virtually no patient will have continuation of the pregnancy. Sequential ultrasonography and frequent examinations to determine both gestational size and lack of cervical dilatation may be in order.

The determination of TSH, T_4, T_3, and T_3 uptake may be indicated, as subclinical hypothyroidism may be responsible for early miscarriage. Coitus during early pregnancy may be inadvisable as the male seminal ejaculate contains prostaglandins in concentrations which can cause uterine contractions in both the nonpregnant and pregnant uterus. Additionally, orgasm is ordinarily associated with increased uterine motility and measurable uterine contractions.

Even if an etiologic cause has been determined and appropriately treated, for instance a double uterus unified or a luteal phase defect supported by progesterone administration, subsequent miscarriage may occur due to a sporadic genetic cause. If 50–60% of all spontaneous miscarriages are caused by random genetic abnormalities, then any single miscarriage may have this etiology. The attempt should be made to culture the fetal tissue from the subsequent miscarriage, to assess its genetic makeup.

Vaginal bleeding, especially if accompanied by cramping, is always of concern. Up to 50% of pregnant women will bleed early in pregnancy and, of those with significant bleeding, about 60–70% will ultimately abort. Bed rest is useful psychologically. Importantly progesterone or a progestational agent administered at this time will not prevent the occurrence of a miscarriage.

Finally, habitual abortion may result from emotional factors, and abruptio placenta is commonly seen in patients under emotional or psychological stress. If no other factors explaining recurrent abortion can be identified, counseling, and the awareness of the importance of emotional factors, may change the outcome in a particular case.

SPONTANEOUS ABORTION

Missed Abortion

When embryonic death occurs, the products of conception are generally expelled within a few weeks. When an early perished embryo is not expelled within 2 months, it is spoken of as a missed abortion.

The diagnosis is not easily made but should be suspected when a woman, apparently pregnant, shows no sign of continued uterine growth. Bleeding of some degree occurs, and this may be slight, muddy, and malodorous; a previously positive pregnancy test will revert to negative. More helpful is ultrasonography which shows a characteristic change in the gestational ring. Severe bleeding due to afibrinogenemia is rarely seen within 6 weeks of fetal death and usually occurs only in the second trimester.

Threatened Abortion

The rate of abortion is estimated to be 10–20% of all pregnancies. One or more missed periods, followed by spotting or bleeding and sometimes cramps, suggests that a pregnancy is threatened. Other causes of bleeding in early pregnancy, including cervical eversion, erosion, or polyp; ectopic pregnancy; and vaginal lesions or infections, must be sought. The symptoms sometimes subside, and the gestation goes on uneventfully to term; about 30–40% of patients with threatened abortions will continue the pregnancy. In other instances, bleeding and cramps may increase with ultimate expulsion of the embryo. Although marked bleeding and cramps are rarely compatible with retention of the fetus, this may nevertheless occur; more than 40% of all pregnancies bleed at some point. If there is no abortion, and the patient goes to term, the expectation of a normal baby is good, although abnormalities of the infant under these circumstances are slightly increased over those seen in an uncomplicated pregnancy.

Patients with threatened abortion can have a realistic prognosis made by monitoring quantitative hCG levels as suggestive of the integrity of the trophoblast and plasma progesterone as reflecting corpus luteum function early on and placental function later. Ultrasonography will show an intact or obliterated gestational ring. There is no effective therapy for a threatened abortion, other than bed rest, and progestational agents may be mentioned only to condemn their use. There is *no* evidence that the administration of progesterone or a progestational agent can improve the prognosis in threatened abortion.

When bleeding and cramps are severe, the cervix is often dilated with the products of conception lying just within the os. This is spoken of as inevitable abortion. Nothing can be done to salvage this pregnancy, as the fetus has already been passed and retained placental fragments are the cause of bleeding.

Incomplete Abortion

An abortion is considered *inevitable* when the internal os admits a finger or is visibly open, and bleeding and cramping are occurring. An abortion is considered *incomplete* when tissue has been passed; if there is continued bleeding, the uterus should be evacuated by sharp or suction curettage, and provisions should be made for blood transfusion, as bleeding may be profuse. An early abortion is frequently complete and requires no therapy. Sometimes an incomplete abortion can be completed medically by intravenous pitocin or ergotrate orally every 4 hours for six doses. More frequently, however, curettage with removal of the retained placental tissue is necessary. Considerable care must be exercised not to perforate the pregnant uterus, which is apt to be soft and mushy. Use of ovum or polyp forceps and a smooth curette is followed by careful sharp curettage, only after intravenous pitocin has been given. The development of the suction curette has avoided some of the problems and increased the speed of procedure.

Where septic abortion is present, the plan of therapy is somewhat different, but should be guided primarily by (1) the degree of infection, and (2) the amount of bleeding. There has always been some difference of thought as to how soon the infected uterus should be evacuated, but the majority opinion favors massive antibiotic therapy followed by curettage. Sepsis with shock and anuria may occur with localized abscesses and thrombophlebitis.

Occasional *Clostridium welchii* infections occur; massive drainage, hysterectomy, and vena cava ligation may be necessary and the prognosis is poor. Supplementary blood, vasopressors, intravenous fluids, antibiotics, cortisone, and other supportive measures are of course necessary and, if there is associated anuria, peritoneal dialysis or hemodialysis may be considered. *E. coli* with gram-negative septicemia may also be associated with extreme sepsis and shock.

Differential Diagnosis: Abortion and Ectopic Pregnancy

When a patient skips a menstrual period and then begins to bleed persistently, the first thought is of early gestation and threatened abortion. It should not be forgotten, however, that ectopic gestation characteristically presents a history of menstrual delay, followed by persistent bleeding, although usually scant in amount. One of the commonest errors in the diagnosis of tubal pregnancy is to mistake it for incomplete or threatened early abortion. In the threatened variety, as with tubal pregnancy, the bleeding may be slight, whereas in the incomplete type it may be rather free. Should there be profuse external bleeding, ectopic pregnancy is unlikely.

In early abortion, pain is not a conspicuous symptom and may be absent. With tubal pregnancy, on the other hand, the bleeding is usually accompanied by attacks of pain in the affected side of the pelvis, sometimes accompanied by nausea, vomiting, or attacks of faintness. Where intra-abdominal bleeding is free, pallor, syncope, and rapid pulse are noted. Pregnancy tests are not usually of decisive importance, as they may be positive or negative in both the tubal and uterine types of pregnancy.

The chief reliance must generally be placed on bimanual examination and ultrasonography. In early uterine abortion one can usually make at least some degree of uterine enlargement, with often softening and patulousness of the cervical canal. Although there is usually no tenderness or palpable enlargement in either adnexal region, occasionally the corpus luteum of pregnancy may be painful to palpation, and occasionally it may bleed. Ultrasonography may reveal an intrauterine gestational ring or show a noncystic mass in the adnexa. In general, the most accurate means of distinguishing an ectopic pregnancy is by culdoscopy or laparoscopy.

With tubal pregnancy, the uterus and cervix may show no noteworthy difference from the normal, whereas an adnexal enlargement—sometimes very slight and indefinite, in other cases large and unquestionable— is present in one side of the pelvis. This very unilaterality of the lesion, combined with the symptoms mentioned above, will usually justify a presumptive diagnosis of tubal pregnancy. Finally, culdocentesis may reveal concentrated, dark, nonclotting blood in the cul-de-sac, which suggests a leaking or rupturing ectopic pregnancy. Decisive help in making the differentiation can be obtained by such diagnostic procedures as culdoscopy, colpotomy, or laparoscopy.

OTHER PROBLEMS OF PREGNANCY

Diagnostic problems involving the question of pregnancy are constantly intruding themselves into the practice of the gynecologist. The possibility of gestation must be considered in the differential diagnosis of amenorrhea, as well as uterine enlargement, abdominal tumors, and uterine bleeding.

Diagnosis of Early Pregnancy

In the early weeks of pregnancy there is insufficient enlargement or softening of the uterus to make a positive diagnosis by palpation, and laboratory tests are essential. Various immunological methods, including slide and tube tests, radioreceptor assays, and specific measures of the β-subunit of hCG may be utilized for the early detection of human chorionic gonadotrophin in urine or serum; the test chosen depends on cost, speed, sensitivity, or specificity considerations.

When there is no urgency for making the diagnosis, the patient can be instructed to return within a few weeks, possibly having recorded her basal temperature. At this time, amenorrhea, frequently associated with such subjective symptoms as nausea and vomiting, soreness of the breasts, and bladder irritability, together with softening of the cervix, Hegar's sign, and symmetrical jug-shaped enlargement of the uterus, leave little doubt as to the existence of early pregnancy.

Coexistence of Pelvic Lesions and Pregnancy

There are many cases in which a pelvic lesion, such as a large uterine myoma or an ovarian tumor, is known to be present but in which there is reason to believe that the patient may also be pregnant. Pregnancy is ordinarily an indication for postponement of the operation. Any patient who has a history of amenorrhea or an abnormal menses, particularly if the cervix is softened, deserves a pregnancy test.

Pseudocyesis

This curious condition of imaginary pregnancy occurs in women who are extremely anxious *to* or *not to* become pregnant. It is characterized by amenorrhea, weight gain and gradual abdominal enlargement, breast enlargement with secretion, morning nausea, and in some cases imagination of fetal movements. Palpation of a small uterus generally clarifies the problem. Hyperprolactinemia, increased LH levels, and other endocrine abnormalities have been reported. During the last 10 years, this interesting psychiatric syndrome has become exceedingly uncommon.

Diagnosis of Pregnancy in Later Stages

In the latter half of pregnancy, diagnosis is usually easily arrived at on the basis of fetal heart sounds, the demonstration of a skeleton by x-ray, and fetal movements. In the obese patient with a questionable uterine or ovarian enlargement, the use of ultrasound has been advocated as a diagnostic technique. As surgery for myomas is rarely an emergency, simple periodic examination with confirmation of a rapidly growing and softening uterus can establish the diagnosis of pregnancy rather than myomas.

Induced Abortion

This procedure has such obvious moral and religious implications that every individual must determine what his own approach should be and should be thoroughly familiar with both national and state laws. Women should be discouraged from using abortion, which carries potential physical and psychological hazards, as a method of family planning. For the true case of rape, abortion also should not be necessary as, under these circumstances, a postcoital contraceptive, estrogen, can be administered or an IUD inserted within 48 hours of the rape and provide protection.

References and Additional Readings

Beck, W. W., Jr.: A critical look at the legal, ethical, and technical aspects of artificial insemination. Fertil. Steril., *27:* 1, 1976.

Byrd, J. R., Askew, D. E., and McDonough, P. G.: Cytogenetic findings in fifty-five couples with recurrent fetal wastage. Fertil. Steril., *28:* 246, 1977.

Czernobilsky, B.: Endometritis and infertility. Fertil. Steril., *30:* 119, 1978.

Davajan, V.: The postcoital tests. J. Reprod. Med., *18:* 132, 1977.

Davajan, V., and Kunitake, G. M.: Fractional in vivo and in vitro examination of postcoital cervical mucus in the human. Fertil. Steril., *20:* 197, 1969.

Decker, A.: *Culdoscopy.* W. B. Saunders Company, Philadelphia, 1952.

Drake, T., Tredway, D., Buchanan, G., Takaki, N., and Daane, T.: Unexplained infertility. Obstet. Gynecol., *50:* 644, 1977.

Franklin, R. R., and Dukes, C. D.: Antispermatozoal antibody and unexplained infertility. Am. J. Obstet. Gynecol., *89:* 6, 1964.

Garcia, J., Jones, G. S., and Wentz, A. C.: The use of clomiphene citrate. Fertil. Steril., *28:* 707, 1977.

Glass, R. H., and Golbus, M. S.: Habitual abortion. Fertil. Steril., *29:* 257, 1978.

Goldenberg, R. L., White, R., and Magendantz, H. G.: Pregnancy during the hysterogram cycle. Fertil. Steril. *27:* 1274, 1976.

Greenberg, S. H.: Varicocele and male infertility. Fertil. Steril., *28:* 699, 1977.

Greenhill, J. P.: World trends of therapeutic abortion and sterilization. Clin. Obstet. Gynaecol. *7:* 37, 1964.

Horta, J. L. H., Fernandez, J. G., Soto de Leon, B., and Cortes-Gallegos, V.: Direct evidence of luteal insufficiency in women with habitual abortion. Obstet. Gynecol., *49:* 705, 1977.

Isojima, S., Koyama, K., and Tsuchiya, K.: The effect on fertility in women of circulating antibodies against human spermatozoa. J. Reprod. Fertil. (Suppl.), *21:* 125, 1974.

Jones, G. S.: World trends of therapeutic abortion and sterilization. Clin. Obstet. Gynaecol. *7:* 37, 1964.

Jones, G. E. S., and Delfs, E.: Endocrine patterns in term pregnancies following abortion. JAMA, *146:* 1212, 1951.

Kibrick, S., Belding, D. L., and Merrill, B.: Methods for the detection of antibodies against mammalian spermatozoa II. A modified macroscopic agglutination test. Fertil. Steril., *3:* 419, 1952.

Kleegman, S. J.: Therapeutic donor insemination. Fertil. Steril., *5:* 7, 1954.

Lauritsen, J. G.: Aetiology of spontaneous abortion. Acta Obstet. Gynecol. Scand., Suppl., *52:* 1, 1976

Lenton, E. A., Weston, G. A., and Cooke, I. D.: Long-term follow-up of the apparently normal couple with a complaint of infertility. Fertil. Steril., *28:* 913, 1977.

14, 1974.

Marshall, J. R.: Induction of ovulation. Clin. Obstet. Gynecol., *21:* 147, 1978.

Moghissi, K. S., Syner, F. N., and Evans, T. N.: A composite picture of the menstrual cycle. Am. J. Obstet. Gynecol., *114:* 405, 1972.

Novak, E. R.: Ovulation after fifty. Obstet. Gynecol., *36:* 903, 1970.

Noyes, R. W., Hertig, A. T., and Rock, J.: Dating the endometrial biopsy. Fertil. Steril., *1:* 3, 1950.

Ornoy, A., Benady, S., Kohen-raz, R., and Russell, A.: Association between maternal bleeding during gestation and congenital anomalies in the offspring. Am. J. Obstet. Gynecol., *124:* 474, 1976.

Pauerstein, C. J., Eddy, C. A., Croxatto, H. D., Hess, R., Siler-Khodr, T. M., and Croxatto, H. B.: Temporal relationships of estrogen, progesterone, and luteinizing hormone levels to ovulation in women and infrahuman primates. Am. J. Obstet. Gynecol., *130:* 876, 1978.

Poland, B. J., Miller, J. R., Jones, D. C., and Trimble, B. K.: Reproductive counseling in patients who have had a spontaneous abortion. Am. J. Obstet. Gynecol., *127:* 685, 1977.

Rock, J. A., and Jones, H. W., Jr.: The clinical management of the double uterus. Fertil. Steril., *28:* 798, 1977.

Ross, G. T., Cargille, C. M., Lipsett, M. B., Rayford, P. L., Marshall, J. R., Strott, C. A., and Rodbard, D.: Pituitary and gonadal hormones in women during spontaneous and induced ovulatory cycles. Recent Prog. Horm. Res., *26:* 1, 1970.

Rubin, I.: Non-operative determination of patency of fallopian tubes in sterility; intrauterine inflation with oxygen and production of a subphrenic pneumoperitoneum. JAMA, *74:* 1017, 1920.

Sherman, Barry M., and Korenman, Stanley G.: Hormonal characteristics of the human menstrual cycle throughout reproductive life. J. Clin. Invest. *55:* 699, 1975.

Smith, C., Gregori, C. A., and Breen, J. L.: Ultrasonography in threatened abortion. Obstet. Gynecol., *51:* 173, 1978.

Steinberger, E.: The etiology and pathophysiology and testicular dysfunction in man. Fertil. Steril., *29:* 481, 1978.

Stray-Pedersen, B., Eng. J., and Reikvam, T. M.: Uterine T-mycoplasma colonization in reproductive failure. Am. J. Obstet. Gynecol., *130:* 307, 1978.

Umezaki, C., Katayama, K. P., and Jones, H. W., Jr.: Pregnancy rates after reconstructive surgery of the fallopian tubes. Obstet. Gynecol., *43:* 418, 1974.

Warburton, D., and Fraser, F. C.: On the probability that a woman who has had a spontaneous abortion will abort in subsequent pregnancies. J. Obstet. Gynecol. Br. Common., *68:* 784, 1964.

CHAPTER 30

Amenorrhea

GENERAL CONSIDERATIONS

Definitions

Amenorrhea is not a disease but a symptom and may be arbitrarily defined as the absence of menses for 3 months or longer. *Primary amenorrhea* is defined as the failure of menses to appear initially and should not be diagnosed before the patient has reached the age of 17 years. *Secondary amenorrhea* implies the cessation of menses after an initial menarche. *Physiological amenorrhea* is the normal absence of menses before puberty, during pregnancy and lactation, and after the menopause. *Cryptomenorrhea* signifies that menstruation actually occurs but does not appear externally because of obstruction of the lower genital canal. *Oligomenorrhea* is defined as a reduction in the frequency of menses; the interval must be longer than 38 days but less than 3 months. This must not be confused with the term *hypomenorrhea*, which is used to designate the reduction in the number of days or the amount of menstrual flow.

Classification

Amenorrhea and oligomenorrhea are symptoms which may be caused by a variety of etiological factors. A single individual with a constant etiological background may show at various times any or all of the pathological manifestations of menstruation, including dysfunctional uterine bleeding, oligomenorrhea, amenorrhea, infertility, and habitual abortion. It is most satisfactory, therefore, whenever possible, to make the classification of these symptom complexes on the basis of the underlying etiological disturbance. The following outline shows the etiological classification of amenorrhea, based on anatomi-

cal location, to be used in the discussion. Eponyms of the most common syndromes are included.

Etiological Classification of Amenorrhea

I. Central Nervous System Lesions
  A. Neurogenic—Hypothalamus and above
    1. Organic—destructive lesions, tumors or scars
    2. Insufficiency-hypothalamic dysfunction
      a. Polycystic ovarian disease (PCO, Stein-Leventhal syndrome)
      b. Deficient prolactin inhibiting factor (hyperprolactinemia, Chiari-Frommel syndrome)
      c. Iatrogenic—drugs
      d. Congenital defects—hypogonadotropic eunuchoidism, anosomic amenorrhea, Kallmann's syndrome
  B. Psychogenic amenorrhea-Functional
    1. Stress
      a. Psychiatric disease
      b. Polycystic ovarian disease (PCO, Stein-Leventhal Syndrome).
      c. Hyperprolactinemia
      d. Anorexia nervosa
      e. Pseudocyesis
  C. Pituitary disease
    1. Insufficiency
      a. Destructive processes (Sheehan's and Simmond's disease)
    2. Tumors
      a. Chromophobe adenoma
        (1) "Non-functioning, partial

gonadotropin or TSH-secreting

    (2) Prolactinomas (Forbes-Albright)

  b. Acidophilic adenoma (acromegaly)

  c. Basophilic adenoma (Cushing's disease)

  3. Congenital defects (Hypogonadotropic eunuchoidism)

II. Gonadal Lesions—Ovarian Amenorrhea

  A. Insufficiency

    1. Congenital developmental defects—hermaphroditism and related conditions

      a. Gonadal dysgenesis (Turner's syndrome)

      b. True hermaphroditism

      c. Male hermaphroditism, (androgen insensitivity syndrome)

      d. Testicular feminization syndrome, (androgen insensitivity syndrome)

    2. Premature menopause

      a. Chromosomal

      b. Destructive

        (1) Iatrogenic—surgical, drugs

        (2) Irradiation, neoplasia, abscesses, viral disease

      c. Autoimmune disease

      d. "Constitutional"

  B. The insensitive ovary

  C. Tumors

    1. Arrhenoblastoma, hilus cells, adrenal rest

    2. Granulosa cell, thecoma

    3. Nonspecific with steroidogenic stroma

III. End Organ Lesions—Cryptomenorrhea

  A. Congenital defects

    1. Imperforate hymen

    2. Absence or atresia of vagina

    3. Septum of vagina

    4. Absence of uterus (congenital absence of Müllerian ducts, Rokitanski's syndrome)

  B. Traumatic

    1. Stenosis of vagina

    2. Stenosis of cervix

    3. Sclerosis of uterine cavity (Asherman's disease)

IV. Diseases of Intermediate Metabolism and Nutrition

  A. Metabolic disease

    1. Thyroid

      a. Hypothyroidism and hyperthyroidism

    2. Pancreas

      a. Diabetes mellitus

    3. Adrenal

      a. Congenital adrenal hyperplasia, adrenogenital syndrome, and related disturbances

      b. Cushing's disease and "stress obesity"

      c. Tumors

  B. Nutritional disturbances

    1. Malnutrition—weight loss and athlete's amenorrhea

    2. Exogenous obesity

  C. Excretory and metabolic organs

    1. Liver, cirrhosis

    2. Kidney, chronic nephritis (?)

  D. Chronic illness

V. Physiologic amenorrhea

  A. Delayed puberty

  B. Pregnancy

  C. Postpartum amenorrhea

  D. Menopause

Clinical Management

As oligomenorrhea and amenorrhea are symptoms of a great variety of difficulties, from organic brain disease to localized disorders in the female generative tract, it is obvious that extensive tests and examinations may be required in order to make a correct etiological diagnosis. Optimal success in the therapy of amenorrhea usually depends upon such a diagnosis. The most careful observer is occasionally confronted with a patient in whom no etiological factor is demonstrable. It is undoubtedly incorrect to classify all such cases as of psychogenic origin, but such a practice is not uncommon and, unti additional evidence is available, no more satisfactory solution can be suggested.

The endometrial findings among a group of amenorrheic and oligomenorrheic patients will show, in the main, atrophic or nonsecretory patterns. However, there will be a moderate number of hyperplastic patterns and a few with endometritis, including tuberculosis and other forms of inflammatory and sclerotic processes, scar tissue, retained placental fragments, and polyps. Having excluded a viable pregnancy, an endometrial biopsy is, therefore, a helpful diagnostic aid early in the investigation of amenorrhea. This is especially indicated in those patients with clinical signs of estrogen stimulation, as they are in a high risk category for endometrial cancer.

Investigative Procedures

There is no substitute for a good history. This must include a careful reconstruction of the setting of the amenorrhea, emphasizing such factors as relate to emotional stress; gain or loss of weight; acute or chronic illnesses; accidents or injuries; relationship to pregnancy; symptoms characteristic of metabolic diseases, such as polyuria and polydipsia for diabetes; susceptibility to temperature changes, changes in bowel habits, and energy for thyroid disease; and a family history relating to menstrual characteristics, fertility, metabolic disease, abnormalities of the immune system, or tuberculosis. In the case of primary amenorrhea the early developmental history, as well as the notation of possible birth trauma, is important.

Although a complete investigation for primary amenorrhea need not be undertaken until after the age of 17 years, a history should be obtained and a physical examination, including a pelvic or rectal examination, should be made whenever the patient, or her family, is concerned enough to consult a physician. If this is done, one can detect congenital anomalies at an early age, when the best psychological adjustment of both child and parents is possible.

In the investigation of secondary amenorrhea, after a viable pregnancy has been ruled out, an endometrial biopsy and, if any suspicion of tuberculosis exists, an acid-fast culture should be taken at the initial visit. This test is often a diagnostic shortcut and will indicate immediately (1) the ovarian-hypothalamic-pituitary function by the observed estrogen effect on the endometrium; (2) the possibility of pregnancy complications, old hyalinized retained placental fragments or shadow villae; and (3) end organ factors such as tuberculous endometritis and traumatic amenorrhea. A Papanicolaou smear with maturation index and cervical mucus study will also help in the evaluation of ovarian function and should be obtained at the preliminary examination. In all patients with primary amenorrhea, a karyotype must be considered and is usually indicated.

Other examinations will depend upon the specific problems involved. If no clue to the diagnosis is found in the history or physical examination, laboratory studies are ordered on the basis of the estimated estrogen milieu, which is indicative of the ovarian-hypothalamic-pituitary function. The estrogen milieu can be judged clinically by (1) the maturation index taken at the time of the pelvic examination, (2) the appearance of the cervix and cervical mucus as described in Chapter 29, and (3) the result of the endometrial biopsy. A low estrogen milieu must alert one to the most serious possibilities of either premature ovarian failure or a pituitary tumor. An FSH/LH assay should be obtained first, as it will usually separate lesions of ovarian origin from CNS (central nervous system), end organ, or metabolic disease. A high value signals a premature menopause. A low value makes a CNS lesion suspect, and a prolactin assay is then obtained followed by the appropriate neurological and radiological examination if prolactin is elevated. A high estrogen milieu is most commonly associated with polycystic ovarian disease (PCO), and the LH may be expected to be elevated. If the LH, but more especially the FSH, is low with a high estrogen milieu, an ovarian estrogen-secreting tumor must be suspected.

General Considerations for Therapy

Each patient must be treated according to the etiological factors involved and such specific therapy will be outlined under the specific headings. Only general considerations will be discussed in the following paragraphs.

Amenorrhea per se is not necessarily an indication for therapy. The production of a regular menstrual flow is possible by the administration of steroid hormones whenever there is a functioning end organ with no obstruction of the lower genital tract. **A single course of steroid therapy**, to assess the uterine competence, **may be justified**. However, the **prolonged use** of ovarian hormones to promote monthly menstrual bleeding is **rarely, if ever, indicated**. Such medication may, in fact, aggravate the condition by causing suppression of the hypothalamic LRH. The appearance of periodic bleeding is also prone to give both the physician and the patient a feeling of false security. The physician must differentiate in his own mind this type of **induced menstruation** from the **induction of ovulation**, which is quite a different matter. Careful analysis must be made of each individual patient to determine if her symptoms warrant treatment for the induction of ovulation. In patients with oligomenorrhea, there is often no necessity for any treatment other than reassurance, since fertility is usually not appreciably impaired. This advice obviously does not apply to those patients who present clear evidence of endocrinopathy of one sort or another, nor does it mean that improvement in general hygiene such as rest and proper food should not be advised whenever necessary regardless of the patient's age.

There are several general methods advocated for the production of ovulation when the amenorrhea is due to factors located in the nervous system, either psychosomatic or neurogenic: (1) Steroid therapy designed to trigger pituitary function. Although the normal hypothalamic pituitary unit will respond to this type of "feedback" control, the amenorrheic patient is not normal. This form of therapy is therefore usually unsuccessful and will not be discussed. (2) Gonadotropic therapy designed to replace pituitary function. (3) Clomiphene therapy which stimulates pituitary activity via the hypothalamus by blocking the estrogen inhibitory effect. (4) Hypothalamic hormone (LRH) stimulation which may directly stimulate synthesis and release of pituitary gonadotropins. This therapy is still in the research area. The dopamine agonist, bromoergocryptine (Parlodel, Sandoz), is specific therapy for those patients with hyperprolactinemia.

Gonadotropin Therapy

For the proper use, rather than abuse, of human pituitary gonadotropin, it is necessary (1) to make an etiological diagnosis in order to select the proper patients for therapy, (2) to arrive at a proper dose schedule, and (3) to be familiar with possible complications which may arise.

Any lesion of central origin (see Etiological Classification of Amenorrhea) will respond to gonadotropic therapy. However, the classic indication is hypogonadotropic eunuchoidism. It is obvious that individuals having pituitary or brain tumors should be carefully excluded and, in consideration of the treatment of patients with psychogenic amenorrhea or Sheehan's disease, factors other than gynecological should play a major role in the selection of suitable patients.

If the patient has a normal pituitary function, this will invalidate the dosage calculation, and complications, ovarian cysts, and multiple pregnancies may arise due to overdosage. The Stein-Leventhal syndrome is specifically important to identify as the polycystic ovary is peculiarly sensitive to gonadotropin stimulation.

A highly purified preparation of gonadotropins (HMG) has been prepared from the urine of menopausal women. This contains a 1:1 ratio of FSH and LH and can be used to stimulate growth of a follicle prior to induction of ovulation by hCG, which is substituted for the pituitary LH surge. Human pituitary extracts are not commercially available.

The dosage schedule which has usually been found satisfactory is 1500–2500 IU equivalents of FSH, standardized against the second European standard menopausal urine preparation (IRP-HMG-2). This is given in two injections daily of 75 IU, or 75 and 150 IU, for approximately 7–10 days. Although patients will respond to less frequent injections, daily administration is more efficient. It is necessary to induce a urinary estrogen level of between 50 and 150 μg/24 hours by the Brown technique to ensure proper maturation of the follicle for induction of ovulation. Estrogen values above 150 μg/24 hours indicate overstimulation and under these circumstances, the ovulatory stimulus of hCG should not be given. When serum estrogen values are used for monitoring ovulation induction, the lowest level compatible with ovulation is 300 pg/ml, and 900 pg/ml the highest level compatible with safety. Most observers agree that a value of over 400 pg/ml is more often associated with successful ovulation. The clinical evaluation, a daily vaginal smear for a maturation index, and observation for the occurrence of cervical dilatation and estrogenic mucus should be used to judge when the serum or urine estrogen assays should be obtained and pelvic examinations made to determine ovarian size. Ultrasonography should be used to confine numbers of follicles and sizes. If no response has been obtained by 14 days, treatment should be discontinued and reinstituted at a higher dose level. It is more efficient to give the highest FSH dose at the beginning of therapy rather than to increase the dosage if no response is seen. At the peak estrogen response, following a 1-day rest period,

10,000 IU of hCG is given. In our experience although 1500–2500 IU HMG is usually an adequate dose schedule to induce follicle maturation in the hypogonadotropic, amenorrheic patient, each patient must be individualized and occasionally a total dose of 3,000 IU or more of HMG will be necessary.

The major complications of gonadotropin therapy are superovulations with multiple follicular cyst formation and subsequent multiple pregnancies. These complications have led to death through rupture of the cysts, or rupture of the uterus during pregnancy.

Indirect Methods of Pituitary Stimulation

Clomiphene

Clomiphene citrate, a derivative of a weak synthetic estrogen, tri-para-anisyl-chloro-ethylene (Tace), is an effective ovulatory drug in the human. It acts as a competitive inhibitor of estrogen, apparently blocking estrogen at the hypothalamic level and thus removing the inhibition of pituitary gonadotropin production and allowing a gonadotropic flood. The increased gonadotropic secretion causes increased ovarian stimulation with excretion of urinary estrogen. The follicular estrogen, after cessation of therapy, induces the LH flood and ovulation with normal or inadaqute corpus luteum function.

The success rate, as with any drug, depends upon the care and skill used in making an etiologic diagnosis when selecting patients suitable for therapy. The classic indication for clomiphene treatment is hypothalamic hypogonadotropism.

The following criteria should be used in selection of patients for clomiphene therapy. There should be some evidence of pituitary function, e.g., the total urinary gonadotropins should be within the low normal range, and clinical evidence of estrogen activity should be present, giving additional evidence that the pituitary FSH and LH function is relatively intact. A normal prolactin assay must preclude a lesion which will respond to specific therapy such as bromoergocryptine (Parlodel). The thyroid and adrenal function should be normal, as should the nutritional status. Radiologic examination of the sella turcica or examination of visual fields should be negative for evidence of intracranial tumors. Those patients who have destruction of the pituitary from tumors, Sheehan's disease, or **primary ovarian failure** (premature menopause) should be specifically excluded from therapy. Except for the unusual patient who has primary amenorrhea and polycystic ovarian disease, most patients with primary amenorrhea will not respond to clomiphene.

The most serious complications reported are the occurrence of multiple ovarian cysts with rupture and multiple pregnancies. As the pathological picture is similar to that seen with pituitary gonadotropin administration, it seems clear that these effects are the results of pituitary overstimulation. If care is taken to use an initial low dosage over a short period and the patient is observed for evidence of ovarian stimulation and not retreated until the initial reaction has subsided, this complication can usually be avoided. Transitory blurring of vision and hot flushes are infrequent symptoms. Liver function studies should be made if there is a history of any liver disease, as clomiphene is excreted through the bile ducts.

Prior to initiation of therapy, the patient should have had an FSH and LH assay, a normal pelvic examination, vaginal cytology, endometrial biopsy, and mucus examinaton and should be on a basal body temperature chart. An injection of 50 mg of progesterone should be given intramuscularly to induce withdrawal bleeding. This not only ensures the integrity of the endometrium but also precludes a pregnancy. If the infertility investigation has not been completed, plans for its completion should be made at this time. Although many dosage schedules of clomiphene have been reported, the following is recommended (Table 30.1).

In the absence of ovulation the schedule can be changed in three ways: (1) increase the amount, (2) change duration of administration of the drug, or (3) give chorionic gonadotropin adjunctively. (Table 30.2). Increasing the amount of clomiphene increases the FSH stimulation; increasing the duration of the administration increases the LH stimulation; and the addition of hCG substitutes for an inadequate LH surge. Unfortunately, there are no clinical criteria which will help in determining which of the first two variations should be necessary; therefore, a systematic trial of variations must be used (Table 30.3).

The third variation of the clomiphene

Table 30.1

Clomiphene Ovulation Induction—Initial Schedule and Monitoring

How?
1. Initial schedule
   Progesterone 50 mg im
    Clomid 50 mg × 5 days, after 5 days
2. Monitor—onset of Clomid therapy is day 1
   Cervical mucus day 14
   BBT day 24
    Biphasic—Endometrial biopsy
    Monophasic
     Check for pregnancy day 35
     Negative
      Progesterone 50 mg im
      5 Days begin different schedule

Table 30.2

Variations of Schedule for Clomiphene Ovulation Induction

1. Increase amount of Clomid—preferentially increases FSH
2. Increase duration of Clomid—preferentially increases LH
3. Add hCG—substitutes for LH surge

Table 30.3

Variations of Dosage and Duration of Clomiphene Therapy

Clomid	Total Amount
mg/day	*mgm*
50 × 5	250
50 × 7	350
100 × 5	500
50 × 10	500
150 × 5	750
100 × 7	700
200 × 5	1,000
100 × 10	1,000
150 × 7	1,050
200 × 7	1,400
200 × 10	2,000

schedule, by the addition of hCG, chorionic gonadotropin, should be made only in those patients in whom a mucus flood is seen 14 days or so after clomiphene therapy is begun. If this mucus flood is seen and either no ovulation occurs, or ovulation with a deficient luteal phase occurs, this is evidence of an inadequate preovulatory LH surge. The administration of 5,000 units of hCG at the time of the optimum cervical mucus and repeated in 5 days will usually substitute for this defect.

With careful manipulation of clomiphene dosage and the indicated addition of hCG, approximately 95% of anovulatory patients can be made to ovulate.

Although most patients who respond to therapy continue to do so in a surprisingly regular manner, there is an occasional patient who responds erratically. Such patients should be checked periodically with serum FSH assays to rule out the possibility of a beginning premature menopause.

Although no adverse effects on the fetus have been reported in humans treated during early pregnancy, clomiphene has produced fetal anomalies in experimental animals. It is therefore recommended that treatment be avoided during pregnancy.

Therapy may be continued as long as desired by the patient if the physician has assured that all other infertility factors are normal. However, all therapy should be interrupted for at least 2 months after six successful cycles. This will determine if normal physiology has been reestablished.

Luteinizing Release Hormone

Schedules of LRH administration developed by Knobil's laboratory using the Rhesus monkey as a model, seem to be successful for induction of ovulation in the human. These investigators found that a low-dose pulse of LRH given every 2 hours was necessary to reproduce the normal FSH and LH patterns seen in a normal ovulatory cycle.

The changes in FSH and LH serum values throughout the cycle depend apparently upon the pulsatile LRH release, the differential FSH and LH circulation times, and the estrogen feedback. The feedback by inhibin on FSH, although not so clear, is also probably important.

Knowledge of these fundamental physiologic mechanisms promises to make LRH a most useful tool in the future for both induction of ovulation and diagnosis of unusual central nevous system causes of amenorrhea. At the present writing, this is still in the developmental stage.

Thyroid

Thyroid has long been advocated as of therapeutic value in the correction of menstrual disorders; however, its empiric and indiscriminate use should be discouraged. It will prove useful only when there is evidence of a low thyroid function as reflected by some reliable thyroid assay.

Nutrition

A good nutritional status is mandatory for the ultimate success of any treatment and must not be overlooked in our zeal for less mundane therapy.

SPECIFIC CONSIDERATIONS

Lesions of Central Nervous System

Lesions of central origin can be subdivided into three major groups: (1) neurogenic, (2) psychogenic, and (3) pituitary. Pituitary amenorrhea may be classified into pituitary insufficiency related to (1) trauma, (2) tumors, and (3) congenital abnormalities of gonadotropic hormone production.

Neurogenic Lesions—Hypothalamic and Above

Organic Brain Disease

The diagnosis of organic brain disease is made with the help of the physical examination and history of encephalitis or related infections, accidents, injuries, or exposure to toxic substances such as lead or carbon monoxide. Laboratory findings are characterized by a low or low normal gonadotropin production, and low estrogen production as indicated by a moderately atrophic vaginal smear, and poor cervical mucus. Depending upon the severity or the position of the neurological lesion, there may be associated abnormalities of laboratory findings related to thyroid, adrenal, or pancreatic functions. The neurologic examination and electroencephalogram are valuable diagnostic aids.

The prognosis in patients with neurogenic amenorrhea is poor except for those following acute trauma. Under these circumstances, recovery may occur.

Adequate pituitary hormone therapy should be successful in bypassing the neurological lesions.

Hypothalamic Dysfunction—Insufficiency

The characteristic pattern of amenorrhea related to idiopathic hypothalamic failure is infrequent, but usually **ovulatory**, menstruations; the menstrual irregularity dates from the menarche and may be associated with a family history of menstrual irregularities. There is no history of psychogenic factors and on physical examination there are no detectable neurological abnormalities. The FSH and LH values are similar to those in patients with organic brain disease.

There is often no indication for therapy among this group of patients, as pregnancy frequently occurs without difficulty. However, if infertility is a problem, regular menstruation with a reasonable expectation of ensuing pregnancy can usually be initiated with clomiphene.

Polycystic Ovarian Disase (PCO, Stein-Leventhal Syndrome). The Stein-Leventhal syndrome, now commonly referred to as polycystic ovarian syndrome (PCO), is defined in this text in reference to an anovulatory patient with a high LH and normal FSH value. In addition to the two symptoms required for the diagnosis, anovulatory menstrual dysfunction and an elevated LH value, bilateral ovarian enlargement and a mild or marked degree of hirsutism are frequently present. One of the most difficult differential diagnoses is between polycystic ovarian disease and Cushing's disease (Fig. 30.1).

Pathology. Macroscopically, the ovaries are pearly white in appearance with multiple cysts beneath the capsule. Microscopically, they are characterized by a capsule formed by hyalinization of the interstitial tissue of the cortex directly beneath the germinal epithelium. This hyalinization may engulf the primordial follicles. There are numerous follicular cysts which characteristically have a thin granulosal lining with a marked luteinization of the theca interna. There are no corpora lutea present, although there may be evidence of old corpora albicantia (occasionally, however, even in a typical Stein-Leventhal syndrome, a sporadic ovulation can occur). As all of these elements are present at times in the normal ovary and the findings represent simply an exaggeration of the normal, there is no **diagnostic** pathological picture. Therefore, one can only report the ovarian findings as "compatible with" those seen with the Stein-Leventhal syndrome. However, although a positive finding is not diagnostic, a negative correlation, e.g., "not compatible with," is good evidence that one is *not* dealing with a Stein-Leventhal syndrome.

Symptoms. The presenting clinical symptoms can be infertility, amenorrhea, oligo-

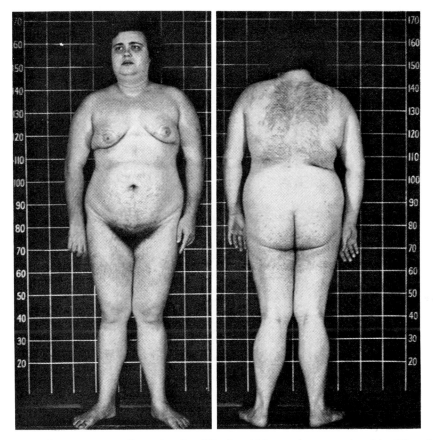

Figure 30.1. A Stein syndrome illustrating the difficulty which may be encountered in differentiating the condition from Cushing's syndrome by the physical appearance of the patient.

menorrhea, or dysfunctional uterine bleeding. Mild or marked hirsutism is usually present and there may be periodic abdominal discomfort from bilateral ovarian enlargement.

Pathogenesis. Although the exact pathogenesis is still not completely understood, the syndrome can be classified as a disease of the neuroendocrine homeostasis control mechanisms. These diseases are characterized by excessive glandular activity in the presence of paradoxical excessive target organ hormones, hyperresponsiveness to stimulation, and decreased responsiveness to suppression in the apparent absence of tumor.

In some patients with PCO disease there is an estrogen insensitivity. As clomiphene, an antiestrogen, will usually correct the problem, it seems to be a dysfunction rather than a true defect. However, one does occasionally see a patient who apparently has a true defect. Such patients usually have delayed menarche and greatly elevated LH values and are re-

fractory to Clomid. It is, therefore, necessary to use gonadotrophic therapy for induction of ovulation in this specific circumstance.

Therapy. Successful therapy of any condition depends upon knowledge of the basic pathophysiology. The intracellular mechanisms concerned in this peculiar disturbance of feedback control are not understood. Clomiphene will temporarily interrupt it but does not cure it. Wedge resection will temporarily "cure" it, apparently by interrupting the synthesis of ADD, but permanent cures are rare. Relapses are the rule. The inciting cause is likewise usually obscure. It would seem from a review of case histories that there may be multiple etiologic factors, therefore multiple therapies might be anticipated.

Steroids, either androgens or estrogens, are blocking agents for hypothalamic neurons. Small estrogen or androgen steroid-producing ovarian or adrenal tumors are occasionally associated with a clinical picture of PCO syndrome. Fifteen percent of patients in our series had such tumors as the primary etiology of the syndrome. Operative removal is a definitive therapy.

Rarely, the excessive androgen is caused by an associated attenuated congenital adrenal hyperplasia. However, by far, the most common factor in our series was chronic emotional stress. An elevated prolactin value may be seen occasionally with PCO disease, perhaps also indicating stress. The indications for therapy are infertility, dysfunctional uterine bleeding, and/or hirsutism.

Infertility. Therapy for infertility by induction of ovulation with clomiphene is successful in 48% of patients. Although one might expect that patients with a high LH would require less Clomid, this is not our experience. Some patients, however, are brittle, with a very small margin of safety between the successful therapeutic dose which causes ovulation and that which causes hyperstimulation. It is, therefore, important if it is necessary to increase the dose, that this be done gradually, alternating monthly with an increase in the duration of therapy. In spite of the endogenously high LH, some patients will require hCG as an additional stimulus for ovulation.

The patients who have specific factors, either adrenal or ovarian, require specific therapy. Those patients with attenuated congenital adrenal hyperplasia (CAH) will respond to cortisone therapy, 50 mg daily of cortisone acetate for 1 month, reduced to 37.5 mg and then to 25 mg as a maintenance dose. Those patients with hyperprolactinemia will respond to bromocryptine, 2.5 mg a day. This, however, is not definitive therapy and microadenomas of the pituitary must always be ruled out.

A bilateral ovarian wedge resection operation, originally recommended by Stein, can be offered to patients who have had six or more courses of Clomid with successful induction of ovulation but no pregnancy or patients who are brittle; those who do not respond with ovulation to one dosage and at the next higher dose increment are uncomfortable with large hyperstimulated ovaries. Surgery has a chance of being definitive therapy; also, the 15% of patients with small steroid-producing tumors of the ovary will be diagnosed by this technique. The recurrence rate is low *if* patients are carefully selected. When surgery is to be done, it must be performed with the same meticulous care used in tubal reconstructive surgery if one is not to produce more damage than one is correcting. The pregnancy rate is between 75% and 85%.

Dysfunctional Uterine Bleeding. Patients with PCO syndrome are in a high-risk category for the development of endometrial cancer. It is, therefore, extremely important to have an endometrial biopsy on all patients when this diagnosis is entertained. One cannot tell by the bleeding pattern what the microscopic appearance of the endometrium will be.

The choice of therapy depends upon the histologic findings. If the pattern is a **simple proliferative** one or **mild endometrial hyperplasia** and hirsutism is not a problem, 5 mg of norethindrone daily for 5 days every 6 weeks will usually induce fairly regular bleeding phases with 6-week intervals. If hirsutism is of concern, the use of cyclic high-dose estrogen oral contraceptives is indicated for both problems. An endometrial biopsy periodically, probably every year, is mandatory with this therapy. If the pattern is **marked** or **atypical hyperplasia**, Megace 40 mg a day for 3 months should be used in an effort to reverse the hyperplastic pattern. The biopsy should be taken at the end of the therapy and dilatation and curettage should be done 1 month after treatment has been discontinued. If the pattern has reverted to simple proliferative endometrium, a progestational drug can be used in a cyclic fashion as described above. To document persistence of a benign pattern, a repeat biopsy must be taken while the patient continues on therapy. If atypical hyperplasia persists and family formation is not of concern, some consideration should be given to hysterectomy. If this is unacceptable or contraindicated for any reason, induction of ovulation by clomiphene is perhaps the best and most physiologic method for reversing the hyperestrogenic endometrial pattern. Under these circumstances, however, if pregnancy is undesirable, barrier method birth control must be practiced.

Hirsutism. If hirsutism is a problem, Givens et al. have recommended the use of oral contraceptive pills. Although theoretically sound, the clinical results are often not dramatic. One must expect an arrest, rather than a regression, of the hirsutism.

Shaving, wax removal, dipilatories, and electrolysis are still the most practical methods of therapy.

Hyperprolactinemic Amenorrhea. *Definition.* With the availability of a specific radioimmunoassay for identification of prolactin and hypercycloidal axial tomography for the identification of pituitary microadenomas, multiple clinical syndromes have merged into one and now are classified as hyperprolactinemic amenorrhea.

Pathophysiology. The pathophysiology of the diverse clinical symptoms of menstrual irregularities and infertility associated with hyperprolactinemia is not completely clear. It is often impossible to establish whether the lesion is in the hypothalamus or a pituitary adenoma. Likewise it is impossible to determine if the menstrual abnormalities are a cause and effect of **excessive prolactin** from the **pituitary** or an association related to a **hypothalamic dopamine deficiency.**

Although patients with hyperprolactinemia usually have normal FSH and lowered LH values, this is by no means consistent. The most consistent finding is a defective "positive estrogen feedback," with failure of the ovulatory LH surge.

Symptomatology. Galactorrhea, defined as any breast secretion which is bilateral, is the only presenting symptom of hyperprolactinemia. However, a substantial minority of patients with galactorrhea have normal prolactin values while an additional group with menstrual irregularities *without* galactorrhea, have hyperprolactinemia (Table 30.4).

Galactorrhea with Regular Menses. Patients with galactorrhea and normal menses have an elevated prolactin in approximately 15% of the cases. If infertility is the problem, and hyperprolactinemia is found, one should suspect anovulatory cycles or a defective luteal phase. The galactorrhea in the remaining 85% of the patients is usually induced by nipple manipulation, but chest wall and spinal cord nerve root tumors must be ex-

cluded. Efforts should be made to prevent nipple manipulation during a 2-month period. If discharge remains a problem, a prolactin assay should be obtained. Bromocryptine is usually helpful in controlling symptoms even in the absence of an elevated prolactin assay.

Secondary Amenorrhea, Oligomenorrhea, Dysfunctional Uterine Bleeding. Approximately 30% of patients with irregular menses will have hyperprolactinemia in the absence of galactorrhea. Therefore, any patient who has protracted secondary amenorrhea with low or low-normal gonadotropins (FSH and LH) requires a prolactin assay. Any patient who has a history of menstrual irregularities, following pregnancy or lactation or associated with response to stress, oral contraception, or phenothiazine usage, should have a prolactin assay after FSH and LH assays are obtained. If the gonadotropin assays are elevated, indicating ovarian failure, or if there is a clear-cut diagnosis of anorexia nervosa, a prolactin assay is not indicated. As prolactin may be elevated in the polycystic ovarian syndrome (PCO), one must consider the possibility of a prolactin assay in patients with this syndrome if response to conventional management is unsatisfactory.

Infertility. As an elevated prolactin is associated with abnormalities of the preovulatory LH surge, infertility patients with a diagnosis of a luteal phase defect or of anovulatory cycles should have a prolactin assay. The so-called "normal infertile couple" also deserves the benefit of this additional test. The infertile male who is impotent, especially if associated with a lowered serum testosterone, a low LH and oligospermia, may also suffer from hyperprolactinemia.

Interpretation of an Elevated Prolactin As-

Table 30.4
Relation of Galactorrhoea to Hyperprolactinaemia and Various Clinical Conditions[a]

	Normal Prolactin Patients	Hyperprolactinaemia Patients	Total Patients
Amenorrhoea			
Galactorrhoea	46 (44.4%)	60 (56.6%)	106
No galactorrhoea	18 (72%)	7 (28%)	25
Regular Menses			
Galactorrhoea	64 (84.2%)	12 (15.8%)	76
Pituitary Tumors			
Galactorrhoea	6 (12.5%)	42 (87.5%)	48
No galactorrhoea	8 (30%)	19 (70%)	27

[a] From Kleinberg et al.: *New England Journal of Medicine,* 296: 589, 1977, and Sepälä et al.: *Lancet, 1:* 1154, 1976.

say. Factors Which Cause Elevations. The normal prolactin values are given in Chapter 2. Factors which elevate prolactin can be classified into three categories:

1. Physiologic Elevations. Prolactin is secreted in a pulsatile pattern with a diurnal variation. A single assay can represent either the apex or the nadir of the pulse. The prolactin rise begins with sleep. The diurnal rise is highest at the end of sleep. It is, therefore, important to obtain an assay at least 2 hours after waking. As any stress can cause an elevation of prolactin, blood should not be taken immediately after a stressful interview or examination, such as a pelvic examination. Pregnancy and suckling are the most potent physiologic stimuli. If an elevated prolactin value is obtained, the assay should be repeated under as optimum conditions as possible.

2. Drugs. A number of categories of drugs can cause an elevated prolactin level: neuroleptics, most commonly the **tranquilizing drugs** such as phenothiazine derivatives; **steroids**, estrogens, and some progestational steroids, including cyproterone and danazol; **opiates**, including β-enkephalin and morphine. Thyrotrophic releasing hormone (**TRH**) also causes elevation of prolactin which may be physiologic. **Anesthesia** is associated with an elevation which may be related to the stress of the operative procedure.

3. Associated Diseases. Two disease states associated with hyperprolactinemia must always be excluded. Severe **hypothyroidism**, usually resulting from Hashimoto's thyroiditis with destruction of the thyroid, can lead to an elevated TRH. Under these circumstances, pituitary thyrotrophic stimulating hormone (TSH) is always elevated. As occult hypothyroidism is an extremely difficult diagnosis to make, TSH should always be obtained when an elevated prolactin is reported. Severely **impaired renal function** is also associated with hyperprolactinemia.

Differential Diagnosis: Prolactinoma or "Hyperplasia." The differential diagnosis of a prolactinoma or pituitary "hyperplasia" is largely determined by the history and the prolactin value. Levels over 100 ng/ml are highly suspicious of tumor. As there is no diagnostic method which will absolutely exclude a tumor, all patients must be regarded as suspect of harboring a tumor unless clinical symptoms and laboratory findings regress spontaneously.

History. The history will decide if one is dealing with a factor known to stimulate prolactin production. A history of long duration is more frequently associated with an adenoma.

Prolactin Values Less Than 40 ng/ml. If (1) the prolactin value is below 40 ng/ml, and (2) the history is of short duration and suggests a postpartum, postlactation, postpill, or postneuroleptic drug association, the possibility of a tumor is slight. Anterior and lateral skull films should be ordered. A tumor with suprasellar extension or a craniopharyngioma may be associated with bony erosion of the adjacent structures. A ballooned or deformed sella may indicate an empty sella syndrome. An ophthalmologic examination with Goldman planimetry and color visual fields will serve as a reference point if future follow-up becomes necessary. If the sella is normal by conventional x-ray, one may feel comfortable in observing the patient and repeating the prolactin in 6 months or, if indicated, treating the patient with a dopamine agonist, bromocryptine, without axial cycloidal polytomography.

If, in the 6-month follow-up, the prolactin is not rising but is still in the range below 40 ng/ml and bromocryptine has not been given, it should now be given. Under both of these circumstances, the patient must understand the necessity and reason for routine follow-up. If a repeat prolactin assay at 6 months shows rising levels, polytomography must be obtained.

Prolactin Values Over 40 ng/ml. If the prolactin is over 40 ng/ml, an ophthalmological examination as described above should be ordered. If this is abnormal, the patient can be referred directly to a neurosurgeon who will order imaging investigations at his discretion. If visual fields are normal, anterior and lateral skull films serve as a screen. If visual fields and skull x-rays are normal, computerized axial cycloidal tomography must be ordered to exclude a microadenoma.

If evidence of sella erosion, irregularity, or ballooning is obtained radiologically, the empty sella syndrome must be ruled out. A pneumoencephalogram or its equivalent must always be done prior to advising a surgical transsphenoidal approach for a micro- or macroadenoma.

Therapy. General Considerations. Selection of therapy is controversial because the underlying pathophysiology of hyperprolactinemia is not firmly established, nor is the life history of the hyperprolactinemia "syndrome" known. There are no dynamic tests or series of tests which will differentiate a pituitary tumor from hyperplasia, or a primary pituitary defect from a primary hypothalamic defect as the source of the prolactinemia. It would seem that a conservative approach would be to treat only those patients surgically who can be shown by radiologic techniques to have a reasonable expectation of a tumor. Medical therapy, such as a dopamine agonist bromergocryptine, might be reserved for all other individuals.

Medical Therapy. As prolactin is inhibited by dopamine, replacement therapy with dopamine agonists, the ergot derivatives bromocryptine (Parlodel) and lergotrile mesylate, is the treatment of choice for those patients without tumors and presumably with some interference in delivery of dopamine to the pituitary lactotrophs.

It has been shown that most prolactinomas will also respond to Parlodel. This indicates that there are dopamine receptors on the tumor membranes. Tumors may therefore be suppressed by medical therapy.

Specific Case Selection for Medication. Patients can be divided into three major categories for establishing a therapeutic approach.

1. Patients with Prolactin Values Below 40 ng/ml. Those patients who have a history (1) suggesting a recent exposure to a prolactin stimulus, e.g., pregnancy, suckling, or drugs and (2) of short duration, can be observed for 3–6 months after cessation of the prolactin stimulus and then the prolactin assay repeated. If the prolactin remains elevated and/or menses have not become regular, bromocryptine is indicated. If prolactin is rising, investigation must be initiated to exclude a tumor.

2. Patients with Prolactin Values above 40 ng/ml without Evidence of Tumor. Having ruled out occult hypothyroidism and discontinued all lactotropic stimulants, bromocryptine should be started at the time the second prolactin assay is taken. If pregnancy is desired, it should be precluded by barrier methods until prolactin has been reduced to normal values and an endometrial biopsy indi-

cates a normal luteal phase. Previously undetected tumors may enlarge rapidly with pregnancy, giving pressure to the optic nerves and causing temporary blindness or occasionally optic atrophy with irreversible changes. However, most pregnancies progress normally without ophthalmologic complications. In the event of pregnancy during drug administration, the drug should be stopped immediately. All pregnant patients must be followed monthly with prolactin assays and visual field examinations. If symptoms of headache or visual disturbance warrant, these examinations should be made more frequently. Although the prolactin value will rise rapidly after discontinuing the drug, it will reach a plateau in 2 weeks and then will parallel the normal pregnancy rise. Therefore, any unusual increase can be detected.

3. With Evidence of Tumor. All patients with evidence of tumor must be considered for neurosurgery. There are indications, however, that the microadenomas can be treated successfully by medical rather than surgical therapy. Radiologic evidence of tumor regression has been described with remodeling and recalcification of the sella similar to that seen in severe, prolonged hypothyroidism after thyroid therapy. If the decision to try medical suppression is made, prolactin assays are requested every month. If no tumor progression is demonstrated, and prolactin is normalized, a pregnancy can be attempted after the third normal menstrual cycle.

Bromergocryptine (Parlodel). Bromergocryptine, a dopamine agonist which acts at the dopamine receptor site on the lactotrophic cell membrane, is the available medical drug for therapy. As dopamine can cause hypotension and nausea, these are the major side effects to be expected. If the drug is given just prior to retiring, and if therapy is begun with a low dose and gradually increased to the therapeutic level, symptoms are rarely a problem. The amount of drug required depends upon the level of the prolactin. One should begin with half a tablet, 1.25 mg at night, and increase in 4 days to 2.5 mg. This is usually a sufficient dose to lower prolactin to a normal level within 2 or 3 weeks if the initial value was less than 100 ng/ml. Delay in increasing the dose is advised if prolactin suppression is occurring satisfactorily. Experience indicates that the first or second menstrual cycle on therapy may be anovulatory or show a deficient luteal phase, while subsequent ones on the same dosage may be normal. If adequate prolactin suppression is not accomplished, or if luteal function remains abnormal, the dose can be gradually increased to 5 or a maximum of 7.5 mg daily. Much larger doses, 20–60 mg a day, have been used to control inoperable tumors, but in the absence of tumor, doses over 7.5 mg/day are usually excessive. Unfortunately, most patients will have a return of hyperprolactinemia and associated symptoms when therapy is discontinued.

Surgical Therapy. When there is radiologic evidence of a tumor, as stated above, neurosurgery must be considered. Macroadenomas should have transsphenoidal surgery if possible. Because of the usual ventrolateral locations, prolactin secreting adenomas are especially amenable to this type of surgical resection.

In spite of apparently complete removal of an adenoma, not all patients attain a normal postoperative prolactin value.

Bromocryptine has been used to suppress tumor growth, apparently successfully, in some but not all cases. Therefore, if tumor has been left behind in an operative procedure, bromocryptine, again, is indicated.

The question of what will happen to a microadenoma if left untreated surgically is still unanswered.

Irradiation. The most satisfactory irradiation therapy is the directed proton beam. This treatment can be delivered at a single therapeutic session on an otpatient basis. As far as is known, it is without sequelae. The effects are not fully realized for 1 year.

Supravoltage cobalt irradiation should be reserved for inoperable tumors. It requires 4 or 5 weeks for completion of therapy and may be associated with damaged pituitary and hypothalamic vasculature, or both, which can result in later development of panhypopituitarism. The reproductive history of patients following this type of therapy is, therefore, understandably poor.

Pregnancy. Although no teratogenicity of bromocryptine has been reported, it would seem wise to monitor patients on bromocryptine carefully. If a pregnancy should occur during therapy, bromocryptine should be stopped.

The major concern in following patients with hyperprolactinemia who have become pregnant is the possibility of the development of a rapidly growing pituitary adenoma during the pregnancy.

Patients who become pregnant must be monitored monthly with prolactin assays and visual field studies during the pregnancy or more frequently if symptoms warrant such. Frequent radiologic monitoring is to be discouraged because of possible irradiation hazard. In the event of acute ophthalmologic symptoms, bromergocryptine may be restarted and frequently will control symptoms. If the visual symptoms are not rapidly relieved by bromocryptine, some type of decompression procedure will be necessary to prevent permanent damage to the optic nerve.

Iatrogenic Drugs. Phenothiazine derivatives and oral contraceptive drugs, corticosteroids, morphine and morphine derivatives, have been referred to above as possible iatrogenic causes of the inappropriate lactation syndrome. Nevertheless, it is important to rule out other causes of amenorrhea before accepting an iatrogenic etiology. The two most severe problems which must be excluded are (1) a pituitary or central nervous system tumor and, (2) a premature menopause. Thus, FSH, LH, and prolactin assays are necessary.

The prognosis in this form of amenorrhea is good and no treatment is necessary if the patient can be persuaded that menses will recur if enough time is allowed. It is indeed unwise, however, to compound the situation by prescribing additional steroid therapy to "regulate" a cycle. Clomiphene therapy is usually effective. If there is an associated hyperprolactinemia, of course, bromocryptine is specific treatment. Exogenous pituitary gonadotrophins are indicated only when all else fails.

Congenital Defects (CNS Lesions, Neurogenic). Anosmic Amenorrhea, (Kallmann's Syndrome), Hypogonadotrophic Eunuchoidism. Isolated hypogonadotropic hypogonadism can be caused by a familial LRH deficiency associated with agenesis or hypoplasia of the olfactory bulb and various other related abnormalities. In addition to this cause of hypogonadotropic hypogonadism, an isolated gonadotropin deficiency possibly related to defective LRH stimulation by defective neurotransmitters, there is the patient who apparently has a congenital absence of LRH or an abnormal LRH, as evidenced by development of LRH antibodies following clinical LRH administration. To be described also in this chapter is the absence of pituitary gonadotropins or the secretion of defective gonadotropins, which are biologically inactive. It is, therefore, both interesting and important to realize that hypogonadotropic eunuchoidism is not a single disease entity, but can be associated with pathology in the adrenergic nervous system, hypothalamus, or pituitary.

All types of hypogonadotropic hypogonadism will respond to ovulation induction by pituitary gonadotropin substitution therapy. However, when a satisfactory mode of LRH stimulation is accomplished, patients with hypothalamic or CNS lesions can be treated by LRH administration.

Psychogenic Amenorrhea—Functional

Psychogenic amenorrhea can be considered, in the broad sense, as the individual's response to stress.

The physician's diagnosis of chronic stress depends upon his evaluation of the patient's interpretation of, and response to, everyday life as "stress." Ordinary life situations can be perceived by a vulnerable individual as stress, and the inability to cope is related to deficient personality characteristics and/or lack of specific social supports. This inability to cope with everyday life situations leads to dysfunctions of the nervous system which are reflected in disturbed physiology. The disturbed physiology, in this case amenorrhea, presents in association with a specific neurogenic pattern, depending upon the individual. This pattern may be polycystic ovarian disease (PCO), amenorrhea/galactorrhea, anorexia nervosa, or more rarely in our experience at the present time, pseudocyesis.

A major point of interest is what determines the length of time from cessation of trauma or stress to subsequent recovery. In acute traumatic episodes, as best illustrated in emotional shock, or physical shock therapy, the usual recovery time, in relation to ovulation and menstruation, is between 6 weeks and 3 months. However, this time can be greatly protracted. In seriously disturbed patients treatment consists of psychiatric care and the therapeutic success is directly related to psychiatric therapy. Pregnancy is contraindicated in patients with severe psychiatric disorders.

Chronic Stress (CNS Lesions, Psychogenic)

As mentioned above, chronic stress without severe psychiatric disorder may be manifest by several specific syndromes: polycystic ovarian disease, the hyperprolactinemic syndrome, anorexia nervosa, and simple hypothalamic amenorrhea manifest by low gonadotropins in the presence of normal weight without hyperprolactinemia or elevated LH. It is extremely helpful to the patient to have the psychogenic stress problems elaborated and explained by the physician. Alleviation of the stress or an adjustment of response to stress will frequently result in regular menstrual periods. In patients who have no serious psychiatric problems, it is quite satisfactory to induce ovulation with clomiphene or specific therapy as indicated. It is neither acceptable nor indicated to "induce regular menses" with steroids such as oral contraceptives. Such a course not only masks the condition but may aggravate the problem.

Anorexia Nervosa. Definition. Anorexia nervosa is a disease of adolescence characterized by severe malnutrition but without an associated lethargy. The most frequent age distribution is between 11 and 21 years and 90% of the patients are female. The nomenclature is poor as the weight loss is purposeful and it is not a true anorexia but a pathologic obsession with body size resulting in inability, or refusal, to recognize hunger. In association with this, there is also inability to recognize body image and inability to interpret fatigue. This latter results in constant restless activity and inappropriate expenditure of energy. The psychiatric problem, although often associated with acute or chronic stress, is thought to be initiated by the struggle of an obsessive-compulsive perfectionist to obtain initiative and self-directed identity. This occurs in a family which has a tendency to either confuse the signals or to continue uncompromising domination of a bright individual who is attempting to develop adult status. The weight fixation is interpreted as the intense desire of these bright, perfectionist individuals to develop complete self-control.

Although most of the physical and laboratory findings are a result of the severe chronic malnutrition, this is secondary to the severe emotional disturbance.

History. The history is often related to an

acute traumatic episode but may be more insidious. The symptom of amenorrhea occurs early in the illness and can, therefore, be used as a marker to determine the duration of the disease, which is helpful in making a prognosis. The patient is obsessed with fear of obesity and this weight fixation is associated with the use of every kind of excess one can imagine to control appetite and weight; bulimia, forced vomiting after binge eating, and excessive abuse of laxatives are not uncommon. Unusual food handling behavior occurs; food hiding, food hoarding, and even garbage scavenging may be present. A history of diabetes insipidus can often be elicited, and although sleep disturbances are always present, a history of this is often difficult to obtain. It is characteristic of the syndrome that the patient is unable to give an accurate account of her food intake and she either willfully or compulsively falsifies the record.

Physical Examination. The physical examination is characterized by emaciation, fine lanugo-type hirsutism, normal axillary and pubic hair, and atrophy of the internal an external genitalia. Additional findings are hypothermia, hypotension, bradycardia, carotinemia, and, as a late finding, nutritional edema.

Laboratory Findings. The weight loss is primarily associated with a carbohydrate deficit and only secondarily, as the condition progresses, with a protein deficiency. Most of the laboratory findings, if not all, are correlated with the attempt of the physiologic mechanisms to compensate for chronic starvation. These can be grouped into two major categories: those related to hypothalamic-pituitary adjustments and those related to liver dysfunction in association with protein malnutrition.

Pituitary gonadotropic function is depressed while the thyrotropic and adrenotropic functions are normal. However, the total T_3, free T_3, and T_4 are low with a normal reverse T_3. These findings, together with the normal TSH, suggest a peripheral hypothyroid effect with normal thyroid and central nervous system mechanisms. The same derangement of thyroid function is seen in simple weight loss amenorrhea and must **not** be interpreted as an indiction of true **hypothyroidism.** Although the ACTH value is normal, cortisol production is usually found to be excessive when 24-hour cortisol pulse studies

are done. This is apparently related to the decreased REM sleep. The decreased sleep is in turn associated with decreased carbohydrate nutrition and may be due to decreased catecholamine synthesis. Prolactin is usually normal but may be elevated, indicating a hypothalamic dopamine deficiency. Growth hormone is frequently elevated, apparently in response to a low somatomedin due to abnormal liver function. Another evidence of disturbed liver function is the shift in estrogen metabolism from the estriol to the catechole estrogen pathway.

Most of the adaptive findings recorded above are the result of chronic carbohydrate and protein starvation; vitamin deficiencies are rarely, if ever, seen. This is probably because of food selection as well as the reduced requirements of vitamins in the starvation state. Carotinemia is often explained on the basis of an intake of large amounts of raw vegetables by patients with anorexia nervosa. However, as there is frequently no history of ingestion of unusual amounts of raw, yellow vegetables, it is also possible that it is related to defective utilization or metabolism of vitamin A due to the abnormal liver function. When carotinemia is present, its disappearence can be a useful laboratory measure of the patient's improved dietary habits. An unexplained finding is a delayed response to LRH or TRH stimulation.

The most interesting development in the syndrome is the finding that patients with anorexia nervosa revert to a gonadotropin pattern characteristic of the prepubertal child. As recovery occurs, the patient repeats the stages of development seen during prepuberty and puberty. First FSH pulses are seen, then LH pulses begin during the night; next the negative estrogen feedback is established, and there is an exaggerated LH response to LRH as in puberty. The circadian LH pulse is converted to a constant 24-hour pulse; finally the excess LRH response is lost and the positive estrogen feedback is recovered as ovulatory menses occur. These findings would seem to indicate that the disturbance may be above the hypothalamus and related to catecholamine input. The disturbances of REM sleep reported above, apparently related to catecholamine synthesis, is perhaps also indicative of this association.

Etiology. The underlying defect which allows development of anorexia nervosa in response to stress is not known, but there are indications that it may be associated with an heritable dysfunction of the central nervous system. Thus, it is not uncommon for two members of a family to be affected. There is an increased incidence of psychiatric and neurotic disease among the families of affected individuals. A genetic defect is also suggested by the association of anorexia nervosa with gonadal dysgenesis, which is more frequent than would be expected from a chance association.

Prognosis. Anorexia nervosa has a serious prognosis. Remissions can occur with or without therapy and relapses are common. Bruch reports that three or four deaths occurred among patients who at one time were considered to be recovered.

Therapy. From a therapeutic point of view, although the nutritional aspect must be corrected as a lifesaving approach, and although even short-term refeeding can reverse most of the abnormal hypothalamic and pituitary laboratory findings, correction of the nutrition alone will not cure the patient. The primary problem is a psychiatric one and requires psychiatric therapy. Prognosis can be made on the basis of (1) the age of the individual when first seen—the younger the age, the worse the prognosis; (2) the duration of the illness, which usually coincides with the amenorrhea—the longer the duration, the more serious the prognosis; (3) the occurrence of recognized psychiatric problems in addition to the anorexia—these make the prognosis worse, and (4) the severity of the weight loss when first seen. The course of recovery can be followed if necessary by LRH stimulation studies. Frisch and MacAuthur published a chart which allows for a fairly accurate prognosis of when menses will return in relation to the height and weight (see Chapter 4).

Pseudocyesis. With changing mores in relation to the view of society and the individual toward the status of pregnancy, **pseudocyesis**, a simulated pregnancy, has become an unusual psychiatric aberration. It will, perhaps, disappear entirely as did the 'Napoleon Syndrome" in the nineteenth century.

Pseudocyesis is characterized by (1) an obsession of pregnancy; (2) weight gain; (3) normal secondary sexual characteristics and pelvic organs; (4) lactation; and (5) absence of ovulation. A corpus luteum cyst, an ectopic

pregnancy, and a missed abortion may be associated with somewhat similar symptoms, and these diagnoses must be excluded.

The laboratory findings are characterized by an increased prolactin and normal gonadotropin values. Clinical assessments of estrogen levels are normal and are substantiated by estrogen assays which vary from midfollicular to early luteal values. A negative serum chorionic gonadotropin assay will assist in the differential diagnosis. Yen postulates that a decreased dopamine secretion is the underlying neuroendocrine pathway for this psychiatric disturbance.

Because the basis of the problem is often the patient's desire to become pregnant and her inability to do so, the gynecologist can sometimes handle the situation without psychiatric help. Thus, a discussion and explanation of the problem together with the initiation of an infertility investigation may suffice. However, each patient must be individualized, as some represent a severe, underlying, chronic psychiatric disease.

Pituitary Disease

Pituitary Insufficiency (Sheehan's Disease)

The most common cause of pituitary insufficiency is necrosis of the anterior lobe due to a traumatic labor or delivery, as classically described by Sheehan. Nassar has inferred from experimental work that the use of ergot to control uterine bleeding may predispose to pituitary thrombosis. However, the pituitary is normally enlarged during pregnancy and may, on occasion, thrombose spontaneously. Depending upon the severity of the thrombosis, there is postpartum collapse and hyperpyrexia. After an immediate recovery there is an absence of lactation and amenorrhea. The initial physical signs are uterine and vaginal atrophy with a moderate, or occasionally marked, gain in weight (Fig. 30.2). Signs characteristic of the late stages are loss of axillary and pubic hair, lowered blood pressure, and loss of weight as initially described by Simmonds for pituitary cachexia. Such patients are susceptible to infections and other forms of stress and thus live in a precarious state.

It is reported that some patients, over a period of years, tend to have an amelioration of the disease, probably due to a compensatory hypertrophy of the few remaining pitui-

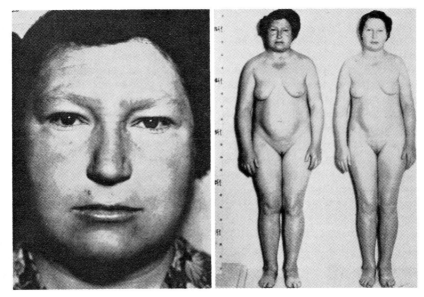

Figure 30.2.   Late stage of Sheehan's syndrome. *Left*, at the age of 35 years. This patient had amenorrhea of 16 years duration. Her last pregnancy, at 19 years of age, was associated with severe postpartum hemorrhage. *Center*, before treatment. Notice mild obesity, puffiness of face (myxedema), and loss of pubic hair. *Right*, after 8 months of treatment with 2 grains of thyroid daily.

tary cells. If satisfactory replacement therapy can be obtained, patients have been reported to have become pregnant. Under these circumstances, however, special care must be observed. Without sufficient pituitary reserve the stress of labor and delivery may cause collapse and death.

The laboratory findings are characteristic of panhypopituitarism: a low growth hormone, a lowered gonadtropin, a low 17-ketosteroid and 17-hydroxycorticosteroid excretion, a low protein-bound iodine and basal metabolic rate, a flat glucose tolerance test, and anemia.

The treatment is replacement therapy, with 25 mg of cortisone acetate or its equivalent, and 0.15 mg synthetic thyroid daily. Replacement estrogen therapy is also indicated. As mentioned in Chapter 32, support tissues require a lower estrogen dosage for maintenance than that required to induce an endometrial bleed. When sterility is a problem, pituitary gonadotropin therapy is the treatment of choice if one has the temerity to care for the pregnancy which may ensue.

Pituitary Tumors

Although pituitary tumors are uncommon in any series of amenorrheic patients, the reverse is not true, as amenorrhea is an extremely common symptom among women with pituitary tumors.

A history of headache and visual disturbances with amenorrhea is suggestive of an intracranial difficulty. However, these are late symptoms and a slow growing lesion can exist for years before their onset. The specific laboratory diagnostic aids are (1) an anterior-posterior and lateral x-ray of the skull and (2) a color visual field examination using Goldman planimetry, as the first diagnostic sign may be the encroachment of the tumor on the optic tracts with an ensuing defect in red perception.

Any type of pituitary tumor can produce amenorrhea. The most common type, the *chromophobe adenoma*, usually has no specific endocrine symptoms and produces amenorrhea through gross destruction of pituitary tissue. With the more frequent use of prolactin assays, it has become obvious that many chromophobe adenomas are in fact prolactinomas.

The prolactinoma is discussed under the heading of hyperprolactinemia. Cushing's syndrome associated classically with a basophilic, ACTH-producing adenoma, is discussed under the adrenal in lesions of intermediate origin.

The acidophilic adenoma is characterized

clinically by symptoms of acromegaly due to excessive growth hormone. Eighty-five percent of young women with acromegaly are said to have menstrual disturbances. The physical appearance of the patient with this condition is usually the best diagnostic aid. There is excessive growth of hands and feet and an increase in coarseness of all the features. This is associated with an increase in the size of the nose and prognathous of the lower jaw. There may be unusual muscular weakness, polyuria, and polydipsia in the later stages. The laboratory findings are characterized by an increased serum growth hormone, decreased gonadotropins, a diabetic type of glucose tolerance curve, and an increased protein-bound iodine. It is important to recognize these tumors before the occurrence of severe visual field defects, as pressure on the optic nerves may cause blindness.

Although eosinophilic adenomas respond to some extent to dopamine agonists and are radiosensitive, if diagnosed while still within the sella the transsphenoidal surgical approach is the best therapy. As growth hormone is a tumor marker, assay of growth hormone allows one to determine if all tumor has been removed and frequent periodic assays will afford early detection of a recurrence. If the assay indicates residual tumor, medical therapy or irradiation should be given immediately. A neurosurgeon must decide on the basis of the radiologic findings which of these three therapeutic approaches is indicated.

Pituitary gonadotropin reserve can be accessed by a double LRH stimulation study given pre- and post 100 mg of clomiphene for 7 days, as described by Rosenwaks et al.

Congenital Deficiency of Gonadotropic Hormones (Hypogonadotropic Eunuchoidism)

This cause of hypogonadotropic hypogonadism is extremely rare. It is theoretically due to a specific failure of the pituitary to produce normal, biologically active FSH and/or LH. One proven case has been reported by Rabin.

The diagnosis is made when primary amenorrhea occurs with a eunuchoid stature and serum FSH or LH values below normal. A familial incidence is reported. The pathology of the ovary shows follicles up to the antrum stage but no evidence of ovulation or corpus luteum formation. Because of the fa-

milial occurrence a protein defect might be suspected. If infertility is a complaint, the treatment of choice is substitution gonadotropin therapy. If pregnancy is not desirable, substitution estrogen therapy as described in Chapter 32 is indicated.

Gonadal Lesions

Ovarian Insufficiency

Ovarian causes for amenorrhea can be classified as follows:

1. Ovarian Insufficiency
   a. Congenital defects, gonadal dysgenesis, and related conditions (see Chapter 8)
   b. Premature menopause, congenital and acquired (see Chapter 32)
2. The Insensitive Ovary Syndrome
3. Ovarian Tumors
   a. Arrhenoblastoma, hilus cell tumor and adrenal rest tumor
   b. Theca-granulosa cell tumors
   c. Dysgerminoma; usually with dysgenetic ovarian development
   d. Nonspecific tumors with steroidogenic stroma (see Chapter 24)

Congenitally Defective Gonads

Gonadal Agenesis (Turner's Syndrome), Pure Gonadal Dysgenesis. In 1938 Turner described a syndrome of "infantilism," congenital webbed neck, and cubitus valgus. Albright et al., in 1942, demonstrated the association of this syndrome with an elevated urinary gonadotropin titer, and Wilkins and Fleischmann, in 1944, described the pathological condition which was characterized by absence of gonads and the presence of normally developed but immature Müllerian ducts. The gonads are represented grossly by a primitive streak, and microscopically by stroma only or by stroma and Leydig cells. In 1954, a number of investigators independently reported that a majority of these patients had a negative or male type chromatin pattern, and in 1959, Ford and Jones reported that at least some patients with negative chromatin patterns represented not an XY but XO configuration of sex chromosomes. These contributions provided the building stones for a satisfactory explanation of the syndrome. Those patients who show a 45,XO chromosomal configuration can be explained on the basis of nondisjunction of the sex chromosomes. Patients who have a normal XX chromosome pattern, **pure gonadal dysgenesis**, are usually of normal height and may represent the result of embryonic oocyte damage prior to the 8th week of development. Patients with mosaic or 46,XY chromosome patterns may present with similar findings but have different etiologic backgrounds (Chapter 8).

Every stage of gonadal developmental defects can be seen in patients with a 46,XY pattern or a Y fragment or Y translocation. These may vary from streak gonads with a few Leydig cells associated with female genitalia and hypertrophy of the clitoris only (first described by Pich in 1937) to almost normal testicular development and male external genitalia with hypospadias. For a complete summary of this abnormal development, see the text by Jones and Scott.

The clinical features of a typical Turner's syndrome are so characteristic that one can recognize such a patient as she walks into the consultation room. There is shortness of stature, webbing of the neck, deformity of the carrying angle, a shield-type chest with nipples placed far laterally, no breast development, and scanty or absent axillary and pubic hair. Two other associated congenital defects have been described which are serious health hazards and should therefore always be checked: coarctation of the aorta and absence of one kidney. From the typical picture of patients with Turner's syndrome and dwarf stature, there are all gradations of gonadal and physical development in patients with pure gonadal dysgenesis.

The laboratory findings are characterized by an elevated gonadotropin assay in all patients and an abnormal chromatin pattern in most; the buccal smear, although often the most rapid and least expensive way to make a diagnosis, is also the least reliable laboratory technique; therefore, a karyotype is important. As autoimmune disease is also associated with Turner's syndrome, it is important to check for both thyroid function and diabetes. The growth hormone is invariably normal.

Until such a time as transplantation of ovaries is feasible, the treatment of this condition will remain as substitution therapy only. Estrogen is given in interrupted dosage, depending upon the amount of drug necessary to induce vaginal bleeding: 0.325 mg–1.25 mg of conjugated estrogen, or its equiv-

lent, daily through the 25th day of each month with the addition of a progestational drug during the last week for its antimitotic action. Treatment should be discontinued and resumed the 1st day of the following month. An endometrial biopsy should be obtained periodically to ensure that there is a normal growth pattern, for endometrial cancer has been reported after long-term estrogen therapy. When full development of secondary sexual characteristics has been obtained, the estrogen dose should be reduced to the lowest one compatible with support of vaginal epithelial growth. This is usually 0.3 mg a day. When the karyotype shows a Y chromosome or fragment, an operation for removal of the gonads is indicated to prevent tumor formation.

True Hermaphroditism. True hermaphroditism is extremely rare. Most true hermaphrodites are raised as men. This indicates, of course, that in a majority of instances the external genitalia are masculine rather than feminine in appearance. The condition should be suspected in patients who show some ambiguity of the external genitalia, associated in the adult with breast development. Minimal hirsutism may occur but has been absent in the majority of the reported cases.

The diagnosis can be suspected by the physical findings, and the laboratory data are of very little assistance. The chromatin pattern can be positive or negative and the 17-ketosteroid serum androgen and gonadotrophin assays are within normal range. The diagnosis, therefore, is made by the pathologist at the time of operation, and the treatment is surgical correction.

Male Hermaphroditism. Male hermaphrodites show ambiguous external genitalia, no breast development, minimal hirsutism, and a negative chromatin pattern. This condition is discussed in Chapter 8 in detail.

Testicular Feminization: Androgen Insensitivity. This interesting form of hermaphroditism is characterized by a normal female appearance with excellent breast development and completely normal female external genitalia. However, in about a third of the patients there is either extremely scanty or no axillary or pubic hair. There is always a short or absent vagina and no cervix. The differential diagnosis must be made between this condition and that of congenital absence of the Müllerian ducts. The family history is important as the androgen insensitivity syndrome is a sex-linked, dominant, heritable disease. At laparotomy, relatively normal testes are present and the uterus is absent. A negative chromatin pattern is confirmatory of a diagnosis of testicular feminization, the androgen insensitivity syndrome, and the karyotype is a normal 46,XY male pattern.

The laboratory findings are bizarre and can vary widely. Some patients show slightly elevated urinary gonadotropins. Others show urinary gonadotropins in the normal range. Most patients have a 17-ketosteroid excretion compatible with a normal male and estrogen excretion compatible with a normal female. Morris and Mahesh have reported a comprehensive survey of experience with this condition. The findings of the testis are described in detail in Chapter 8. The assumption is that this is a heritable developmental defect of the testosterone target organs which lack the protein androgen receptor, causing insensitivity to androgen stimulation.

The treatment is operative removal of the testes after the age of puberty because of the predilection to tumor formation, and vaginal plastic procedure if indicated. Estrogen substitution therapy after operation is usually advisable.

Premature Menopause

Premature menopause is caused by disappearance of oocytes from the ovary, depriving the organ of the stimulus for follicle formation. The etiology can be congenital or acquired. Any germ cell toxin can produce this end result. The insult to germ plasm can occur at any age from the earliest embryo through adulthood. Some factors which interfere with oogenesis or cause damage are known. Anomalies of the X chromosomes make the meiotic division of the germ cell impossible. These defects cause disappearance of germ cells at about the 4th month of life; they are discussed under Gonadal Dysgenesis (Turner's Syndrome) in a previous section and in Chapter 8. Cytotoxins, such as busulfan and methotrexate, and irradiation, specifically damage germ cells as do viral infections, an example of which is mumps. Nonspecific destruction of ovarian tissue from abscess formation by the tubercle bacillus and certain rare tropical diseases, surgical destruction by removal of ovarian tissue or interruption of the normal blood supply,

ovarian torsion, and, finally, autoimmune disease as described by Irvine et al. may all be causes of the premature menopause.

The diagnosis can be suspected when the patient gives a history of hot flushes. As there is a heritable tendency for this anomaly in certain families, a good history of the menopausal ages of all family members is important. The laboratory findings of elevated gonadotropins is strongly suggestive but the absolute diagnostic criterion is the pathologic demonstration of absence of oocytes and follicles in the ovarian tissue. There is no cure for premature menopause and therapy must be substitutional only. This is discussed in Chapter 32.

The Insensitive Ovary Syndrome

There are apparently two forms of this syndrome; one associated with primary amenorrhea and the other with secondary amenorrhea. This very unusual cause of primary amenorrhea is characterized by well developed breasts, axillary and pubic hair, but atrophic vaginal and endometrial mucosa. The serum and urinary gonadotrophins, FSH and LH, are elevated and the estrogens are low. The ovary grossly resembles a prepubertal organ and microscopically shows numerous primordial follicles but none developed past the antrum stage. Ovulation can occasionaly be induced by excessive amounts of exogenous gonadotrophins (3–10 times the dosage used for hypophysectomized patients). It is assumed that this syndrome may be due to lack of FSH receptor protein or an abnormality in the activator proteins in the cell membranes.

When the syndrome is associated with secondary amenorrhea, the diagnosis of a premature menopause can be ruled out only by an ovarian biopsy. Instead of absence of follicles, the biopsy shows numerous primordial and primary follicles. The etiology of this syndrome may be a defective immunologic system with ovarian antibody formation. The association with other autoimmune diseases may alert one to the possibility of this disorder. The presence of ovarian antibodies confirms the diagnosis, but lack of circulating antibodies does not rule it out. The presence of round cell infiltration in the ovarian biopsy is also confirmatory evidence of an autoimmune disease.

There are several reports in the literature

of spontaneous recovery and subsequent pregnancies among patients with this diagnosis. Therefore, the prognosis must be guarded. Replacement estrogen therapy is indicated. Massive gonadotropin therapy might theoretically prove beneficial, but there is no clinical experience to substantiate this.

Ovarian Tumors

Amenorrhea related to ovarian tumors has been discussed in Chapter 24.

End Organ—Uterine and Vaginal Cryptomenorrhea

The conditions embraced under this heading are: traumatic occlusion of the vagina, the imperforate hymen, congenital absence or atresia of the vagina, vaginal septa, congenital absence of the Müllerian ducts, traumatic occlusion of the cervix, and destruction of the endometrium. All of these are discussed in Chapter 8.

Diseases of Intermediate Metabolism and Nutrition

Metabolic Disease

Thyroid

Ovarian hormones apparently play a major, though poorly understood, role in pituitary-thyroid control mechanism. Thyroid disease is most commonly seen during puberty and at the menopause and also occurs much more frequently among women than men. Estrogen increases TSH response to TRH much as it increases LH response to LRH. An increased pulsatile response at the pituitary level could conceivably increase the total TSH by an increased response to the same TRH stimulus. This would, therefore, increase the thyroxin response and cause a negative feedback effect at the pituitary level. The same ability of estrogen to increase the sensitivity of the pituitary gonadotropins to LRH is theoretically the reason for the LH surge at midcycle. The direct feedback of T_3 and T_4 at the pituitary level apparently prevents a midcycle TSH elevation.

Although both hypo- and hyperthyroidism may be associated with menstrual irregularities and amenorrhea, neither of these symptoms will be corrected by the administration of thyroid hormone in the absence of laboratory demonstration of thyroid disease. This diagnosis must be made on the basis of: a thyroid screen, T_3, T_4, and T index (a measure of free thyroxin). If thyroid function is normal, all of these thyroid values should be within limits. A **low normal** value is, nevertheless, still **normal** and does not warrant therapy. It should also be remembered that the diagnosis of hypothyroidism cannot be made in the presence of malnutrition, as low thyroid function invariably exists under these conditions. A TSH assay is probably the most sensitive assay for the diagnosis of hypothyroidism. Minimal TSH elevations may suggest hypothyroidism, and a TRH stimulation study which shows a hyperresponse will confirm the diagnosis. Hyperthyroidism is very rarely due to a pituitary adenoma or a hypothalamic hamartoma. TSH values under these circumstances would be elevated also.O Hyperthyroidism, or thyrotoxicosis, is usually an autoimmune disease associated with antibodies against TSH receptors. These antibodies can stimulate the thyroid to secrete T_4. TSH values are low, as the pituitary function is suppressed by the excess T_4 values.

Hypothyroidism. Hypothyroidism is most commonly related to an iatrogenic cause; removal of the thyroid or irradiation for thyroid adenoma, carcinoma, or hyperthyroidism (autoimmune disease), Hashimoto's thyroiditis associated with anti-thyroid antibodies is the next most common cause of hypothyroidism. Although the classic signs of hypothyroidism are recognized as sensitivity to cold, tendency to constipation, dryness of skin and hair, a slow reflex reaction time, skin changes characteristic of myxedema, carotenemia (giving the characteristic sallow color to the skin), and the croaking, hoarse voice, these may all be late symptoms. In young women particularly, the onset may be insidious and the diagnosis difficult. Probably the best laboratory method for diagnosis is the serum TSH. If this is in the upper limits of normal or just above, diagnosis can be confirmed by a TRH stimulation function study. A hyperresponse will be obtained with hypothyroidism. This test will also help in the rare diagnosis of hypothyroidism due to primary pituitary TSH deficiency, as under these circumstances no increase in TSH will be seen. In hypothyroidism there is a reduced steroid hormone binding globulin and a relative increase in unbound estradiol and testosterone. There is also a shift in the metabolic pathway from the catechole estradiol pathway to the estriol pathway, perhaps influencing the central feedback mechanisms.

Hyperthroidism. The most common cause of hyperthyroidism is Graves' Disease; thyroid adenoma and carcinoma are uncommon; and still rarer is a pituitary TSH-producing adenoma.

As both Graves' disease and hypothyroidism, due to Hashimoto's disease, are autoimmune diseases, one must also consider that the associated amenorrhea may be related to an associated autoimmune disease of the ovary rather than to an ovarian dysfunction due to the thyroid disease. A gonadotrophin assay will answer this question, as with autoimmune disease of the ovary the FSH and LH will be elevated.

Pancreas

Diabetes. Although uncontrolled *diabetes mellitus* is more apt to be associated with dysfunctional bleeding, amenorrhea is occasionally present.

The classic signs and symptoms are obesity followed by weight loss, polyuria, polydipsia, and nocturia. Often, however, it is the monilial vulvovaginitis, commonly associated with diabetes, which brings the patient to the doctor; therefore, the gynecologist may be the first who has the opportunity of making the diagnosis. It should be unnecessary to state that in the presence of these symptoms, an office examination of a urine specimen for sugar must be obtained.

The important laboratory finding is an elevated fasting blood sugar. It has been our experience that when the diabetes is satisfactorily controlled, the menstrual periods become regulated.

Adrenal

Congenital Adrenal Hyperplasia. This unusual and instructive heritable disease has been discussed in Chapter 8 in the section on female hermaphroditism with virilization.

It is now recognized that congenital adrenal hyperplasia is a heritable deficiency of a specific enzyme in the pathway of adrenal steroidogenesis of cortisol from cholesterol. A deficiency of the 21-hydroxylase enzyme is the most usual one. But deficiencies in enzymes at every step, involved in this synthetic pathway, have been observed.

Congenital adrenal hyperplasia (CAH) is an autosomal recessive defect; thus, both parents are carriers. If the defect is in fact related to a structural gene, a series of allelic genes must be involved. All grades of severity of the condition have been described from the **most severe deficiency**, which is associated with **salt loss** and the most marked deformity of external genitalia, the **penile urethra**, to the **mildest form of attenuated**, or **pubertal** onset, adrenal hyperplasia. It is of importance, however, that each form is peculiar to the particular family involved. Genetic studies have shown that patients with attenuated congenital adrenal hyperplasia are not heterozygote carriers for CAH but are actually homozygote individuals with heterozygote parents. Therefore, it seems that the genetic defect is either a series of allelic genes or involves a defect in a modulatory gene.

Depending upon the particular enzyme deficiency which the patient has inherited, excess of certain specific steroids will be present in the serum. Characteristic metabolites of these steroids will be increased in the urine. In the classic form of the 21-hydroxylase defect, 17-hydroxyprogesterone (17-OH prog.) is the steroid which accumulates in serum, and its urinary metabolite is pregnanetriol. The next most common type of CAH is caused by a defect in the 11-β hydroxylase enzyme. This form is associated with less severe virilization, with irregular menses instead of amenorrhea, and with severe hypertension due to excessive serum 11-desoxycorticosterone (DOC), and 11-desoxy-cortisol. The urinary 17-ketosteroid assay in this type of adrenal hyperplasia may not be elevated, as compound S, the tetrohydro derivative of desoxycortisone, may be the major metabolite. This in turn may be further metabolized to androsterone and etiocholanolone without being converted to a 17-ketosteroid metabolite. Unfortunately, the 11-β hydroxylase defect is extremely difficult to recognize clinically because of the unavailability of serum 11-desoxycortisol and desoxycortisone assays and the difficulty in obtaining accurate measurements of the urinary metabolite, compound S. It is, an extremely important syndrome to diagnose because of the hypertensive problem. If not diagnosed and treated prior to the establishment of severe hypertension, the hypertension becomes irreversible. As abnormalities of the external genitalia may be relatively mild this is further reason for the syndrome to go unrecognized (Glenthøj et al.).

There are two early enzymic defects in the biosynthetic pathway. The defect of 20-α hydroxylase, which converts cholesterol to 20-α hydroxycholesterol prior to pregnenolone, was initially described by Prader as the lipoid form of congenital adrenal hyperplasia. It is a lethal defect seen only in newborns. A defect of the 3-β-ol dehydrogenase enzyme, which converts pregnanolone to progesterone, is also usually lethal and is seen most often in newborns. The importance of recognizing both of these defects is in order to give the parents the proper genetic counselling. These infants may be difficult to diagnose, as the external genitalia may appear to be entirely female. However, one may see ambiguous external genitalia in the male infant.

As mentioned above, attenuated congenital adrenal hyperplasia has been shown to be a heritable defect in the gene mechanism controlling the 21-hydroxylase enzyme. One should also remember that there are patients who seem to have a true "acquired" defect of the 11-β hydroxylase enzyme. Bush and Mahesh showed that stress can induce adrenal hyperplasia in some patients by causing a build-up of adrenal androstenedione. Fragachan et al., from Dorfman's laboratory, in 1969 reported that Δ_4-androstenedione inhibited 11-β hydroxylase activity in the adrenal. A patient with a partially defective 17-20 desmolase, when under excessive stress, might increase the rate of synthesis of androstenedione sufficiently to initiate a vicious circle.

Inborn errors of metabolism also have been reported in the adrenal mineralocortical metabolic pathway. A defect of corticosterone methyloxidase which blocks aldosterone synthesis from corticosterone must be differentiated from those salt-losing defects associated with other enzymic deficiencies which interfere with adrenal steroidogenesis and are associated with salt loss. This differential can be made by identifying the specific steroid prior to the enzyme block. The problems are nicely discussed in the article by Veldhuis et al.

A fine line must be followed in the therapeutic steroid control of all forms of congenital adrenal hyperplasia as too little steroid allows increased androgens with virilization and closure of the epiphyses at an early age while too much steroid is also deleterious, producing Cushing features and suppression of linear growth. A dosage of cortisone should be administered which will maintain the urinary 17-ketosteroid value below the level of 3.5 mg/24 hour/meter body squared, or the serum 17-hydroxyprogesterone values within the normal level. The ideal plasma steroid for monitoring the efficiency of therapy should define both the upper and lower limits of adrenal suppression and, therefore, detect either under- or overtreatment. Unfortunately, although several steroids can be used as monitors to define undertreatment, none will define overtreatment. Winter has used 17-hydroxyprogesterone as the glucocorticoid monitor in the serum and is also persuaded that, especially in infants, plasma renin monitoring is important to access the mineralocorticoids. With the use of fludrocortisone acetate, a long-acting steroid, both carbohydrate and electrolyte defects can be controlled. When this is given in conjunction with cortisol, the total dose of cortisol can be markedly reduced because of the prolonged action of the fludrocortisone acetate. This also smooths out the effects of the adrenal diurnal variation and makes control more uniform. However, because of its electrolyte affect, it can cause hypertension, edema, potassium loss and negative sodium balance, if the diet is deficient in any of these electrolytes. Using this combination therapy and monitoring with both plasma renin activity for electrolytes and 17-hydroxyprogesterone, checked occasionally by urinary 17-ketosteroids and pregnanetriol, an adequate control of corticoid dosage should be possible. In lieu of 17-hydroxyprogesterone for monitoring glucocorticoid activity, androstenedione can be used and may be preferable as it is not subject to the marked diurnal fluctuations associated with serum 17-hydroxyprogesterone. Because of the diurnal variation of ACTH, the major cortisone dosage should be given at night to induce the most effective suppressive therapy. If the dosage is adequate throughout life from birth, growth, menarche, and reproductive capacity are usually in the normal range.

Maintenance of proper replacement therapy, depends upon the ability of the **doctor** to **calculate** the **proper dosage** as the child grows and of the **parents** and child to **comply** with **instructions**. However, this ideal situation is not always attained and most of these individuals tend to be shorter than their expected family height and some, even though the control has apparently been ideal, seem to have a delayed maturation and delayed menarche.

Summary. Congenital virilizing adrenal hyperplasia exists as a phenotypic spectrum: at one end the manifestation of the alarming salt losing form of female hermaphroditism, at the other the mildest form of attenuated congenital adrenal hyperplasia. The most common enzymatic defect is of the 21-hydroxylase. An enzyme defect in the pathway between cholesterol and cortisol causes a deficiency of cortisol production; as cortisol is the major steroid feedback at the pituitary level on adrenocorticotrophic hormone, an excessive ACTH production results. This excess ACTH in turn produces abnormal stimulation to the adrenal glands, which secrete, in lieu of cortisol, excessive amounts of all other adrenal steroids, up to the enzyme block. The steroid just prior to the block is the major steroid found in the serum, and the metabolite of this steroid is the major one found in the urine. In the case of the 21-hydroxylase defect, this is 17-hydroxyprogesterone in the serum and pregnanetriol in the urine. The adrenal pathology is characterized by hyperplasia of the zona reticularis and either anatomical absence or failure of steroid accumulation in the zona fasciculata. The androgens and estrogens which are produced as byproducts of the adrenal androgen steroids in turn shut off the pituitary gonadotropins and ovarian insufficiency and amenorrhea ensue.

Cushing's Syndrome. In contrast to congenital adrenal hyperplasia, Cushing's disease represents a hyperfunction of the entire adrenal cortex including the glucocorticoid-secreting zona fasciculata. The pituitary-adrenal homeostatis mechanisms are out of control, as there is excessive ACTH production in spite of excessive cortisol. Cushing, in his initial publication, believed that the syndrome was always the result of a pituitary tumor or pituitary basophilism. Since the initial report, however, it has become clear that bilateral adrenal hyperplasia may occur without a demonstrable pituitary lesion and adrenal tumors are not infrequently responsible for the condition. Heinbecker has implicated

the hypothalamus as the primary disease site in pituitary basophilia without adenoma. Thus, when Cushing's disease exists, the differential diagnosis includes a consideration of a pituitary tumor, bilateral hyperplasia of the adrenals due to hypothalamic stimulation and pituitary "basophilism," or adrenal tumor.

In addition to the three principal primary sites of origin for the syndrome, there is Cushing's disease resulting from an adrenal rest tumor in the ovary (Kepler et al. and Rottino and McGrath) and in this era of corticosteroid therapy for many diseases, the physician should also be alert to the possibility of an iatrogenic factor in the production of a "Cushing-like" picture.

Cushing's syndrome is characterized by centripetal obesity, amenorrhea, moon face, hirsutism, hypertension, purple striae, erythemic acne, and easy bruisability. The pelvic organs are usually normal and there is no enlargement of the clitoris or marked vaginal atrophy. Office findings of help are a positive urinary sugar and a hematocrit indicating polycythemia. When the full blown picture exists, the syndrome is so striking that the diagnosis is blatant; however, in the early stages diagnosis may be extremely difficult.

The laboratory findings are characterized by an elevation of plasma cortisol above 20 ng/dl. The urinary hydroxycorticoid value is also elevated. The free cortisol is the most significant urinary metabolite as it is not affected by obesity or stress. The normal value of 0.03 mg/24 hours should be above 0.1 mg/24 hours. The urinary 17-ketosteroid assay is usually normal, or only moderately elevated; however, if an adrenal tumor is present, it may be markedly elevated. Polycythemia, a diabetic glucose tolerance curve, and X-ray evidence of osteoporosis are also found. A loss of diurnal variation, from the normal 15 mg/dl AM plasma cortisol to 5 mg/dl PM plasma cortisol, is diagnostic. A short screening test is a dexamethasone suppression dose of 1 mg at midnight. If the AM plasma cortisol level is not below 5 mg/dl, Cushing's syndrome should be suspected. The typical response to ACTH stimulation is an over reaction with at least a 3-fold increase of the urinary and blood corticoids. It is usually impossible to suppress the urinary corticoids below 10 mg/24 hours by dexamethasone. When an adrenal tumor is present there is usually no response to ACTH stimulation or cortisol suppression. Unfortunately, however, not all tumors are autonomous and some do show a response.

An ACTH assay is of value, as it is undetectable in patients with adrenal tumors, normal or only slightly elevated in hyperplasia, and grossly elevated in the presence of an ectopic ACTH secreting tumor.

The treatment of the disease depends upon its etiology. If a pituitary tumor can be demonstrated, a transsphenoidal extirpation is the treatment of choice for a microadenoma. In the absence of pituitary disease, adult surgery is advised.

It is often possible to decide at operation, by the appearance of one adrenal, whether or not there is a tumor in the other. If at operation the exposed gland is atrophied, it should be left in situ with a presumptive diagnosis of a contralateral tumor. If, however, the exposed adrenal is hypertrophied, it is removed with all or 90% of the opposite gland. When the partial operation is performed, there is always a possibility that a second operation will be necessary; however, this seems to be a worthwhile risk in an effort to prevent lifelong invalidism with dependence upon prolonged, expensive replacement therapy.

Adrenalectomy is followed in 10–20% of cases by Nelson's syndrome. This is due to a rapidly growing ACTH-secreting tumor which is sometimes malignant. It is characterized by pigmentation due to associated melanophor-stimulating secretion, and by signs of suprasellar expansion, headaches, and optic nerve compression.

Stress Obesity. A borderline clinical picture, with moderately elevated urinary corticoids, occurs more frequently than true Cushing's disease. It is thought that this picture represents the response of certain individuals to the "*stress of obesity.*" Experimental evidence indicates that dilatin will inhibit the hypothalamic releasing factor, CRF, and might therefore be of therapeutic value. The most important therapy is the recognition of stress by the patient and relief of stress factors. This includes, of course, a reduction diet.

Adrenal Tumors. Tumors of the adrenal are usually characterized by marked hirsutism with some associated virilization, e.g., enlargement of the clitoris, fat pad wasting, breast changes, and loss of scalp hair. Voice changes are not frequently present. Amenorrhea is often an early symptom, but occasionally patients menstruate fairly regularly and have even been known to ovulate and become pregnant. The laboratory diagnosis is made on the basis of an elevated 17-ketosteroid assay which does not suppress with dexamethasone. An elevation of dehydroisoandrosterone is the metabolic fingerprint of adrenal tumors, and this assay should always be requested when a neoplasm is suspected. An intravenous pyelogram may show a depression of the renal outline and a suprarenal mass.

As adrenal tumors can be slow growing benign adenomas, the symptoms can be present for many years. As with all tumors, both the symptoms and laboratory findings are also variable. Depending upon the tumor site, one may have symptoms of an adrenogenital syndrome, Cushing's disease, amenorrhea with minor hirsutism, or even marked hirsutism with regular menses and ovulation.

The treatment is operative removal and the prognosis is guarded.

Nutritional Disturbances

Secondary amenorrhea due to simple weight loss and primary amenorrhea associated with constitutional weight/height disparity are associated with the same physical and laboratory findings as anorexia nervosa, but to a lesser degree. Thus, these patients have indications of lowered thyroid function, carotenemia, abnormal thermal regulation, partial diabetes insipidus, and a delayed response to TRH and LRH stimulation tests; sleep aberrations have not been studied. The history and the behavior patterns of these patients are quite different from those of anorexia nervosa, and this usually makes the differential diagnosis easy. The history is one of nutritional weight loss with some goal in mind, such as ballet dancing or modeling, or simple peer pressures. There is no inability to perceive reality either in relation to diet, appearance, or energy. The symptoms are apparently related to a specific body composition with decreased subcutaneous fat and a resulting increased body protein ratio. Competitive athletes, runners and swimmers with severe training schedules, and obsessive joggers show the same body composition of fat in relation to protein. The incidence of amenorrhea among this category of women with all muscle and no subcutaneous body fat is also very high.

The occurrence of amenorrhea in patients

with exogenous obesity is somewhat more difficult to explain. The most obvious reason is that it is secondary to a psychogenic stress, which is the initial cause of the obesity. However, an alternative explanation is that a relative dietary deficiency has occurred associated with an abnormal caloric intake or that the peripheral estrogen metabolism has disturbed the central nervous system mechanisms. Subcutaneous fat increases the peripheral conversion of androstenedione to estrone and decreases the conversion to catechole estrogens.

The treatment of malnutrition and obesity is directed towards improvement of general dietary habits, either weight gain or weight reduction with a well balanced high protein diet. In the patient whose amenorrhea can be directly related to a specific weight gain or weight loss, this type of nutritional therapy is predictably successful.

Excretory and Metabolic Organs

Liver, Cirrhosis

The steroid carrying proteins, as well as conjugation and metabolism of estrogens and progesterone, takes place in the liver; the excretion is accomplished to a large extent through the bile and hepatic portal system to the bowel. In cirrhosis of the liver, impairment of conjugation of estrogen leads to excessive circulating, active "free" estrogens. This may result in dysfunctional bleeding interspersed with periods of amenorrhea. Although this is certainly the most common menstrual aberration associated with cirrhosis, Green and Rubin report 18 patients having amenorrhea as the menstrual symptom. The diagnosis is made on the basis of the physical findings and liver function tests.

The treatment is medical and the prognosis is poor.

Chronic Nephritis

As both ovarian steroid and pituitary protein hormones are at least partially excreted through the urinary tract, it is not surprising that patients with chronic nephritis frequently show abnormalities of the menstrual cycle usually characterized by amenorrhea. Goodwin et al. in 1968 studied the effects of uremia and chronic hemodialysis on the menstrual cycle. These investigators found that the men-

strual irregularities correlated well with the degree of renal failure and that the irregularities began when the uremic symptoms were first detectable, as when the endogenous creatinine clearance fell to between 10 and 15 ml per minute. When this level reached 4 or below, amenorrhea ensued. The findings suggest that the amenorrhea may in fact be due to a central disturbance rather than one of steroid clearance. Hyperprolactinemia also may be associated.

Although chronic hemodyalis may correct the amenorrhea and successful gestation has been reported, serious dysfunctional uterine bleeding may replace the amenorrhea. This further aggravates the chronic renal failure. Steroid therapy, Megace 40 mg a day, will sometimes control the bleeding, but hysterectomy or intrauterine radiation therapy may be necessary.

Chronic Disease

Theoretically, any chronic disease process associated with inanition can be associated with amenorrhea, an example being tuberculosis. Disturbances of the immunologic system are also characteristically associated with menstrual irregularities. Most of the other chronic diseases known to be associated with amenorrhea are related to disturbances of kidney or liver function, and diseases of metabolic endocrine glands, hypo- and hyperthyroidism and diabetes.

Physiological Amenorrhea

Physiologic types of amenorrhea associated with puberty, pregnancy, lactation and the menopause need only be mentioned briefly. In the appropriate setting these diagnoses must always be considered and eliminated.

Delayed Puberty

The diagnosis of delayed puberty might be best included under lesions of the nervous system, as it is now our concept that puberty is initiated by maturation of the adrenergic nervous system. (See Chapter 4).

Statistically speaking, the diagnosis cannot be made until after the age of 17 years, although any delay of menstruation after 14 years is considered delayed over the average age. Investigation is also indicated if development of secondary sexual characteristics has been present for two years or more with no initiation of menarche. The diagnosis is made when the history, physical findings, and laboratory data are all within normal limits, and it is facilitated if there is a family history of delayed menarche. An LRH stimulation may characterize the stage of pubertal development. The causes are numerous, the most important being poor general health, nutrition, or hygiene.

A careful follow-up examination should be made yearly until one is sure that the correct diagnosis has been established.

Pregnancy and Postpartum Amenorrhea

Any patient presenting with amenorrhea is presumed to be pregnant until proved otherwise. If the physical examination is equivocal, a pregnancy test can be performed to exclude the diagnosis. Postpartum amenorrhea is usual, especially if the patient nurses her baby. The normal duration of this amenorrhea is between six weeks and three months if the patient does not lactate. If the patient has nursed, menses usually return within six months of delivery, or six weeks after cessation of lactation; any period of amenorrhea longer than this can be considered as prolonged, lactation amenorrhea. A differential diagnosis must be made between this physiological condition and true Sheehan's disease, pituitary necrosis caused by the destruction of the gland at the time of a traumatic delivery. If there is a history of a postpartum dilatation and curettage, the possibility of endometrial sclerosis must also be entertained. The diagnosis of postpartum amenorrhea is made on the basis of a history of an uncomplicated delivery and normal laboratory findings. However, this differential diagnosis is not to be made didactically for, if destruction of the pituitary (Sheehan's disease) has not been complete, the findings may be identical with those of postpartum lactation amenorrhea. The Chiari-Frommel syndrome is another variant which is associated with elevated prolactin values.

A prolactin assay is necessary to exclude a hyperprolactinemic syndrome. If the prolactin level is normal, time will usually suffice to cure the amenorrhea. In prolonged amenorrhea, clomiphene can usually be used successfully but a dose schedule may be necessary, which is higher and longer than the routine clomiphene schedule.

Summary

In summary, amenorrhea and oligomenorrhea must always be regarded as symptoms, not diseases. The decision as to whether or not these symptoms require investigation or treatment must be made on the basis of the individual case. Investigation is usually indicated if infertility is a complaint, if the patient is anxious or disturbed about the absence of menstruation, or if there are associated signs and symptoms suggestive of a serious physical problem. When primary amenorrhea exists, it is always important to determine if an anatomical abnormality of the genitalia exists. No intelligent approach can be made to treatment until a proper etiological diagnosis has been attained. With the addition of human pituitary gonadotrophins, clomiphene and bromocryptine, to our therapeutic armamentaria, the results of therapy are more encouraging. LRH is being developed as a therapeutic tool and also shows great promise. The other therapeutic advance is the development of transsphenoidal microsurgery for the treatment of pituitary adenomas.

References and Additional Readings

Akande, E. O.: Plasma estrogens in euthyroid and thyrotoxic women. Am. J. Obstet. Gynecol. *122:* 880, 1975.
Albright, F., Smith, P. H., and Fraser, R.: A syndrome characterized by primary ovarian insufficiency and decreased stature; report of 11 cases with digression on hormonal control of axillary and pubic hair. Am J. Med. Sci., *204:* 625, 1942.
Bruch, H.: Death in anorexia nervosa. Psychosom. Med., *33:* 135, 1971.
Bush, I. E., and Mahesh., V. B.: Adrenocortical hyperfunction with sudden onset of hirsuitism. J. Endocrinol., *18:* 1, 1959.
Chang, R. J., Keye, W. R., Young, J. R., Wilson, C. B. and Jaffee, R. B.: Detection, evaluation and treatment of microadenomas in patients with galactorrhea and amenorrhea. Obstet. Gynecol. Surv. *33:* 128, 1978.
Cowden, E. A., Ratcliffe, W. A., Ratcliffe, J. G., Doobbie, J. W., and Kennedy, A. C.: Hyperprolactinemia in renal disease. Clin. Endocrinol., *9:* 241, 1978.
Cushing, H.: The basophil adenomas of the pituitary body and their clinical manifestations (pituitary basophilism). Bull. Johns Hopkins Hosp., *50:* 137, 1932.
Dale, E., Gerlach, D., and Wilhite, A.: Menstrual dysfunction in distance running. Obstet. Gynecol. *54:* 47, 1979.
Ford, C. E., and Jones, K. W.: Sex chromosome anomaly in a case of gonadal dysgenesis (Turner's syndrome). Lancet, *1:* 711, 1959.
Fragachan, F., Nowaczynski, W., and Bertranau, E.: Evidence of in vivo inhibition of 11B-hydroxylation of steroids by dehydroepiandrosterone in the dog. Endocrinology, *84:* 98, 1969.
Frisch, R. E., and McArthur, J. W.: Menstrual cycles: Fatness as a determinant of minimum weight for height necessary for their maintenance or onset. Science, *185:* 949, 1974
Givens, J. R., Andersen, R. N., Wiser, W. L., and Fish, S. A.: Dynamics of suppression and recovery of plasma FSH, LH and androstenedione and testosterone. J. Clin. Endocrinol. Metab., *38:* 727, 1974.
Glenthoj, A., Nielsen, M., and Starup, J.: Congenital adrenal hyperplasia due to 11B-hydroxylase deficiency: Final diagnosis in adult age in three patients. Acta Endocrinol., *93:* 94, 1980.

Glynn, E. R.: The adrenal cortex; its rest and tumors; its relation to other ductless glands and especially to sex. Q. J. Med., *5:* 157, 1911.

Goodwin, N. J., Valenti, C., Hall, J. E., and Friedman, E. A.: Effects of uremia and chronic hemodialysis on the reproductive cycle. Am. J. Obstet. Gynecol., *100:* 528, 1968.

Green, P., and Rubin, L.: Amenorrhea as a manifestation of chronic liver disease. Am. J. Obstet. Gynecol., *78:* 141, 1959.

Hardy, J., Beauregard, H., and Robert F.: Prolactin secreting pituitary adenomas: Transsphenoidal microsurgical treatment. In *Progress in Prolactin Physiology and Pathology,* edited by C. Robyn and M. Harter, p. 361. Netherlands, Elsevier-North Holland, 1978.

Heinbecker, P.: Pathogenesis of Cushing's syndrome. Medicine, *23:* 225, 1944.

Irvine, W. J., Chan, M. M. W., Scarth, L., Kolb, F. O., Hartog, M., Bayliss, R. I. S., and Dury, M. I.: Immunological aspects of premature ovarian failure associated with idiopathic Addison's disease. Lancet, *2:* 883, 1968.

Jagiello, G. M., and Rogers, J.: Amenorrhea and pituitary tumors. Fertil. Steril., *11:* 559, 1960.

Jones, H. W., Jr., and Scott, W. W.: *Hermaphroditism, Genital Anomalies and Related Endocrine Disorders,* 2nd ed. Williams & Wilkins, Baltimore, 1971.

Kepler, E. J., Dockerty, M. V., and Priestley, J. T.: Adrenal-like ovarian tumor associated with Cushing's syndrome (so-called masculinovoblastoma, luteoma, hypernephroma, adrenal cortical carcinoma of the ovary). Am. J. Obstet. Gynecol., *47:* 43, 1944.

Lipson, L. G., Beitins, I. Z., Kornblith, P. D., McArthur, J. W., Friesen, H. G., Kliman, B., and Kjellberg, R. N.: Tissue culture studies on human pituitary tumours: Radioimmunoassayable anterior pituitary hormones in the culture medium. Acta Endocrinol., *88:* 239, 1978.

Lucas, A. R.: Other meanings of laboratory values in anorexia nervosa. Mayo Clin. Proc., *52:* 748, 1977.

Lucky, A. W., Marynick, S. P., Debar, R. W., Cutler, G. B., Glen, M., Johnsonbaugh, R. E., and Loriaux, D. L.: Replacement oral ethinyloestradiol therapy for gonadal dysgenesis: growth and adrenal androgen studies. Acta Endocrinol., *31:* 519, 1979.

MacDonald, P. C., Rombaut, R. P., and Sitteri, P. K.: Plasma precursors of estrogen. J. Clin. Endocrinol. Metab. *27:* 1103, 1967.

Marshall, J. C., and Kelch, R. P.: Low dose pulsatile gonadotropin-releasing hormone in anorexia nervosa: A model of human pubertal development. J. Clin. Endocrinol., *49:* 712, 1979.

Morris, J. M., and Mahesh, V. B.: Further observations on the syndrome "testicular feminization." Am. J. Obstet. Gynecol., *87:* 731, 1963.

Nassar, G., Greenwood, M., Djanian, A., and Shanklin, W.: The etiological significance of ergot in the incidence of postpartum necrosis of the anterior pituitary a preliminary report. Am. J. Obstet. Gynecol., *60:* 140, 1950.

Pich, G.: Über den angeborenen Eierstockmangel. Beitr. Pathol. Anat., *98:* 218, 1937.

Plotz, C., Knowlton, A., and Ragan, C.: Natural history of Cushing's syndrome. Am. J. Med., *13:* 597, 1952.

Prader, V. A., and Siebenmann, R. E.: Nebenniereninsuffizienz beikogenitaler lipoidhyperplasie der nebennieren. Helvt. Paediat. Acta, *12:* 569, 1957.

Rosenwaks, Z., Jones, G. S., and Wentz, A. C.: The use of a repeated LH-RH stimulation for prediction of pituitary reserve function in amenorrhea patients. edited by C. Beling and A. Wentz. *The LH-Releasing Hormone.* Masson Publishing New York, 1980.

Rottino, A., and McGrath, J. F.: Masculinoblastoma primary masculinizing tumor of the ovary. Arch. Intern. Med., *63:* 686, 1939.

Shangold, M., Freeman, R., Thysen, B., and Gatz, M.: The relationship between long-distance running, plasma progesterone and luteal phase length. Fertil. Steril., *31:* 130, 1979.

Sheehan, H. L.: Post-partum necrosis of anterior pituitary. J. Pathol. Bact., *45:* 189, 1937.

Shimoda, Y., and Kitagawa, T.: Clinical and EEG studies on the emaciation (anorexia nervosa) due to disturbed function of the brain stem. J. Neural Transm., *134:* 195, 1973.

Simmonds, M.: Uber embolische prozesse in der Hypophysis. Arch. Pathol. Anat., *219:* 226, 1914.

Swamey, A. P., Woolf, P. D., and Cestero, R. V.: Hypothalamic-pituitary-ovarian axis in uremic women. J. Lab. Clin. Med., *93:* 1066, 1979.

Talbot, L. M., and Sloan, C.: The effect of a low dose oral contraceptive or serum testosterone levels in polycystic ovary disease. Obstet. Gynecol., *53:* 694, 1979.

Teter, J., and Boczkowski, K.: Occurrence of tumors in dysgenetic gonads. Cancer, *20:* 1301, 1967.

Turner, H. H.: A syndrome of infantilism, congenital webbed neck, and cubitus valgus. Endocrinology, *23:* 566, 1938.

Veldhuis, J. D., Kulin, H. E., Santen, R. J., Wilson, T. E., and Melby, J. C.: Inborn error in the terminal step of aldosterone biosynthesis. N. Engl. J. Med. *303:* 117, 1980.

Werder, K. V., Rahlbusch, R., Landgraf, R., Pickardt, C. R., Rjosk, H. K., and Scriba, P. C.: Treatment of patients with prolactinomas. J. Endocrinol. Invest., *1:* 47, 1978.

Whitelaw, M. J., Thomas, S. F., Graham, W., Foster, T. M., and Brock, C.: Growth response in gonadal dysgenesis to the anabolic steroid. Norethandrolone. Am. J. Obstet. Gynecol., *84:* 501, 1962.

Wilkins, L.: *The Diagnosis and Treatment of Endocrine Disorders in Childhood and Adolescence,* ed. 3. Charles C Thomas, Springfield, Ill., 1965.

Yen, S. S., Rebar, R. W., and Queensberry, W.: Pituitary function in pseudocyesis. J. Clin. Endocrinol. Metab., *43:* 132, 1976.

CHAPTER 31

Abnormal Uterine Bleeding

Dysfunctional uterine bleeding is a menstrual disorder that is both poorly understood and managed; its definition is controversial, and there is considerable disagreement as to the proper approach in its evaluation and effective therapy.

Even though uterine bleeding is a normal, physiologic, episodic occurrence for most women, its characteristics vary considerably. This broad range of normal variation causes difficulty in differentiating normal from abnormal. To avoid the semantic problems in distinguishing functional and dysfunctional uterine bleeding, we have preferred to consider as abnormal any bleeding which is excessive in *duration, frequency,* or *amount* for a particular patient. Our approach to its evaluation is stepwise and logical. There are clear-cut goals of management, primarily based on etiologic diagnosis, as finding the etiology of abnormal bleeding is crucial to its proper management and to the prevention of further occurrences.

In the management of abnormal uterine bleeding, there are two goals: (1) arrest of the immediate bleeding if so excessive as to threaten health; and (2) prevention of future similar occurrences and re-establishment of cyclic menses. Although the etiologic diagnosis may not be initially established when achieving the first goal, determining the cause of bleeding is crucial to achieving the second.

CHARACTERISTICS OF NORMAL MENSTRUATION

As described in Chapter 4, Pubertal Development and Menstruation, menstruation is defined as a bloody, vaginal discharge which is spontaneous and periodic and represents endometrial shedding following ovulation. The commonly observed interval between menstrual periods is approximately 24–32 days, with less than one-sixth of cycles being the lunar 28 days. The duration of normal ovulatory menses is ordinarily from 3 to 7 days. The amount of blood loss in a normal menstrual period averages 33 ml, with over 80 ml considered excessive. During the first 2 days of menstruation, fully 78% of the total menstrual blood loss occurs.

INITIAL CONSIDERATIONS

The first problem in evaluating abnormal bleeding is to establish that the bleeding is uterine in origin. Infrequently, patients may mistake slight bleeding from the rectum, bladder, or urethra for bleeding originating in vagina or uterus. A brief list of lesions responsible for such bleeding is shown in Table 31.1.

Once the bleeding has been determined to be uterine in origin, the differentiation between an organic or anatomical cause and a dysfunction of the neuroendocrine system is made. It is diagnostically useful to classify uterine bleeding under two major headings: (1) abnormal bleeding associated with an ovulatory cycle and (2) abnormal bleeding associated with anovulation.

Abnormal bleeding associated with an ovulatory cycle is ordinarily organic in etiology, although polymenorrhea, irregular endometrial shedding, and a persistent corpus luteum (Halban's disease), may be endocrine in etiology. In the reproductive age bracket, bleeding is also more commonly organic, usually a complication of pregnancy or one related to contraceptive measures. Tumor is rare in

Table 31.1
Anatomic Factors Causing Nonuterine Bleeding

Cervical lesions
   Neoplasia, benign and malignant
     Polyps
     Carcinoma
   Cervical eversion
   Cervicitis
   Cervical condylomata

Vaginal lesions
   Carcinoma, sarcoma, or adenosis
   Laceration or trauma
     Abortion attempts
     Coital injury
   Infections
   Foreign bodies
     Pessaries
     Tampons, chronic usage
   Vaginal adhesions
   Atrophic vaginitis

Bleeding from other sites
   Urinary tract and urethra
     Urethral caruncle, infected diverticulum
     Gastrointestinal tract and rectum
   External genitalia
     Labial varices, condylomata
     Labial trauma, inflammation
     Neoplasia, benign and malignant
     Infections
     Atrophic conditions

these individuals, but intrapelvic organic diagnoses such as pelvic inflammatory disease, submucous fibroids, endometriosis, and cervical or endometrial polyps must be considered.

Anovulatory uterine bleeding is primarily a disease of menarcheal and perimenopausal patients. Atypical bleeding patterns and increased cycle length commonly occur at both extremes of menstrual life. The first menstruation is rarely ovulatory, and a year or more may elapse before normal luteal function is established. In the perimenopausal woman, ovulatory menses become less common approaching the menopause and menstrual periodicity becomes less regular. Thus, undue concern about menstrual irregularity is unnecessary, provided the menses are not unduly frequent, prolonged, or excessive; however, the possibility of an endometrial lesion must be strongly considered and compulsively eliminated.

To summarize, first establish the location or source of abnormal bleeding and identify extrauterine causes. With uterine bleeding, an organic cause must be differentiated from a purely endocrine, anovulatory dysfunction. Classify uterine bleeding under two major headings: (1) ovulatory abnormal bleeding and (2) anovulatory abnormal bleeding. The approaches to differential diagnosis will next be considered.

EVALUATION OF ABNORMAL UTERINE BLEEDING

History

The history is foremost in importance. Nonuterine bleeding may often be suspected, and the history ordinarily gives clues as to whether the bleeding is ovulatory or anovulatory. Bleeding accompanied by dysmenorrhea, breast tenderness, weight gain, predictable periodicity, and emotional lability is ordinarily ovulatory. Particular attention should be paid to the general nature of the bleeding, including the interval, duration, amount of flow, association with cramping, and passage of clots or tissue. A number of confusing terms are used to describe patterns of abnormal bleeding. These terms, along with their commonly accepted definition, are shown in Table 31.2.

The age of the patient may assist initial classification. Figure 31.1 is a representation of the causes of abnormal bleeding throughout a woman's life.

The patient's menstrual pattern must be documented, as many factors may induce an isolated instance of anovulatory bleeding. The history should seek any predisposing causes, particularly psychogenic or emotional factors, or transient stressful situations. A family history of bleeding problems may suggest an inherited blood dyscrasia.

The history must include the details of medication for patients may have taken oral contraceptives, estrogens, or progestational agents unknowingly. Patients on oral contraceptives may have breakthrough bleeding or discontinue the medication at unusual times in the cycle. Usage of anticoagulants, digitalis, or vitamins may be associated with abnormal but usually ovulatory bleeding.

Particular attention must be paid to pregnancy exposure, including the number of pregnancies and their result, ages of children,

Table 31.2
Patterns of Abnormal Bleeding

Oligomenorrhea	Infrequent, irregular episodes of bleeding, usually occurring at intervals greater than 40 days
Polymenorrhea	Frequent, but regular episodes of uterine bleeding, usually occurring at intervals of 21 days or less
Hypermenorrhea (Menorrhagia)	Uterine bleeding excessive in both amount and duration of flow, occurring at regular intervals
Metrorrhagia	Uterine bleeding, usually not excessive, occurring at irregular intervals
Menometrorrhagia	Uterine bleeding, usually excessive and prolonged, occurring at frequent and irregular intervals
Hypomenorrhea	Uterine bleeding that is regular but decreased in amount
Intermenstrual bleeding	Uterine bleeding, usually not excessive, occurring between otherwise regular menstrual periods

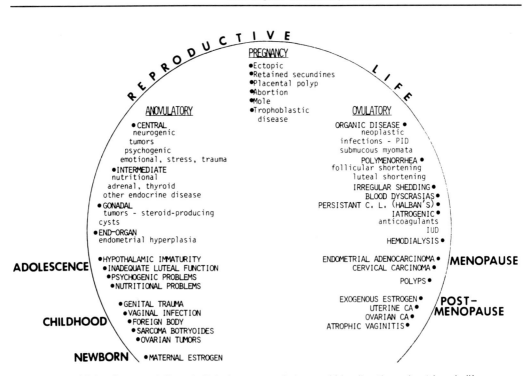

Figure 31.1. Representation of etiologic causes of abnormal bleeding throughout female life.

and contraceptive usage. Nutritional disturbances, including rapid weight loss as well as obesity and rapid weight gain, are commonly associated with abnormal bleeding patterns. Dietary abuses are frequent in patients with anorexia who may ingest large quantities of a particular food stuff to intoxication; hypercarotinemia and vitamin A toxicosis are examples of such dietary indiscretion. A history of lower abdominal discomfort, radiating pain, or distention may provide a clue to benign or malignant abdominal tumors. The history should elicit any chronic illnesses, including essential hypertension, congestive heart failure, chronic nephritis, or liver disease. Chronic diseases, or the drugs used in their therapy, may be associated with anovulation or with abnormal uterine bleeding in the presence of ovulation. Hemodialysis for chronic renal failure is associated with hypermenorrhea.

The excellent history should determine whether the bleeding is anatomic or organic in nature, and whether it is superimposed on an ovulatory cycle or associated with anovulation. In addition, the patient's own expectation is important: the patient interested in fertility will require different therapeutic management than the one interested primarily in having regular bleeding.

Physical Examination

A complete general physical examination is performed with the foregoing etiologic areas in mind. Remember that many of these patients will undergo anesthesia, therefore, their general health is important. The appearance of the patient, whether emaciated or obese, should be noted. Evidence of chronic disease, and signs of blood dyscrasias, such as ecchymoses or splenomegaly, and condition of the skin must be checked. The abdominal examination is important to diagnose either intra-abdominal or intrapelvic tumors. Palpation of the liver edge is helpful in diagnosing cirrhosis, or intrahepatic tumors.

Pelvic Examination

The pelvic examination identifies vaginal and cervical lesions and confirms that blood is indeed coming through the cervical os. Local causes, including benign and malignant neoplasms, infectious diseases of the vagina or cervix, cervical polyps, and ulcerated lesions may be identified. Note the hormonal status of the vagina, whether hyperestrogenic or hypoestrogenic; a Pap smear and maturation index sent to the cytopathologist will be helpful even in the face of bleeding. The presence or absence of cervical mucus gives immediate information about the estrogen milieu. Myomata uteri, ovarian masses and tumors, ectopic pregnancy, complications of an intrauterine pregnancy, foreign bodies, misplaced tampons or pessaries, and partially expelled intrauterine devices (IUD) may be found. The rectovaginal examination is important to exclude pelvic masses in the cul-de-sac, and to palpate nodules suggestive of endometriosis in the uterosacral ligaments, and rectal polyps which could be bleeding.

Cervical Polyps

Bleeding with cervical polyps is characteristically slight and intermenstrual, being provoked by muscular exertion, such as defecation, and especially by coitus (contact bleeding). The slight intermenstrual or postcoital bleeding which often occurs is like that seen in the early stages of cervical carcinoma, and pathological evaluation is essential for diagnosis of a benign polyp, and to rule out the possibility of a prolapsed submucous myoma.

Cervical Erosions or Ectropion

With eversion, erosion, or ectropion, the cervical mucosa may be reddish, granular, and vascular, producing slight bleeding of the type described for cervical polyp. When the tissues are very vascular and bleed on slight touch, there should always be a suspicion of carcinoma, and biopsy is indicated.

Carcinoma of Cervix

The most important cause of uterine bleeding, is uterine cancer, especially of the cervix. Cervical cancer may present with intermenstrual spotting or bleeding, particularly after coitus. The examination, must always include a speculum examination under the best possible light, a Papanicolaou smear, colposcopy where a suspicious lesion can be magnified for better evaluation, and directed biopsy of the identified lesion to determine whether or not cancer is present. The bleeding in cancer is the result of surface ulceration which is seen even in the early stages of malignancy.

Endometrial Polyps

These are much less likely to cause bleeding than are cervical polyps because of their protected position within the uterine cavity. With larger polyps, and especially those which develop pedicles sufficiently long to allow obtrusion of the polyp into the cervical or even the vaginal canal, bleeding is a common symptom. Ulcerative changes and inflammation are common on the dependent surface of the polyp, and necrosis may occur due to interference with the blood supply. Uterine cramping is typical, an attempt to expel the initiative body; cramps at times other than only with menstruation should alert the clinician to the possibility of an endometrial polyp.

Retention of Gestation Products

This is one of the most common of all causes of uterine bleeding, chiefly because of the frequency of abortion, both spontaneous and induced, although placental tissue is not infrequently retained after full-term delivery as well. The bleeding may be slight or it may be exceedingly profuse. The continuance of bleeding after abortion usually indicates retention of gestational products. Occasionally, such retained tissue becomes firmly incorporated within the uterine wall and may form large or small placental polyps (Fig. 31.2). The bleeding is sometimes due to failure or inability of the uterine muscle to contract, but in other cases it is due to the opening up of large venous sinuses when the uterus tries to expel portions of placental tissue still attached to the uterine wall.

Chronic Endometritis

Endometritis is not a common cause of uterine bleeding. Finding chronic endometritis suggests possible upper tract disease (hydrosalpinx, pyosalpinx, or pelvic inflammatory disease), a retained or buried intrauterine device, or retained products of pregnancy following abortion or delivery, or to mycoplasma infection (foci of lymphocytes). Acute endometritis overlies submucous myomata or is found in necrotic endometrial polyps.

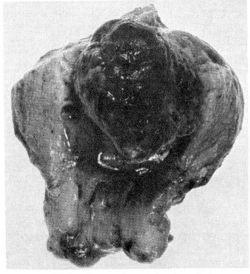

Figure 31.2.   Large placental polyp of uterus.

Subinvolution of the Uterus

This condition is seen with marked retroflexion and retroversion of the acquired type. The incompleteness of the normal involution of the puerperal uterus leaves it large, boggy, and congested, and menstrual excess is not uncommon as a result of the uterine hyperemia.

Carcinoma of the Corpus Uteri

Adenocarcinoma of the uterine body is a common cause of uterine bleeding, especially of the postmenopausal type. In about one-fourth of the cases this disease develops during reproductive life, when the abnormal bleeding may be both menstrual and intermenstrual, the latter being the more significant. In early stages it is only slight and occasional, appearing often as a blood-tinged watery discharge. In patients with adenocarcinoma after the menopause, the bleeding becomes increasingly persistent and more profuse.

Sarcoma of the Uterus

Sarcoma of either the cervix or corpus uteri is far less common than carcinoma, and it produces similar bleeding.

Myoma of Uterus

This exceedingly common cause of uterine bleeding is most likely to occur when the tumors are of the submucous or interstitial variety, not subperitoneal. The finding of myomas in a patient who is bleeding does not justify the conclusion that the tumors cause the bleeding, which may be due to some very different intrauterine condition such as cancer or retained placental tissue.

Hydatidiform Mole and Chorionepithelioma

The bleeding of hydatidiform mole appears in the early months of pregnancy, usually the 3rd to the 5th, and is often associated with a disproportionately large uterus as compared with the duration of the pregnancy. Quantitative serum chorionic gonadotropin assays (β-subunit hCG) are often of value in diagnosis. Chorionepithelioma manifests itself by persistence of bleeding after the evacuation of a hydatidiform mole or after miscarriage or full-term delivery. Quantitative hCG tests may be helpful, but the diagnosis may not be made until later stages, and sometimes not until metastases have appeared (refer to Chapter 27).

Ectopic Pregnancy

The menstrual history suggests the diagnosis in ectopic pregnancy. Menstruation is usually delayed for a few days or several weeks, followed by uterine bleeding which is typically of a spotting character, accompanied by pain in one side of the pelvis. Such a history, together with the finding of a unilateral adnexal mass, should always lead to the suspicion of tubal gestation. Although a definite anatomical lesion is present in such cases, the mechanism of the bleeding is at least partly due to hormonal factors, as discussed in Chapter 26, Ectopic Pregnancy.

Tuberculosis of the Genital Tract

The usual primary seat of genital tuberculosis is in the tubes, but the endometrium is secondarily involved in the majority of cases. Bleeding is frequent but not invariable, and amenorrhea or hypomenorrhea may be noted in some cases, especially in late stages.

Adnexitis

Inflammatory disease of the tubes and ovary may cause not only uterine bleeding but also disturbances of menstrual rhythm, especially in the form of shortened intervals (polymenorrhea). In many cases, the probable immediate factor is ovarian dysfunction rather than pelvic hyperemia.

Tumors of the Ovary

Uterine bleeding is most commonly associated with estrogen-producing ovarian neoplasms. This group includes granulosa cell tumors and thecoma, although others not of the "endocrine variety" may likewise exert a hormonal influence, in most instances by virtue of hyperactive stromal cells. Even large growths of other types, malignant or benign, are most frequently accompanied by no external bleeding.

Tumors of the Tube

These are extremely rare, but the most important of them, carcinoma, is not infrequently associated with bleeding. The blood undoubtedly finds its way into the uterus from the ulcerating intratubal neoplasm, giving a serosanguinous discharge referred to as hydrosalpinx perfluens.

Treatment

The treatment of uterine bleeding due to any of the anatomical causes enumerated above must obviously be directed toward removal or correction of these various etiological factors. Each is discussed under the appropriate chapter heads.

FURTHER DIAGNOSTIC EVALUATION

Further diagnostic evaluation of abnormal uterine bleeding, to exclude organic pathology, divides patients into (1) those with bleeding associated with an ovulatory cycle and (2) those with anovulation. These categories have different etiologic backgrounds and respond to different forms of therapy.

Frequently, the history alone may reveal this distinction, especially if the patient has been keeping a basal temperature chart. Bleeding associated with a secretory pattern of the endometrium must be regarded as anatomical or organic until proven otherwise; the exception to this, ovulatory bleeding associated with an endocrine dysfunction, will be discussed next. Anovulatory bleeding is usually related to dysfunction of the neuroendocrine system but may coexist with an organic cause of the bleeding.

ABNORMAL UTERINE BLEEDING IN ASSOCIATION WITH OVULATION

The causes of bleeding associated with ovulatory cycles are shown in Table 31.3. Diagnosis of ovulation may be difficult, especially when there is no recognizable cycle. The history is important, and a basal body temperature chart is a valuable diagnostic tool under circumstances in which the bleeding is not so severe as to require immediate diagnostic curettage as a therapeutic measure; most cases of ovulatory bleeding fit within this category. Most useful for diagnosis is an *endometrial biopsy* or curettage accomplished *during the bleeding episode.*

Bleeding in an ovulatory cycle due to a *pregnancy complication* is usually due to placental polyps or retained secundines. This may be suspected from the history and

Table 31.3
Abnormal Uterine Bleeding Associated With Ovulatory Cycles

Complications of a past pregnancy
  Retained secundines, placental polyps
Ectopic pregnancy
Organic pelvic disease
  Neoplastic disease (benign or malignant)
    Sarcoma, carcinoma, or myomata of uterine
      fundus, Fallopian tube, and/or ovary
  Infectious disease
    Tuberculosis
    Pelvic inflammatory disease
  Other
    Endometriosis
Bleeding at ovulation (kleine Regel)
Polymenorrhea due to
  Follicular shortening
  Luteal shortening
Irregular endometrial shedding
  Premenstrual staining
  Prolonged menses
Persistent corpus luteum (Halban's disease)
Blood dyscrasias
  ITP, von Willebrand's disease
  Leukemia
Iatrogenic
  Drugs—anticoagulants, progestational agents
  Intrauterine device

proven by an endometrial biopsy or curettage performed during the bleeding. Ectopic pregnancy is the most important diagnosis to be considered if a history of ovulatory cycles preceding the abnormal bleeding episode is obtained. A pregnancy test is positive in less than 25% of the cases, but the constellation of irregular bleeding or spotting, previously normal menses, pregnancy exposure, adnexal tenderness and/or an adnexal mass should alert the clinician. An elevated basal temperature is an additional diagnostic aid. Rarely, the patient may pass a decidual cast. Culdocentesis is a simple diagnostic procedure which will usually reveal blood if present in the cul-de-sac; the hematocrit is greater than that of circulating blood in the case of a leaking ectopic pregnancy and usually less than 10% if blood from the tap is diluted with peritoneal fluid. If an intact intrauterine pregnancy can reasonably be excluded by fundal size, or the amount of bleeding, then an endometrial biopsy may show an Arias-Stella reaction. Diagnostic laparoscopy is frequently necessary for an absolute diagnosis of ectopic gestation.

Other *organic pelvic disease* may be sus-

pected and proven by various diagnostic aids. The endometrial biopsy or curettage at the time of bleeding may reveal endometrial polyps, endometrial neoplasia necessitating further evaluation, or endometritis suggestive of submucous fibroids or tubal inflammatory disease. Hysteroscopy and hyster-osalpingogram may provide valuable diagnostic information about intrauterine pathology. Tuberculosis primarily causes hypomenorrhea but may be diagnosed by repeated culture of the menstrual flow. Endometriosis may be associated with premenstrual staining, usually insignificant from the standpoint of blood loss; the cause is obscure.

Bleeding at ovulation may be easily diagnosed by history and correlation with a basal body temperature chart, especially if it occurs in association with Mittelschmerz or ovulatory pain. An endometrial biopsy may reveal early secretory changes. Usually, periovulatory bleeding is self-limited and rarely requires therapy. If significant, stilbestrol, 0.1 mg from days 1 to 14 may solve the problem, or dilatation and curettage may be curative for reasons not entirely clear.

Polymenorrhea, too frequent menses, is best diagnosed with the aid of a basal temperature chart; the bleeding history is similar to that of anovulatory menometrorrhagia and the basal temperature chart is needed to document the occurrence of ovulation and to give the proper timing for an endometrial biopsy. In polymenorrheic individuals, with cycle lengths from 16 to 22 days, it is important to establish whether shortening of the cycle is follicular or luteal. Follicular shortening responds to ethinyl estradiol, 0.2 mg (20 μg), or stilbestrol, 0.1 mg administered daily from days 1 to 13 of the cycle, usually followed by ovulation on days 14 or 15, with a normal luteal span. Administration of clomiphene citrate may also lengthen the follicular span. Luteal shortening, with an inadequate luteal phase lasting 5–10 days, may be due to inadequate production of progesterone from the corpus luteum. Progesterone cannot be given orally, and intramuscular administration is usually unacceptable, so the use of progesterone suppositories, 25 mg twice daily, is appropriate therapy for patients with infertility. However, in individuals not interested in fertility, a progestational agent (e.g., Norlutin 5 mg) begun after ovulation and continued for 10 days will usually prolong the luteal phase, although the endometrial pattern will show a glandular-stromal disparity. A barrier method of contraception or an IUD should be used. Alternately, a combined oral contraceptive may be chosen, although this is relatively drastic treatment in the patient not needing contraception.

Irregular endometrial shedding, characterized by prolonged menses and theoretically due to a prolonged desquamation phase, must be diagnosed by endometrial biopsy or curettage on the 5th or 6th day of bleeding. The pathologic findings reveal both secretory and proliferative endometrium. The curettage is usually curative. Therapy with a progestational agent is inappropriate, as irregular shedding may be due to persistent luteal progesterone output, but low-dose estrogen begun on cycle day 1 or 2 may be beneficial.

Halban's disease, or a *persistent corpus luteum,* is rare but difficult to differentiate from an ectopic gestation. An endometrial biopsy is a valuable diagnostic aid, but only if there is no intrauterine pregnancy. Both disorders have a secretory endometrium; the pattern in ectopic pregnancy shows hypersecretory glands and the Arias-Stella reaction, whereas in Halban's disease, a pronounced decidual reaction is more common. The presence of an adnexal mass and tenderness on pelvic examination is not useful in differentiating the two entities. Frequently, laparoscopy must be accomplished for accurate diagnosis, although the findings through the laparoscope may be equivocal. The more sensitive and rapidly performed radioimmunologic and radioreceptor hCG assays are extremely helpful in making the differential diagnosis. There is no therapy for a persistent corpus luteum, and even its etiology is unclear. Possibly ovarian prostaglandin synthesis, which may be necessary for luteolysis, is inadequate. Usually the problem is self-limited and not recurrent, terminating in 5–7 days, but bleeding may be excessive.

Blood dyscrasias, which may occasionally present with the symptoms of abnormal but ovulatory uterine bleeding, are usually due to platelet abnormalities. Thrombocytopenic purpura, leukemia, or von Willebrand's disease may be diagnosed by a thorough hematologic evaluation. The diagnosis of von Willebrand's disease should be suspected in all patients who present with a history of recurrent, unexplained menorrhagia, postoperative or postpartum hemorrhage, bleeding following a tooth extraction, easy bruising, epistaxis,

or a family history of bleeding. If menorrhagia is a presenting complaint, it can sometimes be controlled by the use of combined estrogen-progestational compounds. Manifestations of bleeding usually subside as the patient gets older.

Menorrhagia has also been reported in patients with systemic lupus erythematosus, and a lupus cell preparation might be requested if there are other indications of the disease. Iron deficiency anemia has also been reported as associated with ovulatory dysfunctional bleeding, but the reason for this remains obscure.

Chronic renal failure is usually associated with menstrual irregularities and amenorrhea in proportion to the degree of uremia. Women maintained on regular hemodialysis for chronic renal failure may have hypermenorrhea, a relatively unusual form of ovulatory abnormal uterine bleeding. Therapy includes oral progestin-estrogen combinations, but surgical methods and even irradiation may be used. Patients with chronic renal disease who undergo renal transplantation have recovery of regular menses after surgery if the degree of renal function is improved, and approximately 60% of patients establish a normal menstrual pattern.

Finally, iatrogenic causes of abnormal bleeding must be considered. Usually these are related to steroid or anticoagulant ingestion or to an IUD. An adequate history and examination is frequently sufficient to make the diagnosis, but a confirmatory dilatation and curettage or biopsy must be considered.

In summary, diagnosing the presence or absence of ovulation is an important first step in the investigation of abnormal uterine bleeding. A history of menstrual molimina is useful in determining ovulatory cycles, and breast tenderness with uterine cramping is practically pathognomonic. The endometrial biopsy and basal temperature chart are helpful diagnostic aids, provided that bleeding is not of severe extent at the time of initial consultation.

ANOVULATORY UTERINE BLEEDING

Anovulation is frequently associated with bleeding that is excessive in duration, amount, or frequency. Abnormal uterine bleeding is more common during the perimenarcheal and the menopausal years, but at other times, many factors can interrupt or delay normal ovulation with resultant anovulatory bleeding. The causes of the disturbed function can be divided into (1) central, (2) intermediate, (3) peripheral, and (4) physiologic, as shown in Table 31.4. Once the endometrial biopsy taken at the time of bleeding has established the diagnosis of anovulation, it is essential to make an etiologic diagnosis. A careful history will reveal the general area of dysfunction, which is then verified by physical and pelvic examination and documented by selective laboratory, radiologic or therapeutic tests. The management of abnormal anovulatory uterine bleeding will vary depending upon its cause.

It is initially useful to classify patients as pubertal, reproductive age, or menopausal. Etiologic factors tend to cluster according to the three major age groups, although in every group, ovarian tumors must be considered and this diagnosis eliminated. Constitutional factors also tend to cluster in the menstrual age group, probably because this makes up the largest category of women.

The perimenarcheal period is associated with abnormal bleeding due to delayed, asynchronous, or abnormal hypothalamic maturation and is categorized by low FSH, absence of the surge, or a low tonic LH. The most frequent type of bleeding is related to a short menstrual interval, with no real prolongation or increase in flow. Such cycles, if studied intensely, are frequently found to be oligo- or aluteal, with a poor progesterone support of the luteal phase, which is shortened and therefore not truly anovulatory.

True anovulatory cycles are characterized by grossly irregular intervals with prolonged and profuse bleeding phases. These patients may also be manifesting a transient hypothalamic immaturity. If so, lower serum LH assays are observed than in patients who ultimately develop polycystic ovaries, and establishment of a normal ovulatory cycle is to be anticipated within 2 years. Bleeding associated with hypothalamic immaturity is ordinarily self-limited, and if menstrual periods are not overly excessive or prolonged, the adolescent may be reassured that regular function is likely to occur.

However, if the irregular pattern persists, especially if characterized by elevations of serum LH above the levels found in normal cycles during the follicular phase, a polycystic ovarian disease syndrome is suspected. Such stigmata of polycystic ovarian disease as hirsutism or obesity provides a clue that a more severe form of bleeding may be anticipated. The diagnosis is important to make as the reproductive capacity of such patients is jeopardized and they are at higher risk for the development of endometrial hyperplasia or cancer (Fraser et al.). These young patients respond, as do older ones, to clomiphene citrate if ovulation induction is indicated, or to wedge resection in the very rare situation in which bleeding can not be controlled. More typically, pituitary and ovarian suppression with an oral contraceptive, for instance Ortho-Novum 2 mg, is therapeutic and preventive.

In this age group, the ovary may be the primary site of pathology. A karyotype may indicate mosaicism associated with decreased numbers of oocytes and follicles. Transient or persistent elevations of FSH confirm the diagnosis. Visualization of the ovaries is also sometimes helpful, and an open ovarian biopsy is a definitive diagnostic method; the laparoscopic biopsy is usually unsatisfactory.

Table 31.4
Etiologic Classification of Abnormal Uterine Bleeding Associated with Anovulation

Central causes
  Functional and organic disease
    Traumatic, toxic, and infectious lesions
    Stein-Leventhal syndrome
    Immaturity of the hypothalamo-pituitary axis
  Psychogenic factors
    Stress, anxiety, emotional trauma
  Neurogenic factors
  Psychotropic drugs, drug addiction
  Exogenous steroid administration

Intermediate causes
  Chronic illness
  Metabolic or endocrine disease
  Nutritional disturbances

Peripheral causes
  Ovarian
    Functional or inflammatory cysts
    Functional tumors, especially estrogenic
  Premature ovarian failure

Physiologic
  Perimenarcheal
  Perimenopausal

These patients have a compromised ovarian function, and the advisability of any wedge biopsy may, however, be questionable.

In the mature woman, psychogenic causes of abnormal uterine bleeding usually involve marital or sexual life, and a detailed history may reveal significant events preceding the anovulatory episodes. Different age groups are affected by different stressful situations, and the history should probe for factors such as broken family relationships, alcoholism or drug addiction, school or social pressures, all of which seem to be significant in producing anovulation.

A frequent cause of anovulatory bleeding in the reproductive age patient is polycystic ovarian disease (PCOD), and patients with this problem must be identified. Abnormal hormonal feedback at the hypothalamic and/or pituitary level results in the failure of normal follicular development and secondarily in the failure of the normal estradiol trigger of the LH surge. LH stimulation of ovarian steroidogenesis results in the output of the precursor androgenic hormones androstenedione and testosterone, which are peripherally converted to estrone and estradiol. Unopposed estrogen production may induce excessive endometrial stimulation, causing either dysfunctional uterine bleeding or the potential development of hyperplastic or atypical endometrial patterns. These patients tend to be obese and hirsute, and enlarged ovaries may be palpated at physical examination. The characteristic gonadotropin pattern is a persistent pulsatile elevation of LH above the expected normal range for the follicular phase of the cycle and a normal or occasionally suppressed FSH level. These patients are at risk for the development of endometrial adenocarcinoma so the initial examination should include an endometrial biopsy, and subsequent curettage must be considered if any significant abnormality is identified. The pathogenesis of this syndrome of unopposed estrogen stimulation is discussed in Chapter 22. It may be primarily a hypothalamic disease or caused by heritable defects of the nervous system, psychogenic stress factors, obesity, and premature pubarche or early pubertal development due to adrenal causes; rarely, PCOD has been found in association with an ovarian tumor or a dermoid.

Malnutrition and vitamin deficiency states, metabolic disease, and acute or chronic illness, including kidney and liver dysfunction may influence gonadotropin secretion; ordinarily, patients with these diseases are amenorrheic. Hypothyroidism is more frequently associated with menorrhagia, whereas patients with hyperthyroidism are more frequently amenorrheic. Patients with documented thyroid disease commonly have menstrual disorders but the reverse is not true; most patients with anovulatory uterine bleeding have normal thyroid parameters. Mild adrenal hyperplasia and Cushing's syndrome may be associated with anovulation, but frequently menstrual function remains normal until the diagnosis is obvious. Adrenal insufficiency is most commonly associated with amenorrhea. Nutritional deficiencies are less common than in the younger age group, although obesity is not an infrequent finding. The association of obesity with irregular and excessive uterine bleeding is relatively common. Similar to patients with polycystic ovarian disease, obese women tend to have an increased estrogen milieu and are at risk for the development of endometrial hyperplasia. Weight reduction, alone, may result in resumption of normal menses.

Primary ovarian defects may also cause uterine bleeding. Functioning ovarian cysts are not uncommonly seen with anovulation but may be secondary to dysfunction at the central level. Ovarian tumors causing uterine bleeding are usually estrogen producing; the androgen-producing tumors commonly cause virilization and amenorrhea. Some patients with estrogenic tumors will complain of excessive mucus production and abdominal pain, but the diagnosis is usually made at surgery. In the younger patient, a buccal smear may be indicated, as chromosomal mosaicism has been associated with abnormal uterine bleeding. The most common ovarian cause of unusual bleeding is impending ovarian failure or premature menopause, and generally these patients will describe hot flashes.

In the perimenopausal woman, the etiology of menstrual dysfunction is usually related to a failing ovarian function. An increased interval between menses, at least some of which are ovulatory, is normal for the perimenopausal patient. A clue to serious pathology is a history of a shortened interval, or episodic spotting. Elevated gonadotropin values may return to normal, and ovulatory cycles reoccur for a period of time. This pattern seems to represent the ability of the ovary and pituitary to reestablish normal function, probably by regeneration or increased sensitivity of ovarian receptor sites for gonadotropic hormones, or possibly by way of hypothalamic modulation via estrogen.

TREATMENT OF ANOVULATORY DYSFUNCTIONAL BLEEDING

The disturbance of physiology in anovulatory dysfunctional bleeding is the same regardless of the underlying etiology. Therefore, patients can be treated symptomatically to control the bleeding while the primary cause is being investigated. There are two goals in the management of dysfunctional uterine bleeding: (1) control of the acute bleeding episode, and (2) prevention of recurrent bleeding. Although blood loss of life-threatening proportions is fortunately rare, it is important to describe the immediate care of patients so affected.

Management of the Acute Bleeding Episode

When a patient arrives with massive vaginal hemorrhage and deteriorating vital signs, the first step in management is stabilization. As the intravenous route is established, blood is withdrawn for cross-match and initial hematologic studies, which should include a smear done immediately to look for platelets. A Foley catheter and a central venous line are established as necessary. The physical examination seeks an etiology for the bleeding and clearance for probable anesthesia. Pelvic examination is performed, specifically considering the usual causes for such massive blood loss which are (1) a complication or pregnancy, (2) reproductive tract neoplasia, and (3) blood dyscrasia. In the absence of these, the simple technique of office suction curettage may induce almost immediate cessation of bleeding. The uterus is evacuated of clots with suction or, equally simple, with a large 50-cc syringe attached to a Novak curette. Tissue obtained may be sent for immediate diagnosis by frozen section. Dysfunctional uterine bleeding not due to carcinoma or blood dyscrasia will respond to the above measures in almost all cases. The vagina should not be packed, unless a neoplastic

or ulcerating local lesion is the cause, as massive but occult bleeding may continue. Once the acute bleeding episode has been retarded and the diagnosis established, then hormonal therapy is the most logical approach in individuals wishing to maintain fertility.

An acute episode of anovulatory uterine bleeding should be arrested by hormonal therapy in the majority of patients within 48 hours. Ordinarily, the endometrial pattern is proliferative or hyperplastic, although the pathologic specimem may be disrupted by bleeding and repair, and difficult to interpret. Under these circumstances, a potent progestational agent is the treatment of choice. The intramuscular administration of Progesterone-in-oil, 100–200 mg, which may be repeated in 2–4 hours, followed by the oral administration of a progestational compound is acceptable. The choice of the agent and its dose will depend upon the endometrial pattern. The 19-nor progestational agents have acceptable progestational activity, with mild androgenic activity, and are capable of arresting uterine bleeding more readily than the C-21 progestogens. Withdrawal bleeding from a converted progestational endometrium will follow some 3–10 days following discontinuation of the therapy.

Accepted cyclic regimens of oral progestational agents include: for the proliferative or mildly hyperplastic endometrium, Provera 10–20 mg or Norlutin 5–10 mg daily for 5–10 days; for the more hyperplastic or mildly atypical endometrium, the potent progestational agent, Megace, 40 mg a day for a week to 10 days, is useful for conversion. For intramuscular use, Delalutin (17α-hydroxyprogesterone caproate) 250 mg intramuscularly every 3 days for two doses may be effective.

The intravenous administration of conjugated estrogens has been recommended to arrest the acute bleeding episode but has been unsuccessful in our hands. The estrogen is thought to have a direct effect upon capillary bleeding and to produce changes in the blood coagulation scheme. Although these effects provide the rationale for this therapy, using estrogen to treat a potentially hyperplastic endometrium is self-defeating and possibly harmful.

Fortunately, most uterine bleeding is not of an acute and life-threatening nature. Rather, it is of annoyance to the patient and worrisome to the physician because of the implication of an underlying hyperplasia. Uterine curettage is commonly employed in diagnosis and acute management and may be curative in some 40% of patients with a transient or self-limited disorder of ovulation. However, a more chronic etiologic factor may not be corrected and the risk of recurrent dysfunctional bleeding may persist so that projected further management will depend upon the expectation of the patient. Most patients wish to maintain reproductive function. Therefore, the second goal of management, prevention of recurrent bleeding, becomes important.

Treatment of More Chronic Abnormal Uterine Bleeding

Treatment of anovulatory abnormal uterine bleeding in the reproductive age group is based upon the chief complaint of the patient. The physician and the patient have four alternative approaches in management:
1. Observation
2. Cyclic progestational agents, if a barrier method of contraception is used
3. Oral contraceptives; and
4. Ovulation induction, ordinarily clomiphene citrate

If fertility is not an issue and the bleeding pattern is irregular but not profuse, then observation is appropriate and nothing need be done except routine follow-up. These patients normally ovulate irregularly, with 3–4 months between ovulatory menses, and do not have sufficient unopposed estrogen to develop a hyperplastic endometrium. Either endometrial biopsy or curettage must be performed to document this, and the patient warned that even sporadic ovulation may result in unwanted conception.

If the patient is interested in fertility, the induction of ovulation is the treatment of choice. If prevention of a recurrent attack of bleeding and the establishment of cyclic or controlled bleeding is important, the endocrine therapy is chosen.

Endocrine Therapy

Most patients with anovulatory bleeding have either normal or increased estrogen stimulation of the endometrium and, because of anovulation, deficient progesterone. The simplest therapeutic approach, resulting in controlled bleeding from a converted endometrium, is cyclic administration of a progestational agent (Table 31.5). A convenient oral regimen uses Provera, 10 mg a day, or Norlutin, 5 mg a day for the first 7–10 days of each month. In the majority of patients, an acceptable bleeding pattern is produced, but several precautions are necessary. If the patient is sexually active and not interested in pregnancy, she must be warned that this therapy is not contraceptive. Secondly, its efficacy in treating previously diagnosed endometrial hyperplasia must be documented by follow-up biopsy, obtained just before the institution of the progestational agent, at the time of maximal estrogen stimulation. If taken during or shortly after administration of the progestational agent, the mixed secretory pattern with glandular-stromal disparity may mask persistent or recurrent hyperplasia.

As some patients may develop recurrent hyperplasia and others may reestablish normal ovulatory menses while being cycled, it is important to diagnose the cause of any bleeding that occurs at other than expected times. Basal temperature charts and repeat biopsies during bleeding episodes may be diagnostically useful.

The oral contraceptives, including Ortho-Novum 2 mg, and Demulen, result in regular periods, ovulation suppression, decreased FSH and LH output from the pituitary, in-

Table 31.5
Cyclic Progestational Therapy for Anovulatory Uterine Bleeding

Mode of Administration	Generic Name	Trade Name	Monthly Dosage
Intramuscular	Progesterone-in-oil	Lipolutin	50–100 mg
	17α-Hydroxyprogesterone	Delalutin	125 mg
Oral	Norethindrone (Acetate)	Norlutin (Norlutate)	5–10 mg daily for 1st 7–10 days of each month
	Medroxyprogesterone acetate	Provera	10–20 mg daily for 1st 7–10 days of each month
	Megestrol acetate	Megace	40 mg daily for 3 months

creased testosterone-binding globulin, and decreased ovarian steroidogenesis and release. Androstenedione and testosterone levels will decrease, and because of the increase in testosterone-binding globulin, less *free* testosterone will be available for biologic effect (Givens et al.). Certain of the oral contraceptives are associated with a decrease in circulating dehydroepiandrosterone sulfate (DHEA-S), which suggests that this precursor androgen of adrenal etiology is affected by oral contraceptive therapy as well (Madden et al.). Following discontinuation of the oral contraceptive, DHEA-S values have remained suppressed far longer than expected, as ovulatory menses likely resume within a period of weeks. Thus, oral contraceptive administration will result in regularity of menstruation and a decrease in the circulating androgens responsible for hirsutism, and possibly for some element of obesity. Contraception is provided, and the worry of administration of a progestational agent in early pregnancy is avoided.

Induction of Ovulation

Induction of ovulation may be a satisfactory means of controlling anovulatory bleeding. The use of clomiphene citrate is well established, but ordinarily is indicated only when pregnancy is desired. Under special circumstances, especially in the perimenarchial individual, this agent may be used to establish the potential normality of the hypothalamic-pituitary-gonadal axis. In this situation, the patient must be warned that conception can and may occur.

SUMMARY

The management of patients with abnormal uterine bleeding requires a logical, rational approach and an awareness of the etiologic factors. A careful history and examination should attempt to answer these questions: (1) Is the bleeding truly from the uterus? (2) Is the bleeding superimposed upon ovulatory cycles? (3) Is the bleeding anovulatory? The endometrial biopsy *obtained during the bleeding episode* and the basal temperature chart are diagnostically useful. Massive uterine bleeding not due to a complication of pregnancy, neoplasia, or blood dyscrasia usually responds immediately to curettage, done in the operating room or office; follow-up hormonal therapy with progesterone and a progestational agent should control the episode. More chronic forms of abnormal uterine bleeding are approached by identifying and treating the etiologic cause. If the cause is not correctable (e.g., obesity), most patients will respond satisfactorily to the cyclic administration of oral contraceptives or a progestational agent or, if indicated, to induction of ovulation.

References and Additional Readings

Aksel, S., and Jones, G.S.: Etiology and treatment of dysfunctional uterine bleeding. Obstet. Gynecol., *44*:1, 1974.

Evans, P.C.: Obstetric and gynecologic patients with von Willebrand's disease. Obstet. Gynecol, *38*:37, 1971.

Fraser, I.S., Michie, E.A., Wide, L, and Baird, D.T.: Pituitary gonadotropins and ovarian function in adolescent dysfunctional uterine bleeding. J. Clin. Endocrinol. Metab., *37*:407, 1973.

Givens, J.R., Andersen, R.N., Wiser, W.L., and Fish, S.A.: Dynamics of suppression and recovery of plasma FSH, LH, androstenedione and testosterone in polycystic ovarian disease using an oral contraceptive. J. Clin. Endocrinol. Metab., *38:*727, 1974.

Madden, J.D., Milewich, L., Parker, C.R., Carr, B.R., Boyar, R.M., and MacDonald, P.C.: The effect of oral contraceptive treatment on the serum concentration of dehydroisoandrosterone sulfate. Am. J. Obstet. Gynecol., *132*:380, 1978.

Mitch, W.E., Spivak, J.L., Spangler, D.B., and Bell, W.R.: Thrombotic thrombocytopenic purpura presenting with gynecological manifestations. Lancet, *i*:849, 1973.

Perez, R.J., Lipner, H., Abdulla, N., Cicotto, S., and Abrams, M.: Menstrual dysfunction of patients undergoing chronic hemodialysis. Obstet. Gynecol., *51*:552, 1978.

Pugh, M.: Von Willebrand's disease in gynecologic and obstetric practice. Int. J. Gynecol. Obstet., *10*:137, 1972.

Quick, A.J.: Menstruation in hereditary bleeding disorders. Obstet. Gynecol., *28*:37, 1966.

Shane, J.M., Naftolin, F., and Newmark, S.R.: Gynecologic endocrine emergencies. JAMA *231*:393. 1975.

Taw, R.L.: Review of menstrual disorders in which a secretory endometrium was found. Am. J. Obstet. Gynecol., *122*:490, 1975.

Van Look, P.F.S., Hunder, W.M., Fraser, I.S., and Baird, D.T.: Impaired estrogen-induced luteinizing hormone release in young women with anovulatory dysfunctional uterine bleeding. J. Clin. Endocrinol. Metab., *46*:816, 1978.

CHAPTER 32

Management of the Menopause

By definition, the term menopause means the final cessation of menses, whereas the climacteric implies a transitional period in the life of an individual during which the reproductive function is diminished and lost.

It is estimated that, among women of the United States, the average age for the menopause is approximately 48 years, whereas the span of the climacteric lies between the ages of 46 and 50 years. However, many gynecologists are impressed with the frequency with which apparently regular menstruation may persist into the sixth decade.

PHYSIOLOGY

It has been estimated that there are approximately 500,000 available oocytes in the ovaries at the menarche. With every menstrual cycle a certain number of these with their cohort of follicles are expended. This loss of oocytes and follicles ultimately results in a gradual diminution of estrogen and inhibin. The decreased inhibin results in an elevation of FSH, the first laboratory indication of the perimenopause. The increased FSH induces rapid follicular development and the ensuing shortening of cycles is the first clinical evidence of the perimenopause (Sherman and Korenman) (Table 32.1). As the numbers of follicles are further decreased, estrogen production continues to fall, and as levels not compatible with the induction of an LH surge are reached, ovulation may cease or, more frequently, may become irregular. Clinically, this is associated with irregular cycles and a shortened luteal phase or anovulatory cycles with unopposed estrogen

stimulation and endometrial hyperplasia. As ovulation ceases entirely, the LH begins to rise, and the **menopause**, cessation of menses, is at hand. It is nevertheless important to realize that the feedback mechanisms may cause readjustments between the pituitary and ovary as long as there are follicles remaining in the ovary to respond, and over a period of a year or 2, reversal of laboratory findings as well as clinical signs and symptoms may occur.

Although the menopausal ovary may be lacking in follicles, the cells of which normally secrete the major estrogen and progesterone, it should be remembered that many menopausal women are not totally devoid of estrogen. The ovarian stroma cells as well as adrenal cells have a steroidogenic capacity for producing androstenedione, which is converted by the skin and appendages to estrone. The ovaries of approximately one-third of all aging women show "hyperthecosis" of ovarian stroma cells, indicating continued steroidogenic function.

SYMPTOMATOLOGY

Before discussing the symptomatology of the menopause, it is necessary to realize that only 25% of all women have any symptoms which are severe enough to warrant a medical consultation. The other 75% simply stop menstruating and life continues as before with health and happiness unimpaired.

Menopausal symptoms are conveniently divided into two groups: those *acute symptoms* associated with immediate or imminent cessation of menses, and those *later symptoms*

Table 32.1
Characteristics of Menstrual Cycle Length in Normal Women Throughout Reproductive Life and in Disorders of Follicular Maturation[a]

Group	Follicular Phase[c]	Luteal Phase[d]	Total Cycle Length
	days	days	days
Age 18–30	16.9 ± 3.7	12.9 ± 1.8	30.0 ± 3.6
Age 40–41	10.4 ± 2.9	15.0 ± 0.9	25.4 ± 2.3
Age 46–51	8.16 ± 2.8[b]	15.9 ± 1.3	23.2 ± 2.9
Long follicular phase	33.0 ± 2.2	14.2 ± 2.2	47.2 ± 4.3
Short luteal phase	17.2 ± 1.7	7.0 ± 2.4[b]	24.2 ± 3.6
Inadequate luteal phase	71.6 ± 50.5[b]	12.3 ± 0.5	84.0 ± 50.6[b]

[a] Results are means ± SD. (Reproduced with permission from: B. M. Sherman and S. G. Korenman: Journal of Clinical Investigation, 55: 699, 1975.)
[b] $P = <0.05$.
[c] Follicular phase is from first day of menses to the LH peak.
[d] Luteal phase is from LH peak to onset of menses.

which appear after some years of menopause. In a double blind, cross over estrogen/placebo study, the only acute symptom which could be significantly correlated with estrogen deprivation was the hot flush (Cooper). However, we believe that three symptoms may be regarded as truly related to menopause: cessation or irregularity of menses, the hot flush, and insomnia (Schiff et al.). The other host of symptoms sometimes ascribed to the menopause must be regarded as related to either the aging process or anxiety associated with a confrontation of aging. There is nevertheless, a cascade effect which cannot be disregarded. Flushes may be severe enough to impair sleep; loss of sleep impairs energy; lack of energy decreases productivity; decreased productivity impairs interpersonal relationships; and impaired interpersonal relationships cause mood depressions. Late sequelae ascribed to the menopause in association with the long-term lowered estrogen milieu are dyspareunia, urethritis, osteoporosis, and arteriosclerotic cardiovascular disease. As will be discussed later in the chapter, the relationship of arteriosclerotic cardiovascular disease to the menopause is difficult to document.

PATHOGENESIS

The menopause (cessation of menses) is undoubtedly due to failing ovarian function and the associated decreased steroidogenesis. This in turn disturbs the pituitary hypothalamic feedback mechanisms, causing an elevation of pituitary gonadotrophins and hypothalamic LRH. However, although the

ovarian estradiol and progesterone excretion are sharply reduced, as indicated in Chapter 2, the menopausal ovary is nevertheless capable of substantial steroidogenesis. Androstenedione (ADD) is the preferential steroid synthesized by the ovarian stroma, and its production is the characteristic function of the menopausal ovary. Peripheral conversion of ADD to estrone furnishes the major estrogen source at this age. Thus, it would seem that although menopausal women do have an estrogen milieu which is lower than that necessary for **reproductive** function, it is not negligible or absent but is perhaps satisfactory for **maintenance** of **support tissues.** The menopause could then be regarded as a physiologic phenomenon which is protective in nature—protective from undesirable reproduction and the associated growth stimuli.

The etiology of one acute symptom, the hot flush, although dependent upon the estrogen withdrawal, is specifically related to an associated autonomic nervous system instability. Although one would therefore think that the positive input of a specific neurotransmitter must be involved, no such neurohormone has been identified.

DIAGNOSIS

Although the clinical symptoms of vasomotor instability in conjunction with irregularities or cessation of menses are pathognomonic, the laboratory finding which confirms the diagnosis of the menopause is an elevated serum pituitary gonadotrophin assay for FSH and LH. Values for FSH by radioimmunoassay are usually 100 mIU/ml or above, while

LH values are above 75 mIU/ml. These laboratory assays must be used only in conjunction with the clinical findings. Both FSH and LH values should be obtained, as the level of LH can be equally high in the ovulatory phase of the cycle. As indicated in the previous section, the ovarian-hypothalamic-pituitary feedback mechanisms can at times reestablish homeostasis, and these abnormal laboratory values may be normalized for a brief period with reestablishment of cycles. This may also occur in patients with a premature menopause. Therefore, observation over a period of 1 year with repeat hormonal determinations is advisable. In the diagnosis of a premature menopause an ovarian biopsy may be necessary.

Premature Menopause

Diagnosis of the premature menopause, especially in very young girls, is sometimes difficult, and it must be remembered that this condition can occur at any age. The youngest reported patient of whom we are aware was 18 years of age.

If the pituitary FSH values are elevated and the patient complains of hot flushes, the diagnosis is fairly well substantiated. However hot flushes are not always experienced, and if at least two elevated gonadotrophin assays have been obtained, it may be wise to offer the very young patient, an ovarian biopsy prior to making a definitive diagnosis. This is the only way to differentiate a premature menopause, with absence of oocytes and follicles, from the insensitive ovary syndrome (Chapter 30) or a temporary disruption of follicular growth. In the latter two conditions, resumption of normal ovarian function with normal reproductive capacity is a possibility. If a biopsy is done it should be as a minilaparotomy, and a small, full thickness section of the ovaries should be removed. A laparoscopic biopsy affords insufficient material to make this diagnosis.

TREATMENT
General Considerations

As indicated above there is a broad spectrum of symptoms and reaction to symptoms. Patients requiring therapy are those having (1) flushes severe enough to cause discomfort or embarrassment; (2) sweats and resultant insomnia with or without flushes; (3) dyspa-

reunia, a late symptom usually due to senile vaginitis and urethritis; and (4) symptomatic osteoporosis, the latest manifestation of all.

The therapy for acute menopausal symptoms must be individualized, and although estrogen therapy is specific for specific symptoms, the flush and insomnia, or dyspareunia from senile vaginal atrophy, reassurance with minimal sedation may be adequate if the major complaints are those related to psychologic or emotional factors while estrogen dependent symptoms are mild. For those patients in whom estrogens are contraindicated, such as patients who have been treated for estrogen-dependent carcinoma of the female genital tract or for breast tumors, sedation, supplemented by vitamin E and B complex is used, but with only minimal success. Clonidine, an alpha-adrenergic stimulator, has been suggested as an alternative to estrogen therapy, and although not as effective as estrogen, it does ameliorate the symptoms to some extent. Testosterone is of little value and may give rise to more distressing symptoms than relief. Medroxyprogesterone acetate (Provera) has been used by Bullock et al. with some success; however, because of the experimental findings of an increase in breast cancers in Beagle dogs associated with administration of C-21 steroids, some caution should be used in recommending this therapy.

Estrogen Therapy

Regimens of treatment can be divided into four types: (1) those used for menopause occurring at the expected time; (2) those used for the premature menopause; (3) those used when late symptoms of senile vaginitis or urethritis predominate; and (4) regimens used for osteoporosis.

The aim of proper hormonal therapy for acute symptoms is to control these as rapidly as possible with as little medication as possible and to discontinue treatment as soon as possible. If one is able to institute therapy at the onset of symptoms, all of these criteria can usually be met. However, if a patient has been suffering from flushes for many years, a habit pattern has been established which will probably require prolonged therapy.

Types of Estrogen Available

There are three major types of estrogen available: (1) *physiologic*—estradiol, estrone, and estriol; (2) *conjugated natural estrogen*, containing as the major components sulfates or esters of estrone, equilin, and equilenin; and (3) *synthetic estrogens*—ethinyl estradiol, mestranol, and diethylstilbestrol (DES). The synthetic estrogens and mestranol, more so than ethinyl estradiol, are hepatotoxic and, therefore, not to be given to patients with known or suspected liver disease. Conjugated estrogens are the most commonly used in the United States.

Mode of Administration

The mode of administration of estrogens can be oral, vaginal, or subcutaneous by way of pellet implantation or long acting conjugated forms of estrogen. Estrogens administered orally are conjugated, metabolized, and partly excreted by the liver prior to reaching the target organs. The action of estrogens on liver function, stimulation of steroid-binding proteins is, therefore, most efficient by this route. The intramuscular or subcutaneous administration of long acting estrogen conjugates or pellets, although very efficient, has the disadvantage of nonreversability in case of complications. It is therefore not to be recommended.

The vaginal route has several advantages. Steroids are rapidly and reproducibly absorbed from the vagina, medication reaches the target organ prior to circulating through the liver. The conversion of estradiol to estrone, which occurs orally, is decreased by vaginal administration. Serum estradiol levels should, therefore, more accurately reflect the estrogen absorbed and the exposure of the target organs. As the vaginal cornification is increased with estrogen stimualtion, the amount of absorption is decreased as the biological effect is obtained.

Treatment for the Menopause at the Expected Age

Pretherapeutic Interview and Management

Prior to beginning estrogen therapy, a careful history should be obtained to document a family tendency of cancer, hypertension, cardiovascular disease, or osteoporosis. These first two conditions, cancer and hypertension, are potential risk factors and indicate special areas of concern. The last two, cardiovascular disease and osteoporosis, are potential benefit factors. A past history of tumors of the breast, uterus, or central nervous system, including melanomas, is probably an absolute contraindication for estrogen therapy. A history or physical examination indicative of coronary artery disease or stroke is also probably a contraindication to therapy, as sclerotic or damaged vessels are more prone to thrombosis, and estrogen does increase the risk of thromboembolic phenomenon. Although estrogen in doses usually prescribed for menopausal patients has not been shown to be associated with thrombosis, there was an increased rate of coronary thrombosis incidents among men receiving large doses of estrogen in an effort to alleviate arteriosclerotic vascular disease.

The physical examination must include a breast examination to rule out masses or breast secretion and a pelvic examination to rule out pelvic abnormalities and document fibroid tumors. A Papanicolaou smear is obtained not only for routine cervical cancer screening but also for an estrogen index. An endometrial biopsy should be done prior to initiating therapy to rule out any endometrial abnormality. Routine blood chemistries to rule out liver disease, a lipid screen as a baseline for an estimate of possible arteriosclerotic vascular disease, and a blood pressure for future reference must all be obtained.

Specific Estrogen Routine. The patient who is seen initially with **acute** onset of menopausal **symptoms** can usually be managed with the lowest amount of estrogen over the shortest period of time. Estrogen given in a daily dosage, 1.25 mg of conjugated estrogen or its equivalent, should be sufficient to render the patient almost asymptomatic within a 2-week period. As the flush is the most common as well as the most objective symptom of the menopause, patients are asked to record on a large calendar page the number of flushes per day and return to the office within 2 weeks. If this record indicates a sharp reduction of symptoms, the dosage can be reduced by half at this time. If symptoms recur, the reduction has been too rapid and a higher dosage must be resumed at once and continued for another week or until reduction can be accomplished without recurrence of symptoms. The dose of 0.625 mg daily given for 3 weeks with 1 week of rest from therapy can then be maintained for 3 months. Reduction to 0.3 mg daily is then usually possible. Estrogen given in this way can be discontinued, as a rule within 6–9 months, and with such low-dose short duration estrogen, it is usually not necessary to add a progestational drug. However, an endometrial biopsy is always desirable prior to beginning estrogen therapy and, depending upon the pathological picture, progestational therapy may be omitted or started at once. A complete dilatation and curettage, perhaps with hysteroscopy to identify or rule out the presence of a polyp, may be warranted if atypical hyperplasia is present.

As there is a great individual variation in response to estrogen therapy, no scheme can be regarded as infallible but must be used only as a norm from which to deviate. Individualization of therapy is highly desirable. A schedule which is usually successful in patients who present for treatment with **persistent symptoms** is 1.25 mg of conjugated estrogen daily from day 1 through 25 of each month, with a 19-norprogestational drug given from the 12th through the 25th of each month. This dosage is usually not necessary for longer than 2 months. It should then be reduced to 0.625 mg daily of a conjugated estrogen for the next 3–4 months, and finally to 0.3 mg during the next 5 or 6 months. When the conjugated estrogen is reduced to below 0.625 mg daily, it is probably no longer necessary to add the progestational drug, as usually no endometrial growth is stimulated by this amount of estrogen; therefore, no antimitotic drug should be required. One endometrial biopsy should be obtained on this low dose to assure that the endometrium is indeed quiescent.

The vaginal smear with maturation index is a valuable adjunct in controlling the estrogen dosage. A maturation index of over 10% cornified cells is excessive. Complications of too high an estrogen dose, used over too long a period, are headaches, nausea, breast tenderness or swelling, and vaginal bleeding. When bleeding does occur, a curettage is mandatory despite the presumptive diagnosis of bleeding from exogenous steroid therapy.

Testosterone used in conjunction with estrogen is usually unwarranted and should not be given as a combined therapy. Decreased libido is a specific indication for testosterone therapy but for this symptom testosterone should be given as outlined in Chapter 35. The menopausal patient who specifically needs estrogen for vaginitis or urethritis, but who will also benefit from a catabolic drug, should receive a catabolic drug which is not androgenic, and preferably one which will not compete with estrogen binding.

A *progestogen* given at the end of an estrogen course has been used extensively to minimize the estrogen stimulation of the endometrium by its antimitotic effect and to cause *shedding of the endometrium* if proliferation has been induced. The bleeding phase after progesterone withdrawal, however, is not associated with complete sloughing of the functional layer, nor can the histologic appearance of the endometrium be predicted by the bleeding or nonbleeding pattern.

With this knowledge, then, one should add a progestational drug for its antimitotic effects, if a sufficient amount of estrogen to cause endometrial proliferation is to be prescribed for a prolonged period. The progestational drug should be given over a sufficient time, 10–14 days, during the last days of the 21- or 25-day estrogen course, and an endometrial biopsy should be performed periodically, at least once a year, to monitor the effect of medication.

Oral contraception drugs for the treatment of the menopause are usually unsatisfactory estrogen substitution therapy.

Treatment of the Premature Menopause

When the uterus is present, the type of replacement therapy depends upon whether or not it is psychologically advantageous to induce regular menses. Usually, if sufficient time has been taken to educate the patient, this is not necessary. However, when the production of regular menses for psychological reasons seems desirable, as in younger girls living in close contact with others in boarding school, the minimal estrogenic dosage which will induce bleeding should be used. This varies in our experience from between 0.625 mg to 1.25 mg of conjugated estrogen daily or its equivalent given for the first 25 days of each month. Progesterone or one of the synthetic substitutes, 5 mg of a 19-norprogestogen, must be given during the last 14 days of estrogen therapy on the 12th through the 25th day of each month. There should then be an interruption of 5 or 6 days, and pills should be resumed again on the 1st day of the following month. This rest period allows the endometrium to shed and thus usually prevents the occurrence of irregular or profuse bleeding. As stated above, an endometrial biopsy must be taken at the end of one steroid cycle to monitor the histologic growth appearance.

When it is unnecessary to induce a menstrual flow, the amount of estrogen required to produce bleeding is determined and the dosage just under this amount is used in the identical manner as described above; 25 days each month with a 5-day rest period. After regulation is accomplished, patients are checked every 6 months the 1st year and then at yearly intervals, unless bleeding or breast symptoms warrant additional examinations. Again, an endometrial biopsy should be obtained yearly to ensure that an abnormal growth pattern is not being induced.

For the woman under 40 who needs castration, it is possible at laparotomy to insert one or two 25-mg estradiol pellets into the incision, and, at the 6-week postoperative examination, to prescribe estrogen suppositories (stilbestrol, 0.5 mg) or creams during the first 1–3 days each week, depending upon symptoms and vaginal cytology. Such a regimen usually prevents flushes from developing and maintains vaginal pliability and lubrication (Hunter et al.). If estradiol per se is used, a serum estradiol assay will serve for monitoring therapy.

Therapy in all cases should be maintained until the age of 45 or 50 years and then should be discontinued slowly over a year's time. Again, no rule of thumb will prove successful for all women and each must be individualized according to her needs.

Considerable care must be utilized in treating women with estrogens over the course of many years; even though the uterus is removed, it must be remembered that the breasts are also estrogen target organs. The minimal estrogen dosage compatible with prevention of symptoms is therefore still to be recommended (see Chapter 15).

Treatment of Senile Vaginitis and Urethritis

The predominating symptoms of senile vaginitis are discharge, itching, burning, and dyspareunia. The symptoms of senile urethritis are urinary frequency and nocturia unassociated with bladder infection. The most effective therapy for these local symptoms is the vaginal route, the use of estrogen suppositories and/or creams.

If constriction of the vaginal lumen has occurred, this is an additional factor causing dyspareunia, and some form of manual or instrumental dilatation will also be necessary to reestablish normal function and painless intercourse. Plastic test tubes or wax candles in graduated sizes make the most satisfactory dilators. The response of senile urethritis to estrogen vaginal creams in conjunction with estrogen suppositories is frequently dramatic.

OSTEOPOROSIS

Definition

Osteoporosis is characterized by x-ray evidence of decalcification of bone, decrease in stature, kyphosis, and eventually severe joint pain and disability associated with multiple fractures. The term menopausal or, more precisely, senile osteoporosis is used to denote the decrease in bone density which occurs among the general population, with age. This phenomenon is seen in both men and women and in populations of all ethnic groups.

Etiology

It is necessary to understand bone formation in relation to calcium metabolism in order to understand the causes of osteoporosis.

The most significant function of bone is not its role as a supporting structure, but rather its role as a calcium reservoir. As calcium is an essential element for all cell functions, including mentation, and as we are dependent upon ingestion of calcium to supply these needs, this function of calcium storage by bone is critical. For normal cellular activity, the serum calcium level must be maintained at approximately 10 mg/100 ml, and this is done at the expense of bone density, if necessary. The daily calcium requirement in order to maintain this serum calcium level is about 1.5 gr, substantially more than the estimated daily intake of the general population (Jowsey, 1978).

Serum calcium levels and concomitantly, therefore, bone density, are dependent upon three functions: 1) calcium intake, basically dietary calcium; 2) calcium resorption from bone; and 3) serum calcium depletion by bone formation. However, calcium homeostasis is also closely tied to phosphate reserves. As the phosphate goes up, the calcium goes down. Jowsey believes that this may be one of the most important factors in the production of osteoporosis in older American women, as our dietary habit patterns tend to favor a high phosphorus and low calcium intake. Calcium is contained in dairy products only. A high phosphorus diet is one which is high in protein, is eaten by patients who are dieting, is low in cholesterol, and is high in soft drinks and snack foods of all varieties. Absorption of calcium from the gut is also decreased with age. Probably the most important factor associated with this is vitamin D, which may be decreased in older people. However, hydroxylation of vitamin D to its active form 1,25-dihydroxycalciferol, must occur in the kidney (Rasmussen and Bordier). The activator enzyme, 1-α-hydroxylase, which is increased by parathyroid hormone, is also activated by prolactin. Prolactin is decreased in the postmenopausal woman, probably as a result of the decrease in estrogen production, thus further impairing the availability of 1,25-dihydroxycalciferol. The malabsorption syndrome interfers with absorption of calcium from the intestines and a defective lactase enzyme in certain individuals interferes with the availability of calcium from milk or milk products.

Rapid Calcium Exchange From Bone

Rapid calcium exchange between bone and blood serum is effected through the bone canaliculi which connect with the bone lacunae around the osteoclasts. The osteoclast is surrounded by hydroxyapatite, a crystal of calcium and phosphorus which has a water hydration layer. It is the calcium and phosphorus in this hydration layer which can be readily exchanged between bone and serum. The long-term calcium homeostasis is maintained by an exchange of calcium from bone resorption or new bone formation.

Bone Resorption

Bone resorption is controlled by the osteoclast and new bone by the osteoblast, both of which require the action of parathyroid hormone. In the absence of parathyroid hormone, serum calcium decreases from the normal of between 9 and 10 mg/100 ml to 6 or 7 mg/100 ml. Decreased bone resorption and decreased bone formation results. As bone resorption and bone formation are in constant homeostasis, one obviously controls the other. When bone resorption is decreased, then bone formation is also decreased. An elevated parathyroid hormone, hyperparathyroidism, results in increased serum calcium and increased bone resorption but also, therefore, increased bone formation. Mineral bony density is decreased, however. Parathyroid hormone, therefore, produces an increased calcium in the extraskeletal pool. Calcitonin is the counterbalance for parathyroid hormone, but it acts mainly as a rapid control rather than being involved in the long-term homeostasis.

Bone Regeneration

Although, as stated above, bone regeneration is intimately tied with bone resorption, specific factors which influence bone regeneration are relatively poorly understood and the most important one seems to be exercise, which in turn is related to muscle mass.

Summary

In summary, density of bone depends primarily upon the absorption of **dietary calcium**. Decreased density may be associated with (1) a low calcium or a high phosphorus intake, (2) the malabsorption syndrome, or (3) a defective lactase enzyme, interfering with the availability of calcium from milk products. Calcium **absorption** is dependent upon vitamin D; anything which decreases the vitamin D intake or the vitamin D activation by the kidney 1-α-hydroxylase will decrease the calcium absorption. Calcium **resorption** from bone is dependent upon the action of (1) parathormone on the osteoclasts, and this is counterbalanced by the action of (2) calcitonin. Bone formation and resorption are in homeostasis, any factor which increases bone resorption also increases bone regeneration, and vice versa. However, the calcium content of the bone may be decreased thereby.

Muscle mass and exercise are factors known to increase bone regeneration. Nevertheless, it must always be remembered that if the calcium content of the bone is to be maintained or increased, the calcium intake must also be maintained or increased. Bone, which is a reservoir for calcium, will be depleted to provide the calcium necessary for vital intracellular mechanisms which require a serum calcium of about 10 mg/100 ml.

Important factors which also influence bone metabolism are estrogen and fluoride. These decrease bone resorption. Glucocorticoids not only increase bone resorption but prevent new bone formation. Prolaction stimulates the hydroxylation of vitamin D in the kidney, thereby increasing calcium absorption from the gut. Cigarette smoking, apparently by decreasing the exchange of volatile gases, increases bone resorption and therefore osteoporosis.

Diagnosis

Acute Symptomatic Osteoporosis

The diagnosis of acute symptomatic osteoporosis in the postmenopausal woman is facilitated by the examination, which indicates a dowager hump, related to compression fractures of the thoracic spine, and loss of height. Loss of height can be estimated quite accurately by measuring both the height and the span. If the patient's span is substantially greater than the height, this usually indicates that height loss has occurred.

X-ray of the thoracic and lumbar spines is the first diagnostic procedure. One must rule out all other factors which can simulate senile osteoporosis. These are diabetes, hypercorticism, iatrogenic or otherwise, hyperthyroidism, hyperparathyroidism, metastatic carcinoma and multiple myeloma, osteogenesis imperfecta tardas, and osteomalacia. If any of these are suspected, the total urinary hydroxyproline/creatinine and calcium/creatinine ratios, and the serum calcium and phosphate levels should be obtained. In osteoporosis all of these are above normal. If alkaline phosphatase is elevated, one must suspect carcinomatosis or osteomalacia, a vitamin D deficiency. Parathyroid hormone values are normal in osteoporosis and elevated in hyperparathyroidism.

Asymptomatic Osteoporosis

As it is easier to prevent than to reverse the process of osteoporosis, it is desirable to make the diagnosis prior to onset of symptoms which may not occur until late in the disease. If osteoporosis is suspected, one must proceed with the same tests which are done to detect osteoporosis in the symptomatic patient.

The height of all postmenopausal patients should be measured at their yearly examination. The patient with osteoporosis may lose 0.5 cm of height a year, and this should alert the physician to the possibility of osteoporosis early in the disease. It is also possible to identify a population at risk by history. Those patients who are suspect are women who have always been thin with little subcutaneous fat, who are heavy cigarette smokers, and who eat a high protein diet or junk food diet with soft drinks and have a low consumption of dairy products. They are sedentary and have little exposure to sun.

Therapy

All approaches to therapy should be utilized which will serve to maintain the serum calcium at the optimum level of 10 mg/100 ml of blood and at the same time promote new bone formation in homeostasis with bone resorption. Basically, this implies an adequate dietary calcium intake and absorption, exercise to maintain muscle mass and bone regeneration and prevention of increased bone resorption, by estrogen therapy.

Adequate Calcium Intake

To assure a sufficient calcium intake to maintain calcium homeostasis, it has been suggested that between 600 and 1,000 mg of calcium a day is necessary. The usual diet of the menopausal patient contains approximately 450 mg a day. Diet habits should be altered to increase dairy products, decrease junk food and soft drinks, and decrease protein intake, as these foods raise the phosphate content and therefore lower the calcium content. Calcium carbonate, 2.5 gr daily, should also be used as a calcium supplement. Vitamin D can be provided by sunshine, but Avioli has suggested 50,000 units of vitamin D twice a month for 4 months in symptomatic osteoporosis to ensure adequate vitamin D in case of the occurrence of adult osteomalacia.

Stimulation of Bone Regeneration

Alvia and associates advise routine and perhaps supervised exercise for those patients who are physically able to engage in some type of activity. This is in keeping with the results of their investigations which indicate that senile osteoporosis is due not to an increased rate of loss of bone in specific individuals after achievement of bone peak mass but rather to a decreased skeletal mass at maturity. Exercise is the only known therapy for stimulating new bone formation.

Prevention of Bone Resorption

The use of estrogen to prevent bone resorption is pharmacologically sound. Apparently, however, it should not be given without the addition of the above regimes. Without assuring an adequate calcium intake, calcium will not be retained in the bones at the expense of more significant cellular functions. Porcine calcitonin, 1 MRC unit three times a week intramuscularly has also been recommended; however, the documentation of the efficacy of this hormone is scanty. Although fluoride has been advised, this drug is toxic, can produce ligamentous calcifications and exostoses, and can **decrease** skeletal calcium as well as **increase** it. At present it should not be prescribed.

Estrogen Therapy

Gordon reported a study of 220 osteoporotic women who received estrogen therapy over 1864 patient years, and showed that the fracture rate of an expected 40 per 1,000 patient years was significantly reduced to only 3 fractures per 1,000 patient years. The dosage of 1.25 mg of conjugated estrogen for 20–25 consecutive days per month produced no increase in the instance of endometrial cancer, thrombophlebitis, heart disease, or stroke, but reduction of dose or cessation of therapy was promptly followed by recurrent fractures, the rate rising to 25 per 1,000 patient years. If it is necessary to use an estrogen dosage in this range for successful treatment of osteoporosis, this is of some concern. In the Duke study (Chapter 15) on the risk versus benefits of estrogen therapy in the menopause, it was found that patients receiving as little as 0.625 mg of conjugated estrogens a day over a long period of time did develop a significantly increased number of endometrial adenocarcinomas. If one could prevent osteoporosis by administration of the estrogen dosage recommended for the acute symptoms of the menopause, 0.3 mg of conjugated estrogen daily, then estrogen could be recommended for the prevention of **symptomatic** osteoporosis.

Obviously, **symptomatic** osteoporosis is an incapacitating illness, and when this occurs one must use any therapy which can alleviate the symptoms. It has been repeatedly shown that the equivalent of 1.25 mg of conjugated estrogen will relieve symptoms within 1 month. A progestational drug must be given to induce withdrawal bleeding, and an endometrial biopsy must be taken at least every year.

If decreased prolactin, with decreased activation of vitamin D to 1,25-dihydroxy vitamin D, resulting in lowered calcium absorption from the gut, is a major factor in senile osteoporosis, this is additional reason for administering estrogen. Estrogen will raise serum prolactin levels substantially.

Smoking

The topic of smoking should probably be considered also under bone resorption. The decreased exchange of volatile gases because of decreased pulmonary function associated with heavy smoking increases calcium resorption from the bone by changing the acid base balance in the canaliculi around the osteoclasts. Therefore, prohibition of smoking is an important part of therapy for osteoporosis.

Therapeutic Monitoring

Prophylaxis for, or treatment of, symptomatic osteoporosis is obviously long-range therapy. No patient should be placed on any long-range therapeutic regime without some plan being made to monitor the results of therapy. The height of the patient should be recorded at the initial visit and the urinary hydroxyproline and calcium and the serum calcium and phosphate levels obtained. X-ray evaluation of the cortical thickness of the 5th metacarpal of the second finger should also be made. A vaginal smear for maturation index and an endometrial biopsy complete the baseline studies. These should be repeated on a yearly basis.

ARTERIOSCLEROTIC CARDIOVASCULAR DISEASE

Rationale for Association with the Menopause

There have been two major reasons for linking estrogen deficiency to arteriosclerotic cardiovascular disease. First, it has been thought that women, in contrast to men, are "protected" against cardiovascular disease until the menopause. Second, the decreased estrogen is associated with changes of the cholesterol/phospholipid ratio and administration of estrogen reverses this increased cholesterol/phospholipid ratio.

Estrogen Prophylactic Therapy: Theoretical Considerations for Use

Although it was initially inferred that, after cessation of ovarian function, deaths from arteriosclerotic cardiovascular disease increased sharply and the death rate in women approached that of men, Furman has questioned these observations. His interpretation of the facts is that there is no evidence of an increased incidence of cardiovascular disease in women after the menopause, and the death rate climbs in an unbroken line with age. The rate by age in males, however, is not linear, but has two components. These may well represent two population groups: young men with a predilection for cardiovascular disease who die before the age of 55, thus increasing the death rate from cardiovascular accident in young men, and the remaining male population over the age of 55 years who have no increased risk of cardiovascular disease. Therefore, after the age of 55 years, the male death rate approaches that of females. By the age of 75 or 80 the two are almost superimposed. Thus, according to Furman, estrogen does not protect, but rather some factor in certain young males predisposes to cardiovascular disease. As will be discussed later, this factor may be an abnormal oxidation product of cholesterol or a cholesterol metabolite.

Estrogen Effect on Blood Lipids

The blood lipid changes associated with estrogen administration are characterized by an increase in the high density lipoprotein (HDL) cholesterol, and a decrease in the low density lipoprotein (LDL) cholesterol. The increase in HDL after estrogen therapy is particularly marked in patients with elevated cholesterol values and may be unchanged when initial values are normal. Recently the function of the lipoprotein fractions has been recognized as being dependent upon the **protein** part of the molecule which carries the **lipid**, cholesterol, or triglyceride. It is this fraction which is active in lipid metabolism at the target cell. The major lipoproteins, LDL, HDL, VLDL (very low density lipoprotein), and chylomicrons are interrelated in controlling lipid metabolism.

Experimental work by Imai et al. indicates that it is not free cholesterol which causes the intimal vessel damage and therefore the pathology of arteriosclerotic vascular disease, but rather an abnormal oxidation product of cholesterol. It would seem then that there must be some factor in a susceptible population of men and also of women who are estrogen deficient between the ages of 25 and 45, which induces this abnormal oxidation of cholesterol. This would account for early occurrence of arteriosclerotic vascular disease in males and for the increased incidence in young ovariectomized women, described in the Framingham study (Gordon, et al., 1978). If estrogens do then protect against this abnormal oxidation of cholesterol, a specific population might be identified which would benefit from prophylactic postmenopausal estrogen therapy.

Thromboembolic Disease and Hypertension

Because of the known thromboembolic function of estrogen, women who have established coronary artery disease may be at risk with estrogen therapy. Damaged vessels are prone to thrombosis. Estrogen has also been shown to cause hypertension in some susceptible individuals, apparently related to the effect on the renin/angiotensin system (Chapter 34). The blood pressure of patients on estrogen therapy must, therefore, be carefully monitored, and this would be especially true for patients who have a family history of hypertensive disease.

Prophylactic Therapy

Because these considerations tend to negate the theoretical indications for the use of universal estrogen prophylactic therapy for cardiovascular disease, prophylactic estrogen therapy should be given, therefore, only after careful screening. The family history should be consistent with 1) a strong predilection for cardiovascular disease, excluding essential hypertension, and 2) little or no history of tumor formation. The physical examination should exclude breast disease and, as far as possible, existing arteriosclerosis. The laboratory investigation must include a vaginal smear and a lipid screen. The possible benefits and risks must be discussed with the patient and both the physician and the patient should agree that the benefits outweigh the risks. The dosage used must be the lowest one possible to maintain a normal lipid profile and arrangements should be made for systematic follow-up examinations every 6 months. Adverse effects such as vaginal bleeding or breast tenderness are clinical symptoms which indicate excessive estrogen dosage. The patient should be warned about such symptoms and told to report them at once. If they occur, the estrogen dosage should be lowered. The addition of either testosterone or some of the progestational agents to this therapy destroys its efficacy.

As discussed in previous sections, 0.3 mg of conjugated estrogen daily or the equivalent is usually sufficient to maintain the blood lipids within a normal range and insufficient to cause endometrial proliferation. If this dosage is used, it is *probably* not necessary to either give it cyclically or to add a progestational drug. The duration of experience with such therapy is insufficient to be didactic about this advice. It is more customary to interrupt the dosage of estrogen 1 week out of each month and to add a progestagen. Norethindrone, 5 mg a day, given during the last 2 weeks of the estrogen therapy, is an adequate antimitotic stimulus. When the uterus has been removed, progestogens are probably not indicated and may be contraindicated, as progesterone is a growth stimulus for breast tissue.

As stated above, because of the thromboembolic effect of estrogen, the incidence of coronary thrombosis in patients with established arteriosclerotic vascular disease may be increased by estrogen therapy. It is, therefore, contraindicated under these circumstances. Blood pressure must also be checked frequently during the 1st year of therapy to assure one that the patient does not have a predilection for the development of hypertension with estrogen therapy.

POSSIBLE RISKS OF ESTROGENIC THERAPY

Carcinogenic Hazard

The association of endometrial carcinoma with exogenous estrogen therapy has been documented in a number of studies, and the evaluation of them has been examined in Chapter 15. There is no doubt that the association is dose and time related. In the Duke study the risk of endometrial carcinoma was increased at a dose of 0.625 mg or more of conjugated estrogen given over at least 5 years. In this study, cyclic estrogen administration did not seem to protect against carcinoma, while adding a progestational drug did.

In a study of Rosenwaks et al., progestogens did not seem to protect against carcinoma or endometrial hyperplasia. The difference in the two studies may indicate that the dose and duration of the progestogen therapy is critical. It was impossible for Rosenwaks to predict the appearance of the endometrium from the bleeding pattern. Patterns with severe hyperplasia might be associated with no bleeding, regular withdrawal bleeding, or irregular bleeding. The one patient in the series who developed endometrial cancer had had regular withdrawal bleeding. Progestogen withdrawal bleeding is not associated with complete shedding of the functional endometrial layer. Therefore, bleeding does not protect against development of endometrial cancer.

Even when the uterus has been previously removed, one must remember that the breast is also an estrogen target organ. It has been difficult to show a relationship between exogenous estrogen and breast cancer. However, most of the larger studies cover not over 10 years of medication (Gestel et al.). There is some indication from two studies with long follow-up periods that there may be a prolonged latency period between the estrogen administration and the development of breast cancer. Hoover et al. found a suggestion of a minimal risk which was dose related but which was not detected prior to 15 years after initiation of treatment, and Byrd et al. found some increased risk after 10 years of estrogen exposure. Two bits of other persuasive anecdotal evidence have been gathered from the literature. The first is the report of two male transsexuals who developed breast cancer after chronic long-term estrogen exposure. The second is the report by Stamler et al. of the occurrence of bilateral breast cancer in 1 of 500 men who were receiving prophylactic estrogen therapy for cardiovascular disease. Bilateral breast malignancy in males has never been reported to occur spontaneously.

SUPPORTIVE THERAPY

Often the best supportive therapy for the menopausal woman is a sympathetic listener and a doctor who will take the time to explain the normal physiology underlying the menopause. A word of advice, encouragement, or comfort concerning environmental factors which may be aggravating her physiological readjustment may be more valuable than pills. Phenobarbital, 32 mg once or twice a day or only when the patient is under stress, is an old standby but one which is hard to improve upon. Tranquilizers in moderation will also often carry a patient through a particularly stressful episode; however, it is certainly unwise to prescribe these drugs in lieu of an office visit or a little time spent with the patient.

PSYCHOSOMATIC MEASURES

The only treatment necessary for a large proportion of menopausal patients is reassurance and education by the physician. It is surprising how many women, including a good many who are otherwise well educated, have wrong ideas as to the nature and significance of the menopause. Some believe that it means the end of sexual life and of their physical attractiveness to their husbands. On this point they can be reassured, as the function of the ovary in the human appears to have little to do with libido. The psyche and adrenal play far more important roles. Indeed, in many women sexual response may be more highly developed after the menopause than before. Some interpret the hot flush as a symptom of hypertension; other women associate the menopause in a vague way with cancer, and they can, of course, be told that there is no such association. Again, many women are afraid they will become obese after the menopause; although most women do put on some weight at this time, the gain is usually moderate and easily controllable.

Finally, there are still not a few women who fear that the menopause carries with it a hazard of insanity. Psychoses not infrequently develop in middle life in either men or women, most often of the degenerative or involutional types, but it is age and not the menopause per se which is responsible. The slight depressions which a certain proportion of menopausal women exhibit, especially those with severe vasomotor symptoms and those burdened with domestic cares and worries, are not to be mistaken for the actual involutional psychoses. A new intellectual interest—especially if associated with monetary or emotional reward—is the best cure for this type of depression. Many women should be advised, now that families are raised, to refurbish their education and seek employment outside of the home.

SUMMARY

In spite of a healthier attitude among women in general as to the significance of menopause, there is still a considerable substratum of misconceptions on this point, and the physician must take cognizance of this in the management of climacteric women. The majority of women at this phase need no treatment at all, many require only reassurance and education, and in only a comparatively small proportion is endocrine therapy necessary.

Although there is perhaps no gynecological disorder in which the indication for hormone therapy is more rational than in the treatment of typical climacteric symptoms, especially the vasomotor group, it must be remembered that many symptoms frequently observed in menopausal women are not directly due to the endocrine readjustments of this period but are more logically explained as due to environmental and psychogenic factors. The physician who depends upon endocrine therapy alone will fall short of the requirements in many cases, and the indiscriminate use of estrogen should be avoided.

Estrogen therapy is indicated for the control of acute symptoms of the hot flush and insomnia. If treated soon after onset with adequate dosage, the symptoms can usually be controlled rapidly. The hormone then can be gradually withdrawn and discontinued within a year without recurrence of symptoms. As the menopausal woman is not totally estrogen deficient, but only relatively deficient in respect to reproductive capacity, the majority of women will not need constant low-dose estrogen replacement therapy. Chronic low-dose estrogen replacement therapy may be indicated in the premature menopausal patient. Under these circumstances it is sometimes desirable for psychological reasons to give a sufficient estrogen dosage to induce bleeding. If this is necessary, one must of course always add a progestational anti-mitotic drug, and this must be given over a period of at least 10 days in an adequate dosage. Therapy must be monitored by repetitive endometrial biopsies. These may be taken once a year to determine the endometrial pattern. As the histologic endometrial findings are unrelated to the type or time of withdrawal bleeding, a regular bleeding pattern or absence of bleeding cannot substitute for an endometrial biopsy, which is essential.

Indiscriminate prophylactic estrogen therapy for the prevention of arteriosclerotic cardiovascular disease is difficult to justify. For the patient at high risk for osteoporosis, low dosage prophylactic estrogen therapy may be admissable. However, the action of estrogen on bone is to prevent calcium resorption. There is very little evidence that it will stimulate new bone formation. Under normal conditions, bone formation is invariably associated with bone resorption. This mechanism is apparently regulated by a peptide produced in bone which promotes bone regeneration. If this peptide is deficient in some aging patients, this might explain the incidence of symptomatic osteoporosis with fracture formation. Until such a time as more definitive therapy is available, prophylactic estrogen for osteoporosis must be given with caution. Estrogen will decrease calcium resorption rate, but over the years it will not prevent osteoporosis. Bone is a calcium reservoir. Bone will be depleted of calcium if there is a general calcium deficiency. It is therefore important, when estrogen is to be given, to add calcium and vitamin D to the diet, to control the phosphate intake by prescribing a well balanced carbohydrate:fat:protein diet, to prevent cigarette smoking, and to plan a regular exercise program. The progress of the osteoporosis must be monitored with bone density studies, urinary and serum calcium levels at yearly intervals. The two cardinal principles of estrogen therapy are most important in such long-term treatment, "as little as necessary to control symptoms over as short as possible a duration."

References and Additional Readings

Albanese, A.A., Edelson, A.H., Lorenze, E.J., Woodhull, M.L., and Wein, E.H.: Problems of bone health in elderly. NY St. J. Med., 2: 326, 1975.

Albright, F., Smith, P.H., and Richardson, A.M.: Postmenopausal osteoporosis: its clinical features. JAMA, 116: 2465, 1941.

Aloia, J.F., Koh, S.H., Ross, P., Vaswani, A. Abesamis, C., Ellis, K., and Zanzi, I.: Skeletal mass in postmenopausal women. Am. J. Physiol., 235 (1): e82, 1978.

Alvia, J. F.: Prevention of involutional bone loss by exercise. Ann. Intern. Med., 89: 356, 1978.

Arthes, F.G., Sartwell, P.E., and Lewison, E.F.: The pill, estrogens, and the breast: Epidemiological aspects. Cancer, 28: 1391, 1971.

Avioli, L. V.: What to do with "postmenopausal osteoporosis?" Am. J. Med. 65: 881, 1978.

Boston Collaborative Drug Surveillance Program, Boston University Medical Center: Surgically confirmed gallbladder disease, venous thromboembolism, and breast tumors in relation to postmenopausal estrogen therapy. N. Engl. J. Med., 290: 15, 1974.

Brinton, L.A., Williams, R.R., Hoover, R.N., Stegens, N.L., Feinleib, M., and Fraumeni, J.F., Jr: Breast cancer risk factors among screening program participants. J. Natl. Cancer Inst., 62: 37, 1979

Brown, M.S., and Goldstein, J.E.: Low density lipoprotein pathology in human fibroblasts: Relation between cell surface receptor binding and endocytosis of low density liproprotein. NY Acad. Sci., 275: 244, 1976.

Bullock, J.L., Massey, F.M., and Gambrell, R.D. Jr.: Use of medroxyprogesterone acetate to prevent menopausal symptoms. Obstet. Gynecol. 46: 165, 1975.

Byrd, B.F., Jr., Burch, J.C., and Vaughn, W.K.: The impact of long term estrogen support after hysterectomy. A report of 1016 cases. Ann. Surg., 185: 574, 1977.

Cooper, J.: Double blind cross-over study of estrogen replacement therapy, In The Management of the Menopause and Post-Menopausal Years, edited by S. Campbell, p. 159. MTP Press Limited, Lancaster, England, 1976.

Frantz, I. D., Jr., and Moore, R. B.: The sterol hypothesis in atherogenesis. Am. J. Med., 46: 686, 1969.

Furman, R.H.: Gonadal steroid effects on serum lipids. In Metabolic Effects on Gonadal Hormones and Contraceptive Steroids, Plenum Press, New York and London, 1969.

Gordon, G.S.: Drug treatment of the osteoporoses. Ann. Rev. Pharmacol. Toxicol., 18: 253, 1978.

Gordon, T., Kannel, W. B., Hjortland, M. C., and McNamara, P. M.: Menopause and coronary heart disease. Ann. Intern. Med., 89: 157, 1978.

Hammond, C.B., Jelovsek, F.R., Lee, K.L., Creasman, W.T., and Parker, R.T.: Effects of long-term estrogen replacement therapy. I. Metabolic effects. Am. J. Obstet. Gynecol., 133: 525, 1979.

Hoover, R., Gray, L.A., Sr., Cole, P., and MacMahon, B.: Menopausal estrogens and breast cancer. N. Engl. J. Med., 295: 401, 1976.

Howard, G. A., and Baylink, D. J.: In vitro bone metabolism: evidence for coupling of formation and resorption. Pres. in Wash., D. C. Oct. 1979. Cited in Science, 207: 628, 1980. by Jean Marx.

Hunter, D.J.S., Akande, E.O., Carr, P., and Stalworthy, J.: The clinical and endocrinological effects of estradiol implants at the time of hysterectomy and bilateral salpingo-oophorectomy. J. Obstet. Gynaecol. B. Common., 80: 827, 1973.

Hutton, J.D., Jacobs, H.S., Marray, M.A.F., and James, V.H.T.: Relation between plasma oestrone and oestradiol and climateric symptoms. Lancet, 1: 678, 1978.

Imai, H., Werthesen, N.T., Subramanyam, V., LeQuesne, P.W., Soloway, A.H., and Kanisawa, M.: Angiotoxicity of oxygenated sterols and possible precursors. Science, 207: 651, 1980.

Jowsey, J.: Why is mineral nutrition important in osteoporosis? Geriatrics, 33: 39, 1978.

Jowsey, J., and Riggs, B.L.: Bone formation in hypercortisonism. Acta Endocrinol., 63: 21, 1970.

Jowsey, J., Riggs, B.L., Kelly, P.J., and Hoffman, D.L.: Effect of combined therapy with sodium-fluoride vitamin D and calcium in osteoporosis. Am. J. Med., 53: 43, 1972.

Kasper, Yen, and Wilkes: Science, 205: 823, 1979.

Lindsey, R., Aitken, J.M., Anderson, J.B., Hart, D.M., MacDonald, E.B., and Clark, A.C.: Long term prevention of postmenopausal osteoporosis by estrogen. Evidence for an increased bone mass after delayed onset of estrogen treatment. Lancet, 1: 1038, 1976.

Marmorston, J., Magidons, O., Lewis, J., Mehl, J. Moore, F., and Bernstein, J.: Effect of small doses of estrogens on serum lipids in female patients with myocardial infarction. New Engl. J. Med., *258:* 583, 1958.

Meema, S., Bunker, M.L., and Meema, H.E.: Preventive effect of estrogen on postmenopausal bone loss. Arch. Int. Med., *135:* 1436, 1975.

Newcomer, A. D., Hodgson, S. F., McGill, D. B., and Thomas, P. J.: Lactase deficiency: prevalence in osteoporosis. Ann. Intern. Med., *89:* 218, 1978.

Nutik, G., and Cruess, R.L.: Estrogen receptors in bone and evaluation of the uptake of estrogen in bone cells. Proc. Soc. Exper. Biol. Med., *146:* 265, 1975.

Pfeffer, R.I., Kurosaki, T.T., and Charlton, S.K.: Estrogen use and blood pressure in later life. Am. J. Epidemiol., *110:* 469, 1979.

Rasmussen, H., and Bordier, P.: The physiologic and cellular basis of metabolic bone disease. Williams and Wilkins, Baltimore, 1974.

Rosenwaks, Z., Wentz, A.C., Jones, G.S., Urban, M.D., Lee, P.A., Migeon, C.J., Parmley, T.H., and Woodruff, J.D.: Endometrial pathology and estrogens. Obstet. Gynecol., *53:* 403, 1979.

Schiff, I., Regestein, Q. Tulchinsky, D. and Ryan, K.J.: Effects of estrogens on sleep and psychological state of the hypogonadal women. JAMA, *242:* 2405, 1979.

Sherman, B. M., and Korenman, S. G.: J. Clin. Invest. *55:* 699, 1975.

Spanos, E., Pike, J.W., Haussler, M.R., Colston, K.W., Evans, I.M., Goldner, A.M., McCain, T.A., and MacIntyre, I.: Circulating 1-α-25-hydroxy vitamin D in the chicken: enhancement by injection of prolactin and during egg laying. Life Sci., *19:* 1751, 1976.

Stamler, J., Best, M., and Turner, J.: The status of hormonal therapy for the primary and secondary prevention of atherosclerotic coronary heart disease. Prog. Cardiovasc. Dis., *6:* 220, 1963.

Sturdee, D.W., Wilson, K.A., Pipili, E. and Crocker, A.D.: Physiological aspects of menopausal hot flush. Br. Med. J., *2:* 79, 1978.

CHAPTER 33

Dysmenorrhea, Premenstrual Tension, and Related Disorders

DYSMENORRHEA

Dysmenorrhea, or painful menstruation, is the most common of all gynecologic disorders. Over half of all postmenarcheal women have some discomfort and 10% are incapacitated for 1–3 days each month.

The causes and pathophysiology of dysmenorrhea remain poorly understood, although significant strides have been made within the past 5 years.

Definition

Primary dysmenorrhea is menstrual pain observed in the absence of any noteworthy pelvic lesion and due to factors intrinsic in the uterus itself. Characteristically, the pain begins with the onset of menstruation, lasts for a few hours, and has a spasmodic, colicky, labor-like nature. It is centered in the lower midline but may radiate to the lower back or down the thighs. Numerous symptoms may accompany the pelvic pain, including nausea, vomiting and/or anorexia, diarrhea, headache and/or dizziness, tiredness, and nervousness. The pain and its accompanying symptoms may require bed rest of one to several days each month. The first day of menstruation is ordinarily the most severely symptomatic, and some women may be entirely incapacitated from normal activity. Most women with primary dysmenorrhea have a tendency toward spontaneous improvement in the condition with advancing age. Relief from dysmenorrhea after childbirth cannot be relied upon, but dysmenorrhea experienced for the first time after delivery, suggests an identifiable physical cause.

Secondary dysmenorrhea is pain with menstruation noted in the presence of other pelvic disease, including endometriosis, intrauterine or submucous myomata, endometrial polyps, and pelvic inflammatory disease.

Primary dysmenorrhea may appear with the first period but usually is not experienced until many months or even years after the menarche. The initial menstrual cycles in young girls are either anovulatory or oligoluteal in character, and usually painless. When ovulation and normal corpus luteum function begin, primary dysmenorrhea may develop, but this ordinarily does not occur until some 6–12 months after initiation of menses.

On the other hand, dysmenorrhea starting after the age of 20 is usually secondary to another pelvic problem. The history of painful menses occurring later should alert the clinician to the probability of a coexistent pelvic abnormality.

Causative Factors and Their Management

Many theories have been advanced to explain the etiology of primary dysmenorrhea. Some of the more plausible contributing factors and their management are discussed below.

Psychogenic

A moderate amount of pelvic heaviness and some cramping during menstruation may be considered normal, and the line between this normal discomfort and real dysmenorrhea is difficult to draw. The distinction is commonly made subjectively by the patient herself, on the basis of the incapacity produced, and it is this subjective nature of the disorder that has made its study so difficult. When asked to compare the efficacy of two analgesics in the treatment of dysmenorrhea, 20–50% of patients have uniformly shown marked improvement with a *placebo*. Suggestibility is a hallmark of the dysmenorrheic woman.

The psychogenic element, therefore, is one which can never be overlooked in the management of cases of dysmenorrhea. All factors which might accentuate or lessen the subjective element in the particular case must be considered.

The physician can soon learn the importance of the psychogenic factor in the individual case, and thus determine the value or the futility of intensifying the psychotherapeutic approach.

Constitutional

Closely linked with the purely subjective group of causes is the factor of constitutional debility. Anemia, voluntary weight loss, diabetes, chronic illness, and overwork may be associated with a lowering of the threshold of pain. A regimen calculated to raise the patient's general health level may cause disappearance or marked amelioration of the dysmenorrhea.

Obstructive and Anatomical

Mechanical obstruction may have an etiologic role in a small proportion of cases. Cervical stenosis, or acute uterine ante- or retroflexion could result in delayed passage of the menstrual discharge, the formation of clots, and distention of the uterine cavity. Dilatation of the internal os by the passage of a clot causes discomfort; increased systemic absorption of prostaglandin synthesized and released from the endometrium may increase uterine motility and muscular contraction and induce such prostaglandin-associated effects as vomiting, diarrhea, and headache. Pedunculated submucous fibroids or endometrial polyps also can cause dysmenorrhea because the musculature contracts in an effort to expel the space-occupying lesions. This same mechanism is partly responsible for the dysmenorrhea associated with an intrauterine contraceptive device.

Endocrine Factors

Dysmenorrhea is almost always found with normal ovulatory menses and a normal hormonal milieu; there is no associated hormonal imbalance. The cramps characteristic of primary dysmenorrhea are related to exaggerated uterine contractility.

Dysmenorrheic pain is not characteristic of the perimenarcheal individual in whom normal corpus luteum function is not established. Patients with anovulatory dysfunctional uterine bleeding do not have dysmenorrhea, and any cramps are usually associated with passage of clots.

Prostaglandins and Myometrial Activity

Exaggerated uterine contractility is associated with dysmenorrheic pain, and myometrial contractility patterns now have been studied using several different techniques. Electrical activity of the nonpregnant human uterus is highest during menstruation. Direct measurement of the contractility in the nonpregnant uterus has revealed vigorous and labor-like uterine contractility during menstruation, and weak, short duration, small amplitude contractions not ordinarily appreciated by the patient, during the preovulatory phase. A basal tonus of the myometrium greater than 50 mm Hg is usually recorded during cramping episodes. During the luteal part of the cycle, basal pressures increase, and higher amplitude contractions can be recorded. In conditions with estrogen dominance, for instance during anovulatory cycles or during estrogen treatment, the motility pattern is closely similiar to that in the proliferative part of the normal ovulatory cycle, and cramping is not appreciated.

The "labor-like" character of dysmenorrheic pain can be correlated with excessive myometrial contractility. The etiology of the exaggerated uterine contractility was first suggested by the work of Pickles studying prostaglandin production in the endometrium. Most persuasive is recent evidence, obtained through analysis of endometrial tissue, or of tampons as a means of collection of the menstrual discharge, that subjects with primary dysmenorrhea had significantly higher-than-normal concentrations of prostaglandins (PG's) in the endometrium, in endometrial jet washings, and in the menstrual fluid itself. These high concentrations of PG's may be due to increased synthesis, abnormal release, or decreased breakdown; that the concentrations correlate with dysmenorrheic pain virtually solves the puzzle of the etiology of dysmenorrhea. That PG synthetase inhibitors, of which six or seven have now been clinically tested, may relieve the symptomatology of dysmenorrhea is further proof of the etiologic role of PG's in producing increased uterine contractility, the cause of dysmenorrhea.

Treatment

Dysmenorrhea has been treated symptomatically, endocrinologically, and surgically. The advent of PG synthetase inhibitors in the therapy has added a completely new dimension, and a particularly successful one, to the management of dysmenorrhea.

Management begins with taking the history and continues through the pelvic examination, both of which can be made an educational experience for the patient. Hormonal agents, other drugs or even surgery may be used as therapy, but the physician who depends entirely upon these, and does not recognize constitutional or psychogenic factors, is sure to fail in a large proportion of cases. Generally, one therapy is not wholly successful; because causative factors interact, several approaches, including reassurance and specific medical treatment, may be needed.

Symptomatic Management

Treatment of the dysmenorrheic attack depends upon its severity; once the pain begins, it is apt to run its course. Since preventing the pain may be easier than stopping it, any type of medication is more efficient if taken before the dysmenorrheic attack has been established.

Most cases respond to the local use of heat and to mild drugs with analgesic, sedative, or antispasmodic properties. Diuretics have occasionally been employed with marked relief due to the mobilization of fluid and decrease in pelvic congestion. Simple exercise may relieve some of the distress and serve as diversion. Particular care should be taken to avoid the use of habit forming drugs such as morphine and alcohol, which will always relieve the pain. Dysmenorrhea must be regarded as a chronic illness and the possibility of addiction is real.

Endocrine Therapy

The widespread use of steroid contraception has decreased the incidence of dysmenorrhea because of the efficacy of inhibition of ovulation in eliminating dysmenorrhea. However, the use of birth control pills for 21 days to control 1–2 days of dysmenorrhea may be poor medicine, particularly in the woman not requiring contraception, or in one with a relative contraindication to the use of estrogenic steroids. However, some progestational drugs, without estrogen added, can be used to control dysmenorrhea. Unlike estrogens, progestogens can be used in the same dosage month after month with a similar suppression of ovulation and beneficial effects. As little as 2.5 mg of 19-norethisterone (Norlutin), given daily during the first 25 days of each cycle, is a sufficient dose to suppress ovulation. Side effects are minimal with this small dosage.

The treatment is effective only in the cycle of therapy and no permanent relief is attained. However, since experience demonstrates that dysmenorrhea is invariably aggravated by general psychic tension, sometimes a course of 3–6 months of treatment will carry a patient through an unusually difficult time. It then may be possible to control her symptoms with more general measures for several months, after which treatment can be reinitiated if necessary.

Tocolytic Agents

The use of agents to inhibit muscular contraction and increase uterine blood flow is theoretically sound. Unfortunately, the use of β-receptor stimulators such as hydroxyphenylorciprenaline and isoxuprine have proved uniformly ineffective (Osler). Terbutaline, a specific β-2 stimulator, is effective in inhibition of myometrial contractility and increase in blood flow (Hansen and Secher), but its side effects (palpitations, quivering, flushing) and its intravenous route of administration are disadvantageous.

The calcium antagonist, nifedipine, effectively decreases myometrial activity and decreases intrauterine pressure measurements (Andersson and Ulmsten), but flushing, headache, and tachycardia are side effects which limit its clinical usefulness.

Presacral Neurectomy

The operation of presacral neurectomy or sympathectomy is a rational and frequently effective procedure in an occasional patient with unusually severe dysmenorrhea which has proved intractable to more conservative procedures. It gives complete, or almost complete, relief from pain in perhaps 60–70% of cases.

Prostaglandin Inhibitors

Drugs known to inhibit PG synthesis or its action have been developed, and clinical trials show that these drugs provide substantial relief of the painful cramping and other symptoms of dysmenorrhea.

In general, the various prostaglandin synthetase inhibitors are all effective, resulting in alleviation of the symptoms of dysmenorrhea in the majority of patients treated (Budoff, Chan et al., Corson and Bolognese, Boehm and Sarratt, and Csapo et al.). Uterine activity and contractility, resting and active pressures of the uterus, the content of both PG and PG metabolites in the menstrual discharge, and menstrual pain are all decreased. PG synthetase inhibitors available for clinical use are shown in Table 33.1.

Side effects of PG inhibitors and antagonists are relatively mild and quite tolerable (Andersson). Headache, gastrointestinal symptoms, rash, and occasional blurred vision have been reported. Patients with a known history of gastrointestinal ulcer disease should not receive these drugs. Occasionally, patients report a feeling of disorientation or being "spaced out," and others have reported drowsiness, dizziness, and nervousness. If the PG synthetase inhibitors are given before the onset of menstrual flow, patients may report that the flow is delayed or begins with dark brown spotting. One of the advantages of these drugs is the decrease in heavy bleeding and a reduction of generalized menstrual blood loss. In patients with menorrhagia secondary to the intrauterine device, these compounds may be effective in decreasing both the associated discomfort and blood loss.

To summarize, clinical as well as experimental evidence now upholds the PG theory of the etiology of dysmenorrhea. This provides an appropriate and effective method for the management and treatment of this common but distressing disorder.

Summary of Management

No therapy of such a subjective pain disorder as primary dysmenorrhea can be based purely on PG synthetase inhibition, and endocrine, constitutional, or psychogenic factors should not be overlooked. In addition to a general symptomatic approach, reassurance with medical treatment, and the advice to try to remain up and about rather than going to bed during the pain of the attack, seem preferable to the complications and inconveni-

Table 33.1
Prostaglandin Synthetase Inhibitors

	Trade Name	Company	Dosage	Side Effects
Indomethacin	Indocin	Merck	25 mg tid	Dizziness, fatigue, nausea, weakness, gastrointestinal, lightheadedness, headaches, corneal deposits
Naproxen	Naprosyn	Syntex	250 mg q 4–6 hours	Nausea
Naproxen sodium	Anaprox		550 mg stat, then 275 mg q 6 hours	Nausea
Ibuprofen	Motrin	Upjohn	400 mg qid	Nausea, diarrhea, gastrointestinal, visual
Mefenamic acid	Ponstel	Parke, Davis	250 mg qid 500 mg q 8 hours	Gastrointestinal, hematologic toxicity, headache, dizziness
Suprofen		Ortho	200 mg q 4 hours	Dizziness, lightheadedness

ence of endocrine therapy. A low incidence of side effects and problems was encountered by Morrison and Jennings who used a PG synthetase inhibitor taken at half the ordinary dose and with meals in cases of mild dysmenorrhea. When the dysmenorrhea is more protracted and severe, higher doses may be tried, frequently with significant benefit. Endocrine therapy designed to inhibit ovulation should be tried before resorting to more radical measures such as presacral neurectomy. The evidence now clearly indicates what has long been suspected, that primary dysmenorrhea is a disorder of ovulating women and that it is probably relieved by preventing ovulation. This can apparently be done for any one particular cycle by progestogen therapy from the 5th through the 25th day of the cycle. The specific etiologic agent responsible for the dysmenorrhea now seems to be $PGF_{2\alpha}$ synthesized by the endometrial cells under the influence of progesterone. Therefore, specific treatment with inhibition of $PGF_{2\alpha}$ is usually effective, but inhibition of ovulation is another means of decreasing the endometrial content of prostaglandin.

PREMENSTRUAL TENSION AND EDEMA

Definition and Description

Premenstrual tension occurs to a mild degree in over 40% of women, and includes such symptoms as breast discomfort, fluid retention with slight weight gain, and emotional lability or depression. A few women, perhaps 5% at most, experience severe incapacitating symptomatology premenstrually. These premenstrual syndromes usually consist of some combination of nervous tension, irritability, anxiety, bloated feelings of the abdomen and breasts, swelling of the fingers and legs, tightness and itching of the skin with or without skin eruption, headaches, dizziness, and palpitations. Hypersomnia, excessive thirst and appetite, increased sex drive, and an increased tendency to asthma, migraine, vasomotor rhinitis, urticaria, and epilepsy are less commonly observed. All of these symptoms occur in the days before the onset of menstruation. Dysmenorrhea is characteristically not suffered by women with premenstrual tension, nor do patients with premenstrual tension classically have dysmenorrhea although the explanation is unclear.

Although some patients show both preovulatory and premenstrual edema paralleling the ovarian estrogen secretion pattern, premenstrual tension usually occurs in the ovulatory cycle, linking it at least circumstantially to progesterone secretion. As with dysmenorrhea, no abnormality of the ovarian hormone production or metabolism has been demonstrated. The associated edema suggests that the condition may also represent a disturbance of adrenal aldosterone which is increased in normally menstruating women premenstrually.

Premenstrual tension in minor degrees is relatively common; extreme degrees are rare and may be very distressing. The milder forms of the condition are characterized by nervousness, depression, or restlessness whereas the severe types closely approach a psychotic state with striking personality changes and emotional outbursts which make the patient difficult for family and physician alike. The most characteristic complaint may be incapacitating headaches, which on occasion are associated with the sensory or motor symptoms of cerebrovascular spasms.

Etiologic Factors

The premenstrual tension syndrome is characterized by symptoms which increase in intensity 4–10 days prior to menstruation and disappear with its onset. There may be a relationship to excessive tissue hydration and the intensity of the symptoms varies directly with the amount of water retained.

Secondary aldosteronism, described as hypersecretion due to extrinsic factors affecting the adrenal zona glomerulosa, may be associated with increases in ACTH stimulation, potassium, or progesterone, or to changes in body fluid volume, surgical trauma and anxiety states. The accompanying edema seems to be dependent upon the increased aldosterone secretion because, under experimental conditions in animals, adrenalectomy will usually eliminate the edema.

We are able then to picture a harassed housewife, endowed with a reactive nervous system, who by her fourth decade is burdened with more anxiety than she is able to handle. Having ovulated, she is now producing progesterone and increased amounts of estrogen which lead to mild fluid retention. These two factors, the hormones and the fluid retention, stimulate increased aldosterone production, which then causes more fluid retention, thus creating a vicious circle which produces symptoms of headache, irritability, depression, and swelling. The intracellular edema itself causes increased tension, headache, and anxiety. The anxiety further stimulates aldosterone production, and thus the syndrome grows in proportion. It is often difficult to know where the chain begins and how to interrupt it.

The theory of secondary aldosteronism and fluid retention is not the entire answer. Andersch and colleagues studied the total body water, total body potassium, and weight during the follicular and luteal phases in 20 patients with severe premenstrual tension and 20 patients without symptoms. The mean body water and the mean body potassium levels in the premenstrual tension group did not differ significantly from those in the controls. During the late luteal phase the water/potassium ratio in liters/mol of potassium was significantly higher in the patients with premenstrual tension, but the mean body water and weight in the premenstrual tension group were similar in the late luteal and early follicular phases. Andersch et al. found nothing to support the belief that normal women, or women with premenstrual tension, gain weight premenstrually. The absence of substantial weight gain suggests that the symptoms of premenstrual tension may be due to redistribution of fluid rather than increase in total body fluids, and that fluid balance is disturbed. Patients who suffer from premenstrual edema may have a shift of fluid from the intravascular to the extravascular space, with a predilection for abdomen and breasts instead of more dependent body parts. It also has been postulated that hormonal abnormalities, particularly disturbances of the renin-angiotensin system and aldosterone play an important role in premenstrual tension, and these are credited with causing such symptoms as localized edema, weight gain and headaches. The estrogens are thought to be responsible for fluid retention; progesterone, through its sodium-losing action, is believed to stimulate the renin-angiotensin system, and to produce a luteal phase increase in aldosterone secretion contributing to further fluid retention. Most studies, however, have found no significant differences in plasma progesterone and 17β-estradiol; some cycles are anovulatory but still symptomatic, suggesting that caution must be employed when discussing estrogen/progesterone ratios since no particular correlation can be observed.

Aldosterone, by inducing sodium retention, may be the causative agent in the premenstrual syndrome; the aldosterone antagonist spironolactone reduced weight and relieved psychological symptoms in 80% of treated cycles. Progesterone levels were higher postovulation in symptomatic patients and may have contributed to salt retention. Spironolactone has a diuretic action, and is well tolerated. However, other diuretics have not been shown to be more effective than a placebo.

Recently, the involvement of prolactin in the premenstrual tension syndrome has attracted a lot of interest. Serum prolactin levels are elevated during the luteal phase in some women with premenstrual tension syndrome. Whether this indicates a general increase due to stress, or is actually involved in producing some of the symptomatology constituting premenstrual syndrome is unknown; however, increased prolactin levels in the luteal phase have been associated with *decreased* progesterone output, although no difference in estrogen levels has been observed. Elevated prolactin levels may decrease FSH/LH levels, and impair gonadal steroidogenesis; breast enlargement and tenderness may occur. Thus, there is at least theoretical reason to suspect that prolactin may be involved in hormonal changes that may at least subtly be involved in the etiology of the syndrome.

Treatment

The clinical management of the premenstrual tension syndrome is a reminder that medicine is still an art and not an exact science; the therapy is by no means standardized.

In the milder cases and in the younger group of patients, especially when edema is the predominating symptom, a low-salt diet may suffice. For more severe edema problems, Diuril 500 mg can be given once or twice a day for 2 or 3 days during the onset of swelling. Prolonged, continuous therapy is inadvisable, as marked edema will occur on withdrawal of medication. Spironolactone, given cyclically, may prove advantageous.

When severe emotional disturbances exist, these should be treated only in conjunction with a psychiatrist. If recurrent depression is a prominent feature, the use of continuous lithium has proved beneficial. Given as lithium carbonate, 300 mg 2 or 3 times a day, and monitored with blood lithium values, it controls the depressive symptoms remarkably well but is not effective for swelling or headache. As lithium can induce hypothyroidism, thyroid function should be checked periodically. It is also teratogenic for experimental animals and is therefore not to be given during pregnancy.

A combination of belladonna alkaloids, ergotamine tartrate and phenobarbitone (Bellergal), was effective in a placebo-controlled, double blind British study to manage the fatigue, breast symptoms, irritability, and nervousness.

When headache is the major symptom, methyltestosterone 25 mg daily for 2 or 3 days premenstrually will often prove helpful.

Interruption of ovulation, using either combined oral contraceptives or minidose progestational therapy may cure some patients and not help others at all. The patient's age and her specific set of symptoms may determine whether this approach is likely to succeed. Pyridoxine (vitamin B$_6$) has been claimed to be effective in high dose, but no controlled studies have been reported. Bromocriptine or Parlodel, an ergot alkaloid and dopamine agonist, has been used as therapy for the syndrome; although results remain controversial, at least some patients appear to be benefitted compared to placebo administration.

In recapitulation, one can alleviate the symptoms of premenstrual tension and edema by salt restriction and diuretics, by inducing anovulatory cycles, by giving 25 mg of methyltestosterone daily for not over a 10-day period each month, by Bellergal treatment and possibly by treating with bromocriptine. When recurrent depression is a predominant symptom, lithium carbonate has proved very beneficial. Little of permanent value can be expected from any therapeutic regimen without concomitant counselling or even psychotherapy. Let us not resort to operative procedures as a desperate therapeutic attempt. It has been our experience that, especially in those patients with edema, the symptoms may well remain even following a bilateral oophorectomy and hysterectomy. A psychiatrist is a much better recourse.

PREMENSTRUAL EDEMA AND IDIOPATHIC EDEMA

Premenstrual edema was first described by Thomas in 1933. Many normal women show a slight gain of weight during the premenstrual period. Sweeney, for example, found that 30% of a group of normal women showed a gain of 3 or more pounds. In the occasional patient, however, the weight gain may be far greater and is obviously due to retention of fluid. There is often a marked edema with puffiness of the face and eyes and swelling of the feet and ankles. The edema usually begins a few days before the onset of menstruation but may also appear at ovulation time. Toward the beginning of menstruation, or sometime immediately after its cessation, marked polyuria occurs with rapid disappearances of edema. The condition may be noted at any age during reproductive life but is most common during the fourth decade.

Idiopathic edema is a disease affecting almost exclusively women in the reproductive age. Neurogenic and/or emotional stimuli may trigger remarkable swelling, and a weight gain of 9 kg within 48 hours under emotional stress accompanied by extreme polydipsia has been reported. The mechanism of the sudden rise in sodium and water retention is not well understood, and the responsiveness of the renin-angiotensin-aldosterone system is probably not the sole cause of sodium retention. Kuchel and co-workers have suggested that a decrease in urinary dopamine, a catecholamine recently recognized to have natriuretic action, possibly reflects the suppression of the renal dopaminergic system and may contribute to the excessive sodium retention in idiopathic edema, either directly or indirectly, through the renin-aldosterone system.

VICARIOUS MENSTRUATION

This is of historical interest mainly and is the designation applied to certain rare cases in which extragenital hemorrhages of one source or another take place at periodic intervals corresponding to the menstrual cycle. The most frequent site of the bleeding is from the nasal mucous membrane in the form of epistaxis. The local hyperemia and other vascular changes produced by the ovarian hormones would seem to offer a satisfactory explanation.

Vicarious menstruation has been described as occurring from a great variety of other sources: the stomach, intestines, lungs, mammary glands, skin and various skin lesions such as ulcers or nevi, kidneys, abdominal fistulas, umbilicus, external auditory meatus, eyes, and eyelids. Most cases, particularly those of umbilical origin, are no doubt explained by the existence of endometriosis.

Treatment

The treatment of the nasal type of vicarious menstruation is cauterization of the bleeding site. When bleeding occurs elsewhere, an investigation for endometriosis should be made; if confirmed, excision or laparoscopic fulguration of the area when possible is most expedient. Either Danazol, 800 mg daily, or methyltestosterone 5 mg daily, can be used; or a synthetic progesterone in combination with estrogens, as in the commercial oral contraceptive preparations, may provide relief.

INTERMENSTRUAL PAIN (MITTELSCHMERZ) AND BLEEDING

These two conditions may be discussed together, in spite of the fact that the pain often occurs without the bleeding, and vice versa. They are both linked with the phenomenon of ovulation, although little is known as to the exact mechanism.

Intermenstrual pain, occurring usually at approximately the midinterval period, may be slight, or it may be as severe as the more intense forms of dysmenorrhea. The duration may be only a few hours, but in some cases it may last 2 or 3 days. There may be associated bleeding, sometimes so slight as to cause only a brownish discharge, but in other cases sufficiently free and prolonged as to mimic a menstrual flow. To such scanty flows, regularly interpolated between the periods, the Germans have applied the term *kleine Regel* (little period). In the occasional case, this interval type of bleeding is so free that the patient states she menstruates twice a month. Even when there is no macroscopic bleeding with *Mittelschmerz*, blood corpuscles may often be found in microscopic examination of the vaginal discharge. The bleeding may be due to the temporary drop in estrogen im-

mediately following ovulation; since follicular rupture is associated with bleeding, this may be an alternative source. Some have suggested that the pain may be due to slight intra-abdominal hemorrhage, or from ovarian swelling due to follicular growth and development. No treatment is necessary except reassurance and perhaps simple analgesics for any accompanying pain.

MENSTRUAL EPILEPSY

Epileptic seizures occur most frequently at the time of the menstrual period. The seizures are not due to cerebral edema, as there are no differences between water balance studies of epileptic patients and those of normal individuals. A midluteal reduction in the number of epileptic seizures has been documented and may be related to an anticonvulsant action of progesterone, with an exaggeration of seizure activity when the beneficial suppressive effect is withdrawn.

Treatment

The therapy for menstrual epilepsy is similar to that for epilepsy in general. For the occasional patient who suffers severe cyclic seizures and who is either in the older age group or has completed her family, ovariectomy may be advised; major seizures may be greatly reduced or cease entirely, although petit mal is apt to continue. Endocrine therapy for the suppression of ovulation is usually successful, and the progestational compounds are useful.

References and Additional Readings

Abraham, G.E.: Primary dysmenorrhea. Clin. Obstet. Gynecol. 21: 139, 1978.

Akerlund, M.: Pathophysiology of Dysmenorrhea. Acta Obstet. Gynecol. Scand. Suppl., 87: 27, 1979.

Andersch, B., Hahn, L., Andersson, M., and Isaksson, B.: Body water and weight in patients with premenstrual tension. Br. J. Obstet. Gynecol., 85: 546, 1978.

Andersch, B., Hahn, L., Wendestam, C., Ohman, R., and Abrahamsson, L.: Treatment of premenstrual tension syndrome with bromocriptine. Acta Endocrinol. Suppl. 216, 88: 165, 1978.

Andersen, A.N., and Larsen, J.F.: Bromocriptine in the treatment of the premenstrual syndrome. Drugs, 17: 383, 1979.

Anderson, A.B., Fraser, I.S., Haynes, P.J., and Turnbull, A.C.: Trial of prostaglandin-synthetase inhibitors in primary dysmenorrhea. Lancet, i: 345, 1978.

Andersson, K.E.: Side-effects of prostaglandin synthetase inhibitors. Acta Obstet. Gynecol. Scand. Suppl., 87: 101, 1979.

Andersson, K.E., and Ulmsten, U.: Effects of nifedipine on myometrial activity and lower abdominal pain in women with primary dysmenorrhea. Br. J. Obstet. Gynecol., 85: 142, 1978.

Boehm, F.H., and Sarratt, H.: Indomethacin for the treatment of dysmenorrhea—A preliminary report. J. Reprod. Med., 15: 84, 1975.

Budoff, P.W.: Use of mefenamic acid in the treatment of primary dysmenorrhea. JAMA, *241:* 2713, 1979.

Chan, W.Y., Dawood, M.Y., and Fuchs, F.: Relief of dysmenorrhea with the prostaglandin synthetase inhibitor ibuprofen: Effect on prostaglandin levels in menstrual fluid. Am. J. Obstet. Gynecol., *135:* 102, 1979.

Corson, S.L., and Bolognese, R.J.: Ibuprofen therapy for dysmenorrhea. J. Reprod. Med., *20:* 246, 1978.

Csapo, A.I., Pulkkinen, M.O., and Henzl, M.R.: The effect of naproxen-sodium on the intrauterine pressure and menstrual pain of dysmenorrheic patients. Prostaglandins, *13:* 193, 1977.

Hansen, M.K., and Secher, N.J.: Beta-receptor stimulation in essential dysmenorrhea. Am. J. Obstet. Gynecol., *121:* 566, 1975.

Henzl, M.R., Buttram, V., Segre, E.J., and Bessler, S.: The treatment of dysmenorrhea with naproxen sodium. Am. J. Obstet. Gynecol., *8:* 818, 1977.

Kuchel, O., Cuche, J.L., Buu, N.T., Guthrie, G.P., Unger, T., Nowaczynski, W., Boucher, R., and Genest, J.: Catecholamine excretion in "idiopathic" edema: Decreased dopamine excretion, a pathogenic factor? J. Clin. Endocrinol. Metab., *44:* 639, 1977.

Lundstrom, V.: Treatment of primary dysmenorrhea with prostaglandin synthetase inhibitors—A promising therapeutic alternative. Acta Obstet. Gynecol. Scand., *57:* 421, 1978.

Morrison, J.C., and Jennings, J.C.: Primary dysmenorrhea treated with indomethacin. South Med. J., *72:* 425, 1979.

O'Brien, P.M.S., Craven, D., Selby, C., and Symonds, E.M.: Treatment of premenstrual syndrome by spironolactone. Br. J. Obstet. Gynecol., *86:* 142, 1979.

Pickles, V.R.: Prostaglandins and dysmenorrhea. Acta Obstet. Gynecol. Scand. Suppl., *87:* 7, 1979.

Pulkkinen, M.O., Henzl, M.R., and Csapo, A.I.: The effect of naproxen-sodium on the prostaglandin concentrations of the menstrual blood and uterine "jet-washings" in dysmenorrheic women. Prostaglandins, *15:* 543, 1978.

Robinson, K., Huntington, K., and Wallace, M.G.: Treatment of the premenstrual syndrome. Br. J. Obstet. Gynecol., *84:* 784, 1977.

Whittle, B.: Prostaglandin synthetase inhibitors. Acta Obstet. Gynecol. Scand. Suppl., *87:* 21, 1979.

Widholm, O., and Kantero, R. L.: A statistical analysis of the menstrual patterns of 8000 Finish girls and their mothers. Acta Obstet. Gynecol. Scand. Suppl. 14, 1971.

CHAPTER 34

Family Planning

Although the scope of this text will not permit a comprehensive discussion of demographic problems and population control, the topic is of too great importance to omit completely. Family planning is population control reduced to the individual rather than to the national or global level. For a proper perspective in either, it seems necessary to have some concept of the problems in both areas.

Few, if any, informed persons fail to recognize the urgency of the need for control of reproduction at all levels—family, national, and world.

GENERAL CONSIDERATIONS

There are two major considerations in approaching the subject of either family planning for an individual or population control for a society: (1) motivation which determines who will participate, and (2) methodology which determines how. Studies on motivation indicate that this is influenced first by education, e.g., factual knowledge and understanding; second by cultural backgrounds, e.g., religion and traditional ways of life; and third by specific individual needs dependent, perhaps, upon highly personalized situational factors. It has been demonstrated that the physician who is sincerely interested and adequately trained in contraceptive therapy and practice plays an effective role in motivation. The physician's role in methodology, the imparting of technical knowledge or utilization of trained skills in this area, is paramount in making voluntary control of reproduction possible.

Demographers agree that the responsible parent today should plan a family of two or not more than three children in an effort to replace, but not increase, the world population. Those individuals emotionally and financially capable of raising larger families should plan to do so by adoption. It is the physician's responsibility to set the example as well as to disseminate knowledge of the seriousness of the world problem.

Because education is a slow process and motivation apparently depends to a large extent upon education, many observers feel that those methods which require the least motivation offer the most promise for rapid results in population control. Although the ideal method has probably not as yet been developed, those currently available are satisfactory, efficient, and offer such a variety of techniques that any individual couple should be able to achieve satisfactory family planning. It is probable that no method, however ideal, will be universally applicable to all couples.

CONTRACEPTIVE METHODS

General Considerations

As stated, there are presently many approaches to family planning, and these can be suited to the needs and capabilities of the individuals involved. Basically, one must consider if a couple is interested in limiting or spacing children, e.g., have they reached the ideal of two or more children, or are they contemplating additional pregnancies. Next, one must assess the motivation, intelligence, cultural background, financial status, and general health as well as the individual's personal preferences, acceptances, and prejudices. The older mechanical barrier methods—diaphragm, condom, tablets, and foams—replaced still older methods—abstinence, late marriage, coitus interruptus, abortion, and rhythm. The mechanical methods have in turn been supplemented by various forms of oral steroid contraception—long-acting injectable steroids, local vaginal steroids, and the recrudescence of the intrauterine device. Finally, sterilization of either partner has become an accepted means of absolute contraception when the family size is completed, either for socioeconomic or maternal health indications.

Although it has been stressed that each individual should use the method of her choice and, indeed, this must be so if any success is anticipated, nevertheless, there are frequently medical and socioeconomic indications which dictate the preference of one method over another. A skillful and knowledgeable physician can present the evidence in such a way as to ensure that the patient makes the proper selection.

If family planning educational facilities have not been available to the patient before her first pregnancy, the subject should be introduced during the prenatal visits. Initial definitive discussions conducted in the immediate postpartum period have proved ideal, as the patient is most receptive to contraception advice at this time.

Coitus Interruptus

Coitus interruptus, commonly referred to as "withdrawal," is said to be probably the earliest natural method of contraception and is thought to have been the method of effecting population control during the 19th century in Switzerland and France. It is still probably the most frequently used contraception in Europe. As it simply involves withdrawal of the penis from the vagina when ejaculation is imminent, with completion of ejaculation outside of the vagina, there is no expense involved, nor is technical advice necessary. For successful use of this method, however, it is obvious that the man must have good self-control, be highly motivated, and have a strong sense of responsibility to protect his sexual partner.

This method is completely unsatisfactory for men with premature or early ejaculation. It is estimated that the method would be inapplicable to about 50% of all males due to inability to control ejaculation. The use failure rate is quoted as between 6 and 16 per 100 women years. Because coitus interruptus is a method which is always available at no cost, it should be learned for those situations in which no other method is possible.

Condom Contraception

Condom contraception, or the use of a rubber sheath worn over the penis during coitus, is probably the most widely used mechanical contraceptive throughout the world. The only precautions necessary are to leave a dead space in the condom, from which the air has been expelled, to receive the ejaculate, to use proper lubrication if necessary, to effect withdrawal of the penis before cessation of the erection, and to grasp the ring of the sheath at the time of withdrawal to prevent it from slipping off. It has the advantage of protecting both against pregnancy and venereal disease and is, therefore, probably the most useful type of contraception in casual intercourse. Its other advantages are relative inexpensiveness, almost universal availability, and ease of usage. An additional advantage of the condom is found for men who have a tendency to premature ejaculation. The condom may blunt the sensation sufficiently to prolong the intercourse time. The delegation of the responsibility for family planning or for pregnancy prevention to the male may also increase his feeling of responsibility and family importance.

The disadvantages of the method are that it sometimes interferes with coital sensations both for male and female. It may interrupt the mood, as application of the condom requires an erect penis. It is not satisfactory for hot climates because of the deterioration of rubber.

The failure rate is usually given as between 6 and 13 per 100 women years, but some studies show much higher failure rates, the highest being 36 per 100 women years. The failure is largely due to rupture of the condom, with the deposition of the entire ejaculate into the vagina. Such accidents are probably related to failure of proper condom application, usually by failure to leave an adequate dead space. If this type of accident is reported immediately to the physician, a pregnancy can be circumvented by use of a high estrogen dosage recommended by Morris and referred to as the "pill for the morning after" or **pregnancy interception.**

Vaginal Diaphragm and Spermicidal Jelly

This mechanical method for the female partner is, perhaps, the most sophisticated type of contraception and, therefore, is suitable for the better educated patient. The diaphragm is a mechanical rubber device which must fit snugly behind the pubic bone and over the cervix into the posterior fornix. Too large a diaphragm causes pelvic discomfort, whereas too small a diaphragm can be displaced during intercourse. The diaphragm itself is used to prevent the sperm from being deposited directly onto the cervical mucus, allowing the spermicidal jelly, which is used in the diaphragm and also deposited with an applicator in the posterior fornix, time to exert its spermicidal action. The diaphragm should not be removed until 8 hours after the last intercourse. The most satisfactory method for using a diaphragm is to insert it each night with jelly before retiring and to remove it, cleanse it, and reinsert it with jelly the following evening. Thus, the diaphragm is always in place and its use is divorced from the act of intercourse, therefore improving the esthetic aspects.

Diaphragm contraception has the advantage of being locally effective and, therefore, unassociated with systemic side effects. It places the responsibility for pregnancy prevention and family planning entirely on the woman's shoulders and, therefore, perhaps affords her more sense of security. It does not interfere with coital sensations. If properly fitted, it should be completely comfortable and neither partner should be aware of its presence. It has the disadvantage of having to be fitted by a competent gynecologist, and it cannot be used in some patients who have vaginal relaxations, uterine descensus, or occasionally marked retroposition of the uterus. As it should be removed and reinserted each evening, it requires constant motivation.

The diaphragm remains medically the most acceptable form of contraception from the point of view of absence of complications. The use failure rate is between 2 and 3 per 100 women years among a private practice group and 33.6 per 100 women years in a Puerto Rican clinic study.

Vaginal Foam

Vaginal contraceptive foams are available as aerosol vials, jells, creams, or tablets. The spermicidal drug used is usually Nonoxynol-9. The active agents in vaginal foam tablets are tartaric acid and sodium bicarbonate. Although aerosol and jells are effective immediately, for most effective use application should be within one-half hour prior to intercourse. The tablets require some 5–10 minutes to dissolve before effectiveness is achieved. The advantages of this method are that it is inexpensive, easy to use and requires no instruction. Because of these characteristics, the method has been found acceptable in the lower socioeconomic levels. The disadvantage is that the failure rate is somewhat higher than among the previously discussed methods, being between 38 and 42 per 100 women years. It is, therefore, a method which could be recommended for patients who are child spacing or to be used in a combination with some other form of contraception such as rhythm or coitus interruptus.

Vaginal Steroid Therapy

Mishell has reported the successful use of a silastic ring pessary which has been impregnated with a progestational agent. Sufficient absorption can be obtained from the vaginal mucosa in this manner to obtain inhibition of ovulation. The pessary can be inserted by the patient after each menstrual period and removed at the end of a 25-day interval. This form of contraception, of course, requires monthly insertion of the pessary, and, if this is done by a physician, necessitates a monthly visit. It requires less motivation and offers less opportunity for patient failure than daily pill contraception. This technique has not been subjected to a sufficient clinical trial as yet to give any estimate of its effectiveness, but theoretically it seems to offer some advantages in specific circumstances.

Intrauterine Device (IUD)

The great advantage of this method is the lack of necessity for high motivation. Once the device is in situ, no further action on the part of the patient is necessary. It is, therefore, most suitable for the couple with the lowest income, education, and motivation.

The device should be placed in the uterine

cavity by an experienced gynecologist at the time of the menstrual period. This not only allows for ease of insertion when the cervix is relatively dilated, but also assures that the patient is not pregnant at the time of the insertion. Although postpartum insertion is at times theoretically desirable, this type of insertion is associated with a greater number of complications, perforation being the most serious, as well as a higher expulsion rate. However, once the device is retained in the pospartum period, it obtains the lowest expulsion rate of all.

The disadvantages of this method are the menstrual complications which occur—excessive, profuse periods, irregular bleeding between periods, and abdominal cramps.

Additional disadvantages are the failure to protect against ectopic pregnancy and the associated risk of pelvic inflammatory disease. This latter effect can be minimized by clipping the attached string sufficiently short to be retained in the cervix.

Because of the possibility of associated pelvic inflammatory disease and sterility due to tubal infection, many physicians hesitate to recommend an intrauterine device as a contraceptive method for a nulliparous patient. The method is unfortunately also unsuitable for some grand multipara with large uteri or patients who have myomata with irregularities of the uterine cavity, because the expulsion rate is high.

Medicated Devices, Copper, Steroids

Those devices which depend upon copper for effectiveness seem to have two disadvantages; first, the introduction into the system of copper, a potentially toxic metal; second, the necessity for removal and reinsertion periodically.

Contraindication for the use of copper-containing intrauterine devices are either allergy to copper or Wilson's disease, hepatolenticular degeneration, abnormal absorption, and metabolism of copper.

The intrauterine device which contains progesterone, 38 mg, and releases 65 mcg/day during the 1st year is said to have the advantage of decreasing rather than increasing the amount of blood loss during the menstrual period. However, it also is occasionally associated with amenorrhea, which is not common in any other type of intrauterine device. The removal rate for pain and bleeding is said to be between 12.3 and 16 which is somewhat lower than the rate quoted for intrauterine device in general which is, as stated below, 22.6 during the 1st year.

IUD Continuation Rates

The success of any type of contraception must be judged by its acceptability and by the continuation rate, which depends upon the unpleasant complications associated with the method and the inherent successfulness of the method. Failure rates for intrauterine device methods are highest in the 1st month from expulsions and discontinuation rates in the 1st year are 22.6 from both expulsions and removal for medical indications which are mainly pain and excessive bleeding. The pregnancy rate of 2.4 is also highest in the 1st year.

The most serious complications of the intrauterine device are perforations, usually at insertion, and pelvic inflammatory disease. The incidence of infection is increased in those populations at risk for pelvic inflammatory disease—women with prior histories of infection, multiple sex partners, or nulliparous patients under the age of 25 years. If the patient is free from infection when the intrauterine device is inserted, the risk of developing a related pelvic inflammatory disease is about three times that of the control population. Although **morbidity** from an intrauterine device is increased over other types of contraception due to the incidence of pelvic inflammatory disease, ectopic pregnancy, and uterine perforation, the incidence is nevertheless low, 5 per 1000 women years against 1 per 1000 women years of use in women on oral contraceptives. **Mortality**, on the other hand, is lower among intrauterine device users than among users of all other forms of contraception, which, according to Jain, is between 3 and 5 deaths per 1,000,000 women per year.

Oral Contraception

General Considerations

Oral contraceptives can currently be divided into two major categories: (1) *combined steroid therapy* consisting of a pill with an estrogen and a progestogen usually taken for 21 days during each month, beginning on the

5th day after the onset of menses, and (2) *microprogestational therapy*, which is a low dosage of a progestational drug given continuously. The estrogens most commonly used are mestranol and ethinyl estradiol and most of the progestogens are derived from androgens, 19-carbon compounds.

The synthetic estrogen and progestational drugs most frequently used in combined oral contraceptive preparations are shown in Table 34.1. Ethinylestradiol is more predictably absorbed than mestranol, which must be metabolized to ethinylestradiol in the liver. Mestranol is, therefore, almost twice as active but ethinylestradiol is less hepatoxic. Norethindrone is a less active progestogen and, as it is a 19-norsteroid, should be devoid of progestational stimulation of the breast. For this reason, a combined contraceptive with these steroids in low dosage, 35 mcg–50 mcg of ethinylestradiol and 0.5–1 mg of norethindrone might be preferred if tolerated by the

Table 34.1
Synthetic Estrogens and Progestogens Most Frequently Used in Oral Contraception

Estrogens	Relative Potency	Progestogens	Relative Potency	Brand Name	
	µg		*mg*		
Ethinyl Estradiol	2.0	Norethindrone (Antiestrogenic)	1	Ovcon-35	35-.4
				Ovcon-50	50-.1
				Brevicon	35-.5
				Modicon	35-.5
		Norethindrone Acetate	2	Loestrin	20-1
					20-1.5
				Norlestrine	50-1
					50-2.5
		Ethynodiol Diacetate	15	Demulen	50-1
		Norgestrel	30	Ovral	50-.1
					30-.3
		Norethynodrel (Estrogenic)	2	———	———
Mestranol	1.0	Norethindrone		Norinyl	50
					80-1
					100-2
				Ortho-Novum	50-1
					80-1
					100-2
					60-10
				———	———
None		Norethindrone Acetate			
				Ovulen	100-1
		Ethynodiol Diacetate			
		Norgestrel		———	———
				Enovid E	100-2.5
		Norethynodrel		1.5	75-5
		Norethindrone		Micronor	.35
				Nor-Q.D.	.35
		Norgestrel		Ovrette	.075

patient. The very low estrogen combination is, however, often associated with an unacceptable level of bleeding.

Method

The combination steroids are given beginning on the 5th cycle day and continuing through the 24th, starting again on the 5th day after the onset of bleeding, or on the 5th day after cessation of therapy, if bleeding does not begin. It is extremely important for patients to understand this because, unless they reinstitute their suppressive therapy, the hypothalamic escape will allow a pituitary stimulation and ovulation to occur. Unless there is some medical indication, such as treatment of hirsutism in patients with polycystic ovarian disease, it is no longer justifiable to use the combination steroids containing the high dosages of estrogen. The low estrogen preparations should be tried initially. If unacceptable irregular bleeding patterns occur, the higher dose estrogens, 50 or 80 mcg per preparation can be tried. Some preparations are packaged with placebo tablets to take during the days when steroids are discontinued. This is an especially advantageous package for the poorly motivated, poorly educated patient.

Mode of Action

It has been well documented by a number of investigators that the oral steroids exert their action by inhibition of the hypothalamic-releasing hormone, LRH, thus blocking pituitary gonadotrophin activity and causing secondary ovarian atrophy. The lower dose *steroid* pills may disrupt the cycle by disturbing the LH surge and ovulation. The progestational agents preferentially inhibit the preovulatory LH surge, with a lesser effect upon FSH function. The suppression is directly related to the amount and duration of the dosage. The estrogenic component, on the other hand, preferentially inhibits FSH and is also dose-dependent. The longer the period of administration, the more severe the pituitary suppression and ovarian atrophy, with subsequent decreased endogenous estrogen milieu. It is this lowered ovarian estrogen effect that is responsible for the shortened scanty menstrual flow which most women experience after taking oral contraceptives for a number of years. As hyperprolactinemia may also be associated with these symptoms,

a prolactin assay should be considered under this circumstance. Galactorrhea may be initiated only after the steroid suppression at the breast end organ level has been removed by discontinuing the contraception. Therefore, galactorrhea per se cannot serve as a warning symptom.

Advantages

Oral contraception has two great advantages over all other methods of contraception: its remarkable effectiveness and its rather general acceptability. The combined steroid therapy has the theoretical failure rate of zero, and, even if 4 days of medication are missed, the failure rate is only 2 per 100 women years, which is still lower than any other method. The microdosage is less effective, having a failure rate of 3.7 per 100 women years. It also has very little margin of safety, and the failure rate apparently rises rapidly if as few as one or two pills are missed.

The high acceptability of the oral contraception method is probably related to the fact that it is completely divorced from the sex act. As it eliminates self-handling, it is also especially attractive for those women who find this distasteful.

Disadvantages

The greatest disadvantage of the method is that it involves the administration to completely well women of potent drugs which have many diversified systemic effects. The second disadvantage is the time and cost of proper patient supervision. A careful history and complete physical and gynecological examination as well as blood pressure and urine analysis should be made before administration of oral contraception. A gynecological check examination should ideally be made every 6 months or at least yearly, while the individual is on medication. The risk of complications and side effects must be weighed against the possible advantages which will accrue, as well as the advisability and acceptability of some other form of contraception.

Complications

Probably the most serious complication which has been reported in association with oral contraception is thromboembolic disease. Three statistical studies from the United Kingdom seem to have conclusively demonstrated that contraceptive steroid drugs predispose to thrombophlebitis. The annual death rate from embolism attributed to oral contraception was estimated to be about 3 per 100,000 users.

The second serious complication is essential hypertension. It has been suggested that the estrogen component in oral contraceptives causes an increase in plasma angiotensinogen. It has been shown that patients who remain normotensive while on oral contraceptives show a decrease in plasma renin concentration, while those who develop hypertension do not. Angiotensin II and aldosterone both have a feedback at the kidney juxtaglomerular cells to decrease renin production. Patients who develop hypertension on oral contraceptives apparently have an insensitivity or a decreased feedback at this level, making it impossible to lower renin and thereby lower antiotensin II.

The third medical problem is the associated disturbance of carbohydrate metabolism. The evidence indicates that women who have a diabetic tendency may show a diabetic type of glucose tolerance test when on oral contraception. This seems to be because of the effect of **estrogen** on growth hormone, which causes hyperglycemia, demanding a higher insulin level. Patients who are unable to adjust to this changing blood glucose level, because of an inherent pancreatic insufficiency, will develop diabetes.

Spellacy et al., in 1973 showed that the 19-**norprogestational steroids** per se also caused deterioration of carbohydrate metabolism. The most recent work seems to indicate that either high estrogens or high doses of 19-norprogestogens are deleterious to carbohydrate metabolism, causing both increased glucose and increased insulin. Steele and Duncan found a suggestion in a diabetic population that proliferative retinopathy may progress rapidly, resembling the "accelerated retinopathy" of pregnancy, in some patients on oral contraceptive pills. These findings make the selection of the lowest dose estrogens **and** the lowest dose progestogens especially important in the diabetic patient.

Wynn described certain changes in the blood lipids which resemble those found in early arteriosclerotic vascular disease. The suggestion has been made that, in women who have a predisposition to arteriosclerosis, oral contraception may speed the process. This is as yet a theoretical consideration.

Finally, the effect upon the hepatic cells predisposes patients on oral contraceptive therapy to liver adenomas (Terblanche). These adenomas, although not malignant, may cause death from rupture and associated hemorrhage. Rooks et al. report an increased risk of 120 times in women who have used oral contraception for from 3–7 years. In addition to this rather serious but rare liver complication, the incidence of gall bladder disease among patients on oral contraceptive therapy is apparently increased by a factor of approximately 2.

Side Effects

There are certain specific side effects which occur in some women receiving any form of oral steroid contraception. These are residual menstrual irregularities, fluid retention, gastric disturbances, increased varicosities, irritability or depression, changes of libido, either plus or minus, melasma, headache, and migraine. Although none of these are serious, they are of sufficient concern to the patient that an estimated 40% of oral contraceptive users discontinue before the end of 2 years.

From a medical point of view, one of the disadvantages of oral contraception is that it interferes with a number of laboratory diagnostic procedures. Among these are the sedimentation rate, tests for protein-bound iodine or thyroxine, blood corticotrophins, and, on occasion, even a Papanicolaou smear; an endometrial biopsy or cervical biopsy can also present diagnostic difficulties.

Vaginitis

Both yeast vaginitis and trichomonas vaginitis have been reported as frequent complications of oral contraception. Yeast vaginitis might be related to the atrophy of the vagina which occurs due to the low estrogen milieu and also associated with the above mentioned changes in carbohydrate metabolism. This type of vaginitis can, on occasion, be intractable and, although usually it will respond to the recommended therapy, gentian violet and/or nystatin, occasionally oral contraception must be discontinued before the condition can be controlled. Trichomonas vaginitis may be related to multiple sexual partners rather than to the actual steroid effects on the vagina.

Amenorrhea

After discontinuing oral contraception, the majority of patients resume ovulatory cycles within 4–6 weeks. However, it is not unusual for a patient to have 1 or 2 months of amenorrhea before her first menstrual period. The cause and effect relation between more prolonged amenorrhea and contraception is more controversial.

Office or Clinic Visits

Probably one of the greatest disadvantages or deterrents to the use of oral contraception is the necessity for a gynecological consultation before administration of medication and the return for refill of prescription.

In the ideal situation, oral contraception should not be advised without a complete history and gynecological examination, including several laboratory investigations.

Contraindications

Possible contraindications for oral contraception are found in the **family history**; if there is a diabetic family history, a history of essential hypertension, or a history of breast or endometrial cancer steroid contraception may not be the proper choice. Factors in the patient's **past history** which may contraindicate oral contraception are a history of menstrual irregularities, especially long periods of amenorrhea, breast or endometrial cancer, thromboembolic disease, liver disease, cardiac or renal disease, depressive reactions, or migraine headaches. The **physical examination** should exclude thyroid and breast nodules, cardiac or renal disease, cervical polyps, and uterine myomas. Every patient should have a blood pressure, urine analysis for albumin and sugar, and a Papanicolaou smear before beginning oral contraception. Only a history of thromboembolic phenomenon or cancer of the breast is an absolute contraindication to therapy, but abnormalities in any of the areas mentioned require special consideration and attention. Patients who are over 35 years of age or who are heavy smokers are not ideal candidates for oral contraception.

Each patient should return in 2 months from beginning oral contraceptive therapy, at which time the blood pressure and urinary sugar analysis should be repeated, and any factors which signaled special attention at the first visit should be rechecked. Ideally each patient should be seen every 6 months thereafter while on steroid contraceptives and contraception should be discontinued over a month or 6 week period after approximately 2½ years to be sure that the hypothalamic pituitary axis is not unduly suppressed. If this is done, however, it must be remembered that some other form of contraception must be provided during the rest period.

Pregnancy Interception for Postpregnancy Exposure

Morris has described the use of estrogen as a postintercourse protective drug. This method is useful when there has been a single pregnancy exposure, as in rape or method failure. The method has been referred to as "the pill for the morning after." It involves the administration of relatively high amounts of estrogen, 25 mg of stilbestrol or its equivalent, daily. Morris advocates a 4-day administration period but, over the years, we have used a 2-week interval. This ensures the production of an abnormal endometrium which will not sustain a normal implantation and, when the pill is withdrawn, a withdrawal bleeding phase ensues. If given immediately after exposure and during the following 2 weeks, it offers absolute protection. This method has obvious limited applicability and is especially valuable in cases of rape. It can be associated with gastrointestinal complications, nausea and vomiting, and, occasionally, with excessive bleeding. In the rare incident of failure, the pregnancy which results must be aborted because of the known effects of DES (diethelstilbestrol) and estrogen on the early embryonic development.

Long Acting Injectable Steroids

Medroxyprogesterone acetate (Depo-Provera), 150 mg intramuscularly every 3 months, will inhibit ovulation and menstrual function. Erratic spotty bleeding usually occurs during the first 3 months of treatment and sometimes longer. The advantage of this method is the delegation of responsibility for contraception to the physician or the paramedical personnel, requiring a house visit by the Public Health officer or an office or clinic visit by the patient only once every 3 months. The disadvantage of the method is the absence of regular menstrual periods and the presence of irregular bleeding which may be prolonged and inconvenient. In addition, the hypothalamic suppression is so efficient that prolonged anovulation and amenorrhea may occur following cessation of injections. Because of these characteristics, this form of contraception is best suited to those patients who are absolute "limiters," and who, for one reason or another, are unable to take personal responsibility for their birth control. It has been especially useful in patients with serious blood dyscrasias, because complete amenorrhea can be established. It also has a place in the management of patients who have myomata uteri and, therefore, should receive as little estrogen stimulation as possible.

Rhythm Contraception—Periodic Continence

The so-called rhythm method of family planning, as proposed by Ogino is based on three fundamental theoretical concepts, and perhaps the efficacy of this method can best be evaluated by examining the validity of these concepts. These are (1) the fertilizable life span of an oocyte is not over 24 hours after ovulation; (2) sperm survival in the female genital tract is not over 4 days; and (3) ovulation which determines the rhythm of a cycle occurs 14 days before the menstrual flow, and every women will have cycles which vary within a predictable range. Using these assumptions, Ogino calculated the so-called safe period by obtaining cycle records of a woman over a 6-month or, preferably, 1-year period. Fourteen days were subtracted from the longest cycle to obtain the latest ovulation date, 1 day added for ovum survival and 1 more for good measure, and this date was regarded as the end of the fertile period. Fourteen days were then subtracted from the shortest cycle to calculate the earliest ovulation date and 4 days subtracted for sperm survival, 1 additional day was subtracted for good measure, and this date determined the beginning of the fertile period.

Reexamination of the principles upon which the method is based in the light of current knowledge indicates that some of the premises are false. From knowledge based on assumptions derived from animal experimentation, it is probably correct that the life span of the unfertilized oocyte in the female tract is not over 24 hours. However, the second assumption, that human sperm survive with normal fertilizing capacity no longer than 96 hours, seems unjustifiable. Information obtained from donor insemination in the human indicates that 4 days is not unusual and data collected by Marshall during a study on rhythm contraception indicated that 10 days is the probable "cut-off" period. The third premise, e.g., all ovulation occurs at 14 days premenstrually, is also probably incorrect. Studies by Strott et al. indicate that, at least in young women, ovulation may occur much closer to the menses. Thus, it would seem that, instead of a 14-day period, one would, perhaps, need to use a figure of 10 days. The variation of the menstrual cycle is another factor which must be responsible for many rhythm failures. Tietze, in his estimate of the efficacy of rhythm contraception, advised that it can be used for child spacing satisfactorily, but not for child limitation, as within a 2-year period, each woman can be expected to have one cycle which is markedly inconsistent from those characteristic of that individual. This variation is usually caused by factors which disturb the preovulatory cyclic surge of pituitary LH. Such factors are psychogenic stress, acute illnesses, fever, medication, and travel. Women using this method must be alert to these possible interferences and abstain in cycles exposed to such influences. Wade et al. found an 11% pregnancy rate.

The other method for circumventing such problems is by the use of the basal body temperature chart. The findings indicate that there is really no "safe period" before ovulation. When basal body temperature graphs are used to pinpoint ovulation and intercourse is confined to the areas *after the thermal shift*, in a small highly motivated group of patients, the method's success rate, according to Sobrero, approximates 100%. According to Marshall, when used in conjunction with the basal body temperature chart in this fashion, the failure rate is 6.6 per 100 women years, whereas, if even as much as a day is added in the preovulatory phase, the failure rate rises to 19 per 100 women years.

In summary, to make the method acceptable in regard to its effectiveness, one must pinpoint ovulation with the basal body temperature chart and confine intercourse to the immediate postovulatory-premenstrual area. This limits exposure to approximately 10 days per cycle and is, therefore, impractical for younger couples. The method obviously requires the highest degree of motivation but rates among the least expensive. One of the interesting advantages, which has been reported for the method, is that it leads to some increase in libido due to the long periods of continence. On the other side of the coin, one might say it leads to psychological problems due to frustrations.

The ovulation method, described by Billings (Wilson), depends upon the evaluation of cervical mucus. Safe periods are estimated by dryness of the vulva after a menses, when there has been no preceding mucus. Abstinence days are those marked by mucus secretion as observed by examination of vulvar secretions obtained on tissue paper or finger. Abstinence must be maintained throughout the time during which mucus is observed and until 3 days after peak mucus, which is judged as the ovulation day. The ovulation day is recognized by a clear mucus which stretches without breaking and is slippery and sometimes tinted with blood. The method requires careful instruction by dedicated teachers and routine observation with daily recording by participants. The advantage of the method is the absence of necessity for any devices and the theoretical applicability to promotion of fertility as well as prevention of pregnancy. The disadvantages are those recorded above for any of the rhythm methods. In a study of use effectiveness, Wade et al. found fewer than 10% of all couples were continuing to use the method after 1 year. The pregnancy rate was 23%.

Methods for Absolute Limitation

Sterilization: Female

Surgical methods for sterilization of the female are discussed in any gynecological surgical text and range from electrocoagulation and division or mechanical occlusion of tubes at laparoscopy to the more intrusive forms of tubal ligation at minilaparotomy, or laparotomy, to hysterectomy. Hysterectomy for the purpose of sterilization should be performed only when there are other indications for removal of the uterus. Although at one time postpartum laparoscopic tubal ligation was thought to be unacceptable, with wider experience it has become a satisfactory procedure. Failure rates are low for all types of sterilization procedures.

The disadvantages of the laparoscopic fulgeration techniques of sterilization are the complications associated with the abdominal puncture wound and the bowel injuries which may result from burns and which are frequently unrecognized. In addition, due to the extensive destruction of the tube, following fulgeration, the procedure is sometimes irreversible. However, as this method is relatively simple requiring no hospitalization and with a minimal mortality and morbidity rate, it has become medically acceptable to consider sterilization of any patient who requests it. Demand has increased dramatically since 1975. It is now almost as frequent a method of contraception in the older women over the age of 35 as is the pill. It is probably the method of choice for those women who have completed their family and are over the age of 30 years. Because of the possible irreversibility of the procedure, however, it would seem wise to avoid such a final method in relatively young women except for maternal health problems or eugenic considerations.

Sterilization: Male

The same considerations apply to male sterilization as have been discussed in female sterilization. However, the method of sterilization in the male is simpler. It is unassociated with the morbidity and mortality accompanying female sterilization. In addition to these advantages, it also has the advantage of being a permanent procedure and the disadvantage of being probably irreversible. The theoretical failure rate is low, although occasionally the duct will recanalize. Pregnancy exposure must be avoided over the 3- to 4-month period following operation when collecting tubules are being emptied of sperm. It is wise to ask the patient to use precautions until a urologist has declared his ejaculate free of sperm. As in the female, it is probably unwise to sterilize a relatively young male, and likewise a husband should not be sterilized because of medical indications in the wife. The fear of serious medical complications associated with autoimmune disease due to the sperm granulomata has not been substantiated.

Abortion

Induced abortion has been a recognized method for a second line of defenses in failed contraception increasing the efficacy of family and population control throughout the world. The only advantage of the method seems to be its efficacy. However, even aside from the moral and ethical aspects of the procedure, which must not be disregarded, abortion should not be used as a contraceptive method. Every woman who subjects herself to an abortion because of failure to use birth control has risked her life as well as her future reproductive capacity unnecessarily. Albeit small, the mortality from therapeutic abortion is still appreciable, 0.6%, and the morbidity, which is, of course, more difficult to evaluate absolutely, is thought to be approximately 10%. These considerations allow abortion to be viewed only as a backup procedure for contraception method failures, not as a contraceptive method.

Summation

The success or effectiveness of any contraceptive method depends upon its inherent **method** failure rate, (1) **method effectiveness**, as well as its **patient** failure rate, (2) **use effectiveness**. Method effectiveness depends upon the ease with which the method is used and use effectiveness depends largely upon motivation. Motivation is influenced by the maturity and responsibility of the individual but also depends upon the **side effects**, either real or imagined, associated with the method use and the recognized dangers of the method, **morbidity** and **mortality**.

Steroid oral contraception is the most effective method as measured by its inherent method effectiveness. However, because of its relatively high side effects, its continuance rate is not as good as one would hope. The morbidity, especially in relation to vascular disease and hypertension, is also a deterrent, and its mortality, because of its effect on vascular disease, is probably the highest of any type of contraception. These risks increase in relation to the duration of the use of oral contraceptives as well as in relation to the age of the individual. The patient who smokes is at extreme risk. Because of these considerations, oral contraception is probably the contraception of choice for the young nulliparous woman, should be used with caution in the woman who is over the age of 35, and should not be used at all in the woman over the age of 30 who smokes.

The intrauterine device requires the least motivation and therefore has the best continuation rates over long intervals. However, because of its association with pelvic inflammatory disease and because it will not protect against ectopic pregnancy, it is not to be recommended for nulliparous women, particularly women with multiple partner exposures and women known to be exposed to venereal disease. The method effectiveness is lower than that of oral contraception and the morbidity and mortality rates are lower than those of oral contraception. If smoking is a habit pattern which cannot or will not be foregone, the intrauterine device should be seriously considered in any age group. Because of the increasing morbidity and mortality among oral contraception users after the age of 30, the intrauterine device should be the treatment of choice in the mature woman over 30 who has perhaps completed her family.

Barrier methods of contraception are associated with higher failure rates but most of this failure rate is due to patient failure or lack of motivation. If the method is the method of the patient's choice and the individual is well motivated and responsible, the use effectiveness is almost equal to that of the intrauterine device. The diaphragm and condom methods have the lowest morbidity and mortality rate when used with abortion as a back up. If abortion is not used, the complications from the accidental pregnancies which ensue raise the morbidity to equal that of the intrauterine device.

Sterilization should be considered for the woman over 35 years of age who has completed her family or for the patient with a medical contraindication to pregnancy. Sterilization for the male should be considered when medically indicated or when he feels he is no longer willing to undertake the financial, emotional, or intellectual responsibilities of child rearing. If these decisions are to be made in a family situation, both partners should be involved in the decision making. However, the major responsibility for the decision should be borne by the party most affected. Sterilization of either man or woman under the age of 30 years should be evaluated extremely carefully and, if performed, attention should be given to the possible reversibility of the procedure.

References and Additional Readings

Jain, A. K.: Mortality risks associated with the use of oral contraceptives. Stud. Fam. Plann., 8: 50, 1977.

Garcia, R., Pincus, G., and Rock, J.: Effects of three 19-norsteroids on human ovulation and menstruation. Am. J. Obstet. Gynecol., 75: 82, 1958

Ludwig, H.: A position paper on the relation between oral contraceptives and blood coagulation. Contraception, 20: 257,

1979.

Marshall, J.: A field trial of the basal body temperature method of regulating births. Lancet, *2:* 8, 1968

Mayer, J.: Food and population: A different view. Nutri. Rev., *22:* 353, 1964.

Mishell, Daniel R., Jr., and Lumkin, Mary E.: Contraceptive effect of varying dosages of progestogens in silastic vaginal rings. Fertil. Steril., *21:* No. 2, February, 1970.

Morris, G. McL., and Van Wagenen, G.: Compounds interfering with ovum implantation and development. Am. J. Obstet. Gynecol., *96:* 804, 1966.

Ogino, K.: Uber konseptionstermin des Weides und seine Anwendung in der Praxex. ZBL. Gynaek. *56:* 721, 1932.

Rooks, J. B.: The association between oral contraception and hepatocellular adenoma. 1st National Medical Conference on Safety of Fertility Control, Chicago March 6, 1977.

Spellacy, W. N., Buhi, W. C. and Birk, S. A.: Carbohydrate metabolism prospectively studied in women using a low-estrogen oral contraceptive for six months. Contraception, *20:* 137, 1979.

Spellacy, W. N., Carlson, K. L., Birk, S. A., and Schade, S. L.: Glucose and insulin alterations after one year of combination-type oral contraceptive treatment. Metabolism, *17:* 496, 1968.

Steel, J. M., and Duncan, L. J. P.: Serious complications of oral contraception in insulin-dependent diabetics. Contraception, *17:* 291, 1978.

Strott, C. A., Cargille, C. M., Ross, G. T., and Lipsett, M. B.: The short luteal phase. J. Clin. Endocrinol. Metab., *30:* 246, 1970.

Sturgis, S. H., and Albright, F.: Mechanism of estrin therapy in relief of dysmenorrhea. Endocrinology, *26:* 102, 1940.

Terblanche, J.: Liver tumours associated with the use of contraceptive pills. S. Afr. Med. J., *53:* 439, 1978.

Tietze, C., Poliakoff, S. R., and Rock, J.: Clinical effectiveness of rhythm method of contraception. Fertil. Steril., *2:* 441, 1951.

Tietze, C., and Potter, R. G., Jr.: Statistical evaluation of the rhythm method. Am. J. Obstet. Gynecol., *84:* 692, 1962.

Vessey, M. P., and Doll, R.: Investigation of relation between use of oral contraceptives and thromboembolic disease. Br. Med. J., *2:* 199, 1968.

Vessey, M. P., and Mann, J. I.: Female sex hormones and thrombosis. Br. Med. Bull. *34:* 157, 1978.

Wade, M. E., McCarthy, P., Abernathy, J. R., Harris, G. S., Danzer, H. C., and Uricchio, W. A. A randomized prospective study of the use effectiveness of two methods of natural family planning: An interim report. Am. J. Obstet. Gynecol., *134:* 628, 1979.

Wilson, M. A.: *The Ovulation Method of Birth Regulation.* Van Nostrand Reinhold New York, 1980.

Wynn, Y., Doar, J. W. H., Mill, G. L., and Stokes, T.: Fasting serum triglyceride, cholesterol and lipoprotein levels during oral contraceptive therapy. Lancet, *2:* 756, 1969.

Wynn, V., and Doar, J. W. H.: Some effects of oral contraceptives on carbohydrate metabolism. Lancet, *2:* 761, 1969.

Index